# Register Now for Online Access to Your Book!

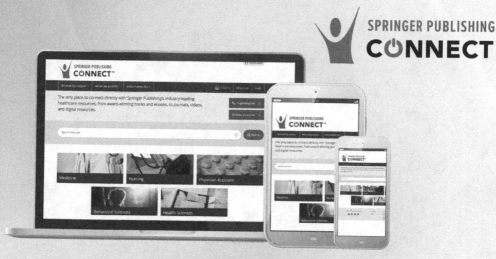

**SPRINGER PUBLISHING**
**CONNECT™**

Your print purchase of *Handbook of Physical Medicine and Rehabilitation* **includes online access to the contents of your book**—increasing accessibility, portability, and searchability!

**Access today at:**
http://connect.springerpub.com/content/book/978-0-8261-6226-7
or scan the QR code at the right with your smartphone. Log in or register, then click "Redeem a voucher" and use the code below.

AE3Y5LA6

*Scan here for quick access.*

**Having trouble redeeming a voucher code?**
**Go to https://connect.springerpub.com/redeeming-voucher-code**

**If you are experiencing problems accessing the digital component of this product, please contact our customer service department at cs@springerpub.com**

The online access with your print purchase is available at the publisher's discretion and may be removed at any time without notice.

**Publisher's Note:** New and used products purchased from third-party sellers are not guaranteed for quality, authenticity, or access to any included digital components.

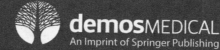

**demos**MEDICAL
An Imprint of Springer Publishing

**View all our products at springerpub.com/demosmedical**

# HANDBOOK OF PHYSICAL MEDICINE AND REHABILITATION

# HANDBOOK OF PHYSICAL MEDICINE AND REHABILITATION

## Editors

### Marlís González-Fernández, MD, PhD

Associate Professor, Physical Medicine and Rehabilitation and Orthopaedic Surgery,
Vice Chair for Clinical Operations, Department of Physical Medicine and Rehabilitation,
Johns Hopkins University School of Medicine, Baltimore, Maryland

### Stephen Schaaf, MD

Assistant Professor, Department of Physical Medicine and Rehabilitation,
Vanderbilt University Medical Center, Nashville, Tennessee

## Associate Editors

### Jennifer M. Zumsteg, MD

Associate Professor, Department of Rehabilitation Medicine,
University of Washington, Seattle, Washington

### Danielle Perret, MD

Associate Clinical Professor, Departments of Physical Medicine and Rehabilitation and Anesthesiology,
University of California, Irvine, Orange, California

### David J. Kennedy, MD

Professor and Chair, Department of Physical Medicine and Rehabilitation,
Vanderbilt University Medical Center, Nashville, Tennessee

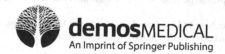

**demos**MEDICAL
An Imprint of Springer Publishing

Springer Publishing Company, LLC
11 West 42nd Street, New York, NY 10036
www.springerpub.com
connect.springerpub.com/

*Acquisitions Editor*: Beth Barry
*Compositor*: Amnet Systems

ISBN: 978-0-8261-6225-0
ebook ISBN: 978-0-8261-6226-7
DOI: 10.1891/9780826162267

21 22 23 24 / 5 4 3 2 1

Medicine is an ever-changing science. Research and clinical experience are continually expanding our
knowledge, in particular our understanding of proper treatment and drug therapy. The authors, editors, and
publisher have made every effort to ensure that all information in this book is in accordance with the state
of knowledge at the time of production of the book. Nevertheless, the authors, editors, and publisher are
not responsible for any errors or omissions or for any consequence from application of the information in
this book and make no warranty, expressed or implied, with respect to the content of this publication. Every
reader should examine carefully the package inserts accompanying each drug and should carefully check
whether the dosage schedules therein or the contraindications stated by the manufacturer differ from the
statements made in this book. Such examination is particularly important with drugs that are either rarely
used or have been newly released on the market.

**Library of Congress Cataloging-in-Publication Data**

Names: González-Fernández, Marlís, editor. | Schaaf, Stephen, editor. |
    Zumsteg, Jennifer M., editor. | Perret, Danielle, editor. | Kennedy, David J., editor.
Title: Handbook of physical medicine and rehabilitation / editors, Marlís González-Fernández,
    Stephen Schaaf ; associate editors, Jennifer M. Zumsteg, Danielle Perret, David J. Kennedy.
Other titles: Handbook of physical medicine and rehabilitation
    (González-Fernández)
Description: First Springer Publishing edition. | New York, NY : Springer Publishing Company,
    LLC, 2022. | Includes bibliographical references and index.
Identifiers: LCCN 2021020924 (print) | LCCN 2021020925 (ebook) | ISBN 9780826162250
    (paperback) | ISBN 9780826162267 (ebook)
Subjects: MESH: Physical and Rehabilitation Medicine—methods | Rehabilitation—methods
Classification: LCC RM700 (print) | LCC RM700 (ebook) | NLM WB 320 | DDC 617/.03—dc23
LC record available at https://lccn.loc.gov/2021020924
LC ebook record available at https://lccn.loc.gov/2021020925

Contact sales@springerpub.com to receive discount rates on bulk purchases.

Printed in the United States of America.

*To the patients with whom we partner as they pursue full lives;
to our colleagues, the rehabilitation physicians, therapists, and
staff with whom we work tirelessly to support our patients' goals;
to family and friends who always support our endeavors;
and to those closest to us for whom we strive to be efficient to get home
every day.*

*"For wisdom will enter your heart, and knowledge will fill you
with joy." Prv. 2:10*

# CONTENTS

## SECTION 4: DIAGNOSTICS, MODALITIES, EQUIPMENT, AND TECHNOLOGY

# CONTRIBUTORS

**Rachel V. Aaron, PhD**   Assistant Professor, Department of Physical Medicine and Rehabilitation, Johns Hopkins University School of Medicine, Baltimore, Maryland

**Lesley Abraham, MD**   Acting Assistant Professor, Department of Rehabilitation Medicine, University of Washington, Seattle, Washington

**Michelle Accardi-Ravid, PhD**   Assistant Professor (Clinical), Division of Physical Medicine and Rehabilitation, Craig H. Neilsen Rehabilitation Hospital, University of Utah Health, Salt Lake City, Utah

**Kevin Alschuler, PhD**   Associate Professor, Department of Rehabilitation Medicine; Director of Psychology MS Center, University of Washington, Seattle, Washington

**Thiru Annaswamy, MD, MA**   Staff Physician and Section Chief, Spine and Electrodiagnostic Sections, Physical Medicine and Rehabilitation Service, VA North Texas Health Care System; Professor, Department of Physical Medicine and Rehabilitation, UT Southwestern Medical Center, Dallas, Texas

**Abana Azariah, MD**   Clinical Chief, Disorders of Consciousness Program, TIRR Memorial Hermann; Attending Physician, McGovern UT Health School of Medicine, Houston, Texas

**Alba Azola, MD**   Assistant Professor, Department of Physical Medicine and Rehabilitation, John Hopkins University School of Medicine, Baltimore, Maryland

**Heather R. Baer, MD**   Associate Professor, Departments of Physical Medicine and Rehabilitation and Neurology, University of Colorado Denver, Denver, Colorado

**Vishal Bansal, MD**   Physician, Department of Physical Medicine and Rehabilitation University of Texas Health Houston, Houston, Texas

**Kevin Barrette, MD**   Associate Professor, Department of Neurosurgery, University of California, San Francisco, San Francisco, California

**Matthew N. Bartels, MD, MPH**   Professor and Chairman, Department of Rehabilitation Medicine, Albert Einstein College of Medicine, Montefiore Health System, Bronx, New York

**Alison M. Bays, MD, MPH&TM**   Assistant Professor, Division of Rheumatology, Department of Medicine, University of Washington, Seattle, Washington

**Allison Bean, MD, PhD**   Assistant Professor, Department of Physical Medicine and Rehabilitation, University of Pittsburgh Medical Center, Pittsburgh, Pennsylvania

**Shauna K. Berube, MS, CCC-SLP** Speech-Language Pathologist, Department of Physical Medicine and Rehabilitation, Johns Hopkins Hospital, Baltimore, Maryland

**Glendaliz Bosques, MD** Chief of Pediatric Rehabilitation Medicine, Dell Children's Hospital; Associate Professor, Department of Neurology, Dell Medical School at University of Texas–Austin, Austin, Texas

**Martin B. Brodsky, PhD, ScM, CCC-SLP, F-ASHA** Associate Professor, Department of Physical Medicine and Rehabilitation, Johns Hopkins University, Baltimore, Maryland

**Aaron E. Bunnell, MD** Assistant Professor, Department of Rehabilitation Medicine, University of Washington, Seattle, Washington

**Philippines G. Cabahug, MD** Director, Spinal Cord Injury Medicine Fellowship, International Center for Spinal Cord Injury, Kennedy Krieger Institute; Assistant Professor, Department of Physical Medicine and Rehabilitation, Johns Hopkins School of Medicine, Baltimore, Maryland

**Scott J. Campea, MD** Clinical Assistant Professor, Department of Rehabilitation Medicine, University of Washington, Seattle, Washington

**John Chan, MD** Resident, Department of Orthopaedic Surgery, Stanford University, Palo Alto, California

**Debra Cherry, MD, MS** Director, Occupational and Environmental Medicine Residency; Associate Professor, Department of General Internal Medicine; Adjunct Professor, Department of Environmental and Occupational Health Sciences, University of Washington, Seattle, Washington

**Cheng-Chuan Chiang, DO** Medical Student, Department of Physical Medicine and Rehabilitation, John Hopkins Hospital, Baltimore, Maryland

**Junghoon Choi, MD** Clinical Instructor, Department of Physical Medicine and Rehabilitation, NYU Langone, Brooklyn, New York

**Tyler Clark, MD** Resident, Department of Rehabilitation Medicine, UT Health San Antonio, San Antonio, Texas

**Deborah A. Crane, MD, MPH** Associate Professor, Department of Rehabilitation Medicine, University of Washington, Seattle, Washington

**Nathan Darji, DO** Brain Injury Medicine Fellow, Spaulding Rehabilitation Hospital, Harvard Medical School, Boston, Massachusetts

**Nickolas A. Dasher, PhD** Assistant Professor, Division of Rehabilitation Psychology and Neuropsychology, Department of Rehabilitation Medicine, University of Washington, Seattle, Washington

**Kate E. Delaney, MD** Acting Assistant Professor, Department of Rehabilitation Medicine, University of Washington, Seattle, Washington

**Madeline A. Dicks, DO**   Resident Physician, Department of Rehabilitation Medicine, UT Health San Antonio, San Antonio, Texas

**Craig DiTommaso, MD**   Medical Director, Post-Acute Medical Rehabilitation Hospital of Humble, Humble, Texas; Attending Physician and Director of Early Career Development, U.S. Physiatry, LLC, The Woodlands, Texas

**Stephanie R. Douglas, MD**   Research Assistant, Boston, Massachusetts

**Rebecca A. Dutton, MD**   Assistant Professor, Department of Orthopaedics and Rehabilitation, University of New Mexico, Albuquerque, New Mexico

**Ashley M. Eaves, MD, MA**   Resident Physician, Department of Rehabilitation Medicine, University of Washington, Seattle, Washington

**Jessica Engle, DO**   Assistant Professor, Attending Physician, Department of Physical Medicine and Rehabilitation, Johns Hopkins University School of Medicine, Baltimore, Maryland

**Daniel Ezidiegwu, DO**   Resident, Department of Physical Medicine and Rehabilitation, Johns Hopkins University School of Medicine, Baltimore, Maryland

**Aubree M. Fairfull, MD**   Resident Physician, Department of Rehabilitation Medicine, University of Washington, Seattle, Washington

**Jesse Fann, MD, MPH**   Professor, Department of Psychiatry and Behavioral Sciences, University of Washington, Seattle, Washington

**Elizabeth Farrell, PT, DPT, PCS, ATP/SMS**   Senior Physical Therapist IV, International Center for Spinal Cord Injury, Kennedy Krieger Institute, Baltimore, Maryland

**Dorianne Feldman, MD, MSPT**   Medical Director, Inpatient Rehabilitation Program; Assistant Professor, Department of Physical Medicine and Rehabilitation, John Hopkins Hospital, Baltimore, Maryland

**Richard Fontánez, MD**   Chief Resident, Department of Physical Medicine, Rehabilitation and Sports Medicine, University of Puerto Rico School of Medicine, San Juan, Puerto Rico

**Amanda K. Gallagher, MA, CCC-SLP**   Speech-Language Pathologist, Department of Physical Medicine and Rehabilitation, Johns Hopkins Hospital, Baltimore, Maryland

**Luis Garza, MD, PhD**   Professor, Department of Dermatology, Johns Hopkins University School of Medicine, Baltimore, Maryland

**Rudy Garza, MD**   Assistant Professor, Department of Anesthesiology, UT Health San Antonio, San Antonio, Texas

**Kayli Gimarc, MD**   Resident, Department of Rehabilitation Medicine, University of Washington, Seattle, Washington

**Caroline T. Goldin, MD**   Instructor/Fellow, Department of Neurology, University of Colorado School of Medicine, Aurora, Colorado

**Marlís González-Fernández, MD, PhD**   Associate Professor, Physical Medicine and Rehabilitation and Orthopaedic Surgery; Vice Chair for Clinical Operations, Department of Physical Medicine and Rehabilitation, Johns Hopkins University School of Medicine, Baltimore, Maryland

**Kevin Hakimi, MD**   Associate Professor, Department of Rehabilitation Medicine, University of Washington, Seattle, Washington

**Shahin Hakimian, MD**   Associate Professor, Department of Neurology, University of Washington, Seattle, Washington

**Chad Hanaoka, BA**   Research Assistant, Shirley Ryan AbilityLab, Chicago, Illinois

**Mark Harrast, MD**   Clinical Professor, Departments of Rehabilitation Medicine, Orthopaedics, and Sports Medicine, University of Washington; Medical Director, University of Washington Medicine Sports Medicine Center at Husky Stadium, Seattle, Washington

**Mark S. Hopkins, PT, CPO, MBA**   Chief Executive Officer, Dankmeyer, Inc., Linthicum Heights, Maryland

**Gloria Hou, MD**   Co-Medical Director, UW Medicine Multiple Sclerosis Center, University of Washington, Seattle, Washington

**Ileana Howard, MD**   Associate Professor, Department of Rehabilitation Medicine, University of Washington, Seattle, Washington

**Irvin J. Huang, DO**   Fellow, Division of Rheumatology, Department of Medicine, University of Washington, Seattle, Washington

**Sarah Hwang, MD**   Director of Women's Health Rehabilitation, Shirley Ryan AbilityLab; Assistant Professor, Departments of Physical Medicine and Rehabilitation and Obstetrics and Gynecology, Northwestern University, Chicago, Illinois

**Sherry Igbinigie, MD**   Sports Medicine Fellow, Department of Rehabilitation Medicine, University of Washington, Seattle, Washington

**Tracey Isidro, MD**   Resident, H. Ben Taub Department of Physical Medicine and Rehabilitation, Baylor College of Medicine, Houston, Texas

**Nitin Jain, MD, MSPH**   Co-Director, UT Southwestern Musculoskeletal and Sports Medicine; Vice Chair, Department of Physical Medicine and Rehabilitation; Professor of Physical Medicine and Rehabilitation, Orthopaedics, and Population and Data Sciences, University of Texas Southwestern, Dallas, Texas

**Prakash Jayabalan, MD, PhD**   Director of Clinical Musculoskeletal Research, Shirley Ryan AbilityLab; Assistant Professor, Department of Physical Medicine and Rehabilitation, Northwestern Feinberg School of Medicine, Chicago, Illinois

**Prathap Jayaram, MD**   Director of Regenerative Sports Medicine; Assistant Professor, H. Ben Taub Department of Physical Medicine and Rehabilitation, Department of Orthopedic Surgery, Baylor College of Medicine, Houston, Texas

**Cherry Junn, MD**   Assistant Professor, Program Director, Brain Injury Medicine Fellowship, Department of Rehabilitation Medicine, University of Washington, Seattle, Washington

**Lesley C. Kaye, MD**   Assistant Professor, Department of Neurology, University of Colorado School of Medicine, Aurora, Colorado

**Anthony Kenrick, MD**   Resident, Department of Orthopaedic Surgery, Stanford University, Palo Alto, California

**Soo Yeon Kim, MD**   Assistant Professor, Department of Physical Medicine and Rehabilitation, Johns Hopkins University School of Medicine, Baltimore, Maryland

**Brian J. Krabak, MD, MBA**   Clinical Professor, Departments of Rehabilitation and Orthopaedics and Sports Medicine, University of Washington, Seattle, Washington

**Matt LaCourse, MD**   Resident, Department of Rehabilitation Medicine, University of Washington, Seattle, Washington

**Ny-Ying Lam, MD**   Assistant Professor, Department of Rehabilitation Medicine, University of Washington, Seattle, Washington

**Jennifer Leet, MD**   Resident, Department of Rehabilitation Medicine, UT Health San Antonio, San Antonio, Texas

**Audrey S. Leung, MD**   Assistant Professor, Department of Rehabilitation Medicine, University of Washington, Seattle, Washington

**Josh Levin, MD**   Clinical Associate Professor of Orthopedic Surgery and Neurosurgery; Interim Director, Physical Medicine and Rehabilitation Residency; Director, Physical Medicine and Rehabilitation Spine Fellowship, Stanford University Medical Center, Palo Alto, California

**Isaiah Levy, MD**   Resident, Department of Physical Medicine and Rehabilitation, University of Pittsburgh Medical Center, Pittsburgh, Pennsylvania

**Ryan Lewis, MD**   Resident Physician, Department of Physical Medicine and Rehabilitation, Johns Hopkins University School of Medicine, Baltimore, Maryland

**Cindy Lin, MD, FACSM**   Clinical Associate Professor, Sports and Spine Medicine, Department of Physical Medicine and Rehabilitation, University of Washington, Seattle, Washington

**Meredith Linden, PT, DPT, ATP/SMS**  Clinical Specialist, International Center for Spinal Cord Injury, Kennedy Krieger Institute, Baltimore, Maryland

**Alexander Lloyd, MD**  Fellow, Department of Rehabilitation and Performance Medicine, Swedish Medical Center, Seattle, Washington

**Carmen E. López-Acevedo, MD**  Residency Program Director, Professor of Physical Medicine and Rehabilitation, Department of Physical Medicine, Rehabilitation and Sports Medicine, University of Puerto Rico School of Medicine, San Juan, Puerto Rico

**Melinda Loveless, MD**  Clinical Assistant Professor, Department of Rehabilitation Medicine, University of Washington, Seattle, Washington

**R. Samuel Mayer, MD, MEHP**  Associate Professor, Department of Physical Medicine and Rehabilitation, Johns Hopkins University School of Medicine, Baltimore, Maryland

**Lakeya S. McGill, PhD**  Postdoctoral Fellow, Department of Physical Medicine and Rehabilitation, Johns Hopkins University School of Medicine, Baltimore, Maryland

**Erin Michael, PT, DPT, ATP/SMS**  Manager, Patient Advocacy and Special Programs, International Center for Spinal Cord Injury, Kennedy Krieger Institute, Baltimore, Maryland

**Manoj Mohan, DO**  Resident, Department of Orthopaedic Surgery, Stanford University, Palo Alto, California

**Brian Mugleston, MD**  Resident, Department of Rehabilitation Medicine, University of Washington, Seattle, Washington

**Ameet Nagpal, MD, MS, Med**  Division Chief of Pain Medicine, Department of Anesthesiology, UT Health San Antonio, San Antonio, Texas

**Tony Nguyen, MD**  Attending Physician, Post-Acute Medical Rehabilitation Hospital of Humble, Humble, Texas; Attending Physician, U.S. Physiatry, LLC, The Woodlands, Texas

**Ryan Nussbaum, DO**  Resident, Department of Physical Medicine and Rehabilitation, Northwestern Feinberg School of Medicine, Chicago, Illinois

**Amanda L. Olney, DPT, GCS**  Rehabilitation Care Service, VA Puget Sound Health Care System, Seattle, Washington

**Jaclyn Omura, MD**  Assistant Professor, Department of Rehabilitation Medicine, University of Washington, Seattle, Washington

**Kentaro Onishi, DO**  Assistant Professor, Departments of Physical Medicine and Rehabilitation and Orthopedic Surgery, University of Pittsburgh Medical Center, Pittsburgh, Pennsylvania

**Melissa Osborn, MD**  Fellow, Department of Anesthesiology and Pain Medicine, University of Washington, Seattle, Washington

**Marisa Osorio, DO**   Division Chief, Pediatric Rehabilitation Medicine; Associate Professor, Department of Rehabilitation Medicine, University of Washington, Seattle, Washington

**Eugene L. Palatulan, MD**   Resident Physician, Department of Rehabilitation and Regenerative Medicine, Columbia University Medical Center, New York, New York

**Bhavesh Patel, DO**   Resident Physician, Department of Physical Medicine and Rehabilitation, Johns Hopkins University School of Medicine, Baltimore, Maryland

**Kristina E. Patrick, PhD, BCBA**   Assistant Professor, Department of Neurology, University of Washington; Division of Pediatric Neurology, Seattle Children's Hospital, Seattle, Washington

**Kelly Pham, MD**   Assistant Professor, Department of Rehabilitation Medicine, University of Washington, Seattle, Washington

**Clausyl (CJ) Plummer II, MD**   Assistant Professor, Department of Physical Medicine and Rehabilitation, Vanderbilt University Medical Center, Nashville, Tennessee

**David Z. Prince, MD**   Director, Cardiopulmonary Rehabilitation; Assistant Professor, Department of Rehabilitation Medicine, Montefiore Medical Center, Albert Einstein College of Medicine, Bronx, New York

**Preeti Raghavan, MD**   Sheikh Khalifa Stroke Institute Endowed Chair, Associate Professor, Departments of Physical Medicine and Rehabilitation and Neurology, Johns Hopkins University School of Medicine, Baltimore, Maryland

**Albert C. Recio, MD, PT**   Aquatics Medical Director, Kennedy Krieger Institute; Assistant Professor, Department of Physical Medicine and Rehabilitation, Johns Hopkins School of Medicine, Baltimore, Maryland

**Katherine C. Ritchey, DO, MPH**   Advance Scholar, Geriatrics Research, Education and Clinical Center (GRECC), VA Puget Sound Health Care System; Clinical Instructor, Division of Geriatric and Gerontology, Department of Medicine, University of Washington, Seattle, Washington

**Duane Robinson, MD**   Medical Director, Air Force Medical Service, Washington, DC

**Verónica Rodríguez, MD**   Professor of Physical Medicine and Rehabilitation, Department of Physical Medicine, Rehabilitation and Sports Medicine, University of Puerto Rico School of Medicine, San Juan, Puerto Rico

**Desiree Roge, MD**   Associate Professor, Department of Rehabilitation Medicine, University of Washington, Seattle, Washington

**David Rothman, PhD**   Assistant Clinical Professor, Department of Physical Medicine and Rehabilitation, Virginia Commonwealth University, Sheltering Arms Institute, Richmond, Virginia

**Cristina L. Sadowsky, MD** Clinical Director, International Center for Spinal Cord Injury, Kennedy Krieger Institute; Associate Professor, Department of Physical Medicine and Rehabilitation, Johns Hopkins School of Medicine, Baltimore, Maryland

**Kendl M. Sankary, MD** Resident, Department of Rehabilitation Medicine, University of Washington, Seattle, Washington

**Caroline A. Schepker, DO** Resident Physician, Department of Rehabilitation and Regenerative Medicine, Columbia University Medical Center, New York, New York

**Mark E. Sederberg, DO** Visiting Instructor, Department of Physical Medicine and Rehabilitation, University of Utah, Salt Lake City, Utah

**Patricia C. Siegel, OTD, OTR/L, CHT** Assistant Professor, Occupational Therapy Graduate Program, University of New Mexico, Albuquerque, New Mexico

**Sarah B. Simmons, MD, PhD** Neuroimmunology Fellow, Mellen Center, Cleveland Clinic, Cleveland, Ohio

**Amos Song, MD** Resident, Department of Physical Medicine and Rehabilitation, Vanderbilt University Medical Center, Nashville, Tennessee

**Bo Song, MD** Resident, H. Ben Taub Department of Physical Medicine and Rehabilitation, Baylor College of Medicine, Houston, Texas

**Amy Starosta, PhD** Clinical Assistant Professor, Department of Rehabilitation Medicine, School of Medicine, University of Washington, Seattle, Washington

**Evan Sweren, BA** MD Candidate, University of Michigan Medical School, Ann Arbor, Michigan

**Ronald J. Sweren, MD** Director, Phototherapy/Photopheresis Program; Assistant Professor, Department of Dermatology, Johns Hopkins University School of Medicine, Baltimore, Maryland

**Lyndly Tamura, MD** Resident, Department of Orthopaedic Surgery, Stanford University, Palo Alto, California

**Adam S. Tenforde, MD, FACSM** Director of Running Medicine, Spaulding Rehabilitation Hospital; Assistant Professor, Department of Physical Medicine and Rehabilitation, Harvard Medical School, Boston, Massachusetts

**Jenna L. Thomason, MD, MPH** Acting Instructor, Division of Rheumatology, Department of Medicine, University of Washington, Seattle, Washington

**Megan Thomson, MD** Emergency Medicine Resident Physician, Medical University of South Carolina, Charleston, South Carolina

**Jeffrey Tsai, MD, PhD** Associate Professor, Department of Neurology, University of Washington, Seattle, Washington

**Elaine Tsao, MD**   Assistant Professor, Department of Rehabilitation Medicine, University of Washington, Seattle Children's Hospital, Seattle, Washington

**Jessica Tse, MD**   Resident Physician, Department of Physical Medicine and Rehabilitation, Loma Linda University Health, Loma Linda, California

**Amy K. Unwin, MD**   Resident Physician, Department of Rehabilitation Medicine, University of Washington, Seattle, Washington

**Holly Vance, RN, BSN, CWON**   Clinical Nurse Educator, Wound, Ostomy, Limb Preservation and Amputee Services, Harborview Medical Center, Seattle, Washington

**Monica Verduzco-Gutierrez, MD**   Professor and Chair, Department of Rehabilitation Medicine, UT Health San Antonio, San Antonio, Texas

**Dominique Vinh, MD**   Assistant Professor, Department of Physical Medicine and Rehabilitation, John Hopkins Hospital, Baltimore, Maryland

**Christopher J. Visco, MD**   Assistant Professor, Department of Rehabilitation and Regenerative Medicine, Columbia University Medical Center, New York, New York

**Gloria von Geldern, MD**   Associate Professor, Department of Neurology, University of Washington, Seattle, Washington

**Kayla Williams, MD**   Resident Physician, Department of Physical Medicine and Rehabilitation, UT Southwestern Medical Center, Dallas, Texas

**Katherine Streeter Wright, PhD**   Clinical Instructor, Department of Rehabilitation Medicine, University of Washington, Seattle, Washington

**Derek Yu, MD**   Neurologist, Kaiser Permanente of Washington, Tacoma, Washington

**Xiaoning Yuan, MD, PhD**   Resident Physician, Department of Rehabilitation and Regenerative Medicine, Columbia University Medical Center, New York, New York

**Jennifer M. Zumsteg, MD**   Associate Professor, Department of Rehabilitation Medicine, University of Washington, Seattle, Washington

# PREFACE

Physical medicine and rehabilitation is a broad field. As such, many focus their practice on specific areas within the specialty while on occasion seeing patients within the broader scope of the specialty. Also, maintaining board certification requires a breadth of knowledge that is often beyond the scope of our day-to-day practices.

*Handbook of Physical Medicine and Rehabilitation* is designed to serve as a real-time clinical manual for rehabilitation providers and trainees. The chapters are written in a concise, evidence-based, and clinically focused manner to provide a meaningful refresher for a practice topic. This can fill in knowledge gaps for subspecialized providers who need to remain up to date on general rehabilitation information, trainees who want an understanding of the specialty, and those wanting a quick refresher in the process of maintenance of certification. We anticipate this clinical quick-reference format will be incredibly useful for all rehabilitation providers and trainees.

The book is divided into four sections: the first covers physical medicine and rehabilitation management by diagnosis, the second reviews musculoskeletal management by body region, the third discusses physical medicine and rehabilitation management by problem, and the fourth will touch upon physical medicine and rehabilitation diagnostics, modalities, equipment, and technology. These sections provide the day-to-day information that rehabilitation providers need for clinical care delivery.

We edited *Handbook of Physical Medicine and Rehabilitation* to be a practical resource that facilitates remaining or becoming knowledgeable in a broad variety of topics and as a guide for clinical care in real time. As such, we hope that this book becomes an often used and important part of everyday practice.

*Marlís González-Fernández, MD, PhD*
*Stephen Schaaf, MD*

# Section 1

# PHYSICAL MEDICINE AND REHABILITATION MANAGEMENT BY DIAGNOSIS

1

# AMPUTATION AND PROSTHETICS

MARK S. HOPKINS AND MARLÍS GONZÁLEZ-FERNÁNDEZ

## CORE DEFINITIONS

Prostheses are an integral part of the rehabilitation of patients after limb loss.

A prosthesis interface is a connection between the user and the prosthesis. The interface is a combination of socket and suspension. A typical interface is passive; however, the interface may include active and sophisticated control elements such as elevated vacuum or myoelectric control. Osseointegration is a complete change in human to prosthesis interface and a radical departure from the traditional socket interface definition.

The construction of the prosthesis includes various materials. Traditionally, prosthesis has referred specifically to either an exoskeletal (i.e., the connection between the various parts of the prosthesis is by an external shell) or endoskeletal (i.e., the parts are connected by an internal system of modular connectors) construction. Endoskeletal systems are typically adjustable and lighter. It is now common to forego an external anthropomorphic covering so that the endoskeletal components are exposed.

The major parts of the prosthesis include the foot, knee, hip, hand, wrist, elbow, and shoulder joints and the various connectors that make a whole functional unit.

---

The full reference list appears in the digital product found on http://connect.springerpub.com/content/book/978-0-8261-6226-7/part/part01/chapter/ch01

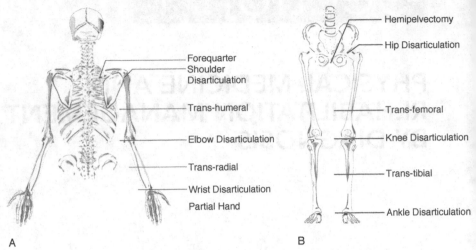

**FIGURE 1.1** Common amputation levels; (A) upper limb, (B) lower limb.

"Accoutrement" is a classic term used to describe the various items that come with the prosthesis but may not be major functional components. They are nonetheless critical for successful prosthesis use. Prosthesis socks, shrinker socks, donning aids, and so forth are often considered accoutrements. In addition to the accoutrements, gel socket inserts (liners) and gel sealing sleeves and some other items are referred to as consumables and are replaced on a regular basis.

The most common amputation levels and components are summarized in Figure 1.1. Prosthesis design and prescription are based on residual limb health (length, strength, skin integrity, sensation, and proximal joint health), the assessed functional ambulatory potential, prior prosthesis use, and the patient's goals and lifestyle.

## ETIOLOGY AND PATHOPHYSIOLOGY

Dysvascular amputations (i.e., due to diabetes or peripheral vascular disease) are the most common, comprising 82% of all amputations; 97% of these affect the lower limb. Traumatic amputations comprise 16% of all amputations, of which 68% were of the upper limb. The remaining 2% of amputations are equally divided between congenital and cancer-related amputation. The majority of congenital amputations (60%) are upper limb, while 76% of cancer-related amputations involve the lower limb.[1]

## DIAGNOSTIC APPROACH

### Rehabilitation Care Plan

Rehabilitation of people with limb loss is a core competency for the physiatrist and the rehabilitation team. A long-term, lifelong rehabilitation care plan including the use of a comprehensive multidisciplinary team and shared decision-making models is required. Rehabilitation of people with limb loss spans the age continuum from prenatal consultation to end of life and spans the care continuum from preoperative to long-term habilitation and all aspects in between. The prescription, provision, training, and long-term management of limb prostheses are typical for the limb loss rehabilitation care plan; however, many individuals will choose not to use a prosthesis at all or choose to use one intermittently over the course of their life. The role of the physiatrist in the limb loss rehabilitation multidisciplinary team is critical and central to successful outcomes bridging the multiple medical, surgical, and therapy specialties and ensuring that the patient and their family remain at the center of the efforts. A detailed working knowledge of the roles, responsibilities, and contributions of the various members of the team is needed so that care is properly coordinated. Rehabilitation of people with limb loss can be viewed as a lifelong and staged care plan.[2]

## Stages of Recovery and Rehabilitation

Preamputation goals include the evaluation and education of the patient in the setting of postamputation expectations, engaging the patient in shared decision-making, and general prehabilitation. The acute postamputation period is focused on residual limb healing, pain management, contracture prevention, and early efforts to promote independence with mobility and activities of daily living (ADLs). The subacute postamputation stage is often focused on the prescription and provision of a prosthesis and the prosthesis use training. It is during this time that return to preamputation duties such as home care, childcare, return to work, and recreation/leisure activities is considered. Lifelong care is critical with this population, as the prosthesis user will need assistance in ensuring proper prosthesis fit and function, assistive device upgrades and replacements, monitoring the health of the residual limb and remaining limbs, and management of secondary conditions related to long-term prosthesis use.

## Prosthesis Provision and Training

The prosthetist is an integral member of the team tasked with the specifics of the evaluation, prescription, provision, maintenance, and replacement of prostheses. They help the patient and team with the details of prosthesis design and the components incorporated into a prosthesis. Physical and occupational therapists usually serve two primary functions: (a) functional assessor tasked with competing outcome measures and documenting change over time and (b) prosthesis use training. The physical therapists typically manage lower limb prosthesis training focusing on gait and mobility. The occupational therapists usually manage upper limb prosthesis training with a focus on dexterity and ADLs. Joint treatments may be required for complex patients with multiple limb loss or complex medical/surgical conditions. Coordination of care with the physicians/surgeons, therapists, and prosthetists is often begun in the preoperative period and extends through the life span.

## Advanced Surgical Options

It is now quite common to consider surgical alteration of the residual limb to address prosthesis fitting problems, improve limb durability for lifelong prosthesis use, and improve function of the prosthesis in the setting of advanced prosthesis designs and components. Surgical limb revision for nerve, soft tissue, and bone reconstruction is fairly common and can be done at multiple life stages. Specific techniques such as targeted muscle reinnervation for motor and sensory control of externally powered prostheses, osteomyoplastic procedures to improve residual limb loading and stability, and osseo-integrated bone-anchored prosthesis (allowing for socket-less fit) have made for significant advances in user–prosthesis interface and improvements in the quality of life of long-term limb prosthesis users.

## TREATMENT

### Lower Limb Prostheses

Medical history, physical examination, and current function are used to determine the patient's functional potential. There are many standardized tests available to assist with this assessment. The most widely utilized system of classification in the United States has been provided by the Centers for Medicare and Medicaid Services (CMS) to assist with lower limb prosthesis knee and foot/ankle selection.[3] Functional categories labeled 0 through 4 describe progressively increasing potential ambulatory function with a prosthesis (Table 1.1).

Prosthesis design reflects the level of limb loss and the intended functional use of the prosthesis. General types of prostheses include immediate and early postoperative prostheses (IPOP/EPOP), preparatory prostheses, definitive prostheses, and specialty or activity-specific prostheses. IPOP/EPOP are provided shortly after amputation, often in the operating room, with the goals of preventing edema, protecting the limb and incision to relieve pain and promote healing, and facilitating early functional independence. Preparatory prostheses are provided as soon as the limb can tolerate the forces of the removable socket and are intended for the achievement of three primary goals: (a) limb maturation (volume reduction, shaping, strengthening, and desensitization), (b) maximizing early functional independence, and (c) assessing for the definitive prosthesis. The definitive prosthesis is provided when the aforementioned goals are achieved

### TABLE 1.1 CENTERS FOR MEDICARE AND MEDICAID SERVICES—FUNCTIONAL LEVELS AND CORRESPONDING PROSTHESIS COMPONENTS

| LEVEL | FOOT/ANKLE ASSEMBLY | KNEE UNITS |
| --- | --- | --- |
| K0 no functional potential with prosthesis | Not eligible for a prosthesis | Not eligible for a prosthesis |
| K1 transfers and limited household distances | SACH or single-axis only | No fluid control allowed |
| K2 household and limited community distances | Flexible keel or multi-axis allowed | No fluid control allowed |
| Community distances; K3 variable cadence; traverse environmental barriers | Any foot/ankle assembly; including energy storage and multiaxial dynamic response | Most knee units include fluid, microprocessor fluid control; no high-activity knee frames |
| High activity, impact and K4 stress; active adult, athlete or child. | Any foot/ankle assembly | Any knee unit |

SACH, solid ankle cushion heel.

and is intended to be used for a longer period of time with the option of a more cosmetic restoration. The definitive prosthesis is modified or replaced when there are significant changes in limb size or volume, significant changes in function, and/or due to wear and tear. Specialty or activity-specific prostheses may be provided for vocational or avocational activities when the primary prosthesis is not appropriate (e.g., aquatics, sprinting or use in extreme environments).

The basic components of lower limb prostheses are the user and machine interface (socket and suspension), construction elements, replacement functional units (foot/ankle, knee, hip), and socks, liners, and accoutrements.

Prosthetic foot/ankle systems are typically passive devices using dynamic materials to accommodate to the ground surface. They can be categorized into two main groups by the presence of a physical hinge and the ability to provide energy return and release. Powered and microprocessor-controlled foot and ankle systems are available.

## Partial Foot Prostheses

General considerations in the design of partial foot prostheses are based on the level of amputation and function of the remaining foot (Figure 1.2). Biomechanically, partial foot prostheses are to support the residual foot structure, control the distribution of forces, replace the lost anterior lever arm, and allow for shoe fit. The prosthesis structure and lever arm control are determined by the height of the device and the materials selected; therefore, typically the shorter the residual limb, the higher the device.

## Syme's Prostheses

A Syme's level amputation is an ankle disarticulation with preservation of the heel pad; thus, it allows distal weight-bearing and reduces proximal loading. A bulbous distal shape reduces need for proximal suspension and a long lever arm, and surface area allows for distribution of force and greater prosthesis control. Conversely, it provides limited space distal to the socket for a prosthetic foot/ankle system, and satisfactory cosmetic restoration is not easily achieved for some patients. The interface is commonly designed for full distal weight-bearing and self-suspension. The socket is typically mounted directly onto the foot (Figure 1.3). A socket window or door is created to allow donning or a cylindrical socket with a soft foam insert is

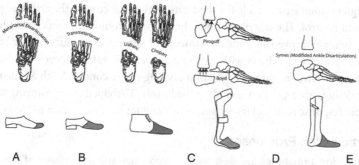

**FIGURE 1.2** Partial foot amputation and suitable prostheses: (A–C) partial foot prosthesis, (D) tibial tubercle height partial foot prosthesis, (E) Syme's prosthesis.

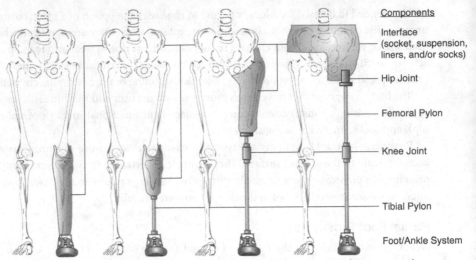

**FIGURE 1.3** Syme's, transtibial, transfemoral, and hip disarticulation prostheses.

used. Socks or gel liners may be used. Due to the available space, a lower profile ankle/foot design is needed; short energy storage feet remain an option.

## Transtibial Prostheses

The design of the transtibial prosthesis creates an interface that optimizes weight-bearing and swing-phase forces (Figure 1.3). The transtibial region extends from the distal Syme's ankle disarticulation to the proximal knee disarticulation level; however, there are surgical considerations that determine optimal length. Leverage and surface area increase with longer limbs, but at the distal levels, soft tissue coverage may be limited, predispose the limb to skin problems, and limit foot/ankle options. Proximally, the extensor mechanism must be maintained to allow for knee control, and the short leverage and surface area may require socket designs that extend above the knee joint resulting in a more cumbersome fitting. Mid-shank lengths around the musculoskeletal junction of the gastrocnemius/soleus muscle group are considered ideal. Distal loading is not generally tolerated so the weight is borne over the entire limb with considerations for pressure sensitive areas.

Many design options are available for the transtibial interface with the ultimate goals being comfort and control. The use of gel liners has become common practice. Gel liners are intended to provide improved suspension, control for sheer and pressure, and loading in a uniform reliable pattern. Gel liners with mechanical locks or sealing sleeves may be used to create suction or elevated vacuum for improving swing-phase control. With an ideal length, all foot/ankle designs are an option including the longer "J"-shaped energy storing feet, multiaxial dynamic response feet, and integrated shock and torque attenuation pylon systems.

## Knee Disarticulation Prostheses

Knee disarticulation prostheses are designed to maximize the advantages of this level of amputation including distal weight-bearing, reduced proximal loading, full hip motor power, a bulbous distal shape allowing for reduced proximal suspension, and a long lever arm and surface area for control of prosthesis. Disadvantages are the limited space distal to the socket for prosthetic knee mechanisms and the difficulty achieving satisfactory cosmetic restoration.

Socket design for the knee disarticulation level prosthesis is relatively simple when compared to the transfemoral prosthesis as the availability of distal limb weight-bearing and self-suspension may eliminate or significantly reduce the need for pelvic weight-bearing, aggressive proximal socket brim designs, or the need for proximal suspension systems (e.g., belts). These advantages make the interface of the knee disarticulation prosthesis less cumbersome for the user and allow for improved comfort in both walking and sitting. Polycentric knee joint mechanisms are commonly prescribed as they allow for the shortest possible thigh length and sitting comfort. Foot and ankle selection is based on the functional potential of the user and is determined along with the function of the knee unit for an integrated foot/ankle and knee system.

## Transfemoral Prostheses

At the transfemoral level, residual length becomes a primary consideration. The shorter amputations result in significantly reduced surface area and leverage for controlling forces. This is of particular concern for prosthetic knee control. Accommodations for short limbs must be made in prosthesis design leading to more cumbersome fitting with aggressive socket brims and pelvic suspension straps for stance and swing-phase control, respectively. Very short transfemoral limbs may be fit with a hip disarticulation style prosthesis. While long residual limbs are desirable for leverage and control, limited room for some knee units may be undesirable.

The primary transfemoral socket shapes are quadrilateral and ischial containment. Both require pelvic weight-bearing on the ischial tuberosity to unload the distal end of the residual limb. The ischial containment socket design is intended to provide greater control of the femur and thereby reduce gait deviations such as lateral trunk lean due to socket instability. Subischial transfemoral socket designs are now possible and increasingly prevalent using hydrostatic gel liners and thigh soft tissue loading or elevated vacuum to create stability and comfort in the absence of pelvic load bearing. The primary goal for the transfemoral socket remains user comfort and control. Knee selection is based on the functional potential of the user and the available residual limb leverage among other factors.

## Hip Disarticulation or Hemipelvectomy Prostheses

The design of the hip disarticulation or transpelvic prostheses is based on the residual pelvic structures and the availability of the ischial tuberosity for weight-bearing and the iliac crest for suspension. Without these two bony anchors, socket control is reliant on soft tissue compression and may be less stable.

The socket interface is most commonly fabricated as a single piece with a rigid attachment to the hip joint and a flexible closure wrapping around and encapsulating the entire residual pelvis for weight-bearing, suspension, and rotational control. Pelvic motions (posterior pelvic tilt) are used to initiate swing phase. Weight-bearing stability is built into the alignment of the prosthesis with extension bias at the knee and hip joints under load. Hip joints are typically single-axis joints with extension assist mechanisms and are aligned with the axis placed on the distal anterior aspect of the socket for maximal extension bias and for sitting comfort. Without active control of the hip joint, knee and foot/ankle component selection is largely based on the need for stance stability and safety.

## Upper Limb Prostheses

The population of upper limb prosthesis users is quite different than lower limb prosthesis users representing a minority of the limb loss population. This is primarily due to the limited number of upper limb amputations and to the much higher prosthesis rejection rate. Unilateral upper limb amputees will quickly become ADL proficient with the remaining limb. There is generally a 3- to 6-month critical period for upper limb amputees to be successfully fitted with a prosthesis, after which time they are much more likely to reject a prosthesis. Bilateral upper limb amputees can become independent in the majority of the essential ADLs with appropriate training. The description of upper limb prostheses mirrors the level of amputation (Figure 1.1). There are six basic options for people with upper limb loss: no prosthesis, passive or static terminal device, body powered, externally powered, hybrid, or specialty prostheses. The term passive refers solely to the terminal device, which may not be activated to open or close; however, the prosthesis is functional as an extension of the residual limb for bimanual activities and for manipulating objects in space. Passive systems are often more cosmetically acceptable. Body-powered systems are cable and harness operated and require the user to provide tension to the cable via biscapular abduction or glenohumeral flexion or abduction (Figure 1.4). Externally powered systems are usually myoelectrically controlled through electromyographic (EMG) signals from the residual muscles.

## Partial Hand Prostheses

Partial hand prostheses are more likely to be rejected than any other level of prosthesis due to their limited function and poor aesthetics. Occupational therapists are critical to successful prosthesis prescription and should be involved as early as possible. General considerations are based on the level of amputation, function of the remaining hand with potential prehension abilities, and unilateral versus bilateral involvement. Levels of amputation include partial or complete digit disarticulation, ray resection, transmetacarpal, and transcarpal.

## Wrist Disarticulation and Transradial Prostheses

The design of the wrist disarticulation and transradial prosthesis is based on the length of the residual limb and the available forearm rotation. At the wrist disarticulation level, the intact radius and ulna allow for improved control, distal pressure tolerance, and full pronation/supination. However, there is limited space at the end of the socket for a wrist and terminal device; thus, the prosthetic limb may be longer than the intact contralateral limb. At the transradial level, the length of the lever arm determines the control system, component, and interface selection. A short residual limb length requires a prosthetic interface that captures more of the limb and may extend above the elbow.

## Elbow Disarticulation and Transhumeral Prostheses

Residual limb length and control of the prosthesis are primary concerns in the design of the elbow disarticulation and transhumeral prosthesis. At the elbow disarticulation level, full

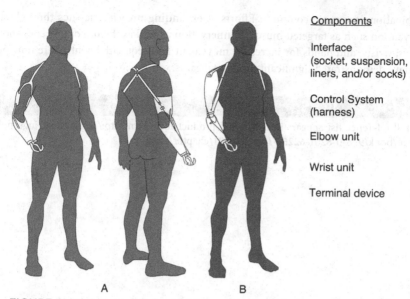

Components

Interface
(socket, suspension,
liners, and/or socks)

Control System
(harness)

Elbow unit

Wrist unit

Terminal device

**FIGURE 1.4** (A) Transradial and (B) transhumeral body-powered prostheses.

humeral length, broad and tolerant distal humeral end, and full leverage allow for improved control of the prosthesis. However, there is limited room for a prosthetic elbow mechanism often requiring the use of external hinges or an elbow unit positioned much lower than the nonamputated limb. At the transhumeral level, the length of the lever arm determines the control system, component, and interface selection. Longer limbs allow the socket trim lines to remain relatively low and end distal to the shoulder joint. At mid-length levels, socket extensions to the pectoralis and scapular areas are common for rotational control. At higher levels with shorter lever arms, the socket may extend over the acromion (i.e., shoulder cap). Patients with a very short residual humerus are fit with shoulder disarticulation level prosthesis. Selection of the elbow unit, wrist unit, and terminal device is based on the control system selected. A common hybrid control system is a body-powered elbow unit and an externally powered hand terminal device.

## Shoulder Disarticulation and Intrascapular/Thoracic Prostheses

General considerations in the design of prostheses at proximal levels involve the availability of the shoulder girdle for control of both the interface and for potential myoelectric sites at the pectoralis, upper trapezius, or scapular muscles. Without the shoulder girdle, control is diminished, and most patients choose to forgo prosthesis fitting. They may be fit with a shoulder cap only, which allows for proper fitting of clothing and protection of the body segment. Passive systems are common at this level and often have manual locking elbow units operated and prepositioned with the contralateral limb. Full body–powered systems are possible but often require the use of inguinal control straps and chin nudge switches, which are cumbersome and increase rejection. Hybrid systems with body power and external power combinations are more common. Efforts at expanding myoelectric sites through surgical intervention such as targeted muscle reinnervation as well as the use of powered shoulders, elbows, wrists, and hands for increased movement and sequential control are now possible and have demonstrated significant functional gains.

## REFERENCES

The full reference list appears in the digital product found on http://connect.springerpub.com/content/book/978-0-8261-6226-7/part/part01/chapter/ch01

# BRAIN TUMORS

NY-YING LAM, ELAINE TSAO, AND JESSICA TSE

## CORE DEFINITIONS

Brain tumors may be primary or secondary (metastatic tumors). Primary brain tumors are a subset of central nervous system (CNS) tumors. In adults, meningioma, a nonmalignant tumor, is the most common (37.1% of adult CNS tumors). The most common malignant CNS tumor in adults is glioma, of which glioblastoma multiforme is the most prevalent type and has the worst prognosis. Metastatic brain tumors are the most frequently diagnosed tumor in the brain with common sources being lung cancer, breast cancer, and melanoma.

In pediatrics (age 0–19), the most common CNS tumor type is glioma (46.5% pediatric CNS tumors), of which pilocytic astrocytoma is the most prevalent type. Embryonal tumors are the second most common brain tumor type in pediatrics (10.4% pediatric CNS tumors) and is most prevalent from ages 0 to 4. Medulloblastoma, a malignant tumor, comprises 63.3% of all embryonal tumors. The location of the brain tumor also differs by age group. In ages 0 to 14, tumors are primarily located in the cerebellum and brainstem (28.4%). In ages 15 to 19, tumors involving the pituitary and craniopharyngeal duct (31.9%) are more common.[1]

Gliomas are classified by the 2016 World Health Organization (WHO) Classification of Tumors of the CNS, which uses histology and molecular parameters obtained from a biopsy. WHO grades indicate the aggressiveness of the tumor with WHO grade I as the least aggressive and WHO grade IV as the most aggressive. Nearly all low-grade tumors (WHO grades I and II) will develop into high-grade tumors (WHO grades III and IV). The molecular profiles included in the classification of gliomas are the presence of isocitrate dehydrogenase (IDH) mutation and chromosome 1p/19q codeletion, each of which have a better prognosis. O[6]-methylguanine-DNA methyltransferase (MGMT) promoter methylation also has a better prognosis and is commonly evaluated but is not part of the WHO criteria.[2]

## ETIOLOGY AND PATHOPHYSIOLOGY

The etiology of primary brain tumors is unknown unless there is an associated genetic condition (e.g., neurofibromatosis, tuberous sclerosis, Von Hippel-Lindau disease, Li-Fraumeni), and HIV/AIDS (primary CNS lymphoma).

Initial presentation of brain tumors varies widely, though most present with nonspecific neurologic signs and symptoms such as headache, seizure, altered mental status, or loss of balance. Focal neurologic deficits may be present depending on tumor size and location.[3]

---

The full list of resources and references appear in the digital product found on http://connect .springerpub.com/content/book/978-0-8261-6226-7/part/part01/chapter/ch02

## DIAGNOSTIC APPROACH

Initial workup for brain tumor includes imaging with head CT. If an intracranial mass is noted, contrast-enhanced brain MRI can better evaluate the lesion. Lesion characteristics on imaging such as location and composition may be suggestive of a specific tumor type; however, pathological diagnosis is crucial for accurate identification and WHO classification. The goals of surgery are to obtain tissue for pathology as well as to reduce tumor burden and mass effect while preserving or improve neurological status. Surgical options include stereotactic biopsy, subtotal resection, or gross total resection.

Workup for tumor recurrence may be initiated in the setting of new or worsening neurologic findings. Head CT can quickly evaluate for complications from brain tumor treatment such as hydrocephalus, edema, or bleeding. Contrasted brain MRI and PET scans may help differentiate tumor recurrence from radiation necrosis.

## TREATMENT

Treatment plans differ depending on tumor type and staging. Malignant brain tumors are treated with a combination of surgical resection, chemotherapy, and radiation. Surveillance or complete resection may be sufficient to treat benign tumors. A select sampling of typical treatment protocols is listed in Table 2.1.

Radiation therapy may be used as primary or adjuvant therapy. External beam radiation is typically delivered over multiple fractionated doses for days to weeks until the target therapeutic dose is reached. Proton beam therapy delivers more localized radiation to minimize damage to surrounding structures and usually requires fewer dose fractions. Stereotactic radiosurgery delivers a high dose of radiation with precision to small well-circumscribed lesions with minimal effect to nearby structures and is most effective in treating lesions less than 4 cm in size.

Steroids are commonly used in brain tumor patients to reduce symptoms related to mass effect from vasogenic edema. Functional decline may occur during steroid tapers, so slowing of the taper should be considered if a functional change is noted. The lowest steroid dose to treat symptoms should be prescribed in order to minimize steroid-related side effects. Patients with brain tumor who experience seizures generally require anticonvulsant therapy; however, the duration of treatment is not well defined. Seizure prophylaxis is not indicated in those who have not seized.

Rehabilitation interventions for brain tumor patients can target the impairments arising from the cancer itself and/or sequelae of treatment. If available, neurorehabilitation programs for acquired brain injury can be carefully tailored to address the patient's individual needs. A clear understanding of the brain tumor type, staging, and associated prognosis is necessary for appropriate goal setting. Therapy frequency and intensity may be adjusted to accommodate cancer treatment plans, treatment-related side effects, and fatigue. Patients with advanced brain tumors or poor prognosis still benefit from rehabilitation services with the goal to improve quality of life (QOL) via increasing functional independence and reducing caregiver burden. However, the possibility of further functional decline due to treatment effects or tumor progression must be considered as part of the rehabilitation plan.

## TABLE 2.1 TREATMENT PROTOCOLS FOR SELECTED BRAIN TUMOR TYPES

| BRAIN TUMOR TYPE | TREATMENT PROTOCOL |
|---|---|
| Glioblastoma | Surgical resection if possible<br>"Stupp protocol" = radiation therapy + six cycles of adjuvant temozolomide |
| Anaplastic oligodendroglioma | Surgical resection if possible<br>Radiation therapy + six cycles of adjuvant chemotherapy PCV (procarbazine, lomustine, vincristine) or temozolomide (Temodar®) |
| Recurrent glioblastoma | Bevacizumab, temozolomide, lomustine |
| Metastatic brain tumor | Surgical resection if possible<br>Chemotherapy targeted to primary tumor type<br>± Radiation therapy if radio-responsive tumor type |

Neurocognitive dysfunction is common in brain tumor patients, either due to direct tumor effects or as a treatment sequela. Cognitive dysfunction is especially challenging for survivors of malignant glioma, with cognitive decline found in 50% of patients with glioblastoma 6 years after diagnosis. Neurostimulants such as methylphenidate and modafinil are safe to use in this patient population to address fatigue and cognitive dysfunction, but research is limited regarding true efficacy.[4,5]

Depression is prevalent in all cancer patients, while changes in behavior or mood are more frequently seen in brain tumor patients. Screening for mood disorders should be implemented and monitored over time. Psychotherapy can address both adjustment to cancer diagnosis and coping with new impairments or disability while providing skills to combat fatigue or sleep disturbance. Chaplain services may provide spiritual support. Palliative care consultations provide additional support for defining goals of care, distress with poor prognosis, and symptom management in patients with life-threatening illness.

## COMPLICATIONS

### Brain Tumor-Related Complications

Cancer-related fatigue, cancer-associated cachexia, deep venous thrombosis (DVT), syndrome of inappropriate antidiuretic hormone secretion (SIADH), vasogenic edema, tumor progression or recurrence, hydrocephalus, seizure, headache, focal neurologic deficits, neurogenic bladder, neurogenic bowel, spasticity, dysphagia, sleep disturbance, cognitive impairment, delirium, reactive mood and adjustment disorders, depression, and anxiety.

### Treatment-Related Complications

Corticosteroid-related: Iinsomnia, psychosis/agitation, myopathy, hyperglycemia

Surgery-related: Surgical site infection, bleeding, infection, cerebral salt wasting, posterior fossa syndrome

TABLE 2.2 RADIATION-RELATED COMPLICATIONS

| RADIATION-RELATED COMPLICATIONS | TIMING | SYMPTOMS | PATHOPHYSIOLOGY TREATMENT |
|---|---|---|---|
| Acute radiation encephalopathy | Immediate to 4–6 weeks | Headache, nausea, vomiting, focal neurologic signs | Vasogenic edema *Tx: steroids* |
| Early delayed | 6 weeks to 6 months | Fatigue or somnolence, focal neurologic signs, encephalopathy | Demyelination of irradiated tissue *Tx: steroids* |
| Late delayed | 6 months to years | Dementia, ataxia, incontinence, focal neurologic signs | Radiation necrosis, vascular abnormalities *Irreversible* |

Chemotherapy-related: Fatigue, peripheral neuropathy, nausea, anemia, leukopenia, thrombocytopenia, "chemo-brain"

Radiation-related: See Table 2.2

## FUNCTIONAL PROGNOSIS AND OUTCOMES

The 5-year survival rates for the most common brain tumor types by age group are noted in Table 2.3.[13] Functional prognosis varies significantly based on tumor size, location, post-surgical complications, and treatment-related complications.

### Survivors of Pediatric Brain Tumors

Survival rates of pediatric brain tumors are increasing, with relative 5-year survival rate of 88.3% for children diagnosed in 2011 compared to 76.5% in 1990. With improved survival rates, there are associated long-term morbidities in survivors of childhood brain tumors across several outcome measures, including neurocognitive function, general health, vocation, and social and psychological adjustment. Neurocognitive deficits include problems with attention, working memory, processing speed, and visuospatial skills. Risk factors for neurocognitive dysfunction include cranial or craniospinal irradiation, surgery, chemotherapy, and the effect of the tumor itself. Survivors are also at higher risk of depression, anxiety, suicidal ideation, and behavioral and social adjustment issues compared to the general population. Long-term general health issues may include physical performance limitations, neurosensory deficits, neuroendocrine dysfunction, and neurologic complications such as strokes or late-occurring seizures. These deficits may also result in adverse educational and vocational outcomes for adult survivors of pediatric brain tumors.[6]

### Survivors of Adult Primary Brain Tumors

Adult patients with malignant gliomas report lower function in all domains of QOL including physical or functional status, emotional well-being, and social well-being compared to age- and sex-matched healthy controls. Patients with low-grade gliomas also report lower overall

## TABLE 2.3 FIVE-YEAR RELATIVE SURVIVAL RATES

| HISTOLOGY | CHILDREN (0–14 YEARS) | ADOLESCENT, YOUNG ADULT (15–39 YEARS) | ADULTS (40+ YEARS) |
|---|---|---|---|
| Pilocytic astrocytoma (WHO grade I) | 96.9% | 93.2% | 79.7% |
| Anaplastic astrocytoma (WHO grade III) | 21.9% | 55.7% | 19.8% |
| Glioblastoma (WHO grade IV) | 19.6% | 22.7% | 4.3% |
| Medulloblastoma (WHO grade IV) | 72.8% | 75.1% | 69.0% |
| Meningioma (WHO grades I–III) | – | 89.0% | 61.5% |

QOL with more complaints of fatigue, cognitive dysfunction, and altered mood compared to healthy patients and those with non-CNS cancers.

Fatigue is the most significant symptom for patients with gliomas and may be independently predictive of poorer overall survival in high-grade glioma. Another common problem is pain, with headache as the most common type of pain experienced by >50% of patients with high-grade glioma.[7]

While literature regarding efficacy of rehabilitation for patients with brain tumors is limited, there is evidence to suggest that patients make functional gains in the inpatient and outpatient settings.[8–11] Most studies evaluating inpatient rehabilitation demonstrated that patients with brain tumors make functional gains that can be maintained post-discharge. Furthermore, their functional gains are comparable to those made by patients with stroke and brain injury and are achieved across different tumor types and locations or presence of metastases.[12]

## BASIC ORDER SETS

### Workup for Altered Mental Status or Acute Neurologic Change in the Brain Tumor Patient

Laboratory orders:

- Complete blood count (CBC), chemistry panel ± liver function tests (LFTs)
- Urinalysis with reflex culture
- Consider blood cultures or lumbar puncture for cerebrospinal fluid (CSF) evaluation if concerned for systemic infection, meningitis, encephalitis
- If on seizure medication, check antiepileptic medication level

Imaging: Head CT

- If negative for hemorrhage, enlarged ventricles, or increased tumor burden, consider brain MRI with contrast

Other: Consider EEG

Consults: Neurosurgery and/or neurology and/or neuro-oncology

Differential diagnosis: Vasogenic edema, SIADH, infection (urinary tract infection [UTI], pneumonia, bacteremia, intracranial abscess, meningitis, encephalitis), hydrocephalus, hemorrhage, tumor progression, seizure, radiation effect (acute, early delayed, necrosis), delirium, medication effect (opioids, sedating meds), stroke, elevated intracranial pressure, chemotherapy-associated central neurotoxicity (methotrexate, ifosfamide, cytarabine), posterior reversible encephalopathy syndrome.

## RESOURCES AND REFERENCES

The full list of resources and references appear in the digital product found on http://connect .springerpub.com/content/book/978-0-8261-6226-7/part/part01/chapter/ch02

# CANCER REHABILITATION

RYAN LEWIS, BHAVESH PATEL, AND JESSICA ENGLE

## CORE DEFINITIONS

Cancer rehabilitation is a continuously evolving field that may be defined as "medical care that should be integrated throughout the oncology care continuum and delivered by trained rehabilitation professionals who have it within their scope of practice to diagnose and treat patients' physical, psychological and cognitive impairments in an effort to maintain or restore function, reduce symptom burden, maximize independence and improve quality of life."[1] One important aspect of this definition is the continuum of care along which rehabilitation interventions may be integrated. This is best represented by the widely accepted Dietz classification,[2,3] which divides the continuum into the following four phases:

**Prehabilitation:** Early intervention after diagnosis but prior to treatment with the focus on establishing a functional baseline and identification and prevention of potential impairments.

**Restorative rehabilitation:** For patients with potential curable cancer and reversible deficits, the focus is on regaining complete functional recovery.

**Supportive rehabilitation:** For patients with chronic cancer and potentially irreversible deficits, the focus is on maximizing functional independence.

**Palliative rehabilitation:** For patients with terminal cancer refractory to treatment, the focus is on maximizing comfort and quality of life.

While cancer rehabilitation comprises a wide breadth of diverse disease processes with various pathologies, the harmonizing focus is addressing functional impairments utilizing a multidisciplinary and holistic approach with the overarching goal of optimizing quality of life.

## ETIOLOGY AND PATHOPHYSIOLOGY

Cancer is the second leading cause of death in the United States. As of 2019, 16.9 million Americans had cancer at some point in their lives. In the United States, lung, colorectal, breast, and prostate cancer are the most frequently occurring malignancies. There is an association of cancer with aging, and 80% of all cancers are diagnosed in people over 55 years old. Cancer prevention can be achieved through lifestyle changes, increased physical activity, and unhealthy behavior mitigation as well as early screening and detection. Due to

The full list of references appears in the digital product found on http://connect.springerpub.com/content/book/978-0-8261-6226-7/part/part01/chapter/ch03

these factors, the 5-year cancer survival rate has increased since the 1960s. Cancer survivors are more likely to acquire various musculoskeletal impairments and comorbidities from the natural aging process, further complicating cancer-related impairments and disabilities.[4]

## DIAGNOSTIC APPROACH

Evaluation of patients in cancer rehabilitation may utilize a wide variety of investigations to help identify the etiology of functional impairments and guide a safe treatment plan. Commonly used diagnostic tests can be divided into three categories—physiologic, psychologic, and functional—as outlined here:

### Physiologic

*Imaging*: MRI, CT, PET, or bone scans are used to evaluate for disease progression and new metastases. Ultrasound (US) or MRI may be used to evaluate for musculoskeletal, soft tissue, and vascular pathologies. Chest x-ray may be used to evaluate for pulmonary and cardiac pathologies.

*Laboratory studies*: General medical laboratory studies (e.g., complete blood count [CBC], comprehensive metabolic panel [CMP], Hgb A1c, thyroid stimulating hormone [TSH], lipid panel) are used to establish a baseline, identify treatable comorbidities (i.e., diabetes mellitus [DM], hyperlipidemia [HLD], thyroid dysfunction), and monitor treatment-related side effects (i.e., anemia, thrombocytopenia). Tumor markers are used to evaluate disease progression and treatment response. When neuropathy is present, TSH, vitamin $B_{12}$, blood glucose, folate, serum protein electrophoresis (SPEP) and creatine kinase (CK) should be evaluated to rule out reversible causes.

*Electrodiagnostics*: Nerve conduction velocity studies (NCVS) and electromyography (EMG) are helpful in the evaluation of neuropathies.

*Lymphatic evaluation*:Documentation by direct size measurement, bioimpedance spectroscopy, or lymphoscintigraphy (gold standard) is important for monitoring lymphedema.[5]

*Cardiopulmonary evaluation*: Used as part of the pre-exercise assessment in high-risk patient groups.[6]

### Psychologic

*Mood*: Formal evaluation with patient-reported scales, such as Patient Health Questionnaire 9 (PHQ-9) and Beck Depression Inventory (BDI) , should be used to screen for depression.

*Cognitive*: Screening of cognitive function should be performed with validated tools such as the Functional Assessment of Cancer Therapy-Cognitive Function (FACT-Cog), Montreal Cognitive Assessment (MOCA), Mini-Mental Status Examination (MMSE), or Mini-Cog. Positive screening should be followed by neuropsychological testing, the gold standard for diagnosis.[7]

### Functional

General functional evaluation should be carried out using validated tools such as the Eastern Cooperative Oncology Group (ECOG) Performance Status, Karnofsky Performance Scale (KPS), Short Form-36 (SF-36), or Functional Independence Measure (FIM). The 6-Minute Walk Test (6MWT), Timed Up and Go (TUG), Tinetti balance score, and Berg balance scale are important to evaluate mobility and balance. Pain can be documented using tools like the

Brief Pain Inventory (BPI) or visual analogue scales among others. Fatigue is an important problem in this population. The Functional Assessment of Chronic Illness Therapy-Fatigue (FACIT-F), Piper fatigue scale, or visual analogue scales may be used for evaluation.

## TREATMENT

### Medical

Medical management in cancer rehabilitation focuses on pharmacologic management of functional impairments and cancer treatment side effects. Treatment is typically administered in conjunction with nonpharmacologic rehabilitation interventions. Comorbidity and risk factor management is done in coordination with oncologic, surgical, and primary medical teams. While not directly managed by the rehabilitation physician, awareness of potential oncologic emergencies is important to allow for prompt referral and minimization of sequelae. Common components of the medical management plan are detailed here.

*Pain Management* (per WHO pain ladder)[8]

1. Non-opioids: Tylenol, non-steroidal anti-inflammatory drugs (NSAIDs) tailored to patients' comorbidities
2. Opioids: For pain refractory to non-opioids
3. Adjuncts: Anticonvulsants (i.e., gabapentin, pregabalin), antidepressants (i.e., tricyclic antidepressant [TCA]/serotonin norepinephrine reuptake inhibitors [SNRI]), topicals (i.e., lidocaine patch, diclofenac gel, capsaicin cream), corticosteroids, bisphosphonates
4. Interventional Procedures: Joint/epidural steroid injections, nerve blocks, radiofrequency ablation (RFA)

*Spasticity*: Most commonly managed with baclofen and localized chemodenervation (i.e., botulinum toxin injections). Other agents (e.g., tizanidine, dantrolene, diazepam) may be considered as indicated.

*Peripheral neuropathy*: The use of duloxetine for the treatment of peripheral neuropathy has the most robust evidence.[9] Other neuropathic agents (i.e., gabapentin, pregabalin, TCAs) are commonly used in practice. Topical medications such as menthol or combination amitriptyline and ketamine may be used.[9,10]

*Cognitive impairments*: Neurostimulants such as methylphenidate and modafinil have shown mild to moderate evidence in some studies and are used in clinical practice, though are not Food and Drug Administration (FDA) approved.[7]

*Mood*: Mood-related disorders such as depression and anxiety are common in the cancer patient population and managed with appropriate psychotropic agents, often under the guidance of a psychiatrist or general medical team.

*Sleep disturbances*: Most commonly managed with melatonin or trazodone. Prescribers must be cautious of cognitive effects of other sedative and hypnotic agents.

*Anorexia/cachexia*: Appropriate dietary supplements are used to provide adequate nutrition and replete metabolic deficiencies. Progesterone analogues and glucocorticoids have been found to be potentially beneficial for appetite stimulation, though there is no FDA-approved agent due to lack of sufficient evidence.[11]

*Gastrointestinal:* A bowel regimen is started with stool softeners and laxatives to manage constipation, with the use of suppository and enemas for neurogenic bowel. Antiemetics may be initiated to control nausea. Mucositis may be treated with oral mouthwashes and appropriate pain medications as indicated.

*Genitourinary*: Urinary incontinence and retention is managed with the use of appropriate agents (e.g., oxybutynin, tamsulosin). It may require referral to a urologist for urodynamic studies. Patients should be monitored for anticholinergic side effects, particularly in regard to cognition.

*Sexual function*: Common complaints such as erectile dysfunction and vaginal atrophy or dryness can be managed with phosphodiesterase inhibitors (e.g., sidenafil) and topical vaginal lubricants, respectively. Nonhormonal topical agents may be used when patients have hormone-sensitive cancers.[12]

*Dermatologic*: Rashes/skin irritation may be treated with appropriate topical or oral agents and may require referral to a dermatologist for further workup and management. Pentoxifylline and vitamin E have shown some benefit for prevention of radiation-induced fibrosis, but currently there is no consensus on treatment.[13]

*Secondary cancer prevention*: Treatment should focus on management of comorbidities and risk factor reduction (e.g., smoking cessation, alcohol consumption reduction).

*Some Common Oncologic Emergencies*[14]

1. Spinal Cord Compression—Requires emergent neurosurgical evaluation for decompression.
2. Deep Venous Thrombosis (DVT)/Pulmonary Embolism (PE)—Emergent workup (i.e., venous duplex ultrasound, CT with PE protocol) is needed with prompt initiation of therapeutic anticoagulation.
3. Malignant Pericardial Effusion—Emergent cardiology or cardiac surgery evaluation is required.
4. Superior Vena Cava Syndrome—Emergent vascular surgery evaluation is needed.
5. Tumor Lysis Syndrome, Neutropenic Fever—Usually requires emergent hospitalization for medical management, typically under the guidance of the primary oncology teams.
6. Infection—Clinicians must have a low threshold for infectious workup if there is any change in function and/or mental status.

## Rehabilitation

Comprehensive cancer rehabilitation aims to address the four pillars of survivorship care, as defined by the Institute of Medicine.[15,16]

1. Surveillance: To detect primary cancer recurrence, development of additional cancers, and for late effects
2. Intervention: For treatment-related complications
3. Prevention: Of recurrence, new cancers, late effects, and comorbidities
4. Coordination: With primary care, oncology, and other specialists

One comprehensive cancer rehabilitation model proposed by the American Society of Clinical Oncology (ASCO) expands on the best practice prospective model of surveillance. It provides a framework for rehabilitation that includes the following levels of stepped outpatient care[16]:

1. General Conditioning Activities, Unspecialized: Exercise counseling for patients without any specific functional impairments and who do not require the supervision of a specialist (i.e., physical therapy [PT]).
2. General Conditioning Activities, Specialized: Specialist supervised exercise program for patients without any specific functional impairments.
3. Impairment Directed Care, Uncomplicated: Focuses on impairment driven interventions for patients with functional deficits but without any severe symptoms/systemic concerns (e.g., radiation fibrosis, chemotherapy-induced peripheral neuropathy [CIPN]). This level may also involve psychosocial counseling for mood and coping.
4. Impairment Directed Care, Complicated: Focuses on patients with severely symptomatic functional impairments or complications that may be refractory to first-line interventions. This is the most resource-intensive level that requires coordination among the cancer rehabilitation physician and other members of the multidisciplinary team (i.e., PT, occupational therapy [OT], speech and language therapy [SLP], psychology).

The model describes inpatient rehabilitation as an important aspect of comprehensive cancer rehabilitation care since this is where the majority of impairments, especially in advanced cancers, are identified.[16] Goals of care are similar to level 4 of outpatient rehabilitation and employ a multidisciplinary approach (PT, OT, SLP, case management [CM]/social work [SW], psychology, dietician).

*Exercise* is the one component of any cancer rehabilitation program that is integrated into each level of care.[16] The importance of this simple intervention stems from its positive effect on a wide variety of symptoms and functional impairments as well as the potential morbidity and mortality benefit in cancer survivors. Systematic review of exercise guidelines resulted in the following recommendations.[6,12]

*Duration*: Moderate intensity aerobic exercise is recommended at least 3 days each week practiced in at least 30-minute intervals. Resistance exercise should be done at least 2 days per week including major muscle groups. Long-term exercise (i.e., 18 weeks) has been shown to have positive effect on quality of life and muscular/aerobic fitness.

*Intensity*: The goal would be to reach moderate intensity, described as three to six times the baseline metabolic equivalent (MET). It should include a warm-up and cooldown during each session. Moderate intensity can also be defined subjectively as "the ability to talk during exertion to the point where one cannot sing."[17]

*Setting*: Group or supervised exercise sessions are recommended as this provides motivation and education with potential for improved outcomes in quality of life and fitness.

*Safety*: Use of pre-exercise medical assessments allows for appropriate risk stratification, identification of comorbidities, disease, and treatment effects. While exercise is generally safe across all cancer types and treatment phases, it is important to be aware of specific safety considerations that require activity modifications (Table 3.1).[14,18]

Other impairment-driven interventions that are common components of the rehabilitation management plan are outlined here.

**TABLE 3.1 COMMON REHABILITATION SAFETY CONSIDERATIONS AND RECOMMENDATIONS IN CANCER SURVIVORS**

| CRITERION | RECOMMENDATION |
|---|---|
| $FEV_1$ or FVC <50% predicted; pulse ox <90% | Limit aerobic exercise and consider oxygen supplementation |
| HR >80% maximum; LVEF <20% | Limit aerobic exercise |
| Unstable arrhythmia | Exercise only with cardiac monitoring |
| >50% cortical involvement of bone malignancy; risk of pathologic fracture | Non–weight-bearing precautions |
| 25%–50% cortical involvement of bone malignancy | Partial weight-bearing precautions |
| <25% cortical involvement of bone malignancy | No high-impact activities or sports |
| Any grade of lymphedema | No restrictions for exercise or weight-lifting |
| Uncontrolled emesis or diarrhea | No strenuous activity |
| Platelets <20,000 | Limited ambulation, no high-fall risk activities |
| ANC <1,000 | Neutropenic precautions |
| Hgb <8 | Low-intensity, symptom-limited intervention |

ANC, absolute neutrophil count; LVEF, left ventricular ejection fraction; $FEV_1$, forced expiratory volume in 1 second; FVC, forced vital capacity; HR, heart therapy.

## Referrals

*PT*: For supervision of formal exercise program, functional mobility, strengthening, gait and balance training, and specialized treatments (i.e., lymphedema complete decongestive therapy, pelvic floor strengthening, peripheral neuropathy desensitization, and mirror therapies)[12]

*OT*: For activities of daily living (ADL) and safety training, use of adaptive equipment, and recommendations on home modifications

*SLP*: For speech, swallowing, and cognitive evaluation and treatment

*Recreation therapy*: For relaxation strategies (i.e., music therapy), leisure activities, and social integration

*Psychology*: For comprehensive neuropsychological testing and therapies (i.e., cognitive behavioral therapy [CBT]) to address impairments in adjustment, mood, and cognitive function

*Dietician*: For recommendations on both enteral (oral vs. tube feeds) and parenteral nutrition to ensure adequate caloric and nutrition intake

*Prosthetist/orthotist*: For appropriate prosthesis/orthoses to maximize functional mobility

*Sexual therapist*: For evaluation, education, and nonpharmacologic treatment of sexual dysfunction (e.g., low libido)

*Skilled nursing*: For patients who require continued medical management or monitoring in the home environment (i.e., lab draws, IV infusions, tube feeds, drain/line management, wound care)

*Home health aide*: For assistance with ADLs at home

*SW*: For assistance with access to resources

**Modalities**[12,14]: Although limited evidence exists in the cancer patient population, the following methods may be used in practice, with appropriate precautions, with the aim of improved functional mobility. Deep heat methods, such as therapeutic US, are typically contraindicated due to the potential risk of potentiating tumor spread. Modalities should generally not be used directly over a tumor site/radiation area or severely damaged skin (i.e., open wounds, severely impaired sensation, peripheral vascular disease [PVD]/ischemia).

1. *Superficial heat*—May be used for myofascial pain
2. *Cryotherapy*—Beneficial for pain or acute inflammation
3. *Transcutaneous electrical nerve stimulation (TENs)*—May also be used for sensory pain management
4. *Functional electrical stimulation (FES)*—For restoration of muscle contraction (requires intact nerve conduction)
5. *Manual therapy or massage*—Soft tissue manipulation for improving pain and range of motion and lymphatic stimulation; complete decongestive therapy is the mainstay of lymphedema treatment, which includes manual lymphatic drainage and compression[19]
6. *Low- level laser therapy*—May be used in the treatment of oral mucositis and lymphedema
7. *Spinal stimulation*—Is contraindicated with bone fragility (i.e., metastasis, osteoporosis) and spinal pathology (i.e., cord compression, spinal stenosis, myelopathy, radiculopathy)
8. *Bracing*—May be beneficial for skeletal instability or vertebral compression pain
9. *Acupuncture*—May be beneficial for treatment of musculoskeletal pain; it is still being investigated for its role in the treatment of neuropathic pain[10]
10. *Scrambler therapy*—Emerging treatment for CIPN[10]

## Counseling

1. *Physical activity* is recommended for all patients and functional impairments, with restrictions as mentioned earlier. Activities such as yoga and aquatic therapy have also been shown to be beneficial.[12]
2. All patients should receive education on appropriate *sleep hygiene* to help mitigate effects of fatigue and cognitive dysfunction.
3. It is important to provide education on *fatigue* expectations and monitoring for concerning symptoms, promoting regular exercise, and discussing energy conservation techniques.
4. It is recommended to provide education on potential treatment-related *cognitive effects* and give guidance on mental stimulation, relaxation, stress management, and adaptive

strategies. SLP and neuropsychology can be helpful with teaching and implementing these strategies.

5. Regular screening for mood-related disorders (i.e., depression/anxiety), evaluation of social support, and appropriate neuropsychology referral for nonpharmacologic therapeutic interventions (e.g., CBT) should be performed as needed.

6. General age-appropriate health counseling for lifestyle modification should include regular exercise, balanced diet, weight management, and smoking or alcohol cessation.

## REFERENCES

The full list of references appears in the digital product found on http://connect.springerpub.com/content/book/978-0-8261-6226-7/part/part01/chapter/ch03

# CEREBRAL PALSY

MARISA OSORIO, KELLY PHAM, JACLYN OMURA, AND DESIREE ROGE

## CORE DEFINITION

Cerebral palsy (CP): "A group of permanent disorders of the development of movement and posture, causing activity limitation that are attributed to nonprogressive disturbances that occurred in the developing fetal or infant brain."[1]

## ETIOLOGY AND PATHOPHYSIOLOGY

CP is caused by a static lesion to the brain in the prenatal, perinatal, or postnatal periods. The etiology of the brain injury in some instances is hypoxic ischemic, inflammatory, due to a genetic disorder, or related to a congenital malformation in brain development.

Risk factors in the prenatal period include multiple gestations, congenital infection (hepatitis B, syphilis, HIV, streptococcus B, and TORCH infections [toxoplasmosis, rubella, cytomegalovirus, herpes]), maternal disease (seizures, intellectual disability, thyroid disease, coagulopathy), brain malformations (schizencephaly, polymicrogyria, etc.), and placental complications.[2] The understanding of the genetic etiology of CP is in its infancy, but early research suggests that there is a link between iNOS-231 T allele and the apoE ε4 allele and development of CP.[3]

In the perinatal period, prematurity, low gestational age, low birth weight, large for gestational age, premature rupture of membranes, maternal infection, thrombophilia (resulting in perinatal stroke), hyperbilirubinemia, placental complications, and birth hypoxia are risk factors.[2,4] Prematurity is a significant risk factor for brain injury as the vascular system is immature and predisposed to hemorrhage with disturbances in cerebral blood flow and changes in perfusion pressures.[5] Germinal matrix hemorrhage and intraventricular hemorrhage have the potential to lead to long-term neurologic sequelae, regardless of the severity of the hemorrhage. However, more severe hemorrhage and development of hydrocephalus can result in more significant neurologic impairments.[6]

Postnatal brain injury can include infection (meningitis), trauma (nonaccidental trauma, motor vehicle accident, fall, etc.), hypoxic-ischemic encephalopathy (HIE; near drowning, cardiac arrest, etc.), and stroke.

---

The full list of resources and references appears in the digital product found on http://connect .springerpub.com/content/book/978-0-8261-6226-7/part/part01/chapter/ch04

## DIAGNOSTIC APPROACH

When considering a diagnosis of CP, a thorough history including birth, development, medical, and family histories is important. Consider the risk factors mentioned previously when obtaining a birth history. A history consistent with prematurity or congenital infection, for example, can be supportive of a diagnosis of CP. Developmental history may demonstrate delays in some or all areas of development. Any history of regression in development should prompt the examiner to consider other diagnoses as CP is static and a loss of skills is unexpected. A family history can give context to the possibility of a genetic etiology of CP or another diagnosis entirely. Medical history can help to rule out other diagnoses as well.

A physical examination including a thorough neurological examination can evaluate for both the positive signs of CP (hyperreflexia, spasticity, dystonia, etc.) as well as the negative signs (hypotonia and weakness) representative of a central nervous system injury.

In preterm infants, cranial ultrasound is the standard of care and may show evidence of intraventricular hemorrhage or white matter injury. In term infants, MRI of the brain is standard and most commonly demonstrates periventricular leukomalacia (PVL) in the setting of prematurity and hyperintensity in the deep brain in the setting of HIE. Imaging findings are not diagnostic but can be helpful in the overall clinical picture. Of note, normal imaging does not preclude the diagnosis of CP, but other etiologies for the constellation of symptoms should be explored.

Diagnosis of CP is dependent on meeting the criteria that define CP, notably that there is a permanent disorder affecting movement and posture due to a nonprogressive lesion to a developing brain.[7] There is a growing body of evidence in support of early diagnosis using the Prechtl General Movements Assessment (GMA) and the Hammersmith Infant Neurological Examination (HINE) in infants at risk for CP.[8,9]

## TREATMENT

The management of a child with CP requires a multidisciplinary team that understands the primary and secondary conditions associated with CP and its multisystem involvement. The family and child should be active team members when setting goals within the context of the level of impairments and the child's age.

There is no cure for CP. Rehabilitation care consists of physical therapy (PT), occupational therapy (OT), speech and language therapy, feeding, and vision and behavioral therapies. These therapies facilitate treatment of motor and communication impairments and other comorbidities. Therapies should be child active, repetitive and structured practice of gross motor, hand function, and learning tasks.[9] The intensity and frequency of therapies is often higher in the early years. As the child grows, goal-oriented models of sporadic intensive burst of therapies are most effective.[10]

Early intervention services are government-sponsored programs under the Individuals with Disabilities Education Act available to infants and toddlers with developmental disabilities from birth to 3 years old. The goals of early intervention are to maximize early neuroplasticity that will result in improved motor, cognition, and communication outcomes and reduce secondary comorbidities.[9]

Stretching and strengthening are part of most OT and PT programs. In CP, therapy interventions with evidence supporting improvement in motor function are constraint-induced movement therapy (CIMT), bimanual therapy, goal-directed training, home programs, and OT following botulinum toxin (BoNT).[10] Additional therapy interventions with insufficient evidence include hippo therapy, robotic-assisted training, treadmill training, and pool therapy. Craniosacral therapy, hyperbaric oxygen, neurodevelopmental therapy, and sensory integration have shown to be ineffective in children with CP.[10]

Environmental modifications such as orthoses and adaptive equipment that includes walkers, gait trainers, wheelchairs, canes, standers, and bath equipment help to promote inclusion and independence by accommodating the child's developmental stage and disability. Augmentative and alternative communication devices compensate for limited or lack of verbal speech. Examples include communication symbol boards and electronic speech output devices.

Contracture prevention and tone management are important in CP. If untreated these may worsen over time, affecting quality of life and interfering with activity and participation. Dystonia and spasticity are common tone abnormalities found in CP.

There is limited research about the efficacy of tone-modulating medications in CP.[11,12] Diazepam is the only medication with evidence, recommended for the short-term treatment of spasticity in children with CP.[12] Other medications often used but with limited evidence are baclofen, trihexyphenidyl, and levodopa.

BoNT is often used in conjunction with oral agents and/or phenol or alcohol blocks. BoNT treatment should start at a young age when gait patterns and motor function are still flexible, allowing for gross motor function learning. The structure of the muscles changes with growth leading to development of fixed contractures. BoNT is effective in the management of focal spasticity in CP.[10] There is inadequate data on reducing dystonia in CP.[11] BoNT must be used in combination with other modalities such as therapies, bracing, and serial casting.[10,13,14] Pediatric dosing guidelines recommend a lower range of dosing of 12 to 16 U/Kg body weight, particularly for patients of Gross Motor Function Classification System (GMFCS) level V and patients with dysphagia or pulmonary problems.[14]

Intrathecal baclofen therapy (ITB) is used to treat generalized spasticity and/or dystonia. ITB is possibly effective in the management of dystonia and spasticity in CP with goals of care comfort, pain reduction. There is no evidence that it improves function.[10-12]

Selective dorsal rhizotomy (SDR) is a surgical procedure aimed to reduce spasticity in CP. It involves a laminectomy exposing the L2 to S2 nerve roots and selectively cutting a percentage of the dorsal rootlets with abnormal response with electrophysiologic monitoring. Eliminating the abnormal reflex arcs in the sensory roots reduces spasticity without affecting the motor nerves.[15] An SDR is ideal for a child between the ages of 4 and 8 years with diplegic CP, PVL on brain MRI, GMFCS levels I to III, predominantly spastic tone, with little upper limb involvement, good underlying strength and selective motor control, and minimal contractures. Most research demonstrates a reduction in spasticity, but evidence of functional gains is limited and inconclusive. Some studies have shown improved mobility, endurance, and balance which translates to decreased falls and improved independence with activities of daily living (ADLs) and less functional decline with age.[15] Some studies claim less need for orthopedic intervention in children who undergo an SDR at a young age; other studies show no differences in this rate. The reduction of spasticity unmasks muscle weakness. Therefore, an intensive rehabilitation program for strengthening and gait training following the procedure is needed to promote positive outcomes. SDR can also be considered in children who are at GMFCS level IV or V for palliative reasons.

## Orthopedic Surgery

In children with CP, the combination of hypertonia, muscle weakness, impaired motor control, and growth leads to development of contractures and lever arm disease (LAD) or bone torsion abnormalities. Biarticular muscles such as iliopsoas, hamstrings, rectus femoris, and gastrocnemius are commonly contracted. The contractures and LAD may worsen over time leading to unwanted compensatory gait deviations and deterioration. Instrumented 3D gait and motion analysis is helpful in identifying these issues and aids in surgical planning. Surgeries aimed at improving gait in ambulatory children help correct these deformities. Soft tissue lengthenings, muscle transfers, osteotomies, and arthrodesis are used in combination and often simultaneously as part of a single-event multilevel surgery (SEMLS). SEMLS has the advantage of requiring one hospital admission and one period of rehabilitation. There is limited research about SEMLS outcomes.[10]

In the nonambulatory group, the goal of lower limb orthopedic surgery is to facilitate positioning, promote ease of caregiving, prevent skin breakdown, and avoid hip dislocation. Examples include lengthening of hamstrings, hip flexors, and adductors. Larger hip surgeries may be needed in the setting of hip dislocation.

The incidence of hip displacement in children with CP is reported to be 35% and is the result of abnormalities in muscle and bony development.[16] For most children, there is abnormal tone and muscle imbalance between the hip adductors, hamstrings, and hip flexors. In children with limited or no ambulation, there is often a shallow acetabulum and coxa valga that increases the risk of subluxation. The risk of progression is directly related to the GMFCS level with up to 90% in the GMFCS level V group.[17] For ambulatory children, the goal of preserving ambulation requires a contained and stable hip. In the nonambulatory group, hip dislocations may lead to pain, difficulties with sitting balance, and perineal care. Early identification and orthopedic intervention prevent hip dislocation and avoid the need for salvage surgery.[16] Hip surveillance guidelines in CP rely on a combination of serial physical examination and pelvis x-rays.[17] Surgical intervention depends on the degree of subluxation and structural abnormalities.

The incidence of scoliosis is linearly related to the GMFCS level with GMFCS V approaching 100% of incidence. Spinal deformities vary and may contribute to pelvic obliquity. The classic presentation is a long, C-shaped levokyphoscoliosis. Curve progression is gradual with rapid progression during puberty or increased time spent in a wheelchair.[17] Annual or biannual posterior-anterior (PA) and lateral complete spine rays, standing when possible or sitting are recommended for surveillance.[17] Flexible curves under 40° with good sitting balance are observed. Bracing has proven not to be effective in treating neuromuscular scoliosis.[18,19] Spinal instrumentation and fusion is considered when there is significant curve progression and loss of sitting balance.[18,19]

Goals for upper limb surgery include improved function, facilitation of care, and improved cosmesis. Patients with significant athetosis and dystonia tend to have unpredictable and poorer outcomes.[20]

## LIST OF COMORBIDITIES OF CEREBRAL PALSY

- Mobility impairment—nonambulatory, abnormal gait
- Fine motor impairment
- Spasticity
- Dystonia
- Chorea, athetosis or choreoathetosis
- Contractures
- Hip dysplasia/dislocation
- Neuromuscular scoliosis
- Osteopenia/osteoporosis/fragility fractures
- Pain
- Sleep disorders/sleep apnea (obstructive and central)
- Epilepsy
- Intellectual disability
- Learning disabilities
- Attention problems
- Behavior problems
- Communication problems
- Vision problems (strabismus, cortical vision impairment, nystagmus)
- Hearing impairment
- Dysphagia
- Sialorrhea
- Reflux
- Constipation
- Voiding difficulties/neurogenic bladder
- Pulmonary problems/aspiration pneumonia/chronic lung disease
- Sensory impairment

## FUNCTIONAL PROGNOSIS AND OUTCOMES

In 1997, the GMFCS was established as a way to describe the mobility level of children with CP.[21] However, the functional prognosis for mobility in children with CP was limited to observations in clinic, including presence of primitive reflexes and gross motor milestone achievement at the age of 2. In 2002, a longitudinal cohort study of children with CP collected data over 5 years using a standardized measure of functional abilities (Gross Motor Functional Measure 66 [GMFM-66]) and compared this with GMFCS level (see Figure 4.1), concluding that age and GMFCS level are the best tools we have to predict gross motor function in a child with CP.[22] Since then, multiple studies have demonstrated GMFCS levels are stable over time, helping to provide anticipatory guidance for patients with CP and their families. Other classification systems have also been created to describe hand function and communication.

Studies have shown that children with CP rate their quality of life among the lowest in children with chronic illnesses including asthma, diabetes, and cancer. This is a surprising finding but one that can potentially be explained by the impact CP has on all five domains of

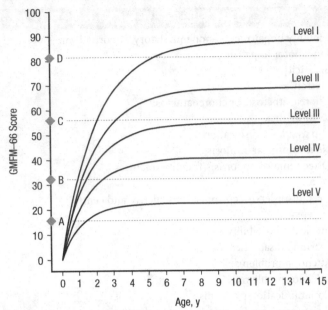

**FIGURE 4.1** Predicted average development by the Gross Motor Function Classification System levels.

The diamonds on the vertical axis identify four GMFM-66 items that predict when children are expected to have a 50% chance of completing that item successfully. The GMFM-66 item 21 (diamond A) assesses whether a child can lift and maintain their head in a vertical position with trunk support by a therapist while sitting; item 24 (diamond B) assesses whether when in a sitting position on a mat, a child can maintain sitting unsupported by their arms for 3 seconds; item 69 (diamond C) measures a child's ability to walk forward 10 steps unsupported; and item 87 (diamond D) assesses the task of walking down four steps alternating feet with arms free.

*Source*: Reprinted by permission from Rutz E, Thomason P, Willoughby K. Integrated management in cerebral palsy: musculoskeletal surgery and rehabilitation in ambulatory patients. In: *Cerebral Palsy: A Multidisciplinary Approach*. Springer Nature; 2018.

the International Classification System of Functioning, Disability and Health (body structure and function, environment, activity, participation, personal factors).

## BASIC ORDER SETS

### Outpatient Clinic Visit

*Diagnosis:* CP

*Diagnostics*

- MRI brain without contrast
- MRI spine without contrast

*Therapies*

■ PT: Evaluation of lower extremity strength, balance, coordination, gait training home stretching program
  ❏ Consider referral for durable medical equipment (DME) evaluation: Assistive device, manual wheelchair, power wheelchair, stander
  ❏ Consider referral for aquatic therapy
■ OT: Evaluation of upper extremity strength, fine motor skills, and age-appropriate self-care skills
  ❏ Consider referral for DME evaluation: Activity chair, adaptive car seat, bath chair, commode chair, hand/wrist splints
■ Speech therapy: Evaluation of verbal and/or nonverbal communication skills, swallow evaluation, cognitive skills
  ❏ Consider referral for augmentative communication device
  ❏ Consider referral for Videofluoroscopic Swallow Study
■ Orthotics/prosthetics referral for ankle foot orthoses (AFOs) to maintain ankle ROM and promote optimal gait mechanics
  ❏ Consider daytime and/or nighttime AFOs

*Medications*

■ Constipation
  ❏ Polyethylene glycol
  ❏ Lactulose
  ❏ Senna
  ❏ Bisacodyl suppository
■ Sialorrhea
  ❏ Glycopyrrolate
  ❏ Scopolamine patch
  ❏ BoNT
■ Spasticity management
  ❏ Baclofen
  ❏ Diazepam
  ❏ Dantrolene
■ Dystonia management
  ❏ Baclofen
  ❏ Trihexyphenidyl
  ❏ Diazepam
  ❏ Carbidopa/levodopa
■ Sleep aides
  ❏ Melatonin
  ❏ Trazodone
  ❏ Clonidine
■ Pain management
  ❏ Tylenol
  ❏ NSAIDs

### Health maintenance

■ XR pelvis, two views (anteroposterior [AP] and frog leg)
■ XR spine, two views (scoliosis)
■ Vitamin D level
■ Influenza vaccine

## RESOURCES AND REFERENCES

The full list of resources and references appears in the digital product found on http://connect
.springerpub.com/content/book/978-0-8261-6226-7/part/part01/chapter/ch04

# CARDIAC REHABILITATION

MATTHEW N. BARTELS AND DAVID Z. PRINCE

## CORE DEFINITIONS

The primary focus of cardiac rehabilitation is the treatment of diseases related to the heart with an aim at secondary prevention and restoring function after a cardiac event. Classically, cardiac rehabilitation focused on ischemic heart disease, but with the advances in the management of cardiac conditions, this has expanded to include heart failure as well as post-surgical and heart transplant-related rehabilitation. The basic terminology that needs to be understood for an informed discussion of cardiac rehabilitation is included in Table 5.1. Cardiac rehabilitation is one of the most effective forms of secondary prevention for individuals with ischemic heart disease, reducing coronary events by up to 20% to 30% with Class Ia evidence.[1]

## ETIOLOGY AND PATHOPHYSIOLOGY

With inactivity, obesity, and poor lifestyle, cardiovascular disease is the leading cause of morbidity and mortality in the United States. The 2017 National Health Interview Survey showed a prevalence of 10.6% for all heart-related diseases, with a higher prevalence in males than females.[2] The leading cardiac disease is ischemic heart disease, with heart failure contributing the majority of the rest of patients. Valvular heart disease, arrhythmias, stroke, peripheral arterial disease, and venous disease are the remainder of cardiovascular disease.

### Atherosclerotic Heart Disease

This category includes subclinical disease, stable angina pectoris, acute coronary syndrome, and coronary heart disease. Acute disease can result in a myocardial infarction and is associated with sudden death. Survivors of a myocardial infarction (MI) need to have secondary prevention to modify lifestyle and limit recurrent cardiac disease as well as recover from the injury of the infarct. Cardiac rehabilitation has a role in disease modification and also in improving outcomes after an infarct.

### Cardiomyopathy and Heart Failure

This category includes individuals with injured myocardium (cardiomyopathy) who have a reduced ejection fraction (HFrEF), and individuals with a preserved ejection fraction but

The full list of resources and references appears in the digital product found on http://connect.springerpub.com/content/book/978-0-8261-6226-7/part/part01/chapter/ch05

**TABLE 5.1 BASIC TERMINOLOGY FOR CARDIAC REHABILITATION**

| TERM | DEFINITION |
|---|---|
| Heart failure | A condition of insufficient cardiac output |
| HFpEF | Heart failure in the presence of preserved ejection fraction (EF) |
| HFrEF | Heart failure in the presence of reduced EF |
| End systolic volume (ESV) | Volume of the left ventricle at end of systole |
| End diastolic volume (EDV) | Volume of the left ventricle at end of diastole |
| Ejection fraction (EF) | Percentage of end diastolic volume ejected each beat (EDV-ESV)/EDV |
| Stroke volume (SV) | Volume of blood pumped in a single heart beat |
| Heart rate (HR) | Number of beats of the heart per minute |
| Systolic and diastolic blood pressure (SBP, DBP) | Usually expressed in mmHg |
| Mean blood pressure (MBP) | The calculated value of mean BP is MBP = (2 × DBP + SBP)/3 |
| Exercise capacity | Maximum ability to perform exercise. Usually assessed with a stress test |
| $VO_2$ max | Maximum volume of oxygen consumed. Usually reported in mL $O_2$/kg body weight/minute. Can be reported as liters $O_2$/minute |
| CPET | Cardiopulmonary exercise test—method to assess the maximal exercise capacity of an individual |
| Exercise stress test | Exercise test done to determine if there is myocardial ischemia, can be done with echocardiography, 12-lead EKG, or nuclear imaging. |
| Primary prevention | Medical and rehabilitation efforts to prevent a condition from arising in an individual |
| Secondary prevention | Medical and rehabilitation efforts to prevent a reoccurrence of a condition in an individual, reducing morbidity and mortality |

decreased cardiac output (HFpEF). Cardiac rehabilitation has a role in disease modification and improvement of quality of life, as well as a role in helping to decrease morbidity and mortality.

## Valvular Heart Disease

This is a category of individuals with valvular heart disease who are often treated in rehabilitation like individuals with heart failure. Often these patients are also seen following surgery or percutaneous interventions to restore function.

## Post-Cardiac Surgery

These patients are often individuals with valvular or ischemic disease, seen after a surgical intervention. The focus is on restoration of function and secondary prevention.

## Heart Transplant

This group of patients have rehabilitation before transplantation focused on maximizing function in preparation for transplant. Post-transplant rehabilitation focuses on restoring function, providing education and reversing post-operative deconditioning following transplantation surgery.

## DIAGNOSTIC APPROACH

The diagnostic evaluation of most patients in cardiac rehabilitation includes the need for basic evaluation of their underlying cardiac condition as well as an assessment of exercise capacity in order to allow for exercise prescription and safety guidelines. Basic tests are outlined in Table 5.2.

## TREATMENT

### Medical

The medical management of patients with cardiac disease in cardiac rehabilitation is to optimize their anti-ischemic or heart failure management. It is also focused on the maintenance of the medical regimen focused on secondary prevention. Table 5.3 has the

**TABLE 5.2 DIAGNOSTIC ELEMENTS FOR CARDIAC REHABILITATION**

| TEST | PURPOSE |
|---|---|
| EKG | - Provide baseline for comparison during CR<br>- Allow identification of old pathology, arrhythmias |
| Echocardiogram | Assess EF and assess for pulmonary hypertension |
| Cardiac stress test | - Assess myocardial ischemia<br>- Obtain a peak HR |
| CPET | Functional laboratory exercise test done on maximal medical management to assess safety, rule out lingering disease, and set exercise parameters |
| Field exercise test (6-minute walk test, shuttle walk test, others) | Functional field exercise test done on maximal medical management to assess safety and set exercise parameters |
| Right heart catheterization | To rule out pulmonary hypertension in individuals at risk, also done to assess cardiac output in individuals with heart failure |
| Coronary angiography | To evaluate and potentially treat coronary disease, common in patients with ischemic heart disease |
| Chest radiograph | To assess for heart failure or coexisting lung disease |

CPET, cardiopulmonary exercise test; CR, cardiac rehabilitation; EF, ejection fraction; HR, heart rate.

**TABLE 5.3 MEDICAL MANAGEMENT FOR ISCHEMIC HEART DISEASE IN CARDIAC REHABILITATION PROGRAMS**

| ELEMENT | COMMENT | LEVEL OF EVIDENCE |
|---|---|---|
| Cardiac stress test prior to rehab | This is usually done prior to rehabilitation starting | Class I for symptomatic Class IIa for low probability |
| Weight management | Aim to achieve target BMI or waist circumference | Class I |
| Smoking cessation | | Class I |
| Management of psychological issues | Depression and anxiety are at high levels in cardiac patients | Class IIa |
| Management of alcohol consumption | Referral to outside management programs | Class IIb |
| Antiplatelet medication | Coordinate with primary medical team | Class I for aspirin Class III for dipyridamole, not recommended |
| Beta-blocker | Coordinate with primary medical team | Class I for all patients LVEF >40% Class IIb for other chronic coronary disease |
| Renin-angiotensin-aldosterone blocker | Coordinate with primary medical team | Class I for CAD with HTN, DM, LVEF <40% |
| Influenza vaccine | Coordinate with primary medical team | Class I |
| Hormone replacement therapy | Coordinate with primary medical team | Class III—no clear benefit, not recommended |
| Nutritional supplements | Vitamins C and E, beta-carotene, B6, B12, garlic, coenzyme Q10, selenium, chromium | Class III—no clear benefit, not recommended |
| Symptomatic anti-ischemic treatments | Beta-blockers, calcium channel blockers, long-acting nitrates, sublingual nitroglycerine | Class I |
| Lipid management | Lifestyle modification, dietary therapy, statin therapy | Class I |
| Adjuvant lipid management | Bile sequestrants, niacin | Class IIa |
| Long-acting calcium channel blocker or ranolazine | | Class IIb |

(continued)

**TABLE 5.3 MEDICAL MANAGEMENT FOR ISCHEMIC HEART DISEASE IN CARDIAC REHABILITATION PROGRAMS (continued)**

| ELEMENT | COMMENT | LEVEL OF EVIDENCE |
| --- | --- | --- |
| Blood pressure management | Lifestyle management, weight control, activity, drug therapy for BP >140/90, angiotensin converting enzyme inhibitor (ACE-I), beta-blocker, diuretic, combination therapy | Class I |
| Diabetes management | Maintain HgA1c <7.0 | Class IIa |
| Diabetes management | Use of pharmacotherapy | Class IIb |
| Diabetes management | Rosiglitazone therapy should be avoided | Class III (harm) |

BMI, body mass index; BP, blood pressure; CAD, coronary artery disease; DM, diabetes mellitus; EECP, enhanced external counter pulsation; HEP, home exercise program; HTN, hypertension; LVEF, left ventricular ejection fraction.

most important elements of medical management that should be included in a cardiac rehabilitation program for ischemic heart disease. These interventions are often started by the primary medical/cardiac team; however, the cardiac rehabilitation specialist should confirm that every patient's medical regimen is appropriate and consistent with secondary prevention guidelines in preparation for an exercise-based cardiac rehabilitation program.[3-6]

## Rehabilitation

Cardiac rehabilitation is divided into three phases: phase 1 is in the acute hospital until discharge after a cardiac event and phase 1b is for individuals with a prolonged inpatient rehabilitation. After discharge, or after revascularization, patients undergo an outpatient phase 2 program. Phase 3 cardiac rehabilitation is lifelong maintenance of the secondary prevention and conditioning gained during rehabilitation.[7] The phase 2 program of rehabilitation is usually composed of three sessions a week of cardiac rehabilitation over a 12-week period, for a total of 36 sessions. A major challenge for fully realizing the efficacy of cardiac rehabilitation is limited access.[8] Modern programs can be spread over a year, and there is now also investigation of home-based phase 2 programs for low-to-moderate risk patients and it appears this may be an acceptable alternative.[9] Exercise in cardiac rehabilitation consists of aerobic exercise such as a treadmill or ergometer, strength training, education, and risk factor modification. Exercise is prescribed to achieve target HRs in a zone appropriate for the risk level of the patients. There are many standards that describe the benefits of the core components of the exercise, of educational program, and the appropriate timing of interventions.[3-7] The rehabilitation interventions and levels of evidence are outlined in Table 5.4.

## FUNCTIONAL PROGNOSIS AND OUTCOMES

It has been demonstrated that patients referred to cardiac rehabilitation have decreased morbidity and mortality.[10] Participation with outpatient cardiac rehabilitation reduces

**TABLE 5.4 ELEMENTS OF REHABILITATION MANAGEMENT FOR ISCHEMIC HEART DISEASE IN CARDIAC REHABILITATION PROGRAMS**

| ELEMENT | COMMENT | LEVEL OF EVIDENCE |
|---|---|---|
| Patient involvement | This is gaining patient self-efficacy, shared responsibility | Class I |
| Physical activity | Aerobic exercise such as treadmill or ergometry, 30 to 60 minutes for 5 days a week | Class I |
| Resistance training | Moderate to low intensity for at least 2 days a week | Class IIa |
| Stress reduction/relaxation | | Class IIa |
| Counseling to avoid air pollution | Managed with education | Class IIa |
| EECP | Used in patients with refractory angina | Class IIb |
| Acupuncture | Used for pain relief in refractory angina | Class III—no clear benefit, not recommended |
| Patient education | Regarding disease process, medications, exercise, and disease self-efficacy | Class I |
| Education and training in independent HEP | Create independent exercise program to sustain exercise (phase 3 cardiac rehab) | Class I |

EECP, enhanced external counter pulsation.

likelihood of future events and can reduce intensity of angina symptoms as well as assist with improvement of coronary artery disease risk factors.

## BASIC ORDER SET

### Inpatient

The most likely application of an inpatient order set for cardiac rehabilitation would be following admission for an acute coronary syndrome or status post-cardiac surgery. Due to the wide variability in clinical status and preadmission function, universal parameters cannot be determined. It is recommended that limiting parameters and patient selection for acute rehabilitation be discussed with the primary team when physical medicine and rehabilitation (PMR) is providing consultation or confirmed with cardiology consultants when patients are admitted for acute rehabilitation to the PMR service. The following example order set is a framework for data collection intended to drive conversation and collaboration among all members of a multidisciplinary team.

- Activity: Out of bed to chair.
- Diet: Low sodium/low cholesterol. Fluid volume max (if relevant).

- Nutrition consultation: Review recommendations for low cholesterol, low-sodium diet. Encourage increase in plant-based dietary content.
- Obtain baseline vital signs daily prior to treatment including SBP/DBP, HR, $SpO_2$, RR, weight.
- Continuous telemetry monitoring while undergoing mobilization, ambulation, and activities of daily living (ADL) training.
- Repeat vital signs at max exertion and following conditioning sessions for comparison to baseline.
- Frequent rests as needed—noted in medical record to establish baseline level of conditioning.
- Progressive mobilization and ambulation as tolerated. Record daily progress for comparison to baseline.
- Monitor fingerstick blood sugar (FBS) as per protocol and observe for post-conditioning decrease.
- Example of limiting parameters:
- Rest for increase/decrease in SBP/HR/RR/$SpO_2$ of _____ compared to daily baseline.
- Hold therapy for SBP/DBP/HR/RR/$SpO_2$ of _____.
- Inform primary provider for increase/decrease in SBP/DBP/HR/RR/$SpO_2$ of _____ while undergoing therapy.
- Refer to outpatient cardiac rehabilitation and provide patient with date and time of appointment prior to discharge.

## RESOURCES AND REFERENCES

The full list of resources and references appears in the digital product found on http://connect .springerpub.com/content/book/978-0-8261-6226-7/part/part01/chapter/ch05

# LYMPHEDEMA

CARMEN E. LÓPEZ-ACEVEDO, RICHARD FONTÁNEZ, AND VERÓNICA RODRÍGUEZ

## CORE DEFINITIONS

Lymphedema is an abnormal collection of lymphatic fluid in tissues just beneath the skin. This swelling commonly occurs in the arm or leg, but it may also occur in other body areas including the breast, chest, head and neck, and genitals (National Lymphedema Network Definition).[1]

## ETIOLOGY AND PATHOPHYSIOLOGY

Lymphedema originates when there is an imbalance of the interstitial fluid with the systemic circulation from an increase in inflow or decrease in outflow of the fluid. The lymph is a protein-rich fluid in which white blood cells, macromolecules, and proteins are delivered.[2] The lymphatic system is composed of lymphatic capillaries that arise within the interstitial spaces of the dermal papillae possessing no valves and draining into subdermal channels. These continue to deeper channels at the epifascial system with valves that run along the smooth muscle.[3] An 80% reduction in flow initiates a cascade of inflammation, dilation, and backflow which promotes fibrosis and stasis within the lymphatic vessels.

The most common cause of lymphedema worldwide is filariasis. In the United States, it is most commonly secondary to cancer treatment, particularly breast cancer.[2] Lymphedema can be a progressing and incapacitating condition with clear effects on self-image and physical appearance. Infrequent forms of lymphedema are described in Table 6.1.

Lymphedema can be classified as primary or secondary. Primary lymphedema may be suspected in patients with congenital or hereditary conditions. In congenital conditions, lymphedema is present at birth or by age 2. Milroy disease presents with lymphedema at birth or shortly thereafter. Meige disease occurs during puberty after a minor lower extremity injury with subsequent swelling of the ankle or foot. Girls are usually more affected than boys. Lymphedema tarda is similar to Meige disease but observed after the third decade of life.[2]

Secondary lymphedema can be the result of a cancer treatment, cancer itself, radiation therapy, chronic venous insufficiency, morbid obesity, lipedema, trauma, infection, immobility, or other systemic conditions.

---

The full list of resources and references appears in the digital product found on http://connect .springerpub.com/content/book/978-0-8261-6226-7/part/part01/chapter/ch06

**TABLE 6.1 INFREQUENT FORMS OF LYMPHEDEMA[2,4]**

| Head/neck | Present with serious complication and functional impairment. Therapy must be started as soon as possible; measurement techniques are poor. Treatment is based on education, skin care, MLD and CDT. |
|---|---|
| Genital lymphedema | Associated with abdominopelvic cancer, urogenital infection, and congenital conditions. Also presenting with lower extremity lymphedema. Education about skin care is important. Emotional and functional status must be assessed. For men, two-layer compression bandages are recommended due to simple use and comfort (e.g., Coban™ two-layer compression system). |
| Congenital | Present at an early age. Associated with vascular malformation and genetic disorder such as Turner, Noonan, Neurofibromatosis Type 1, hemangiomas, trisomy 13, 18, 21, and Klinefelter syndromes.[5] |

CDT, complete decongestive therapy; MLD, manual lymphatic drainage.

## DIAGNOSTIC APPROACH

Lymphedema is a clinical diagnosis that depends on history, physical examination, and psychological evaluation. Physical examination may include techniques to measure volume and questionnaires to measure the grade of functional and psychosocial impairment.

### History

A good history will elicit possible causes or triggers. If a history of cancer is present, information about the specific diagnosis, treatment (including chemotherapy, radiotherapy or surgery), and timing should be obtained. Chronicity is also important. Acute symptoms cue to infection, deep venous thrombosis (DVT), or complex regional pain syndrome (CRPS). Chronic symptoms are usually associated with chronic systemic disease such as congestive heart failure (CHF), chronic venous insufficiency, lipedema, or chronic kidney disease (CKD). The underlying diagnosis is important to direct treatment; there is a relative contraindication for decongestive therapy in CHF or CKD.

Associated symptoms (i.e., paresthesia, pain, heaviness on involved anatomical region), comorbid conditions (e.g., diabetes mellitus, CHF, CKD, rheumatoid arthritis, and thyroid disease), and body mass index (BMI) should also be obtained.

### Physical Examination

#### Inspection

Asymmetries of the involved limbs, localized swelling, and skin appearance (i.e., gray, dark, shiny, ulcers, or malformation), skin folds, muscle bulk, and presence of lymphorrhea should be described.[2]

#### Palpation

Assess temperature changes in the area, change in deep tissue (i.e., fibrotic, thickened, rubbery), and superficial texture. *Stemmer's sign* may be used to evaluate skin thickness. It is performed by pinching and lifting the skin on the dorsum of the middle finger or second toe. It is positive if unable to pinch or lift the skin easily. Stemmer's sign is important to diagnose lymphedema and provide staging. Edema should be described as pitting or non-pitting. Lymph node palpation and description should also be included.

## Neurological Examination

Evaluation of strength (e.g., painless weakness may be secondary to post-radiation damage), sensation (at least soft touch), deep tendon reflexes (e.g., hyperreflexia may be due to upper motor neuron [UMN] or spinal cord injury [SCI]), and cranial nerves should be performed.

A thorough physical examination allows the clinician to distinguish entrapment neuropathy, post-radiation neuropathy/plexopathy, metabolic disease, or extension of the primary disease as potential causes of lymphedema. Painless weakness usually occurs in the context of post-radiation-induced neuropathy. Weakness with pain may be associated with malignant invasion.[2]

## Specific Tools
## Volume Measurements

Volume measurements are important for diagnosis, disease progression, and treatment response. It is important to measure both the affected and unaffected limb using the same technique every time the patient is evaluated. Measurement techniques are detailed in Table 6.2. Volume differences between limbs range from 2% to 13% in healthy patients.[2,6] The following measurement differences are diagnostic of lymphedema:

- >2 cm by tape circumference
- >200 mL or >10% by volumetric measurement
- Impedance ration between arms of >3 standard deviations.[2,7–9]

## Quality of Life and Functional Assessments

Formal assessments can be used to objectively evaluate limb function. Lower limb evaluation can be performed using the lower extremity functional scale (LEFS) and upper limb using the disability of arm shoulder and hand (DASH).[2] Informally, quality of life and lymphedema-related limitations should be addressed. Lymphedema-specific instruments to assess function

**TABLE 6.2 VOLUME MEASUREMENTS USED IN THE EVALUATION OF LYMPHEDEMA[2]**

| | |
|---|---|
| Extremity circumference | Describe a region but typically does not include the foot or hand. The excess of volume is calculated as the difference from the affected side compared with the other. |
| Water displacement | Not commonly used as it is not practical due to equipment needs and hygiene. |
| Perometry | Using a squared frame of beam light with perpendicular direction. This equipment is expensive and use more for research purposes. |
| BIS | Evaluates lymph accumulation. Inexpensive, fast, and noninvasive method that can be used unilaterally or bilaterally. Can help diagnose early lymphedema and can be used serially for follow-up. Contraindicated if the patient has an implantable cardiac device. |

BIS, bioelectrical impedance spectrometry.

and quality of life include the upper limb lymphedema-27, the Lymphedema Quality of Life Inventory, and the Lymphedema Life Impact Scale, among others.[10,11]

## Lymphedema Staging

The stage of lymphedema should be described to guide treatment (Table 6.3).

## Laboratory Tests and Imaging

There are no specific laboratory tests in the diagnosis of lymphedema. Common test such as complete blood count (CBC) with differential, basic metabolic panel, urine analysis, sedimentation rate, liver function tests, and lipid profile may be obtained based on the suspected underlying diagnosis. Specific imaging tests to be considered are detailed in Table 6.4.

### TABLE 6.3 LYMPHEDEMA STAGES[2,8]

| 0 | Impaired lymphatic movement with no edema present. Important for secondary prevention of lymphedema |
| 1 | Pitting edema reversible with limb elevation. No tissue damages |
| 2 | Edema is irreversible, skin changes. Stemmer's sign positive. Predispose patient to multiple infections |
| 3 | Volume is very notable, elephantiasis observed, and marked skin changes. Stemmer's sign (+) |

### TABLE 6.4 IMAGING TESTS TO CONSIDER IN LYMPHEDEMA EVALUATION

| IMAGING | DESCRIPTION |
| --- | --- |
| Lymphoscintigraphy | A preferred method for the evaluation of lymphedema. A radioisotope-labeled tracer is injected into the web space of the foot. The movement to the proximal lymph nodes is recorded. Slow movement, backflow, and reflux can be seen. It has 92% sensitivity and 100% of specificity for the diagnosis of lymphedema.[2] |
| ICG lymphography | Diagnogreen 0.5% is injected and tracked as it flows through the lymphatic system using an infrared camera. Can be used for early diagnosis, staging, and follow-up. Is less expensive and generally safer than lymphoscintigraphy.[12] |
| US | Allows visualization of compartments and allows evaluation of thickening and subcutaneous fluid accumulation. Characteristic appearance has been described as a Marshall's cleft (subcutaneous changes) and snowstorm for lipedema.[9] |
| Doppler US | Evaluate other possible causes of lymphedema such as DVT or chronic venous insufficiency. |
| MRI or CT scan | Used for differentiation of stages, MRI can be useful for early stages,[3] and evaluation of cancer recurrence or invasion. |

DVT, deep venous thrombosis; ICG, indocyanine green; US, ultrasound.

## TREATMENT

A multidisciplinary team is needed for best outcomes in the treatment of lymphedema. A comprehensive team should include physiatrists, dermatologists, complete decongestive therapy (CDT)-certified therapists, vascular and plastic surgeons, and psychologists/psychiatrists. Treatment should focus on improved quality of life and daily function as primary goals of therapy.

### Complete Decongestive Therapy

CDT has two phases: intensive phase and long-term phase. The goals during the intensive phase are to control swelling, decrease tissue pressure, provide education, reinforce skin care, and develop a lymphedema exercise program. Multilayer bandages and manual lymphatic drainage (MLD) are used. After tissue volume stabilization, the long-term phase is reached. The mainstays of this stage are compression garments, self-drainage techniques, and exercise to maintain the gains achieved during the previous phase. CDT is found to have good results with the combination of MLD and compression bandages.[2,13,14] Relative contraindications of CDT include edema secondary to cardiac failure, arterial disease, liver diseases, renal failure, active skin infection, DVT, and metastatic disease.

### Skin Care and Weight Loss

Adequate skin care is critical for patients with lymphedema. Moisturizers, proper clothing to protect the skin from abrasion, and avoidance of extreme heat or cold are recommended. pH-neutral skin lotions with no soap are recommended. BMI of >50 can lead to lymphedema.[12] Weight loss is encouraged to reduce complications and lymphedema volume.

### Manual Techniques and Equipment

*MLD*: Soft distal to proximal stroking movements are used for 30 to 45 minutes. These can be taught to patients for in-home use. MLD can decrease symptoms particularly pain or heaviness of the extremity. It is safe and typically well tolerated. Good results have been reported when used for the treatment of upper extremity lymphedema secondary to breast cancer.[2,4]

*Bandaging*: Compressive bandaging is important in the management of lymphedema. Bandages are applied distal to proximal on the affected extremity and are used at least 23 hours a day. A foam padding is used to avoid direct contact with skin.[2]

*Compression garments*: These are used in the intense phase of CDT. The material, size, and design must be included in the order of prescription for individualized use. Custom-fit garments are preferred, but cost may limit availability. Typically, they are used during the day.

*Physical modalities*: Pneumatic compression pumps can be used at home as an adjuvant to compression garments. Compression can usually be adjusted to 25 to 60 mmHg. The use of laser therapy has been promoted for lymphangiogenesis and to stimulate motility of lymphatic fluid. Moderate to strong evidence exist for the use of this modality in patient with breast cancer-related lymphedema.[10,15] Far infrared radiation, extracorporeal shockwave, stellate ganglion blocks, and kinesio taping have also been used.

*Surgery*: Reserved for patients who fail conservative management. Surgical procedures used include vascularized lymph node transfers, lymphoticolymphatic bypass, and

**TABLE 6.5 PHARMACOLOGIC INTERVENTIONS FOR LYMPHEDEMA MANAGEMENT[5]**

| | |
|---|---|
| Benzopyrones | Include coumarin and flavonoids. They bind to interstitial proteins inducing degradation. May decrease edema and decrease secondary infections. Overuse has been associated with liver damage. Limited evidence of effectiveness. |
| Retinoids | Help to decrease inflammation and fibrosis. |
| Topical agents | Ammonium lactate, urea, and salicylic acid can improve epidermal changes. |
| Long-term infection prophylaxis | May use penicillin, cephalexin, or erythromycin if recurrent cellulitis or lymphangitis. |
| Diuretics | Not effective when used for lymphedema. |

suction-assisted protein lipectomy. Use of CDT before and after surgery improves outcomes. More invasive methods include radical excision and debulking; used only in severe or recalcitrant forms.[2]

*Exercise*: Isometric, aerobic, and gentle progression-resistive exercises are usually recommended with emphasis on abdominal breathing control and adequate posture.[2] Recent reports suggest that resistance exercise has positive effects on arm function and strength particularly in breast cancer patients.[2,4]

*Self-management:* Patients should be educated about the use of the garments, equipment, and home MLD and exercise programs.[2]

## Pharmacologic Intervention

The most common pharmacologic interventions are summarized in Table 6.5.

## ASSOCIATED IMPAIRMENTS AND COMPLICATIONS

The most common complications of lymphedema are skin infections. Cellulitis or fungal infection requires treatment with antibiotic or antifungal therapy. Treatment of skin infections needs to be accompanied by education on proper hygiene, skin care, and careful self-examination of the affected extremity. Patients with lymphedema may develop papillomatosis, lymph cyst, or elephantiasis. The most feared and serious complication of chronic lymphedema is Stewart–Treves syndrome, an angiosarcoma originating from chronic lymphedema. This complication has poor prognosis and is associated with purple macular skin lesions. Axillary web syndrome occurs when there is scarring of the tissue from the axilla down. Can be diagnosed by palpating or visualizing a tensioned cord. Treatment includes decongestive therapy and scar tissue massage or collagenase clostridium histolyticum (Xiaflex®).[16]

## FUNCTIONAL PROGNOSIS AND OUTCOMES

Evidence on the effects of lymphedema on quality of life particularly after cancer is scarce. There is some evidence to suggest that MLD may be associated with better emotional function, improvement on dyspnea, and reduced sleep disturbance in women with breast cancer-related lymphedema.[4]

## RESOURCES AND REFERENCES

The full list of resources and references appears in the digital product found on http://connect .springerpub.com/content/book/978-0-8261-6226-7/part/part01/chapter/ch06

# MOTOR NEURON DISEASE

ILEANA HOWARD

## CORE DEFINITIONS

Motor neuron disease is a group of diseases including:

**Acute flaccid myelitis (AFM):** A polio-like clinical presentation involving rapid onset of flaccid paralysis following infection with an enterovirus.

**Amyotrophic lateral sclerosis (ALS):** The most common motor neuron disease presenting with mixed upper and lower motor neuron signs.

**Hirayama's disease (monomelic amyotrophy):** Nonprogressive, single upper limb, predominantly distal weakness due to anterior horn cell disease.

**Kennedy's disease (X-linked spinobulbar muscular atrophy):** Slowly progressive lower motor neuron inherited disorder.

**Poliomyelitis:** Acute flaccid paralysis resulting from an enterovirus infection.

**Primary lateral sclerosis (PLS):** Upper motor neuron variant of ALS which may progress to ALS over time.

**Progressive muscular atrophy (PMA):** Lower motor neuron variant of ALS.

**Spinal muscular atrophy (SMA):** Autosomal recessive inherited lower motor neuron disease. Subtypes based on functional levels of survival motor neuron (SMN) protein with types 1 and 2 presenting earlier with more severe weakness than types 3 and 4. Typically involves proximal greater than distal and lower greater than upper extremity symmetric weakness and hyporeflexia.

## ETIOLOGY AND PATHOPHYSIOLOGY

Apart from inherited motor neuron diseases (SMA, Kennedy's disease, familial ALS [fALS]) and postinfectious motor neuron diseases (AFM, poliomyelitis), the etiology of most of the diseases in this category is largely unknown. There have been breakthroughs in the understanding of common factors in the cascade of events, which results in motor neuron disease. The number of genes associated with familial ALS has rapidly expanded over the past 5 to 10 years. Currently, the most common genetic mutation associated with ALS is an expansion on chromosome 9, open reading frame 72 (C9orf72), which accounts for 34% cases of familial ALS in European populations. Despite the breakthrough in identifying this

---

The full list of resources and references appears in the digital product found on http://connect
.springerpub.com/content/book/978-0-8261-6226-7/part/part01/chapter/ch07

specific mutation, the pathway from mutation to clinical phenotype of ALS remains to be elucidated. The etiology of PLS, PMA, and Hiramaya's disease remains elusive.

## DIAGNOSTIC APPROACH

### History and Physical Examination

Motor neuron disease should be considered in the differential diagnosis when the patient presents with painless progressive weakness. An acute presentation in a person with history of recent febrile infectious illness may be suggestive of AFM. A positive family history for similar symptoms can be informative for familial/genetic forms of motor neuron disease as outlined previously.

Physical examination typically reveals weakness without sensory abnormalities (with exception of Kennedy's disease). Cranial nerve examination may reveal tongue fasciculations, dysarthria, or dysphagia. The presence of perioral fasciculations or gynecomastia could suggest Kennedy's disease. Patterns of weakness, such as symmetric proximal or distal limb weakness, may indicate "motor neuron disease mimics" (Table 7.1). Abnormal reflexes, such as Babinski and jaw jerk, may be present.

### Laboratory Testing and Imaging

Laboratory testing should be driven by the patient's clinical presentation to either confirm the diagnosis or assess for alternative diagnoses. The following laboratory studies may be ordered:

- TSH, serum protein electrophoresis (SPEP) vitamin B12, methylmalonic acid, homocysteine, serum copper and zinc, hexosaminidase A
- Cerebrospinal fluid (CSF) antibody panel (to exclude paraneoplastic syndrome or infections)
- Acetylcholine and muscle-specific kinase (MuSK) antibodies (to exclude possible myasthenia gravis)
- Ganglioside M1 (GM1) antibodies (to exclude multifocal motor neuropathy)
- Twenty-four-hour urine for heavy metals or very long-chain fatty acids
- Serology for suspected infections, including human T-cell lymphotropic virus 1 (HTLV1), HIV, West Nile virus, or Lyme disease
- Muscle biopsy for suspected myopathy
- Genetic screening: for suspected SMA, Kennedy's, or fALS.

### TABLE 7.1 MOTOR NEURON MIMIC DISEASES

| | |
|---|---|
| Multifocal motor neuropathy with conduction block | Cervical/lumbosacral radiculopathy or myelopathy |
| Inclusion body myositis | Chronic inflammatory demyelinating polyneuropathy |
| Myasthenia gravis | Other myopathy |
| Hereditary spastic paraplegia | |

Imaging studies are generally used to exclude competing diagnoses, such as cervical myelopathy or intracranial abnormality. MRI of the brain and spinal cord is most often used for this purpose. A few exceptions exist, including displacement of the posterior cervical dural sac with neck flexion reported in Hiramaya's disease and spinal gray matter changes reported in AFM.

## Electrodiagnostic Testing

ALS is a clinical diagnosis; however, electrodiagnostic studies may provide supportive evidence of subclinical lower motor neuron involvement not readily apparent on physical examination. The currently accepted framework for diagnosis of ALS is the El Escorial–Awaji criteria,[1] which modified the original El Escorial criteria to include electromyography (EMG) evidence of denervation on par with physical examination evidence of lower motor neuron signs, thereby increasing the sensitivity (see Table 7.2).[2] One caveat to consider is that the El Escorial–Awaji criteria was designed to provide guidance on diagnosis of ALS for clinical research studies. Therefore, it should not be used rigidly due to limited sensitivity.

## TREATMENT

### Disease-Modifying Therapies

There are currently two disease-modifying treatment (DMT) options for ALS and two for SMA. Riluzole and edaravone are the two Food and Drug Administration (FDA)–approved therapies for ALS. Serum glutamic pyruvic transaminase (SGPT)/serum glutamic-oxaloacetic transaminase (SGOT) and complete blood count (CBC) should be monitored during use of riluzole. Nusinersin was the first FDA-approved disease-modifying medication for the treatment of SMA. It is an antisense oligonucleotide that targets the SMN2 mRNA, blocking the excision of exon 7, resulting in increased production of full-length SMN protein.[3] A second medication for SMA, onasemnogene abeparvovec, was approved by the FDA in 2019. This drug delivers an intact copy of the *SMN* gene via an adeno-associated virus (AAV1) vector. Table 7.3 details the doses and administration of these agents.

### TABLE 7.2 AWAJI ELECTRODIAGNOSTIC CRITERIA DIAGNOSTIC CATEGORIES[1]

| DIAGNOSTIC CATEGORY | REQUIREMENTS |
| --- | --- |
| Clinically definite ALS | Clinical or electrophysiologic evidence of LMN and UMN signs in the bulbar region and at least two spinal regions **or** the presence of LMN and UMN signs in three spinal regions |
| Clinically probable ALS | Clinical or electrophysiological evidence of LMN and UMN signs in at least two body regions with some UMN signs rostral to (previously) the LMN signs. |
| Clinically possible ALS | Clinical or electrophysiologic evidence of UMN and LMN signs in one body region, or UMN signs (alone) in two or more body regions, or LMN signs rostral to UMN signs, and neuroimaging and clinical laboratory studies will have been performed and other diagnoses must have been excluded. |

ALS, amyotrophic lateral sclerosis; IV, intravenous; SMA, spinal muscular atrophy.

**TABLE 7.3 DISEASE-MODIFYING THERAPIES FOR AMYOTROPHIC LATERAL SCLEROSIS AND SPINAL MUSCULAR ATROPHY DOSING AND ADMINISTRATION**

| DRUG | DOSE AND ADMINISTRATION |
|---|---|
| Riluzole | 50 mg PO BID |
| Edaravone | 60 mg IV daily × 14 days then<br>60 mg IV Monday to Friday × 2 weeks then<br>14 days drug free |
| Nusinersin | 12 mg intrathecally every 14 days × 3 doses, then<br>Fourth dose of 12 mg intrathecally 30 days after third dose<br>Maintenance: 12 mg intrathecally every 4 months |
| Onasemnogene abeparvovec | Single IV dosage based on patient weight |

## Medical and Rehabilitative Management

Rehabilitative management of motor neuron disease follows the key principles of prevention of secondary complications, remediation of impairments, and compensatory strategies.[4] Clinical practice guidelines have been published by the American Academy of Neurology for the management of ALS.[5,6] Similarly, practice guidelines exist for the management of SMA.[7,8] These guidelines provide a broad framework for multidisciplinary care, medical management, respiratory assessment and therapies, symptom management, and prevention of secondary complications.

## Prevention of Secondary Complications

The greatest risk to health for persons with motor neuron disease is respiratory infections or respiratory failure; therefore, it is paramount for the physiatrist to ensure routine and adequate assessment and risk reduction through use of respiratory supports, pulmonary hygiene, vaccination, and caregiver education.[9]

Despite the preservation of protective sensation, persons with advanced state of motor neuron disease are at increased risk of complications related to immobility, including contracture, pain, and wounds. Persons with motor neuron disease and their caregivers must be instructed in range of motion exercises, protective orthoses, and the use of positioning wedges and supports to facilitate repositioning when indicated. A hospital bed with pressure-relieving mattress may facilitate position changes, although this will not obviate the need for a caregiver to assist with repositioning.

ALS is a hypermetabolic disease. This fact, coupled with decreased ability to prepare and self-feed due to weakness, spasticity, and fatigue, often results in progressive weight loss. Literature notes worse prognosis for persons with weight loss at the time or following diagnosis of ALS. Early and adequate nutritional support with supplemental nutrition or enteral feeds through a gastrostomy tube can often stabilize weight or minimize weight loss.

## Remediation of Impairments

Given the progressive, degenerative nature of motor neuron disease, the main focus of rehabilitative management is to slow progression/deterioration. Literature demonstrates that moderate exercise is safe for persons with motor neuron disease and may help slow declines in both functional abilities and respiratory parameters. Adequate evaluation and treatment of secondary symptoms to promote comfort and quality of life are paramount in motor neuron disease (see Table 7.4).

## Compensatory Strategies

A unique consideration for motor neuron disease that distinguishes it from other neurorehabilitation populations is the change expected over time. In ALS, rapid deterioration necessitates the interdisciplinary team plan for future needs to ensure durable medical equipment will be appropriate as needs evolve over time. In pediatric motor neuron disease, changes are compounded by growth and development of the child over time as well as by progression of disease.

## Other Complications/Symptoms and Common Management Interventions

**TABLE 7.4 SYMPTOMS AND MANAGEMENT STRATEGIES**

| SYMPTOM | PREVALENCE[10,11] | MANAGEMENT STRATEGIES[12–15] (FOR ADULT PATIENTS) |
|---|---|---|
| Fatigue | 76%–90% | Methylphenidate 5 mg BID qAM and noon<br>Modafinil 200 mg qAM or BID[16]<br>Amantadine 100 mg BID |
| Sialorrhea | 52% | Atropine drops 2 gtts sublingual QID<br>Amitriptyline 10 mg QHS, increase to 20 mg QHS after 1 week<br>Gycopyrrolate 1 mg TID<br>Scopolamine patch q72h<br>Botulinum toxin injections: bilateral parotid glands (30 units each), submandibular glands (20 units each) |
| Spasticity | 84% | Baclofen 5 mg BID, titrate up to 20 mg QID<br>Tizanidine 2 mg QHS<br>Botulinum toxin injections<br>Intrathecal baclofen pump (particularly for PLS) |
| Muscle cramps | 74% | Mexiletine 150 mg qday × 7 days, then BID[17] |
| Pain (nociceptive > neuropathic) | 40%– 59% | Nociceptive pain: acetaminophen, NSAIDs, opioids, intraarticular steroid injections<br>Neuropathic pain: amitriptyline, gabapentin, pregabalin |

*(continued)*

**TABLE 7.4 SYMPTOMS AND MANAGEMENT STRATEGIES (*continued*)**

| SYMPTOM | PREVALENCE[10,11] | MANAGEMENT STRATEGIES[12–15] (FOR ADULT PATIENTS) |
|---|---|---|
| Anxiety | 55% | SSRI<br>Benzodiazepine |
| Depression | 29%–52% | Amitriptyline (in particular if sialorrhea, pain, or insomnia present)<br>SSRI |
| Bladder dysfunction<br>*Urgency > retention<br>*(More common in PLS)<br>*Compounded by mobility limitations<br>*Autonomic dysfunction is possible | | Same as non-ALS<br>Condom catheter |
| Bowel dysfunction/constipation<br>*Compounded by mobility limitations<br>*Autonomic dysfunction is possible | 51% | Docusate 250 mg BID<br>Polyethylene glycol ½–1 capful qday<br>Docusate suppository/enema<br>Bowel program |
| Orthopnea/dyspnea | 45%–66% | Noninvasive ventilatory support<br>Maximum insufflator/exsufflator (cough assist) |
| Insomnia | 39%–60% | Noninvasive ventilatory support[18]<br>Amitryptiline 10 mg (if pain or sialorrhea present) |
| Cachexia compounded by dysphagia hypermetabolic state is possible | 29% | Oral nutrition supplement (shakes)<br>Tube feeds |
| Itching | 35%[13] | Hydroxyzine 25 mg QID PRN<br>Gabapentin 300 mg TID |
| Aspiration pneumonia | Bronchopnemonia or respiratory failure as cause of death in ~75%[19,20] | Routine swallow evaluation<br>Routine dental care<br>Careful oral hygiene<br>Portable suction device<br>Annual influenza vaccine<br>Pneumonia vaccine |
| Pressure ulcers | | Pressure-relieving mattress and hospital bed |
| Pseudobulbar affect | 38% | Amitriptyline 10 mg QHS<br>Fluoxetine 20 mg qday<br>Dextromethorphan 20 mg/quinidine 10 mg 1 capsule qday × 7 days, then 1 capsule BID |

ALS, amyotrophic lateral sclerosis; NSAIDs, non-steroidal anti-inflammatory drugs; PLS, primary lateral sclerosis; SSRI, selective serotonin reuptake inhibitor.

## FUNCTIONAL PROGNOSIS AND OUTCOMES

There is currently no cure for ALS and PMA; average length of survival is 3 to 5 years after onset of symptoms. The most common cause of death is aspiration pneumonia. PLS that fails to progress to "classic" ALS after 4 years connotes a better prognosis and life span. Persons with Kennedy's disease and brachial amyotrophy have a better prognosis. Prior to the advent of DMT and gene therapy, average length of survival in individuals with spinal muscle atrophy is on the orders of years in those severely affected to nearly normal life span with late-onset disease.

## BASIC ORDER SET

### Consults

- Respiratory therapy
  - ❑ Spirometry for ALS, please include forced vital capacity (FVC), maximum inspiratory pressure (MIP), maximum expiratory pressure (MEP), and peak cough flow (PCF)
  - ❑ Initiate cough assist/pulmonary hygiene
  - ❑ Initiate/follow-up noninvasive ventilatory support
- Pulmonology for evaluation and management of hypoventilation due to neuromuscular respiratory weakness
- Palliative care/hospice for assistance with advance care planning, life-sustaining treatment discussion, end-of-life care planning
- Assistive technology for consideration of alternative computer access, environmental control units (ECUs), augmentative and alternative communication (AAC)
- Interventional radiology or gastroenterology consult for Radiographically Inserted Gastrostomy (RIG) or Percutaneous Endoscopic Gastrostomy (PEG) tube placement
- Dietician: Malnutrition screening/assessment, diet recommendations/education, nutritional supplements, enteral nutrition, home enteral nutrition (HEN) teaching/orders
- Social work: Advance care planning, advance directive education and completion

### Respiratory Treatments

- Cough assist: Three cycles of five inhalations/exhalations each, starting pressure (−40/+40 mmHg)
- Noninvasive ventilatory support: Bilevel noninvasive ventilatory support: initial settings 12 cm $H_2O$ inspiratory positive airway pressure (IPAP), 6 cm $H_2O$ expiratory positive airway pressure (EPAP) backup rate 10 with titration as needed
- ALS hypoxia protocol: For $O_2$ saturation <95%, please:
  - ❑ Sit patient as upright as possible
  - ❑ Perform cough assist/mechanical insufflator-exsufflator (MI-E) for three cycles of five inhalations/exhalations each
  - ❑ Place patient on noninvasive ventilatory support (bilevel)
  - ❑ Do not administer $O_2$ by nasal cannula without specific physician order
  - ❑ Contact primary team if $O_2$ sat remains <95% despite these measures.

## RESOURCES AND REFERENCES

The full list of resources and references appears in the digital product found on http://connect
.springerpub.com/content/book/978-0-8261-6226-7/part/part01/chapter/ch07

# MULTIPLE SCLEROSIS

SARAH B. SIMMONS AND GLORIA HOU

## CORE DEFINITIONS

Multiple sclerosis (MS) is often a devastating illness striking those in the prime of life, affecting approximately 1 million people in the United States.[1] It can attack any part of the central nervous system (CNS) leading to a myriad of symptoms, such as vision loss, transverse myelitis, facial pain, bladder dysfunction, and crippling fatigue. It is characterized by CNS plaques that are distributed throughout the brain and spinal cord and develop across multiple points in time. Patients with MS may have a relapsing and/or progressive clinical course, and these subtypes have highly variable responses to disease-modifying therapies (DMTs). See Figure 8.1.[2]

### Multiple Sclerosis Clinical Subtypes

*Relapsing-remitting multiple sclerosis (RRMS)*: Course characterized by episodic relapses (i.e., "attacks" or "exacerbations") with stable neurological disability between episodes.

*Secondary progressive multiple sclerosis (SPMS)*: A progressive course (steady accumulation of disability independent of relapse activity) following an initial relapsing-remitting course.

*Primary progressive multiple sclerosis (PPMS)*: A progressive course from disease onset with no initial relapsing-remitting phase.

### Multiple Sclerosis Disease Modifiers

*Active versus inactive disease (can apply to RRMS, SPMS, or PPMS)*: Disease is considered active if there has been clinical relapse or MRI lesion activity (i.e., new or enlarging T2 or gadolinium-enhancing lesions) over the previous year.

*With progression versus without progression (can apply to SPMS or PPMS)*: Disease is categorized as "with progression" if there has been documented clinical worsening over the past year that occurs independently of relapse activity.

### Syndromes That May Develop Into Multiple Sclerosis

Radiologically isolated syndrome occurs when MRI findings are strongly suggestive of MS in a patient with no neurological manifestations.

---

The full list of resources and references appears in the digital product found on http://connect .springerpub.com/content/book/978-0-8261-6226-7/part/part01/chapter/ch08

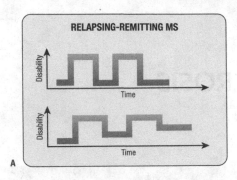
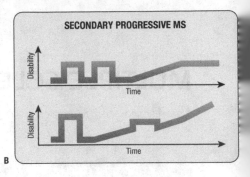
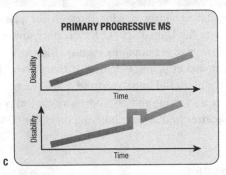

**FIGURE 8.1** MS clinical subtypes. (A) The flat baseline between relapses is consistent with relapsing course without progression. (B) The top picture shows progression (up-sloping baseline) beginning after two relapses. The bottom picture shows progression occurring in between relapses. (C) With primary progressive MS, the baseline slopes up from the start.

*Source*: Reprinted by permission from Lublin FD, Reingold SC, Cohen JA, et al. Defining the clinical course of multiple sclerosis: the 2013 revisions. *Neurology*. 2014;83(3):278–286.

Clinically isolated syndrome (CIS) is a clinical episode corresponding to an inflammatory demyelinating event in the CNS similar to a typical MS relapse. CIS can be thought of as the first attack if a patient is then subsequently diagnosed with MS.

## Relapse Versus Pseudorelapse

It is important to distinguish between pseudorelapse and relapse, as relapses are often treated with steroids, whereas pseudorelapse symptoms improve with treatment of the underlying cause.

Relapse (i.e., attack or exacerbation) is a clinical episode with symptoms and objective findings typical of MS, reflecting an inflammatory demyelinating event in the CNS with a duration of at least 24 hours.

Pseudorelapse is a return or worsening of previous neurologic symptoms that are not caused by new or worsened lesion activity in the CNS. Instead, a pseudorelapse is often associated with stress, medication side effect, heat sensitivity, or infection (often urinary tract or upper respiratory tract infection).

## ETIOLOGY AND PATHOPHYSIOLOGY

MS is an immune-mediated disease characterized by demyelinating lesions located throughout the brain and spinal cord. In addition to demyelination, axonal loss is a key feature. Relapses are hypothesized to be caused by an immune-mediated attack on myelin antigens, and both the adaptive immune system (T and B cells) and innate immune system (particularly microglia and macrophages) contribute to disease pathogenesis. In progressive types of MS, disability accumulation is thought to be caused by neurodegeneration and axonal loss, although the underlying mechanisms are unclear.[3]

MS is caused by a mix of complex genetic and environmental factors. Genome-wide association studies implicate genes involved in the adaptive and innate immune system as well as vitamin D metabolism. Some hypothesize that an infectious agent may also predispose to development of MS, potentially via molecular mimicry.[3]

## DIAGNOSTIC APPROACH

The diagnosis of MS is made based on clinical evidence of lesions, which demonstrate dissemination in space and time, with exclusion of potential mimickers (such as neuromyelitis optica, anti-myelin oligodendrocyte glycoprotein (MOG) syndrome, or neurosarcoidosis). Although imaging is not strictly required, diagnosis is often supported with MRI findings. MRI is also used to assess overall disease severity, to identify the presence of active and inactive plaques, and to establish a baseline for future monitoring of disease activity and response to therapies. Lumbar puncture (for presence of oligoclonal bands) and less frequently, optical coherence tomography, may be requested if diagnosis is otherwise unclear.

### Diagnosis of Relapsing–Remitting Multiple Sclerosis

For patients whose clinical history does not demonstrate two or more distinct clinical attacks reflecting lesions in two or more distinct anatomical locations, the diagnosis of MS can be made by fulfilling McDonald's criteria (see Table 8.1). These were formed (and subsequently revised in 2017) to allow for MRI and cerebrospinal fluid (CSF) findings to fulfill criteria for dissemination in space and time, in hopes that this would lead to earlier diagnosis and treatment for patients.

### Diagnosis of Primary Progressive Multiple Sclerosis

Diagnosis of PPMS can be made (either retrospectively or prospectively) based on clinical evidence of steady disability progression without relapses over a period of at least 1 year. In addition, two of the three following criteria should be fulfilled: one or more T2 lesions in at least one of three brain areas (periventricular, cortical/juxtacortical, or infratentorial region); at least two or more spinal cord lesions; or positive oligoclonal bands.[4]

### Diagnosis of Secondary Progressive Multiple Sclerosis

Currently there are no good radiologic or serologic markers to identify the transition from RRMS to SPMS. Thus, SPMS is a clinical diagnosis based on a steady progressive course following an initial relapsing-remitting course. The transition to SPMS is gradual, and there is often an overlapping period with a progressive course that is also punctuated by relapses.

**TABLE 8.1 DIAGNOSTIC CRITERIA FOR RELAPSING-REMITTING MULTIPLE SCLEROSIS USING MRI/CEREBROSPINAL FLUID FINDINGS IN PATIENTS WITH UNCLEAR CLINICAL HISTORY**

| 2017 MCDONALD CRITERIA FOR DISSEMINATION IN SPACE USING MRI | 2017 MCDONALD CRITERIA FOR DISSEMINATION IN TIME USING MRI/CSF |
|---|---|
| • Two or more T2 lesions in at least two of the following CNS regions typical for MS: periventricular, cortical–juxtacortical, infratentorial, and spinal cord. | • Presence of new T2 or gadolinium-enhancing lesions on follow-up MRI<br>-OR-<br>• Simultaneous gadolinium-enhancing and non-enhancing lesions at any point in time (indicating both active and inactive plaques, respectively)<br>-OR-<br>• If criteria for dissemination in space is met, the presence of CSF-specific oligoclonal bands allows a diagnosis of MS to be made |

CNS, central nervous system; CSF, cerebrospinal fluid; MS, multiple sclerosis.
*Source*: Adapted from Thompson AJ, Banwell BL, Barkhof F, et al. Diagnosis of multiple sclerosis: 2017 revisions of the McDonald criteria. *Lancet Neurol.* 2018;17(2):162–173.

### Diagnostic Approach to Relapse

Relapse is diagnosed based on clinical history and typically presents as new or worsening symptoms attributable to CNS pathology that present over the course of days to weeks. MRI of the brain, cervical spine, and thoracic spine can support diagnosis of a relapse when new, enlarging, or enhancing lesions are identified. However, not all disease activity is capturable by current MRI technology, and it is not always necessary to order MRI prior to treatment with steroids. MRI is most crucial in situations when there is uncertainty about the MS diagnosis, when a change in DMT is under consideration, and when an unclear clinical history makes it difficult to distinguish between a relapse and pseudorelapse.

In addition, certain "red flag" situations should not be missed:

- Stroke: In older patients with vascular risk factors, sudden onset of neurological symptoms should trigger a prompt stroke workup.
- Cervical/lumbar stenosis: In older patients, compressive myelopathy is a common cause of extremity weakness and neurogenic bowel and bladder.
- Progressive multifocal leukoencephalopathy (PML): People taking highly active immunosuppressive therapy for MS (especially natalizumab) can develop a life-threatening infection of the brain from John Cunningham virus (JCV). People on natalizumab presenting with new neurological symptoms should receive an urgent brain MRI to rule out PML.

## TREATMENT

### Pharmacologic Management—Relapse

Corticosteroid treatment is considered the first-line therapy for treatment of relapses. Corticosteroids have been shown to decrease duration of relapse,[5] although there is no conclusive evidence that they improve long-term outcomes[6]; they come with their own risks for which patients should be counseled (including osteonecrosis, osteoporosis, infection, insomnia, irritability, gastrointestinal symptoms). Either oral or intravenous (IV) corticosteroids can be used and have been shown to be equally effective.[7] Typical treatment regimens include IV methylprednisolone 1 g/day for 3 to 5 days or a bioequivalent dose of oral methylprednisolone. If corticosteroids are ineffective or contraindicated, plasmapheresis or intravenous immunoglobulin (IVIG) is sometimes used.

### Rehabilitation

Significant recovery often occurs in the first 2 to 3 months after a relapse, although can take up to 1 year, and approximately ⅓ to ½ of all relapses result in residual disability.[8] Thus, a comprehensive rehabilitation assessment and plan should be made following relapses. Often, patients will benefit from an inpatient rehabilitation stay for intensive therapy and symptom management as outlined in sample order set.

### Disease-Modifying Therapies
### Relapsing-Remitting Multiple Sclerosis

DMTs are used to reduce the recurrence of future relapses and slow disability accumulation but do not reverse disability due to past relapses.[9] See Table 8.2.

### Secondary Progressive Multiple Sclerosis

There are no specific markers that differentiate RRMS from SPMS; thus, many of the same DMTs that are approved for RRMS are often used in patients who transition to SPMS (particularly if they have evidence of disease activity). However, siponimod and cladribine have been approved by the Food and Drug Administration (FDA) specifically for use in patients with active SPMS.

### Primary Progressive Multiple Sclerosis

Options for disease-modifying treatments in patients with progressive MS are limited. Ocrelizumab was the first drug to be approved by the FDA for treatment of PPMS, although it appears to be more efficacious in people with PPMS with active disease.[10]

### TABLE 8.2 DISEASE-MODIFYING THERAPIES FOR PATIENTS WITH RELAPSING-REMITTING MULTIPLE SCLEROSIS

| IMMUNOMODULATORY DMTS | IMMUNOSUPPRESSIVE DMTS |
| --- | --- |
| Interferon-beta (injectable) Glatiramer acetate (injectable) | Fingolimod (oral) Siponimod (oral) Ozanimod (oral) Teriflunomide (oral) Dimethyl fumarate (oral) Diroximel fumarate (oral) Ofatumumab (injectable) Natalizumab (infusion) Ocrelizumab (infusion) Alemtuzumab (infusion) Cladribine (oral) |

DMTs, disease-modifying therapies; RRMS, relapsing-remitting multiple sclerosis.
*Source*: Adapted from Rae-Grant A, Day GS, Marrie RA, et al. Comprehensive systematic review summary: disease-modifying therapies for adults with multiple sclerosis. *Neurology*. 2018;90(17):789–800.

## Disease-Modifying Therapy—Clinical Pearls

People taking highly active immunosuppressive therapy for MS (especially natalizumab, but also fingolimod, rituximab, ocrelizumab, and dimethyl fumarate) are at risk for PML. People on natalizumab are at higher risk after 2 years on therapy or with increasing JCV antibody titers.[11]

Immunosuppressive medications may increase the risk of opportunistic infection and malignancy, especially with prolonged use.

With teriflunomide treatment, there may be a risk of teratogenicity for male sperm, which could last for 2 years after treatment cessation if the patient is not treated with chelation therapy.

Mitoxantrone is an infused DMT that is rarely used anymore due to cardiotoxicity. Patients exposed to mitoxantrone should be evaluated yearly with echocardiogram for monitoring.

**Diet:** Specific diets have been touted as the cure for MS, but evidence on overall efficacy is limited. In general, it is recommended to avoid high sodium and processed foods. Mediterranean diets promoting vascular health (including fish, omega 3, fruits, and vegetables) are generally recommended.

**Immunizations**: Patients with MS should receive vaccines according to standard guidelines; however, vaccinations should be delayed in patients with active relapse. In addition, patients on immunosuppressive medications should avoid live-attenuated vaccines.[12]

**Facilitating Access to Treatment**: Persons with MS often have difficulty navigating the healthcare system due to limited finances, lack of transportation, lack of insurance, depression/anxiety, and cognitive impairment. Where available, people with MS are best served at a multidisciplinary MS center. These centers often have expert, dedicated social work and nursing teams who facilitate access to care in innumerable ways. These teams know how to access drug assistance programs for costly disease-modifying therapies, arrange transportation to appointments, facilitate applications to hospital financial assistance programs, advocate for housing and job accommodations, provide counseling specific to coping with the MS diagnosis, etc. The National MS Society (NMSS) also has excellent tools for finding resources, programs, and support for persons with MS.

## Pregnancy Considerations

Patients with RRMS can be counseled that pregnancy has no negative effect on long-term prognosis, and disease activity often decreases during pregnancy, particularly in the third trimester. Certain DMTs may require a washout period prior to conception. There is evidence that glatiramer acetate (category B for pregnancy) and interferon-beta (category C) are safest. Controversy exists as to whether first-trimester steroid exposure is associated with cleft lip and palate abnormalities, although short-term corticosteroids are commonly used throughout pregnancy to treat relapse (dexamethasone in particular crosses placenta and should be avoided).[13]

## Others

Dalfampridine (Ampyra) has been approved for patients with MS to increase speed of walking.[14] Contraindications include history of seizures or moderate-to-severe renal disease.

## Complications

*Neurological fatigue*: Neurological fatigue affects 78% of people with MS. Fatigue tends to occur daily especially in the afternoon and evening and often worsens other MS symptoms.[15]

*Sleep disorders (obstructive sleep apnea, central sleep apnea, restless legs)*: Sleep disorders are common; thus, consider sleep study for fatigued patients.

*Uhthoff's phenomenon*: Increases in body temperature may cause conduction block in demyelinated nerves, leading to temporary worsening of MS symptoms, for example, blurred vision in a patient previously diagnosed with optic neuritis. Consider cooling vests or air-conditioning for management.

*Osteoporosis*: People with MS have a 1.7-fold increased risk of osteoporotic fracture and a 4-fold increased risk of hip fracture.[16] Dual-energy x-ray absorptiometry (DEXA) scan may be ordered for those patients who are post-menopausal, require an assistive device to walk, have a history of fracture, have significant steroid exposure, or take antiepileptic medication.[17]

*Spasticity*: Physical examination findings of spasticity may at times be subtle in persons with MS and fluctuate with fatigue. Nevertheless, treatment with medications such as baclofen or tizanidine based on history (in the absence of physical examination findings) often still proves to be of great symptomatic benefit.

*Gait disorders*: Falls are very common and may be related to a combination of weakness, foot drop, vertigo, imbalance, altered sensation, fatigue, and impaired multitasking ability.

*Neuropathic pain, including trigeminal neuralgia*: For the most part, neuropathic pain in MS is treated with typical medications and behavioral interventions. However, there is an increased incidence of episodic lancinating pain syndromes such as trigeminal neuralgia which may respond relatively better to anti-seizure medications such as oxcarbazepine or carbamazepine.

*Migraines*: Vestibular migraines that cause vertigo and balance impairment may mimic an MS relapse.

*Neurogenic bladder and bowel*: Overactive bladder and detrusor sphincter dyssynergia are common. However, MS bladder has many presentations, and clinical manifestations can fluctuate over time even within the same person. Constipation and urge bowel incontinence can both be seen in patients with MS.

*Respiratory impairments*: Truncal muscle weakness (more common in wheelchair users) can contribute to weak cough and decreased lung volumes. Consider pulmonary function testing and referral to pulmonary if symptomatic.

*Cognitive impairment*: Information processing, memory, complex attention, executive function, verbal fluency, visuospatial perception, and social cognition may be affected.[18]

*Visual impairment*: Internuclear ophthalmoplegia, optic neuritis, and/or cranial nerve palsies may be present.

*Others*: Dysphagia, mood disorders (depression, anxiety), pseudobulbar affect, and sexual dysfunction may be present.

## FUNCTIONAL PROGNOSIS AND OUTCOMES

Older age at disease onset, male gender, ethnicity (African-American, North-African, and Hispanic-American people accumulate disability faster), smoking, and low vitamin D levels are associated with faster disability accumulation. Clinical factors associated with faster disability accumulation include diagnosis of PPMS (compared to diagnosis of RRMS), high relapse rate, lesion localization (brainstem, spinal cord, or cerebellar onset), high T2 lesion volume, high cortical lesion volume, and motor symptoms at disease onset.[19]

**Smoking**: There is a significant, dose-dependent association between smoking (both passive and active smoking) and risk for MS. Smoking increases the risk of developing MS, the rate of disability accumulation and transition to progressive MS, and degree of cortical atrophy.[20]

**Vitamin D**: Reduced vitamin D levels are associated with an increased risk of developing MS. Although there are no clinical guidelines regarding target serum levels of 25-hydroxy-vitamin D, clinicians often recommend a high normal supplementation goal (e.g., 50 ng/mL).

**Exercise**: Exercise in MS is important and may alleviate symptoms (particularly fatigue and cognitive impairment). Data is also emerging that progressive resistance training may slow overall brain atrophy in MS.[21] Canadian exercise guidelines for MS recommend at least 30 minutes of moderate-intensity aerobic activity two times per week and strength training two times per week.[22]

**Vascular**: Multiple vascular comorbidities (diabetes, hypertension, dyslipidemia, or peripheral vascular disease) are associated with more rapid disability progression in MS.[23] Appropriate management of vascular comorbidities is likely to improve long-term functional outcome.

## BASIC ORDER SETS

**Precautions:** Fall precautions, pacing (avoid overfatigue), aspiration precautions
**Activity:** Progress functional mobility as able. Include aerobic, resistance, stretching, balance components.
**Diet:** May need dysphagia diet.
**Nursing:** Catheter care, turning as needed.
**Therapies:**
    **Physical therapy:** ROM, sitting balance, transfers, gait training, fall prevention and recovery, pacing, vestibular therapy, home exercise program.
    **Occupational therapy:** ROM, activities of daily living (ADLs)/IADLs, energy conservation, evaluation for adaptive equipment
    **Speech language pathology:** Cognitive communication evaluation, swallowing evaluation
    **Psychology:** Coping with disability, anxiety, depression
    **Rehabilitation/vocational counseling:** Discussion of disclosure versus nondisclosure of disease, relapse management, accommodations, Family and Medical Leave Act (FMLA), disability resources
    **Social work:** Discharge planning, financial resources (housing, food, transportation)
**Prophylaxis**
    **DVT prophylaxis**
    **Constipation:** Colace, miralax, suppository as needed.
    **Bladder:** Check post-void residual.

**Medications**

   DMT (may need to bring from home with pharmacy approval)

   Neurostimulants (modafinil, methylphenidate, amantadine)

   Dalfampridine (may need to bring from home)

   Neuropathic pain medications

   Spasticity medications

   Antidepressant or antianxiety (such as selective serotonin reuptake inhibitor [SSRI] and serotonin norepinephrine reuptake inhibitor [SNRI])

**Labs**

   Complete blood count (CBC) and comprehensive metabolic panel (CMP).

## RESOURCES AND REFERENCES

The full list of resources and references appears in the digital product found on http://connect .springerpub.com/content/book/978-0-8261-6226-7/part/part01/chapter/ch08

# OSTEOPOROSIS AND METABOLIC BONE DISEASE

CRISTINA L. SADOWSKY, PHILIPPINES G. CABAHUG, AND ALBERT C. RECIO

## CORE DEFINITION

Osteoporosis is a skeletal disorder characterized by compromised bone strength predisposing a person to an increased risk of fracture.[1]

## ETIOLOGY AND PATHOPHYSIOLOGY

The etiology of spinal cord injury/disease (SCI/D-related bone loss and osteoporosis is multifactorial, including:

- Loss of weight loading and immobilization related to paralysis[2,3]
- Sensory and sympathetic denervation of the bone[4,5]
- Decrease/loss of anabolic factors (i.e., testosterone, growth hormone)[6]
- Increased catabolism related to systemic inflammation, administration of drugs like steroids at the time of injury[7]
- Factors locally influencing bone metabolism (i.e., paracrine influences from atrophied muscles)[8]
- Chronic administration of drugs known to negatively affect bone metabolism (antidepressants, anticonvulsants, opioids, proton pump inhibitors, anticoagulants)[9]

### Pathophysiology

SCI/D-related osteoporosis is characterized by decreased bone mass mostly in weight-unloaded limbs, thus legs more than arms. Massive bone loss occurs early in the course of paralysis, followed later by significant decrease in bone deposition.[8] Bone loss is dependent on time from and extent of neurologic injury, with most bone loss occurring in the first year after complete motor paralysis.[10]

## DIAGNOSTIC APPROACH

The diagnosis of SCI/D-related bone loss and osteoporosis can be clinical based on the occurrence of low impact, pathologic fractures occurring most frequently around the knee (distal femur, proximal tibia).[11] The 2019 International Society for Clinical Densitometry

---

The full list of resources and references appears in the digital product found on http://connect .springerpub.com/content/book/978-0-8261-6226-7/part/part01/chapter/ch09

Position Statement in SCI establishes that dual-energy x-ray absorptiometry (DXA) can be used to both diagnose osteoporosis and predict lower extremity fracture risk in individuals with SCI/D.[12] Imaging should include DXA of total hip, distal femur, and proximal tibia performed in densitometry centers with knowledge in SCI/D.

The traditionally used lumbar spine site to asses bone mineral density (BMD) yields normal or elevated values in individuals with SCI/D, possibly secondary to increased osteoarthritic changes in that region.[13] Sometimes, the lumbar spine site cannot be used because of metallic artifacts from spinal stabilization. It is also advised to measure BMD in both hips as utilizing only one of the hips can lead to underdiagnosis of abnormally low bone mass, especially if there is asymmetric neurologic deficit.

DXA evaluation yields two scores: Z-score, which compares BMD of an individual with age-matched, gender-matched, and ethnic-matched controls, and T-score, which compares BMD of an individual with reference values for peak bone mass, usually achieved between 20 and 30 years of age. In individuals older than 50 years of age, T-score should be used to diagnose primary osteoporosis; normal bone mass is characterized by a T-score of −1.0 SD or higher; T-score between −1.0 and −2.5 SD is indicative of osteopenia, and a T-score equal to or lower than −2.5 SD is indicative of osteoporosis (WHO), For individuals under 50 years of age, the Z-score is used to evaluate bone density, with a Z-score lower than −2.0 indicating low bone mass according to chronologic age. As the average age at injury for traumatic SCI is 43, the diagnosis of osteoporosis in patients with SCI is typically made when they sustain a low-impact fracture. Diagnosis of low bone mass in children 6 to 21 years of age is done utilizing lumbar or total body Z-scores; in children 3 to 6 years of age, only DXA of the whole body is feasible and provides reproducible measures of bone mineral content and BMD.[14]

DXA can also be used to assess response to therapy[12]; testing should include evaluation of BMD at the total hip, distal femur, and proximal tibia, following a minimum of 12 months of therapy at 1- to 2-year intervals. In order to allow for meaningful comparison in BMD values, DXA testing should be done in a densitometry unit that has an established accuracy index (least significant change [LSC] index).

SCI/D-specific risk factors should be used to identify individuals at risk for low-impact fractures rather than the Fracture Risk Assessment Tool (FRAX), which has not been validated in individuals with paralysis.[15,16]

## TREATMENT

The aim of osteoporosis treatment in individuals with SCI/D-related paralysis is dual: prevent ongoing bone loss and reduce the risk of fractures. Not all drugs used in the treatment of primary osteoporosis, like bisphosphonates (alendronate, risedronate, ibandronate, zoledronate), calcitonin, synthetic parathyroid hormone (teriparatide, abaloparatide), anti-RANKL human monoclonal antibody (denosumab), and anti-sclerostin human monoclonal antibody (romosozumab) have been studied in SCI/D-related bone loss. Administration of bisphosphonates (alendronate, zoledronate) and the anti-RANKL monoclonal antibody denosumab can decrease the rate of bone loss in the lower limbs in individuals with SCI/D.[17-20] Proving that bisphosphonate administration increases bone mass at the knee in individuals with SCI/D is harder to do, with some studies showing no significant benefit[21] and others showing slight bone mass increase.[22,23] Teriparatide, postulated to increase osteoblastic activity, thus bone deposition has been shown to increase bone density of the spine, hip, and knee,[24] but its efficacy in fracture prevention was not assessed.

While individuals with SCI/D-related paralysis have been found to have low vitamin D level, there is no evidence that vitamin D supplementation influences fracture rate in them or able-bodied men and premenopausal women.[25,26]

Several physical modalities were shown to have some benefit on bone mass in individuals with SCI/D: standing and ambulation,[27] functional electrical stimulation (FES),[28-31] pulsed electromagnetic fields, and low-intensity ultrasound.[32] There is no established threshold BMD value below which weight-bearing activities are absolutely contraindicated,[12] and no correlation between exercise, modalities, and fracture rates has been established.[33,34] Clinicians should individually assess fracture risk factors prior to recommending engagement in weight-bearing activities for all individuals with SCI/D-related paralysis.

## ASSOCIATED IMPAIRMENTS AND COMPLICATIONS

Fragility fractures are the dreaded complications related to low bone mass and density. In the presence of abnormal sensory function, a great degree of clinical suspicion should be employed as a fracture may present with localized swelling, exacerbation of autonomic symptoms, spasticity, neuropathic pain, or new onset of limb deformity. Treatment may be conservative (padded splints, bivalved casts to allow for frequent skin inspection) or surgical stabilization may be required.

## FUNCTIONAL PROGNOSIS AND OUTCOMES

Fractures in this population are frequently complicated by development of significant comorbidities, like heterotopic ossification, nonunion, or delayed union, malalignment, limb length discrepancy, increased likelihood for venous thromboembolic disease, infection, skin lesions/ulcerations, harder-to-manage spasticity and neuropathic pain, difficulties with seating and positioning in the wheelchair, and overall decrease in mobility and quality of life.[35]

## BASIC ORDER SETS

1. DXA of total hip, distal femur, and proximal tibia.
2. Bone metabolism sample order set: 25 HO vitamin D level, comprehensive metabolic panel (CMP) and phosphorus, C telopeptide (to assess bone resorption), and osteocalcin and P1NP (to assess bone formation).
3. Zoledronic acid infusion sample order: Zoledronic acid 5 mg in 100 mL normal saline (NS); infuse over 30 minutes. Premedicate with Ibuprofen 600 to 800 mg and advise continuation of Ibuprofen 600 to 800 mg every 8 hours for 24 to 30 hours to prevent flu-like symptoms.

## RESOURCES AND REFERENCES

The full list of resources and references appears in the digital product found on http://connect
.springerpub.com/content/book/978-0-8261-6226-7/part/part01/chapter/ch09

# PARKINSON'S DISEASE

HEATHER R. BAER AND CAROLINE T. GOLDIN

## CORE DEFINITION

Parkinsonism: Bradykinesia with rest tremor and/or rigidity.[1]

## ETIOLOGY AND PATHOPHYSIOLOGY

The etiology of Parkinson's disease (PD) is a complex interaction between genetics and the environment. Sporadic cases make up the vast majority, with only 10% of newly diagnosed persons with PD (PwP) reporting a family history.[2] Pathologically, PD is characterized by progressive loss of striatal dopamine, which occurs through interrelated mechanisms, including oxidative stress, mitochondrial dysfunction, excitotoxicity, inflammation, and apoptosis.[2] Accumulation of the abnormal protein alpha-synuclein into Lewy bodies was long thought to be the pathognomonic histologic feature of the disease; however, in some genetic forms, postmortem evaluation has revealed alternative pathways to neurodegeneration,[3] suggesting that PD may be best characterized as a syndrome rather than a distinct illness.

## DIAGNOSTIC APPROACH

PD is a clinical diagnosis. The involvement of a specialist is essential. The diagnosis of PD by an experienced clinician, using specific historical and examination criteria, may be more accurate than current formal diagnostic criteria.[1] The International Parkinson and Movement Disorder Society Clinical Diagnostic Criteria for PD (MDS-PD Criteria) were designed for use in research and to guide clinical diagnosis.

PD has two diagnostic categories based on certainty: clinically established PD (>90% certainty) and clinically probable PD (>80% certainty). A patient with parkinsonism (i.e., bradykinesia with rest tremor and/or rigidity) and supportive criteria, and with no absolute exclusion criteria or red flags, is diagnosed with clinically established PD.[1] The diagnosis of clinically probable PD allows for the presence of some atypical features but no absolute exclusion criteria. Red flag symptoms that suggest an alternative diagnosis include unequivocal early bulbar symptoms (e.g., severe dysphagia or dysphonia), rapid progression of

The full list of resources and references appears in the digital product found on http://connect.springerpub.com/content/book/978-0-8261-6226-7/part/part01/chapter/ch10

gait impairment, recurrent falls within 3 years of onset, and severe autonomic dysfunction within the first 5 years. Unequivocal cerebellar signs, downward vertical supranuclear gaze palsy, and documentation of an alternative condition known to produce parkinsonism are examples of absolute exclusion criteria. No biomarkers have been established for the diagnosis of PD.

Neuroimaging can be supportive of the diagnosis of PD. Specialized PET scans can detect reduced dopaminergic neuronal integrity in the striatum. These PET scans, also called dopamine transporter (DaT) scans, show similar abnormalities in other Parkinsonian disorders (e.g., multiple systems atrophy and progressive supranuclear palsy), but they are normal in patients with medication-induced Parkinsonism, essential tremor, dystonic tremor, and vascular Parkinsonism. Standard MRI sequencing of the brain is typically normal in PD. High field strength MRI can show T2 lucency in the substantia nigra and increased diffusion-weighted imaging signal in the olfactory tract; however, these are not available in clinical practice at this time.

The extent of neuroimaging abnormalities, if present, does not correlate with the severity of the illness, and so several clinical rating scales have been validated for this purpose. The MDS- Unified Parkinson Disease Rating Scale (UPDRS) is commonly used. It quantifies (a) nonmotor experiences of daily living (e.g., cognitive impairment, hallucinations, sleep problems), (b) motor experiences of daily living (e.g., speech, swallow, dressing, tremor), (c) motor examination (see Box 10.1), and (d) motor complications (e.g., dyskinesias, motor fluctuations, painful dystonia).[1] In addition to the MDS-UPDRS, the Hoehn–Yahr staging scale can be used to rate the severity of the disease based on unilateral versus bilateral disease involvement, postural instability, and the need for assistive devices for ambulation.[1] Other validated scales exist to more precisely quantify other vital considerations for PwP, including quality of life and nonmotor symptoms.[4,5]

---

## BOX 10.1

### MOTOR EXAMINATION DOMAINS (MDS-UPDRS)

- Speech
- Facial expression
- Rigidity (in the neck and limbs)
- Bradykinesia (global, hands, and feet)
- Leg agility
- Arising from a chair
- Gait (impairments and use of assistive device)
- Freezing of gait
- Posture
- Postural stability
- Tremor (postural, kinetic, and rest)
- Dyskinesia
- Hoehn and Yahr stage

## TREATMENT

### Medical Treatment and Management: Acute and Chronic

Current medical treatments improve the motor (and some nonmotor) symptoms of PD but do not alter its progressive pathology. Because of this, medications are only started when symptoms are functionally limiting or bothersome. The most commonly used (and most effective) oral medication is carbidopa/levodopa.[2] Levodopa is metabolized to dopamine, which supplements the low dopaminergic action in the striatum in PwP while carbidopa, a dopamine decarboxylase inhibitor, prevents peripheral metabolism of levodopa so it may cross the blood–brain barrier. Dopamine cannot cross the blood–brain barrier. Other oral medications act centrally at the dopaminergic neuron and include agents that inhibit the breakdown of levodopa in the brain, such as catechol-o-methyl transferase (COMT) inhibitors (entacapone, tolcapone, and opicapone) and monoamine oxidase B inhibitors (selegiline, rasagiline, and safinamide), medications that increase dopamine availability (amantadine); and dopamine agonists (ropinirole, pramipexole, rotigotine, and apomorphine).[2] More recently, istradefylline, an adenosine A2A receptor (mechanism of action uncertain) has been approved for the treatment of motor fluctuations.

PwP taking dopaminergic medications should be monitored for impulse control disorders. For patients with a high pill burden or difficulty controlling motor symptom fluctuations, treatments such as deep brain stimulation (DBS), carbidopa–levodopa continuous enteral suspension provided through a gastrostomy–jejunostomy tube, or focused ultrasound cerebral ablation are available.[6] Inhaled levodopa and injectable apomorphine are used for sudden dose failures (i.e., times when patients experience abrupt return of parkinsonian symptoms while on dopaminergic medications for PD). New delivery methods for carbidopa/levodopa (such as subcutaneous pump) are currently in phase 3 clinical trials. Agents to address complications of treatment (such as medication-induced dyskinesias) are also under investigation. At this time, amantadine is the only oral agent proven to address dyskinesias.

Nonmotor symptoms (e.g., anxiety and neurogenic orthostatic hypotension [OH]) impact quality of life and sometimes are the most problematic features of PD. Patient education is key for identifying and managing these issues. Nonmotor symptom questionnaires (e.g., MDS-NMS) can also help identify these problems. While some motor symptoms are responsive to adjustments of dopaminergic medications, most require other treatment approaches (see the following).

### Rehabilitation Management

Although heterogeneous in its presentation and course, anticipatory treatment is based on common features of PD. Both motor and nonmotor symptoms should be considered.

### Early Stages

Start activity-based exercise-oriented treatments to improve mood, activity tolerance, and timely performance of activities of daily living (ADLs) at the time of diagnosis when deconditioning and considerable slowness may already be present.[7] Treatment targets include reducing the impact of tremor and bradykinesia, improvement of balance/gait, and enhancement of quality of life.[8] Apathy is a common symptom in PD, and strategies to support adherence (e.g., group exercise or classes) are required to sustain benefits.[7] Moderate-intensity aerobic exercise 3 to 5 days per week is recommended, starting with 20 minutes and increasing to 60 minutes per session.[8] The exercise intensity target is 40–60% of peak heart rate or a 13 on a 20-point perceived exertion scale. Evidence-based activities include ergometry, walking (including weight-supported treadmill), and aquatics. Progressive resistance exercise targeting large muscle groups 2 to 3 days per week, alternating with days of rest, has also been shown to be beneficial.[8] Even early in the disease, postural abnormalities may be present and should be addressed.[7] If tremor is medication resistant and functionally limiting, or very bothersome to the individual, adaptive strategies or devices (e.g., tremor-canceling spoons) and botulinum toxin injections could be considered.[9,10]

Vocal changes may be problematic, particularly for those still working. Referral to a speech and language pathologist (SLP) can be beneficial.[7,11] Many therapists incorporate principles from the Lee Silverman Voice Training (LSVT®) program. Continuing group sessions (e.g., SPEAK OUT® and The LOUD Crowd®) are available in some regions to help PwP maintain gains.

Nonmotor symptoms can be significant and debilitating for PwP. Anxiety and/or depression are frequently present.[12] Along with oral medications (particularly pramipexole, venlafaxine, nortriptyline, and desipramine), cognitive behavioral therapy has shown benefit for PD-related mood disorders.[12] The involvement of a palliative care expert is recommended to help establish goals of care shortly after the time of diagnosis and to follow for care through later stages of the disease.[7]

## Middle Stages

The exercise prescription is tailored to the individual and should be revised as the disease progresses. Aerobic conditioning, strength, postural integrity, flexibility, safe transfers, gait, and balance should be targeted.[7] Exercise generally should be performed during the best time of symptom control ("ON" medication time). Supervision is recommended for safety, and visual or auditory cues can help with coordination during activity.[8] There appears to be a progressive disturbance in the self-perception of verticality that contributes to postural deformities, postural instability, and balance impairment, so postural correction and balance exercises should be incorporated into treatment.[13] Continued participation in activities that help PwP maintain flexibility and balance, such as Tai Chi or yoga, should be encouraged. Dystonic posturing of the face, neck, or limbs can be painful or functionally limiting. When noninvasive measures (e.g., stretching, strengthening, or oral medications) fail, botulinum toxin injections can be helpful.[9]

Interventions to sustain safety and independence with ADLs are also recommended and become increasingly important over time.[7] Referral to occupational therapy (OT) should be considered. Surveillance for the emergence of functionally limiting nonmotor symptoms (particularly dysautonomia and cognitive impairment) should be stepped up during this stage. If resources are available, annual driving assessments should be considered and a discussion about planning for retirement from driving should be initiated.[6]

## Late Stages

Later stages of the disease are complicated by dopamine-resistant symptoms (e.g., postural instability, dementia, psychosis, and freezing of gait) and a higher susceptibility to side effects of medications. PwP who have undergone DBS may have less bradykinesia, rigidity, and tremor but will still display similar dopamine-resistant late-stage symptoms. Hence, rehabilitation strategies and non-dopaminergic approaches become more important. Serial review of fall risk and updates of safety interventions are required. Cueing-based therapies (e.g., rhythmic auditory stimulation) and other activity-based approaches may be helpful for gait impairments. Efforts should be made to identify effective adaptive strategies (e.g., taking wide turns, shifting weight) and equipment (e.g., laser walker).

As the disease progresses, PwP should be monitored and, when necessary, treated for dysphagia.[7] Sialorrhea, which often accompanies the emergence of dysphagia, can be treated with anticholinergic medications, but botulinum toxin injections are preferred due to side-effect profiles of available oral and topical medications.[7,9,12] Individuals also need to be monitored regularly for the emergence of OH, as this is both a primary symptom of PD and is aggravated by PD medications. If left untreated, OH can result in fatigue, confusion, and falls. Along with nonpharmacologic measures (e.g., compression stockings), medication adjustments and the addition of salt tablets, midodrine, fludrocortisone, and/or droxidopa may be required.[7] PwP should learn to perform orthostatic measurements and be asked to report the emergence of supine hypertension, which may require adjustment of medications and/or administration of antihypertensives at bedtime. Other common nonmotor symptoms that benefit from rehabilitation management include depression, mild cognitive impairment, dementia, psychosis neurogenic bowel (often constipation, but one can see fecal incontinence in later stages), neurogenic bladder (urinary retention, frequency, and/or incontinence), pain, and sleep disorders.

## ASSOCIATED IMPAIRMENTS AND COMPLICATIONS

- Autonomic dysfunction
- Drooling
- Dysautonomia/OH
  - Erectile dysfunction
  - Neurogenic bowel
  - Neurogenic bladder
- Balance impairment
- Communication impairment
  - Hypophonia
  - Hypokinetic speech
  - Micrographia
- Disorders of sleep and wakefulness
  - Excessive daytime sleepiness
  - Insomnia
  - REM sleep behavioral disorder
  - Sleep fragmentation
- Dysphagia
- Dystonia
- Fatigue
- Neuropsychiatric symptoms
  - Anxiety
  - Apathy

- ❏ Cognitive impairment
  - ❏ Mild cognitive impairment (MCI) and dementia
- ❏ Depression
- ❏ Impulse control disorders
- ❏ Psychosis
- ■ Olfactory dysfunction
- ■ Pain
- ■ Postural deformities
- ■ Visual/visuospatial impairment
- ■ Weight loss

## FUNCTIONAL PROGNOSIS AND OUTCOMES

PD is heterogeneous, leading to tremendous variability in the rate of progression of the disorder and the functional outcomes. In general, individuals who present initially with an akinetic–rigid form of PD have a more rapid symptom progression and a shorter life expectancy than those with a tremor-predominant or mixed onset.[14] Significant cognitive impairment and a high burden of autonomic symptoms are also associated with a more rapid progression of neurodegeneration.[7] Serial evaluations by a PD specialist are required to review the diagnosis and identify disease patterns, as atypical Parkinsonism disorders may not be recognized until several years after initial diagnosis and are associated with a rapid course and a shortened life span.[7]

## BASIC ORDER SETS

Common activity-based recommendations/orders for PD:

1.  Physical therapy (PT): Evaluate and treat (including the provision of a home exercise program):

    i.   Postural deformity: Enhance strength, flexibility, and awareness of body position.
    ii.  Balance impairment: Improve postural stability, including recovery from posteriorly directed perturbations. Assess for and train with adaptive devices. Train family/caregivers in strategies for safe transfers and gait.
    iii. Gait asymmetry or slowness: Utilize cueing strategies (such as rhythmic auditory stimulation and BIG therapy techniques).
    iv.  Freezing of gait/start hesitations: Identify strategies to prevent or manage events. Assess for and train with adaptive equipment (such as laser walker or cane).

2.  OT: Evaluate and treat (including the provision of a home exercise program):

    i.   Transfers: Including control of sit-stand transfers. Assess for and train with adaptive equipment (such as laser walker or cane).
    ii.  Dexterity: Provide exercises to try to improve amplitude and speed of movement. Identify adaptive equipment (such as voice-activated software for computers).
    iii. Tremor: Identify adaptive strategies and equipment (such as tremor-canceling spoons and gloves).

iv.   Driving: Assess reaction time, peripheral awareness, dexterity, and cognition/judgment. Consider adaptive driving equipment.

3.   SLP: Evaluate and treat (including the provision of a home program):

i.   Speech impairment: Enhance the audibility and comprehensibility of speech (possibly incorporating LSVT). Assess for and train with augmentative devices. Train family/caregivers in communication techniques.

ii.   Swallow dysfunction: Assess swallow safety and provide recommendations.

iii.   Cognition: Provide exercises for attention and problem-solving. Teach adaptive techniques for memory impairment and word finding difficulties.

## RESOURCES AND REFERENCES

The full list of resources and references appears in the digital product found on http://connect.springerpub.com/content/book/978-0-8261-6226-7/part/part01/chapter/ch10

# SPINA BIFIDA

VISHAL BANSAL AND GLENDALIZ BOSQUES

## CORE DEFINITIONS

Spina bifida (SB) is one of the most common forms of neural tube defects (NTDs) resulting from incomplete closure during embryonic development. With multiple phenotypic expressions, spina bifida can be further classified anatomically. Protrusion of neural or membrane elements exposed through a bony defect from an NTD with absent skin covering is referred to as open spina bifida. The most prevalent forms of open spina bifida are myelomeningocele (MMC) and myelocele.[1] Closed spina bifida best describes a presentation with protrusion of neural or membrane elements through a bony defect with intact skin covering. The most prevalent forms of closed spina bifida are meningocele and lipomyelomeningocele.[1] Caudal regression syndrome is an uncommon complex closed type due to abnormal development of the most distal end of the fetal spine.[2]

## ETIOLOGY AND PATHOPHYSIOLOGY

Spina bifida is a complex birth defect that is hypothesized to be a result of environmental, maternal, nutritional, and genetic risk factors.[3] Individuals with spina bifida have a survival rate of approximately 75% to 85%; a noteworthy change from a mortality rate of 38% prior to the 1970s in part due to advances in rehabilitation care.[4]

To understand NTDs it is imperative to understand the primary disturbance during the first month of embryonic development. Appropriate closure of the neural tube occurs approximately 21 to 27 days after conception in utero. The exact mechanism behind disruption in the appropriate closure is not fully understood. In MMC, the open NTD leads to prolonged exposure of underlying neural tissue to amniotic fluid. In the initial stages, the neural epithelium continues to undergo the appropriate neuronal differentiation; however, progressive exposure of amniotic fluid eventually causes it to hemorrhage leading to neuronal death.[5]

Potential risk factors for NTDs include[5] the following:

*Maternal nutrition*: Alcohol or caffeine use, **Low folate intake***, suboptimal nutrition

*Environmental factors*: Disinfectants by-products in drinking water, nitrate-related compounds, organic solvents, pesticides, polycyclic aromatic compounds

*Other Maternal Factors*: Hyperthermia, low socioeconomic status, ***pregestational insulin-dependent diabetes, pregestational obesity, use of valproic acid, and other medications***

---

The full list of resources and references appears in the digital product found on http://connect.springerpub.com/content/book/978-0-8261-6226-7/part/part01/chapter/ch11

*which may alter folate metabolism, phenotypic predisposition* (*most important risk factors are bolded).

## DIAGNOSTIC APPROACH

### Screening and Diagnostic Evaluation

The primary screening tool used to detect spina bifida is a second-trimester fetal ultrasound in conjunction with a quad-screen. The screen allows for evaluation of maternal levels of alpha-fetoprotein (AFP), human chorionic gonadotropin (HCG), estriol, and inhibin-A. Elevated levels of AFP support a presumptive diagnosis of spina bifida or other NTDs. Ultrasound allows the clinician to perform fetal intracranial and spinal imaging to detect the anatomical abnormality indicative of spina bifida and other open/closed NTDs (anencephaly, encephalocele). Ultrasound features that support the diagnosis of SB may include the *banana sign* (compressed cerebellar hemispheres) or *lemon sign* (concavity of the frontal bones compared to the expected convex shape of frontal bones in the typically developing fetus).[5]

Positive screening prompts referral to maternal-fetal medicine experts for further evaluation. Diagnostic imaging (advanced ultrasound or MRI) and amniocentesis (fetal karyotype, amniotic AFP, and acetylcholinesterase levels) are typically performed. A fetal echocardiogram may be warranted since previous studies have documented a relationship between NTDs and congenital heart disease.[6]

### Genetic Screening

Most cases of spina bifida are sporadic with no clear genetic inheritance pattern. Mutations in *methylenetetrahydrofolate reductase (MTHFR)* genes have been documented in some clinical studies to be a risk factor for NTD. Homozygous expression of the *MTHFR 677 C/T* variant gene leads to elevated levels of homocysteine leading to reduced plasma levels of folate.[7] Other genetic defects have been documented to alter folate metabolism and contribute to the development of NTDs.[8] Chromosomal aneuploidy (trisomy 21 and 13) are reported to account for a minor percentage of NTDs.[9]

### History
### Prenatal History (Environmental Exposures, Risks, Care)

Assess for the appropriate use, dosing and timing of folic acid supplementation, exposure to known environmental toxins, history of NTDs, and other known maternal risk factors.

### Birth History

Delivery type, Apgar scores, surgical interventions, complications, length of stay, pertinent imaging studies.

### Childhood History

Assess nutritional status and physical activity levels to mitigate onset of obesity. Record level of spinal cord involvement to correlate the potential dermatomal and myotomal distributions, sensation, and motor function. This is important to evaluate complications later in life. Any declines in social, mental, and physical functioning and overall neurological development should be documented.

## Complication-Specific History

*Bowel and bladder function:* Continence status and details for bladder and bowel programs should be documented.

*Hydrocephalus:* For infants younger than 12 months (open fontanelle), symptoms suggestive of hydrocephalus may include bulging fontanelle, cranial nerve dysfunction, upward vertical gaze palsy (*sundowning*), decreased feeding, lethargy, macrocephaly, and poor developmental progress. For children older than 12 months with a closed fontanelle, symptoms differ and may include nausea, vomiting, headaches, changes in behavior, irritability, diplopia, drowsiness, and papilledema. Children with hydrocephalus and a ventriculoperitoneal (VP) shunt may develop symptoms of hydrocephalus as a sign of shunt infection or malfunction. Shunt revision history should be recorded (aggregate, last time).

*Chiari II malformation:* Presenting symptoms can include changes in swallowing patterns, choking, hoarseness, central apnea, abnormal breathing patterns, opisthotonos, or sudden death.

*Tethered cord syndrome:* May present with back pain, changes in gait, changes in bowel/bladder patterns, new onset of spasticity, contractures, and rapid scoliosis progression.

*Syringomyelia:* History may include worsening of function above the level of lesion, slower progression of developmental motor milestones, and rapid scoliosis progression.

*Skin breakdown:* Elicit history of prior wounds or ulcers and their state. If current, assess if improving or worsening treatments or home remedies used. Assess for contributing factors.

## Physical Examination

A complete physical examination should include the following components appropriate for the patient's age:

Evaluate skin integrity with a focus on commonly affected sites to include ischial tuberosities, feet, sacrum, and greater trochanters. Skin compromise has also been reported over gibbus deformities in children with thoracic-level lesions.[10]

Serial measurements of head circumference over the first few years should be recorded. Macrocephaly is defined as two or more standard deviations above the average and can be indicative of hydrocephalus.

A complete neurological examination should be performed on a regular basis. Document the affected level and monitor neurological functioning in both upper and lower limbs, including muscle strength and tone. Subtle discrepancies can be indicative of complications such as tethered cord, hydrocephalus, progression of Chiari II malformation, or syringomyelia.

Comprehensive evaluation should also include musculoskeletal assessment. There is a higher risk of developing scoliosis or kyphosis or both as the presence of congenital vertebral anomalies is associated with the development of spinal curvature. Evaluate for contractures, hip dislocation, and foot deformities that will interfere with gait optimization.

## TREATMENT

Therapies and treatment for management of spina bifida are geared toward optimizing the patient's physical, mental, and social well-being while promoting independence and minimizing disabilities. Planned cesarean section delivery is recommended to mitigate risks of spinal cord damage during vaginal delivery. Closure of open NTDs in the natal and postnatal period is usually performed using a staged approach to maintain neurological function. One randomized control trial showed superior outcomes (motor scores, lower rates of death, and incidence of shunt placement at 12 months) for children with prenatal NTD repair compared to postnatal repair.[11]

### Multidisciplinary Approach

Multidisciplinary clinics can facilitate care during the prenatal and childhood periods. Patients will benefit from rehabilitation interventions throughout their lifetime to optimize development and function, ameliorate obesity, optimize nutrition, prevent contractures, and assist with social integration.

Spina bifida is complex with wide variability in phenotypic expressions; rehabilitation issues may include:

### Central Nervous System

Neurologic impairments may be a result of the NTD and presence of other complications such as concomitant hydrocephalus, hindbrain herniation (Arnold Chiari malformation type II), syringomyelia, or tethered cord. Early detection and appropriate intervention mitigate neurologic decline. Patients may require neurosurgical interventions such as endoscopic third ventriculostomy (ETV), VP shunt for hydrocephalus, posterior brain decompression for hindbrain herniation, and pleural shunt for syrinx decompression or release of tethered cord. Cognitive or psychological dysfunction may be present with brain involvement. Monitoring for executive dysfunction, intellectual disability, and depression is important. Therapeutic interventions with physical, occupational, and speech therapy will be required throughout childhood. Neuropsychological testing is recommended for optimization of academic success. Behavioral psychology, play-based therapy, and additional counseling may be necessary to improve social skills, participation, integration, and transitions.

### Neurogenic Bowel and Bladder

Appropriate bladder management mitigates risk of urinary tract infections (UTIs), allows for appropriate bladder growth, decreases damage to renal system, and promotes independence and continence. It is important to note the patient's bowel continence status and details of bowel program (time, frequency, presence of hemorrhoids or bleeding). Renal abnormalities (linked to caudal regression syndrome), external genital abnormalities or anorectal stenosis (linked to caudal regression syndrome), and sexual dysfunction (males) may also be present. Bowel and bladder programs need to be developmentally appropriate. Most patients will need intermittent straight catheterization programs. Some patients may require pharmacological interventions such as anticholinergic oral medications or intravesical botulinum toxin injections. Advanced urologic surgical interventions to assist with independent continence programs may include continent stoma with or without bladder augmentation procedure (Mitrofanoff procedure). Routine bowel programs will require the use of oral stool softeners and/or laxatives. It may require per rectum interventions, such as suppositories, enemas, or rectal irrigation systems. Surgical interventions to assist in fecal continence may include stoma creation for antegrade colonic enema (ACE). Colostomy may also be an option for very severe cases.

## Musculoskeletal

Musculoskeletal abnormalities are typically a result of neurological dysfunction. Spine deformities (scoliosis, kyphosis) may be present. Lower extremity paresis may contribute to joint contractures, acetabular dysplasia (hip subluxation/dislocation), rotation deformities, and Charcot joints. Stretching programs, bracing, and positioning are essential in mitigating the development of these deformities. Orthopedic interventions may be required for severe club feet and other deformities which may impact function and developmental progression.

## Childhood-Onset Osteoporosis

Children living with SB may experience lower bone mineral density and higher occurrences of fractures. Associated risk factors for fracture risk in this population include higher levels of neurological involvement, obesity, non-ambulatory status, limited physical activity, hypercalciuria, contractures, and history of spontaneous fracture.[12]

Adult patients living with SB are subject to the aforementioned risk factors in addition to osteoporosis risk factors for the general adult population. Optimization of nutrition, including vitamin D levels, is essential. Incorporation of standing program may aide stretching and bony deposition. Some patients may benefit from bisphosphonate infusions.

## Skin Breakdown

Sensation disturbances and deformities may contribute to pressure ulcers. Heightened awareness and surveillance are required for prevention, early identification, and management. Patients may require occasional wound care. Wounds may take longer to heal and may recur. Nutritional and equipment status may need to be re-evaluated with nonhealing wounds and recurrences. Some patients may require plastic surgery consult.

Other relevant comorbidities may include the presence of cardiac abnormalities and allergies (latex allergies or latex-fruit syndrome).

## FUNCTIONAL PROGNOSIS AND OUTCOMES

Most patients present with involvement of bowel and bladder function. Skin sensation and muscle weakness level will be dependent on the location of NTD.

Due to the presence of muscle weakness, motor development may be delayed.

Motor function and ambulation potential will depend on the level of defect (thoracic, upper lumbar, lower lumbar, sacral) and the muscles affected. Patients will require different bracing and equipment depending on the potential gross mobility to be achieved (Table 11.1).[13]

The best predictor for ambulation is the presence of quadriceps strength (at least full antigravity).[12]

TABLE 11.1 LEVELS OF MYELOMENINGOCELE DEFECT AND EXPECTED DEVELOPMENTAL MILESTONES AND AMBULATION POTENTIAL

| MOBILITY SKILL | LEVEL OF LESION | | | |
|---|---|---|---|---|
| | T12 AND ABOVE | L1 TO L2 | L3 TO L4 | L5 TO SACRAL |
| ROLLING OVER | Delayed (can be achieved by 18 months by compensation) | Delayed (can be achieved by compensation) | Delayed | Minimal delay |
| SITTING | Delayed (can sit with propping and equipment) | Delayed (can be achieved, has balance issues) | Delayed (can be achieved) | Minimal delay |
| FLOOR MOBILITY | Rolling, combat crawling, bottom scooting | Rolling, combat crawling, bottom scooting | Modified crawling | Crawling |
| AMBULATION | Adaptive equipment and bracing may be required. Poor probability of ambulation. HKAFO, KAFO, RGO, dynamic and static standers | Adaptive equipment and bracing may be required. Household ambulation. KAFO, RGO, dynamic standers. | Bracing may be required. Household and community ambulation. KAFO, GR-AFO, AFO, walkers and crutches. | Community ambulation, AFO, FO |

AFO, ankle foot orthosis; FO, foot orthosis; GR-AFO, ground-reaction ankle foot orthosis; HKAFO, hip ankle foot orthosis; KAFO, knee ankle foot orthosis; RGO, reciprocal gait orthosis.

Equipment and interventions should be introduced to follow expected developmental sequences. Independence in mobility should be encouraged to optimize environmental engagement. Early introduction to wheelchairs should be provided for any patient who will potentially require one for primary or secondary mobility needs. Priority in mobility options and efficiency will most likely change with age.

Approximately 75% to –85% of individuals living with MMC are able to live to young adulthood. These individuals face secondary complications and are at risk of subpar outcomes when the transition of care from pediatric care is not thorough and there is a lack of comprehensive follow-up in multidisciplinary clinics during adulthood.[10]

## Cognition

Children with MMC have reported lower intelligence quotient (IQ) levels, difficulty with math, and difficulty with visual perceptual tasks compared to their able-bodied peers. Lower IQ scores have been reported in those with thoracic-level lesions compared to lumbar- or sacral-level lesions. They also report higher levels of verbal IQ compared to performance IQ. Individuals who experience central nervous system infections, multiple VP stunt revisions display a trend of lower IQ.

**Education and Lifestyle**

Most patients complete high school and about ~50% continue to further education.[10] In the United States, independent living is achieved by 14% to 41%. Employment rates of 25% to 62% have been reported, dependent on intelligence, academic achievements, behavioral functioning, continence status, and severity of physical disability.[10] Limited data has been published concerning educational status, employment status, and living situation.

On average, patients may have lower energy expenditure levels and metabolic rates that could predispose to obesity, metabolic syndrome, diabetes, heart disease, and functional decline in physical activity tolerance.

## BASIC ORDER SETS

Basic order sets to consider in rehabilitation settings include:
- Brain imaging.
- Imaging of the spine.
- Annual renal ultrasound and cystourethrography if necessary.
- Hip imaging.
- Neuropsychological testing at school entry and transition periods.
- Lab workup for cystatin C, 25-hydroxyvitamin D in addition to the routine lab work for well child visits and annual checkups.

## RESOURCES AND REFERENCES

The full list of resources and references appears in the digital product found on http://connect .springerpub.com/content/book/978-0-8261-6226-7/part/part01/chapter/ch11

# SPINAL CORD INJURY

ALBERT C. RECIO, PHILIPPINES G. CABAHUG, AND CRISTINA L. SADOWSKY

## CORE DEFINITIONS

Spinal cord injury (SCI) is an insult to the spinal cord resulting in a permanent or temporary change in sensory, motor, or autonomic function.[1-3] The International Standards for Neurological and Classification of Spinal Cord Injury (ISNCSCI) is a widely accepted system describing the level and extent of injury based on a systematic motor and sensory examination of neurologic function.[1] The following terminology has developed around the classification of SCIs:

### Spinal Cord Injury Clinical Syndromes (Patterns of Incomplete Injuries)

*Central cord syndrome*: Clinically presents with greater weakness of the arms than the legs, bowel, and bladder dysfunction and varying sensory loss below the injury level. It is the most common of the incomplete injury patterns often occurring in patients with underlying cervical spondylosis who sustain severe neck hypertension (most commonly from a fall).[1,4]

*Anterior cord syndrome*: Occurs as a result of interruption of the blood supply to the anterior two-thirds of the spinal cord. The clinical symptoms include a loss of motor function, pain, and temperature sensation at and below the injury level with preservation of light touch and position sense transmitted through the dorsal columns.[1,4]

*Brown-Sequard syndrome*: Results from an asymmetric cord lesion and is historically related to a knife wound injury mechanism; it is classically thought of as a hemisection of the cord although pure hemisection is uncommon with traumatic injuries. The syndrome presents with ipsilateral loss of proprioception, vibration, and motor function with contralateral loss of pain and temperature sensation.[1,4]

*Posterior cord syndrome*: Presents clinically with bilateral deficits in proprioception and vibration. Two pathological mechanisms are vitamin B12 deficiency (subacute combined degeneration) and syphilis (tabes dorsalis).[1,4]

*Cauda equina syndrome*: Involves injury to the lumbosacral nerve roots (the cauda equina or horses' tail) below spinal level lumbar L1. Injury to the nerve roots will present clinically as flaccid paralysis of the muscles in the lower limbs and areflexic bowel and bladder. All sensory modalities are similarly impaired. Sacral reflexes such as bulbocavernosus and anal wink will be absent.[1,4,5]

---

The full list of resources and references appears in the digital product found on http://connect
.springerpub.com/content/book/978-0-8261-6226-7/part/part01/chapter/ch12

*Conus medullaris syndrome*: May be clinically similar to cauda equina syndrome, but the injury is more rostral, involving the distal tip of the cord at the inferior aspect of L1 to L2 area. Injury to the lumbar nerve roots and conus usually results in areflexic bladder and bowel and lower limbs weakness. If it is a high conus lesion, bulbocavernosus reflex and micturition reflexes are preserved.[1,4]

## ETIOLOGY AND PATHOPHYSIOLOGY

In the United States, most epidemiologic and demographic data have been collected by the Model Spinal Cord Injury Care Systems and are published by the National Spinal Cord Injury Statistical Center.[6,7] The causes of traumatic SCI are:

- Motor vehicle crashes are the leading cause of SCI in the United States, about 37% of cases in the database.
- Falls, 29%, are the leading cause of SCI among the elderly.
- Violence as a cause for SCI peaked in the 1990s but has since declined to 14% (most are gunshot wounds).
- Sports injuries are reported to be 9% (most commonly: diving).
- Other causes are reported to be 11%.

Spinal cord injuries usually occur in association with injuries to the vertebral column. These can include any one or more of the following: fracture of one or more of the bony elements, dislocation at one or more joints, tearing of ligaments, and disruption and/or herniation of the intervertebral disc.[8,9]

### Primary Injury

The initial tissue disruption and damage to the spinal cord that occurs at the time of impact is the primary injury.[8,9] This refers to the immediate effect of trauma, which may include:

*Flexion/hyperflexion injury*: Odontoid fracture, tear drop fracture, simple wedge fraction, anterior subluxation, bilateral locked facets, anterior disc space narrowing, widened interspinous distance, clay-shoveler's fracture.

*Hyperextension injury*: Hangman's fracture, subluxation (anterior/posterior), neural arch fracture of C1, anteriorly widened disc space, prevertebral swelling.

*Flexion-rotation injury*: Unilateral locked facets.

*Vertical compression*: Jefferson fracture, burst fracture.

*Lateral flexion/shearing*: Lateral vertebral compression, uncinate fracture, isolated pillar fracture, transverse process fracture.

*Distraction*: Transverse fracture through vertebra (chance fracture; most commonly seen in patients wearing lap seat belts).

### Secondary Injury

Damage occurs due to pathophysiologic processes that follow SCI.[9,10]

Possible mechanisms of secondary injury include ischemia, edema, microvascular perfusion alterations, free radical generation, lipid peroxidation, excitotoxicity (massive glutamate release), calcium overload, inflammatory and immunologic response, and cell death (both necrotic and apoptotic—programmed cell death).

## DIAGNOSTIC APPROACH

### Clinical Diagnosis

Traumatic SCI may not only be obvious from the history or initial examination but also must be excluded in patients with altered mental status (unconscious, confused, or inebriated) when the history regarding trauma is unknown. Physical examination may reveal local and radicular pain, step-off or spinal tenderness, weakness in a radicular or myelopathic distribution, sensory loss, absent tone and reflexes, and urinary retention. The presence and extent of injuries should be confirmed with spinal neuroimaging.

Documenting impairments in SCI patients is best determined by performing a standard-ized neurological examination as developed by the ISNCSCI. The international standards examination used for neurological classification has two components (sensory and motor). The American Spinal Cord Injury Association (ASIA) Impairment Scale (AIS) designation is used in grading the degree of impairment (Table 12.1).[1,4]

### Imaging Diagnosis

Radiographic evaluation following spinal trauma is essential for diagnostic assessment in order to determine further care and plan for surgical decision-making. Plain x-rays of the spine may reveal fractures or dislocation. Although plain x-rays do not image the spinal cord itself, they are used to describe bony structures and alignment. Multi-slice CT is supplanting plain x-rays in spinal trauma, due to its speed, convenience, and markedly superior sensitivity to fracture detection. MRI is the imaging modality of choice for spinal cord imaging. Myelography improves spinal cord resolution when coupled with CT. CT-angiography (CTA) demonstrates the vertebrate and carotid arteries simultaneously with spinal CT if IV contrast bolus is given. Ultrasound has been helpful intraoperatively to assess the parenchyma.[11]

## TREATMENT

### Medical

The basic principles for early hospital management of traumatic SCI include the ABCs (airway, breathing, and circulation) and spinal protection. In addition, diagnostic assessments for clinical care; assessment for associated injuries, pain, nutritional support; and management of complications such as respiratory, cardiac, genitourinary, gastrointestinal (GI), venous thromboembolism, and skin are essential. There are published guidelines recommending management following acute SCI which are included in the Consortium for Spinal Cord Medicine clinical practice guidelines on Early Management in Adults with SCI.[12,13] Prevention and treatment of hypotension as soon as possible is recommended with efforts to maintain mean arterial blood pressure (MAP) greater than or equal to 85 mmHg.[12,13] The guidelines state that no clinical evidence exists to definitively recommend the use of any neuroprotective pharmacologic agent including steroids in the treatment of acute SCI for functional recovery.[14,15] The use of IV methylprednisolone (MP) in acute non-penetrating traumatic SCI was supported by the National Acute Spinal Cord Injury Studies (NASCIS).[16] However, the results of the NASCIS trials have been challenged. The administration of MP for the treatment of SCI is not recommended.[17]

**TABLE 12.1 THE AMERICAN SPINAL CORD INJURY ASSOCIATION IMPAIRMENT SCALE**

| LEVEL | NAME | DESCRIPTION |
|---|---|---|
| A | COMPLETE | No sensory or motor function is preserved in the sacral segments S4–S5 |
| B | SENSORY INCOMPLETE | Sensory but not motor function is preserved at the sacral segments S4–S5, and no motor function is preserved more than three levels below the motor level on either side of the body |
| C | MOTOR INCOMPLETE | Motor function is preserved at the most caudal sacral segments on voluntary anal contraction or the patients meet the criteria for sensory incomplete status with sparing of motor function more than three levels below the motor level on either side of the body. This includes key or non-key muscle functions. For AIS C, less than half of key muscle functions below the single NLI have a muscle grade ≤3. |
| D | MOTOR INCOMPLETE | Motor function is preserved below the neurologic level, and most key muscles below the NL1 have a muscle grade that is greater than or equal to 3. |
| E | NORMAL | Sensory and motor functions as tested with the ISNCSCI are graded as normal in all segments, and if the patient has prior deficits, then the AIS grade is E. Someone without an SCI does not receive an AIS grade. |

AIS, Association Impairment Scale; ISNCSCI, International Standards for Neurological and Functional Classification of Spinal Cord Injury; NLI, neurological level of injury; SCI, spinal cord injury.

## Surgical

Surgical intervention involves realigning the spinal structural elements, stabilizing the spine, and decompressing compromised neural structures. The optimal timing for surgery after SCI remains a controversial topic although there is emerging evidence to suggest that early surgical decompression is safe and possibly associated with better outcomes; the Surgical Timing in Acute SCI Study (STASCIS) for cervical SCI concluded that decompression prior to 24 hours after SCI can be performed safely and is associated with improved neurological outcomes.[18]

## Rehabilitation

An interdisciplinary team approach is important for the optimal care. Transfer to an SCI unit should be made as soon as the patient's spine is stabilized. Skilled physical and occupational therapies are geared to help the patient achieve his or her optimal level of self-care and mobility. An integrated program encompassing range of motion (ROM), strengthening, mat activities, and activities of daily living (ADL) functional training is recommended. In recent years, there has been great excitement for activity-based restorative therapy (ABRT) to achieve activity-dependent neural plasticity driven by repetitive activation of spinal cord pathways located both above and below the level of injury. ABRT is intended to optimize neuromuscular function and offset the rapid aging, physical deterioration, and secondary complications associated with neurological deficits. The five key components of ABRT are weight-bearing activities, functional electrical stimulation (FES), task-specific practice, massed practice, and locomotor training which includes body weight-supported treadmill walking and water treadmill training.[19] Weight-bearing activities include a wide variety of activities, including tall kneeling, weight-bearing on arms while seated (sides, front, and back), quadruped (all four limbs), standing using frames or other supportive devices, and a variety of locomotor activities. FES includes upper- and lower-limb cycling and resistive exercise training via electrical stimulation of individual muscle groups. FES can also be utilized to assist movements during gait training, standing, transferring, and various other activities. Task-specific practice is key to learning a specific skill that begins with repetition of the same movement multiple times in order to develop a motor pattern. The fifth vital component of ABRT is locomotor training which includes body weight-supportive treadmill training (BWSTT) during which the participant is secured from an overhead support via an upper-body harness and trained on a moving treadmill.[19]

## Investigational Strategies

A number of investigational strategies[20] are being studied as potential treatments, and these include autologous macrophages, granulocyte colony-stimulating factor, neuroprotective agents (basic fibroblast growth factor, minocycline, riluzole), neuronal growth factors, thyrotropin-releasing hormone, and spinal cord cooling.

## ASSOCIATED IMPAIRMENTS AND COMPLICATIONS

Patients with SCI are at risk for a number of medical complications which may include:

### Respiratory

Pulmonary complications may include ventilatory failure, pulmonary edema, atelectasis and mucus plugs, sleep-disordered breathing (most common is obstructive sleep apnea), pulmonary embolism, and pneumonia. Pulmonary complications contribute substantively to early morbidity and mortality. Pneumonia is the leading cause of death among SCI patients.[21]

### Autonomic Nervous System

Issues may include bradycardia, orthostatic hypotension, spinal shock, thermal dysregulation, and autonomic dysreflexia (AD). AD is a condition that is unique to SCI patients. It can occur in about 48% to 90% of SCI patients with neurologic injury at T6 or above. It is secondary to the loss of descending central sympathetic control and hypersensitivity of baroreceptors below the level of lesion.[22] It's a constellation of symptoms that may include headaches, sweating, facial flushing, piloerection, irritability, or crying (in the pediatric population) associated with blood pressure elevation of 20 to 40 mmHg higher from the baseline (15–20 mmHg for adolescents and children) and bradycardia. It is due to a noxious stimulus below the level of the lesion such as bladder overdistention or infection (most common), bowel impaction, abdominal emergencies (appendicitis, cholecystitis, pancreatitis), pressure injuries, in-grown toenails, fracture, and infections.

## Cardiovascular

Cardiovascular consequences may include ischemic heart disease, peripheral vascular disease, thromboembolism, and deep venous thrombosis.

## Genitourinary

Complications include urinary tract infections (UTIs), neurogenic bladder, hydronephrosis, vesicoureteral reflux, urinary stones (commonly magnesium ammonium phosphate or struvite), and pyelonephritis. UTI is the leading cause of rehospitalizations among SCI patients.

## Gastrointestinal

Complications include neurogenic bowel, gastric atony, ileus, chronic constipation, fecal impaction, colonic distention, gastroesophageal reflux, cholecystitis, pancreatitis, and superior mesenteric artery (SMA) syndrome. SMA syndrome is a condition in which the third portion of the duodenum is intermittently compressed by overlying SMA resulting in GI obstruction. Gastric atony and ileus are the most common GI complication during the acute phase. Cholecystitis is the most common cause of emergency abdominal surgery in SCI patients.

## Metabolic and Endocrine Issues

Glucose intolerance, hyperglycemia, hypogonadism, altered calcium metabolism (i.e., hypercalciuria, hypercalcemia), osteoporosis, altered energy consumption, and body composition are all associated with SCI. Bone health is discussed in detail in another chapter.

## Musculoskeletal

Spasticity, shoulder impingement syndromes, overuse, degenerative joint disease (DJD), rotator cuff inflammation, carpal tunnel syndrome (CTS), epicondylitis, tendinitis, bursitis, Charcot spine, myofascial pain, and heterotopic ossification. The clinical practice guideline on the preservation of upper limb function provides great information.[23]

## Pain

The International Spinal Cord Injury Pain (ISCIP) classification organizes SCI pain into three tiers: Tier 1 categorizes pain as follows: nociceptive, neuropathic, other, and unknown. Tier 2 includes various subtypes for nociceptive (visceral and musculoskeletal), and neuropathic (at level and below level). Tier 3 is used to specify the primary source and/or pathology (e.g., bursitis, CTS).[24]

## Skin

According to the National Pressure Ulcer Advisory Panel (NPUAP), approximately 25% of acute SCI patients will develop a pressure injury, with up to 80% of patients developing one at some point during their lifetime. Local soft tissue damage results when prolonged pressure over bony prominences exceeding supracapillary pressure (70 mmHg) continuously for 2 hours. Pressure injuries are classified according to the extent of tissue damage with new revisions as of 2016. Long-standing ulcers of 20 years or longer in duration may develop squamous cell carcinoma (Marjolins ulcers).

## FUNCTIONAL PROGNOSIS AND OUTCOMES

When predicting outcomes after an SCI, motor level is superior to the neurologic or sensory level in predicting function. Using the data from the U.S. Model Spinal Cord Injury System, about 13% of patients with AIS grade A admitted within 1 week post-SCI converted to incomplete status by 1 year.[25,26] In patients with complete tetraplegia, more than 95% of key muscles with grade 1 or 2 at 1-month post-SCI will reach grade 3 at 1 year.[26] About 25% of the most cephalad grade 0 muscles at 1 month recover to grade 3 at 1 year.[26] In patients who have complete paraplegia 1 week post-SCI, 73% are found to have neurologic level of injury that remains unchanged at 1 year, 18% improve by one level, and 9% improve more than two levels.[26] In a study done by Waters, only 5% with complete paraplegia achieve community ambulation.[27]

In comparison to complete injuries, the recovery is often more substantial following incomplete injuries; greater than 90% of incomplete injuries gained at least one motor level in the upper extremities compared to 70% to 85% of complete injuries. Waters reported that 46% of individuals with incomplete tetraplegia recover sufficient motor strength to be able to ambulate at 1 year post-SCI.[27] Crozier reported that partial preservation of pinprick sensation below the zone of injury was predictive of eventual functional ambulation.[28] The neurologic evaluation done at 72 versus 24 hours post-injury is better at predicting recovery according to a study done by Maynard et al.[29]

## RESOURCES AND REFERENCES

The full list of resources and references appear in the digital product found on http://connect .springerpub.com/content/book/978-0-8261-6226-7/part/part01/chapter/ch12

# STROKE

DANIEL EZIDIEGWU AND PREETI RAGHAVAN

## CORE DEFINITIONS

The term "stroke" includes all of the following[1]:

**Central nervous system (CNS) infarction:** CNS infarction is brain, spinal cord, or retinal cell death attributable to ischemia, based on (1) pathological, imaging, or other objective evidence of cerebral, spinal cord, or retinal focal ischemic injury in a defined vascular distribution or (2) clinical evidence of cerebral, spinal cord, or retinal focal ischemic injury based on symptoms persisting ≥24 hours or until death, and other etiologies excluded. (Note: CNS infarction includes hemorrhagic infarctions, or hemorrhagic transformation of an infarction, types I and II which are characterized by lack of mass effect. Type I consists of petechiae along the margins of the infarction, whereas type II has confluent petechiae within the infarction but without a space-occupying effect.)

**Ischemic stroke:** An episode of neurological dysfunction caused by focal cerebral, spinal, or retinal infarction. (Note: Evidence of CNS infarction as defined previously.)

**Silent CNS infarction:** Imaging or neuropathological evidence of CNS infarction, without a history of acute neurological dysfunction attributable to the lesion.

**Intracerebral hemorrhage:** A focal collection of blood within the brain parenchyma or ventricular system that is not caused by trauma. Parenchymal hemorrhage is characterized by the presence of mass effect in contrast to a hemorrhagic infarction. Parenchymal hemorrhage type I is a confluent hemorrhage limited to ≤30% of the infarcted area with only mild space-occupying effect, and type II is hemorrhage >30% of the infarcted area and/or that exerts a significant space-occupying effect.

**Stroke caused by intracerebral hemorrhage:** Rapidly developing clinical signs of neurological dysfunction attributable to a focal collection of blood within the brain parenchyma or ventricular system that is not caused by trauma.

**Silent cerebral hemorrhage:** A focal collection of chronic blood products within the brain parenchyma, subarachnoid space, or ventricular system on neuroimaging or neuropathological examination that is not caused by trauma and without a history of acute neurological dysfunction attributable to the lesion.

**Subarachnoid hemorrhage:** Bleeding into the subarachnoid space (the space between the arachnoid membrane and the pia mater of the brain or spinal cord).

---

The full list of resources and references appears in the digital product found on http://connect .springerpub.com/content/book/978-0-8261-6226-7/part/part01/chapter/ch13

**Stroke caused by subarachnoid hemorrhage:** Rapidly developing signs of neurological dysfunction and/or headache because of bleeding into the subarachnoid space (the space between the arachnoid membrane and the pia mater of the brain or spinal cord), which is not caused by trauma.

**Stroke caused by cerebral venous thrombosis:** Infarction or hemorrhage in the brain, spinal cord, or retina because of thrombosis of a cerebral venous structure. Symptoms or signs caused by reversible edema without infarction or hemorrhage do not qualify as stroke.

**Stroke, not otherwise specified:** An episode of acute neurological dysfunction presumed to be caused by ischemia or hemorrhage, persisting ≥24 hours or until death, but without sufficient evidence to be classified as one of the preceding conditions.

## ETIOLOGY AND PATHOPHYSIOLOGY

In the United States, approximately 85% of strokes are ischemic, and the rest are hemorrhagic.

Ischemic strokes are more prevalent in developed countries and may be caused by embolism, thrombosis, or lacunar pathology. Common cardiac sources for embolism include atrial fibrillation (AF), sinoatrial disorder, recent acute myocardial infarction (AMI) causing left ventricular (LV) dilation, LV wall mural thrombi, marantic or subacute bacterial endocarditis, cardiac tumors, and valvular disorders, both native and artificial. Thrombotic strokes are caused by atherosclerotic disease commonly due to diabetes, carotid artery stenosis, and dyslipidemia. Vasculitis (e.g., from granulomatous angiitis, giant cell arteritis, systemic lupus erythematosus, or polyarteritis nodosa) causes inflammation in the blood vessel wall leading to thrombosis and may lead to thromboembolic disease. Injury to the carotid arteries, such as carotid dissection, and hypercoagulable states also predispose individuals to thromboembolic disease. Lacunar strokes result from occlusion of the small penetrating branches of the middle cerebral artery, vertebral or basilar artery, or the lenticulostriate vessels. Typical causes of lacunar strokes include microemboli, fibrinoid necrosis secondary to vasculitis or hypertension, amyloid angiopathy, and hyaline arteriosclerosis. Perfusion failure affects the most distal areas of perfusion or the "watershed zone" causing infarction.

Hemorrhagic strokes are caused by hypertension, aneurysm rupture, arteriovenous malformations, venous angiomas, bleeding due to illicit drugs like cocaine, hemorrhagic metastasis, amyloid angiopathy, and other obscure etiologies and are more prevalent in developing countries and in younger individuals.[2]

### Pathophysiology

Atherosclerosis is a leading cause of vascular disease, including stroke, worldwide. Major modifiable risk factors for atherosclerosis include high blood pressure (BP), diabetes mellitus (DM), hyperlipidemia, physical inactivity, obesity, and smoking. Both ischemia and hemorrhage cause reductions in cerebral blood flow (CBF) (total CBF at rest is about 800 mL/min—15%–20% of total cardiac output). Cerebral perfusion is a high-flow low-pressure system that supplies the brain with oxygen for aerobic metabolism of glucose. Ischemia leads to almost total CBF arrest in the central core region, which dies within minutes due to failure of the Na+/K+ ATPase pumps, depolarization of cells, massive influx of calcium, and release of excitotoxic neurotransmitters, primarily glutamate.[3] CBF may fall below functional thresholds but be above the threshold of cell death in the area surrounding the core, called the penumbra. The penumbra is potentially salvageable tissue, which is the target for acute stroke therapies.

## DIAGNOSTIC APPROACH

Key elements of history should include:
- Determining time of symptom onset or last known normal and family contact information.
- Description of symptoms (facial droop, limb weakness, sensation deficits, vision changes, headache).
- Medications, recent hospitalizations, surgeries, traumas that indicate risk for arteriosclerosis, and cardiovascular disease—diabetes, smoking, AF, drug abuse, migraine, seizures, infection, or pregnancy.

Key elements of physical examination should include:
- Assessment of airway, spontaneous breathing, and circulation.
- Level of consciousness, eyes open or closed, verbal output, command following, gaze deviation, limb posturing, purposeful movement.
- CNII-XII testing, motor strength testing, sensation testing, coordination testing for cerebellar signs and symptoms.
- NIH stroke scale (NIHSS) for assessment of stroke severity. This is an 11-item scale, where the score for each item or ability is a number between 0 and 4, 0 being normal functioning and 4 being completely impaired. The patient's NIHSS score is calculated by adding the number for each item of the scale; 42 is the highest score possible—a higher score indicates greater impairment likely due to proximal vessel occlusion. Tissue Plasminogen Activator (tPA) can be administered with any score on the NIHSS. However, the NIHSS score should be 6+ to be eligible for endovascular therapy.

Diagnostic testing should include the following:
- Basic metabolic panel (BMP), complete blood count (CBC), cardiac markers, coagulation profile (prothrombin time, international normalized ratio [INR], and activated partial thromboplastin time [aPTT]), lipid panel, hemoglobin A1C.
- Stat noncontrast head CT or a combination of head CT, CT angiography, and CT perfusion imaging to examine the vasculature and perfusion. See Table 13.1 for advantages and disadvantages of neuroimaging modalities.
  - On noncontrast CT head, the ASPECTS (Alberta Stroke Program Early CT Score) quantifies early ischemic change in the middle cerebral artery (MCA) territory. The 10-point pretreatment score divides the MCA territory into 10 regions and identifies patients with stroke who are unlikely to have good outcome from thrombolysis. ASPECTS of 10 represents a normal CT scan. Subtract 1 point on evidence of early ischemic change in each territory. ASPECTS of 0 represents diffuse ischemic involvement throughout the complete MCA territory.
- A transthoracic echocardiogram, telemetry monitoring, and neck vessel imaging are necessary to elucidate the etiology of stroke.

## TABLE 13. 1 NEUROIMAGING MODALITIES FOR STROKE

| NEUROIMAGING MODALITY | ADVANTAGES | DISADVANTAGES |
|---|---|---|
| **PARENCHYMA** | | |
| Noncontrast CT | Fast acquisition time, widely available, sensitive to hemorrhage (specificity of 56%–100% and poor sensitivity (20%–75%) for detecting early ischemic changes (within a 6- to 8-hour window) | Limited sensitivity to infarct size and location of early ischemia |
| Diffusion-weighted MRI | Sensitive to early ischemia, fast acquisition time, high conspicuity of lesion (within less than 6 hours from onset has a sensitivity of 91%–100% and specificity of 86%–100%) | Lack of availability, patient contraindications (e.g., metals, claustrophobia), long acquisition time |
| **VASCULATURE** | | |
| CT angiography | Quantifies vascular disease burden (e.g., degree of stenosis, length of clot, characteristics of plaques), fast acquisition time | Potential renal toxicity, allergy to contrast agents; radiation exposure; provides no information on direction or velocity of flow |
| MRA | No contrast | Overestimates stenosis, sensitive to motion and other technical artifacts, long acquisition time, patient contraindications (e.g., metals, claustrophobia) |
| Ultrasound (carotid or transcranial doppler) | Flow data, portable, low cost | User dependent, time consuming, technical constraints |
| **TISSUE PERFUSION** | | |
| CT perfusion | Fast acquisition time | Potential renal toxicity, allergy to contrast agents; radiation exposure; qualitative |
| Magnetic resonance perfusion | Good spatial resolution | Qualitative; patient contraindications (e.g., metals, claustrophobia), requires gadolinium |
| PET | Gold standard for cerebral blood flow measures, provides quantitative measures of physiologic parameters (oxygen extraction fraction and metabolism) | Requires multiple radiotracers with very short half-lives, thus impractical in acute settings; low resolution, limited availability |

MRA, magnetic resonance angiography; PET, positron emission tomography.

## TREATMENT

### Medical Treatment for Acute Ischemic Stroke

- Alteplase (IV recombinant tPA) within 4.5 hours of stroke onset is the standard of care. Exclusions for tPA include patients presenting between 3 and 4.5 hours and are >80 years, have a severe stroke (NIHSS score >25), have a history of diabetes and prior stroke, and are on oral anticoagulant medication regardless of INR.[4] Tenecteplase may be chosen over IV alteplase in patients without contraindications for IV fibrinolysis who are also eligible to undergo mechanical thrombectomy.

- Mechanical thrombectomy with a stent retriever is indicated in patients within 6 hours of stroke onset who are >18 years of age, have minimal pre-stroke disability, have occlusion of the internal carotid artery (ICA) or proximal MCA with an NIHSS of ≥6, and an ALBERTA score of ≥6 on review of the noncontrast head CT.[4] The recent DAWN trial showed that the window for mechanical thrombectomy for large vessel occlusion can be extended up to 24 hours.[5]

- Maintain normothermia: Temperatures <37°C and >39°C are associated with increased risk of in-hospital death compared with normothermia.

- Treat hypoglycemia (blood glucose <60 mg/dL) and hyperglycemia (140–180 mg/dL).

- Delay placement of nasogastric tubes, indwelling bladder catheters, or intra-arterial pressure catheters if the patient can be safely managed without them.

- Obtain a follow-up CT or MRI scan at 24 hours after IV alteplase before starting anti-coagulants or antiplatelet agents. Hemorrhagic transformation is a potential complication after thrombolytic therapy. Symptoms and signs include severe headache, acute hypertension, nausea or vomiting, or worsening neurological examination. Obtain emergent CT scan. Predictive factors include increased infarction area, gray matter stroke, AF and cerebral embolism, acute hyperglycemia, low platelet count, and poor collateral circulation.[6]

- Aspirin is recommended within 24 to 48 hours after stroke onset. It can be delayed for 24 hours in patients treated with IV tPA. Mono/dual antiplatelet therapy is not a contraindication for receiving tPA.

- For patients with a minor ischemic stroke or high-risk transient ischemic attack (TIA), treat with an initial loading dose of clopidogrel (Plavix) followed by 75 mg daily for 90 days and aspirin 50 to 325 mg daily (162 mg daily for 5 days, followed by 81 mg daily). The POINT trial showed that a combination of clopidogrel and aspirin had a lower risk of major ischemic events but a higher risk of major hemorrhage at 90 days than those who received aspirin alone. Secondary analysis from the POINT trial suggests benefit of just 21 days of combined therapy with clopidogrel.

- Anticoagulation is indicated in patients with AF and is started in 7 to 14 days post-stroke but may be delayed by a few weeks in patients with a small hemorrhagic transformation.[7]

- Seizures occur in about 15% of patients within the first few days of the stroke. Those who develop chronic seizures need treatment with antiepileptic medication.

- Although elevated BP is common during acute ischemic stroke, especially among patients with a history of hypertension, the BP often decreases spontaneously in the first 90 minutes. Management of BP should be individualized to maintain cerebral perfusion.

Early initiation or resumption of antihypertensive treatment is indicated only in specific situations: (1) patients treated with tPA, and (2) patients with systolic BP >220 mmHg or diastolic BP >120 mmHg. A long-term goal of BP <130/80 is reasonable.[8]

## Treatment of Acute Hemorrhagic Stroke

■ The Glasgow coma scale (GCS) score should be obtained and monitored to assess severity. Patients may need to be admitted and monitored in the medical ICU or the neurosurgical ICU. Patients with cerebellar hemorrhage who are deteriorating neurologically or who have brainstem compression and/or hydrocephalus from ventricular obstruction should undergo surgical evacuation and decompression as soon as possible.

■ Determine cause of bleed. Any medications ingested or doses missed such as anticoagulants, antiplatelets, antihypertensives, stimulant medications, sympathomimetic medications should be noted. Anticoagulants should be held. Take note of any recent trauma or surgery like carotid endarterectomy or stenting as these may result in hyperperfusion. A concomitant history of dementia may lead one to suspect amyloid angiopathy. Alcohol or illicit drug use such as with cocaine or other stimulants must be documented. Patients with liver disease, cancer, or hematologic disorders may have associated coagulopathy that may be correctable.

■ Patients with severe coagulation factor deficiencies or severe thrombocytopenia should receive appropriate factor replacement therapy. Patients on warfarin may require fresh frozen plasma (FFP) and vitamin K replacement to correct INR. Prothrombin complex concentrates (PCC) and other recombinant factors may be used in place of FFP. Activated charcoal can be used for recent (<2 hours) dosing of dabigatran, apixaban, or rivaroxaban. Hemodialysis may be used for dabigatran. Protamine sulfate can be used to reverse heparin. Deep venous thrombosis (DVT) prophylaxis should be initiated with compression devices.

■ BP should be controlled in all patients with intracerebral hemorrhage (ICH). Lowering systolic BP to 140 mmHg is safe in patients who present with systolic BP between 150 and 220 mmHg.

■ Most patients who die of ICH do so during the initial acute hospitalization, and these deaths usually occur in the setting of withdrawal of support because of presumed poor prognosis. Aggressive care and postponing DNR orders until the second day of hospitalization is recommended due to this.[9]

■ Cortical involvement in patients with ICH is the most important risk factor for early seizures. Any clinical seizures should be treated with anti-seizure medications. A formal screening procedure for dysphagia before initiating diet is important to prevent aspiration pneumonia.

■ Avoidance of long-term anticoagulation with warfarin as a treatment for non-valvular AF is recommended after warfarin-associated spontaneous lobar ICH because of the relatively high risk of recurrence. The optimal timing to resume oral anticoagulation after anticoagulant-related ICH is uncertain. Avoidance of oral anticoagulation for at least 4 weeks in patients without mechanical heart valves might decrease the risk of ICH recurrence.

## Rehabilitation

- Patients should undergo comprehensive assessment of body structures and function, activity limitations, and participation restrictions by an interprofessional team under the leadership of a Physiatrist or specialist trained in rehabilitation medicine, ideally within 48 hours of admission.[10] The rehabilitation team may include a nurse, physical therapist, occupational therapist, speech/language therapist, psychologist, social worker, and others (e.g., dietician, orthotist).
- During the acute hospital stay, the focus of rehabilitation should be on early mobilization and prevention of complications such as aspiration pneumonia, pressure sores, shoulder pain, and DVT. Patients should begin rehabilitation therapies (physical therapy [PT]/ occupational therapy [OT]/ speech and language therapy [SLT]) as soon as the patient is ready and can tolerate it. Time spent upright in the first week[11] and the frequency rather than the amount of time of out-of-bed activity are critical to a favorable outcome. Increasing the frequency of out-of-bed sessions improves the odds of favorable outcome by 13% and improves the odds of walking 50 m unassisted by 66%.[12]
- Patients with multiple disabilities requiring daily nursing services, regular medical interventions, specialized equipment, or interprofessional expertise require multidisciplinary inpatient rehabilitation in a designated inpatient rehabilitation facility.[13]
- Upon discharge from inpatient rehabilitation, therapy may be continued at one of several locations depending on resource availability and patient considerations including hospital-based "day" programs, community-based programs, or home-based programs. Any form of continuing rehabilitation therapy is superior to no additional therapy.[14]
- Patients with mild–moderate disability may benefit from early supported discharge if provided by a well-resourced, coordinated specialized team.[15]
- Use standardized, validated assessment tools to evaluate the patient's stroke-related impairments, functional activity limitations, and role participation restrictions throughout the rehabilitation continuum to measure and monitor physical, cognitive, and emotional issues that interfere with participation in usual life roles.[10,13] Patients may be started on fluoxetine 20 mg daily for 90 days to improve motor recovery.
- Consider use of the Post-Stroke Checklist (see Resources at the end of the chapter).
- Patients with visual deficits may benefit from vision rehabilitation including the use of eye exercises for convergence insufficiency, and yoked prisms for visual field deficits. Driving is a significant factor in return to work. Depending on state regulations, patients with stroke may be required to report their diagnosis. State law determines whether someone with stroke is eligible to drive. Physicians should assess a patient's physical, visual and/or mental impairments that might affect their driving ability. Return to driving is contingent upon successful completion of functional capacity testing and/or on-the-road testing as determined by the state department of motor vehicles.[12]

## ASSOCIATED IMPAIRMENTS AND COMPLICATIONS

Complications to look out for include aspiration pneumonia, chronic regional pain syndrome, depression, DVT, heterotopic ossification, spasticity, muscle stiffness, neuropathic pain, shoulder pain, shoulder subluxation, and urinary tract infection.

Rehabilitation issues to look out for include agnosia, amusia, apraxia, aphasia, cognitive impairment, dysarthria, dysphagia, visual, and vestibular dysfunction.

## FUNCTIONAL PROGNOSIS AND OUTCOMES

- Patients with a smaller diffusion core (70 mL or less) treated with IV/intra-arterial thrombolysis have a significantly better outcome than patients with a larger core.[16]
- The THRIVE score estimates prognosis after an acute ischemic stroke. The patient's age, initial stroke severity as measured by the NIHSS score, and the presence or absence of hypertension, DM, or AF are used to create a 0 to 9 point scale; lower scores predict better outcome (Table 13.2).[17]
- Upper extremity motor recovery can be predicted using the Predict REcovery Potential (PREP2) algorithm. In this algorithm, the outcome of a patient's upper extremity recovery on the Action Research Arm Test (ARAT) is predicted based on three diverse measures (physical movement ability, age, and motor evoked potential) at 3 to 7 days after stroke into excellent, good, limited, or poor recovery categories. Movement ability is measured using the Shoulder Abduction Finger Extension (SAFE) score, which is the combined strength at these two joints on the five-point Medical Research Council (MRC) scale. A SAFE score of ≥5 on day 3 poststroke in a person under the age of 80 years, or a score of ≥8 in a person over the age of 80 years predicts excellent upper extremity motor recovery at 12 weeks poststroke with 78% accuracy.[18]
- Return to work is associated with younger age, less severe impairments, independence in activities of daily living (ADLs), good communication skills, good higher-level cognitive skills and processing speed, and a white-collar profession.

## BASIC ORDER SETS

### Rehab Admission Order Set

- Admit to inpatient PM&R service.
- Monitor vitals q8h. Notify provider if heart rate <50 BPM or >120 BPM, respiratory rate less than 12 RPM or >26, systolic <90 or >180, diastolic <50 or >110, SaO$_2$ <93%.

### TABLE 13.2 THE THRIVE SCORE

| Age (in years) | <60 | 0 |
|---|---|---|
| | 60–79 | 1 |
| | >80 | 2 |
| NIHSS score | <11 | 0 |
| | 11–20 | 2 |
| | >21 | 4 |
| Comorbidities: HTN, DM, AF | None | 0 |
| | 1/3 | 1 |
| | 2/3 | 2 |
| | 3/3 | 3 |
| Total score | | /9 |

AF, atrial fibrillation; DM, diabetes mellitus, HTN, hypertension; NIHSS, NIH stroke scale.

- Isolation: Contact precautions are required if patient is positive for extended spectrum beta-lactamase (ESBL) producing organisms, Methicillin-resistant Staphylococcus aureus (MRSA) or other multidrug-resistant bacteria.
- Activity: As tolerated with assistance. Mobility restrictions if any underlying fractures. Helmet may be required for patients after craniectomy when out of bed. Consider maintaining head of bed >30° for patients at risk of aspiration. Fall precautions or aspiration precautions may be placed for patients at risk.
- Diet: Consider heart-healthy diet for patients with hypertension or carbohydrate-controlled diet if diabetic. Nutrition consult may be placed for education on improving food choices during the inpatient stay or as an outpatient. Due to the prescribed diet in the hospital, BPs and blood sugars may be lower than they typically may be at home.

Dysphagia diet: Start with the best tolerated International Dysphagia Diet (IDD) or that shown to be safe on Modified Barium Swallow as per speech therapy evaluation. Liquid options include thin (IDD 0), slightly thick (IDD1), mildly thick (nectar/IDD2), or moderately thick (honey/IDD3). If no liquids are shown to be safe, no liquid diet is appropriate and hydration/feeding via nasogastric or PEG/G-tube may be sufficient. Consistency of solid diet may be pureed (IDD4), minced and moist (IDD5), soft and bite sized (IDD6), or easy to chew (IDD7). Food consistency may be free of modification if cleared by a swallow evaluation.

Feeding assistance: Patients may need tray setup or even feeding assistance depending on the severity of weakness.

Nutrition consult: Patients with poor appetite may benefit from nutritional supplements such as Glucerna, Ensure, Boost Pudding, or Nepro. Patients should be weighed on admission to assist pharmacy with weight-based medication dosing. Patients with cardiac disease, liver disease, those on dialysis, and those with other fluid balance issues may need to be weighed more frequently.

- Skin: Monitor wounds per nursing. Patients with poor bed mobility should be turned q2h to prevent bed sores. If wounds are complex or severe, a wound care specialist consult may be warranted.
- Smokers should receive tobacco cessation education and possibly be started on nicotine patch or gum PRN for symptoms.
- Labs: On admission, CBC with differential, comprehensive metabolic panel (CMP), international normalized ratio (INR)/prothrombin time may be ordered to obtain a baseline.
- Bowel management: Stool softeners such as docusate sodium given twice a day or osmotic laxatives such as polyethylene glycol given daily as prophylactic dosing may be appropriate for patients with constipation or for those on opioids for pain management.

## Therapy Orders
- PT: Evaluate and treat for impaired mobility, gait/ambulation, strengthening, endurance, and functional mobility: PT for 1 to 2 hours/day for 5 days/week.
- OT: Evaluate and treat for improvement of ADLs/iADLs, transfers, ROM, functional mobility, coordination training, and fall risks: OT for 1 to 2 hours/day for 5 days/week.

- Speech therapy: Evaluate and treat for speech/language and swallowing deficits as well as evaluate for high-level cognitive dysfunction and offer appropriate strategies: SLP for 1 hour/day for 5 days/week.
- Rehabilitation psychology/neuropsychology: Evaluate the patient's current psychological status/coping mechanisms and evaluate for any underlying issues that negatively impact the patient's recovery. Appropriate for patients with mood or adjustment disorders, cognitive impairments, and aphasia.

## RESOURCES AND REFERENCES

The full list of resources and references appears in the digital product found on http://connect.springerpub.com/content/book/978-0-8261-6226-7/part/part01/chapter/ch13

# TRANSPLANT

R. SAMUEL MAYER

## CORE DEFINITIONS

Transplantation is the replacement of a damaged, missing, or dysfunctional organ or body part to restore proper function. The organs used are obtained through donations from living donors (e.g., kidneys) or deceased donor. Since the first successful kidney transplant in 1954, advances in immunosuppressant therapies and tissue typing helped improve outcomes and prolong survival. Given that transplant patients are surviving longer, the ultimate goal of organ transplantation, recovery, and rehabilitation is to return these patients to the highest level of functioning and livelihood as possible.[1] It is estimated that between 1987 and 2012, transplants added 2.1 million life years in the United States.[2]

The most commonly transplanted organ in the United States is the kidney, followed by liver, heart, lung, pancreas, bowel, and multivisceral transplants. The most successful transplant procedures (kidney, heart, liver) have 5-year survival rates around 70% to 80%, compared to other organs (lung, pancreas, intestine, or multivisceral transplants) whose survival rates are closer to 40% to 50%. Vascular composite allografts (VCAs) include upper extremity, facial, and genital allografts. VCAs can be thought of as free flaps: complex, multi-tissue anastomotic grafts that rely on gradual reinnervation for actual function beyond the graft's survival. The combined European and U.S. upper extremity graft survival rate is 90%, most with at least some functional improvement.[3]

## ETIOLOGY AND PATHOPHYSIOLOGY

A myriad of diseases lead to organ failure requiring transplantation. Uncontrolled hypertension and diabetes are the primary reasons for kidney failure. Liver failure is typically the result of alcoholic liver disease, primary liver cancers, cirrhosis, or nonalcoholic steatohepatitis. Heart failure is considered the end stage of all diseases of the heart, most prominently, myocardial infarction-coronary artery disease, valve disease, cardiomyopathy, and congenital heart disease.

## EVALUATION APPROACH

Patients in need of an organ transplantation have significant functional deficits amenable to rehabilitation. A systematic approach to address these deficits before and after transplantation is of paramount importance.

The full list of references appears in the digital product found on http://connect.springerpub.com/content/book/978-0-8261-6226-7/part/part01/chapter/ch14

## Preoperative Rehabilitation

Preoperative rehabilitation ("pre-hab") has received strong support in patients awaiting solid organ transplantation. This patient population is prone to muscle weakness, fatigue, extended hospitalizations, and decreased functional mobility. A recent meta-analysis demonstrated that a walking intervention prior to transplant improved cardiorespiratory fitness, self-reported physical function, and pain. Furthermore, a training exercise program for patients awaiting solid organ transplantation has been recommended based on evidence demonstrating improvement in physical condition and quality of life before and after transplant.[5]

## Early Postoperative Rehabilitation

Rehabilitation should begin as soon as possible. Early rehabilitation in the ICU by a multidisciplinary team should focus on reducing heavy sedation and making therapy available. This strategy has been shown to increase the number of therapy sessions per patient and shorten ICU and overall hospital stay. Rehabilitation in the ICU helps to reduce pulmonary complications, preserve strength and range of motion, and prevent functional loss in the critically ill. This philosophy has been successfully applied to the transplant population.[6]

## Inpatient Rehabilitation

Some patients may require intensive therapy in an inpatient setting to improve mobility and self-care skills to transition home. An inpatient rehabilitation unit equipped with skilled medical, nursing, social work, and therapy staff is the most appropriate environment for medically complex patients including individuals recovering after transplant. One small study of inpatient rehabilitation after heart transplant showed 82% of patients were discharged to the community after significant improvements in daily function.[7]

Transplant patients will commonly have decreased activity tolerance, multifactorial weakness, and active medical issues that require diagnostics and specialty visits. These can delay or interrupt therapy sessions unless they are scheduled around therapy time. A multidisciplinary approach with involvement of the transplant team is essential. Important psychosocial factors that influence patients' participation in rehab include pain, fear of movement, symptom distress, and low physical self-efficacy.[8]

## Community Reintegration

Due to improving survival rates, an increasing number of post-transplant patients return to the community and seek employment. For example, despite their complex courses, the majority of liver transplant patients are alive at 1 year post-transplant having resumed their normal activities without restrictions.[9] Vocational rehabilitation helps all patients affirm their professional self-efficacy and independence. A successful vocational rehab program for transplant patients takes a multidisciplinary approach that addresses neurocognitive concerns, maintains mobility, and plans for workforce integration. A number of studies have been done on reemployment trends in the transplant population.

One cross-sectional study revealed that the majority of kidney transplant patients who were randomly selected and responded to a mailed questionnaire were interested in vocational rehabilitation and felt emotionally and physically ready to work after their transplant. Interestingly, employment rate decreased significantly (68% pre- versus 38% post-transplant), while retirement rates increased (8.3% pre- versus 18% post-transplant).[10]

## Diagnostic Approach

The care or patients after a transplant should focus on the evaluation of common deficits and identification of specific functional impairments amenable to rehabilitation. Transplant patients present with their own set of functional impairments that differ from those patients with more traditional rehabilitation diagnoses. Whether as a consultant or primary provider, a physiatrist must incorporate complex medical history, physical examination findings, and deficits from baseline into a plan for functional progress. Following are important functional impairments that are common to many transplant patients.

## Cognition

Delirium is a very common complication in inpatient and postoperative period. For example, decreased perfusion pressure during lung transplantation operations is associated with increased incidence, duration, and severity of delirium.[11] With any mental status change in a transplant patient, organ function should be evaluated in case of acute rejection or graft failure. Transplant pharmacists can be a key resource, and caution should be taken with hepatotoxic and nephrotoxic medications and doses adjusted accordingly. Medication administration schedules should be checked, and centrally acting medications should be avoided unless absolutely necessary.

## Mood

Prolonged hospitalizations can result in mood disturbances for all solid organ transplant recipients and are not specific to any particular organ. Patient experiences are variable and depend on many factors. Although depression can occur, overall mood generally improves after transplantation. Anxiety regarding falls, shortness of breath, weakness, and pain are common.[12]

## Balance

Transplant medications, neuropathy of critical illness, and cardiovascular complications can all contribute to sensory deficits that present as gait and balance abnormalities.[13]

## Strength Deficits

Immobility and prolonged bed rest can lead to decreased strength and endurance. However, one should not assume that this is the exclusive cause of weakness in transplant patients.[14]

## Peripheral Neuropathies

Transplant patients are at high risk for peripheral neuropathy because of the neurotoxic effects of some transplant medications. Additionally, medications such as tacrolimus can lead to tremor.

### Focal Neuropathies

Single nerve injuries (axillary, radial, ulnar, median, peroneal, or femoral nerves) or even brachial plexus injuries are not uncommon. Injury can result from surgical positioning, invasive line placement, compression from immobility, or edema.

*Myopathies*: Frequently patients have significant proximal muscle weakness. Important potential contributors that should be considered are steroids, statins, transplant medications, and critical illness myopathy.

### Activity Intolerance

The ability to tolerate a full inpatient rehabilitation schedule may be challenging for this population. Many struggle with symptomatic orthostasis which can be due to a multitude of factors including severe deconditioning, autonomic dysfunction, cardiac insufficiency, fluid status, or polypharmacy.

Monitoring weight, input, and output is particularly important with cardiac, renal, and liver transplant patients due to cardiac output, renal clearance, or portal venous congestion, respectively. Orthostasis and dysautonomia symptoms may require additional time for accommodation, compression devices, or, as a last line, medication management such as midodrine, pyridostigmine, or fludrocortisone. Specialty services are often required due to complexity.

### Dysphagia and Dysphonia

Possibly caused by superior and recurrent laryngeal nerve and/or vagus nerve injuries, multiple or traumatic intubations, and/or difficult airway due to varices, obesity, or dental considerations. Independence with feeding and tolerance of an adequate oral diet requires speech language pathology and occasionally consultation with interventional radiology or gastroenterology for alternative routes of nutrition.

### Nutritional Deficits

Optimal nutrition is critical to ongoing surgical and functional recovery. Poor nutrition can lead to a variety of impairments including activity tolerance, strength, cognition, and impaired healing. Careful caloric monitoring and working closely with a hospital nutritionist is critical to insure adequate intake. In cases of poor oral intake, identifying the cause is important. Nausea and constipation should be treated aggressively, obstruction ruled out, and intra-abdominal complications such as infection considered. If appetite is thought to be an issue, consider minimizing medications such as opioids and adding stimulants such as dronabinol or mirtazapine. In addition to following functional gains, labs such as prealbumin electrolytes should be monitored regularly. Intestinal transplants will require close conversations with the primary transplant team.

## TREATMENT

### Neurologic

Up to 10% of cardiac transplant patients have perioperative stroke.[14] In cases where there is significant hemiparesis, rehabilitation will be challenging due to sternal precautions as one cannot use the upper limbs for transfers or weight-bearing. Chronic kidney disease (CKD) and kidney transplant patients have decreased performance in verbal memory and executive functioning skills compared to healthy controls. A small prospective study demonstrated that poor performance in neuropsychology testing associated with end-stage renal disease (ESRD) can be quantifiably reversed at 6 months after kidney transplant.[15] Liver cirrhosis has also been associated with poor cognitive performance. When retested after liver transplantation, cognitive scores improved significantly such that they matched healthy controls, which suggests cognitive deficits in cirrhosis are reversible.[16] Signs and symptoms such as altered mental status, agitation, itching, and asterixis may be warning signs that graft function has been compromised prompting alert to the primary transplant team.

## Cardiovascular

Approximately 60% of patients can develop dyslipidemia after renal transplantation (even when absent preoperatively). It is important to ensure that these patients receive a heart-healthy diet tray and cholesterol-lowering medications as appropriate.

Heart transplantation surgery involves sternotomy. This requires postoperative precautions for 6 to 8 weeks, during which time the patient should avoid significant upper limb weight bearing or overhead reaching. These precautions can make bed mobility, transfers, and sit to stand difficult, especially if the patient has lower limb impairments as well. Vagal and parasympathetic innervation of the heart are compromised in transplantation. As a result, heart transplant recipients tend to have a higher resting heart rate (90–100 bpm). Additionally, the heart's response to and recovery from exercise is dependent only on circulating catecholamines, which take longer to influence heart rate. Rest breaks should be scheduled in between therapy sessions, as heart transplant patients have reduced exercise tolerance and require longer warm-up and recovery time. Vagal denervation also results in insensitivity to typical symptoms of angina or palpitations.

## Gastrointestinal, Endocrine, and Nutrition

Patients who have underweight or overweight/obese BMIs before kidney transplantation have higher mortality. Early post-transplant, they have increased protein requirements due to elevated catabolism/steroid use; later, excess dietary protein should be avoided especially in chronic allograft nephropathy or insufficiency. There is evidence that at 1-year post-renal transplant, up to 20% of patients will develop new-onset diabetes often a result of post-transplant weight gain and choice of immunosuppressive regimen (i.e., tacrolimus).[16] Liver transplant patients will have hypoalbuminemia. They will have increased protein requirements that can be met with dietary supplements. In cases of hypovolemia, intravenous albumin can be used for acute but transient resuscitation.

Lung transplant patients may have impaired cough reflex, poor secretion clearance, dysphagia, and phrenic nerve injury. These patients should be on aspiration precautions, and their rehabilitation sessions should focus on respiratory muscle strengthening. Speech and language pathology involvement is essential in early postoperative care to address communication, nutrition, and airway protection.

Intestinal transplantation occurs after patients have failed both enteral and parenteral nutrition. As a result, they have severe nutritional deficits contributing to overall functional decline. Throughout recovery and inpatient rehabilitation, providers should monitor visceral transplant recipients' weight and overall nutritional status.

## MUSCULOSKELETAL

Osteoporosis and osteopenia are common after kidney, liver, and lung transplantation. High-level evidence recommends daily supplementation with calcitriol (vitamin D3) and calcium to preserve bone density. Weight-bearing exercises should be encouraged to promote bone density, and bisphosphonate therapy may be considered.

## ASSOCIATED IMPAIRMENTS AND COMPLICATIONS

### Immunocompromise Considerations

The post-transplant patient is immunocompromised and at significant risk of developing opportunistic infections. These are a leading cause of morbidity and mortality in this population. Fever, leukocytosis, and altered mental status in a transplant patient should trigger a thorough infectious workup to rule out infections that are otherwise rare (e.g., mycobacterium or fungal species). Consultation with transplant infectious diseases specialists is key for determining appropriate antibiotic selection and duration. In the first 30 days following transplant, bacteria and yeast most commonly cause infections, which are frequently associated with premorbid or surgical site infections. Infections in the intermediate period (30 days to 6 months) are often related to opportunistic or latent infections such as cytomegalovirus, Epstein-Barr virus, pneumocysitis pneumonia, adenovirus, aspergillus, or toxoplasmosis. Late complications include common community-acquired infections (pneumonia) and rarely but most severely post-transplant lymphoproliferative disease and other malignancies.[17]

### Rejection

Hyperacute rejection occurs a few minutes after the transplant when the antigens are completely unmatched. This complication is life-threatening, and tissue must be removed right away. Acute rejection may occur any time 1 to 12 weeks after transplant. All recipients have some amount of acute rejection that is usually managed pharmacologically (see Table 14.1). Chronic rejection can take place over many years. The body's constant immune response against the donor organ slowly damages the transplanted tissues. The diagnosis of rejection requires a biopsy, and the threshold for treating rejection is low. Other conditions can mimic rejection. For example, diffuse lymphocytic infiltration of the kidney can be seen with rejection or lymphoproliferative disorder, and recurrent hepatitis C in the liver can resemble rejection.[18]

## FUNCTIONAL PROGNOSIS AND OUTCOMES

Moderate evidence supports that post-transplant cardiac rehabilitation improves quality of life, morbidity, and mortality. Despite this, less than half of eligible Medicare beneficiaries who

## TABLE 14.1 TYPICAL ANTIREJECTION MEDICATIONS, ADVERSE EFFECTS, AND MONITORING

| MEDICATION | ADVERSE EFFECT | MONITORING |
|---|---|---|
| Azathioprine | Bone marrow suppression, hepatoxicity, pancreatitis, risk of subsequent malignancy | CBC, CMP, aldolase as indicated, clinical course |
| Corticosteroids | Acne, avascular necrosis, cataracts, fluid retention, gastritis/ulcer, hirsutism, insomnia, myopathy, osteoporosis, psychosis, steroid-induced diabetes | CBC, BMP, glucose monitoring, clinical course, and physical examination |
| Cyclosporine | Diabetes, gingival hyperplasia, hepatotoxicity, hirsutism, hyperkalemia, hypertension, hypomagnesemia, myopathy, neuropathy, renal dysfunction, risk of subsequent malignancy | Drug levels, CBC, BMP, CK as indicated, glucose monitoring, Mg, clinical course and physical examination |
| Everolimus and sirolimus | Bone marrow suppression, fluid retention, GI upset, hyperlipidemia, hypertension, interstitial lung disease, poor wound healing, renal toxicity | Drug levels, CBC, BMP, lipids, CXR and PFTs as indicated |
| Mycophenolate | Bone marrow suppression, GI upset, headache, hepatoxicity, hypotension, pleural effusion, progressive multifocal leukoencephalopathy, renal toxicity | Drug levels, CBC, CMP, CXR as indicated, MRI brain as indicated |
| Tacrolimus | Anorexia, diabetes, GI upset, hepatotoxicity, hirsutism, hyperkalemia, hypertension, hypomagnesemia, myopathy, neuropathy, progressive multifocal leukoencephalopathy renal dysfunction, risk of subsequent malignancy, tremor | Drug levels, CBC, CMP, Mg, CK as indicated, clinical course and physical examination, MRI brain as indicated |

BMP, basic metabolic panel; CBC, complete blood count; CK, creatine kinase; CMP, comprehensive metabolic panel; CXR, chest x-ray; GI, gastrointestinal; PFT, pulmonary function test.

received heart transplant patients participated in cardiac rehab programs.[19] Lung transplant patients have improved outcomes with a comprehensive pulmonary rehabilitation program.[20] Liver transplant patients who undergo exercise training increase their distance walked and their resting energy expenditure, suggesting an increase in exercise and functional capacity in spite of impaired aerobic capacity prior to transplant (particularly in those who had liver cirrhosis).[21]

## REFERENCES

The full list of references appears in the digital product found on http://connect.springerpub.com/content/book/978-0-8261-6226-7/part/part01/chapter/ch14

# TRAUMATIC BRAIN INJURY

JENNIFER M. ZUMSTEG AND MELINDA LOVELESS

## CORE DEFINITIONS

- Traumatic brain injury (TBI) is "an alteration in brain function or other evidence of brain pathology caused by an external force."[1]
- Sports-related concussion is "a type of TBI induced by biomechanical forces."[2] It is important to note that the signs/symptoms cannot be explained by other injuries (e.g., cervical spine); drug, alcohol, or medication use; or other comorbidities (e.g., psychological factors or other medical conditions).

## ETIOLOGY AND PATHOPHYSIOLOGY

### Diagnostic Approach

TBI is a clinical diagnosis and must include a reasonable mechanism of injury, altered consciousness at the time of injury (i.e., loss of consciousness, dazed/confused, and/or amnesia), and signs/symptoms consistent with TBI.[2,3] Mechanisms of injury are typically categorized as blunt, penetrating, acceleration/deceleration, and blast forces.

Secondary injury to the brain can occur from hypoxia, cranial hypertension, hypercarbia, hyponatremia, seizures, effects of bleeding in/around the brain, cerebral edema, infection, hydrocephalus, and excitotoxicity. The framework for onset of symptoms caused by TBI is often recommended as 3 days or less,[3] although many clinicians recommend a longer timeframe or no specific time limitation, especially for severe TBI.[2-4]

After the diagnosis of TBI is established, the severity of TBI can be classified by using the Glasgow Coma Scale (GCS) score at a time early after injury but after immediate resuscitation has occurred (e.g., time of presentation to ED or about 30 minutes after injury) as summarized in Table 15.1.[3] Duration of post-traumatic amnesia (PTA) may also be used for severity classification.[3] Imaging findings alone are not utilized for classifying severity.

Many classic symptoms in TBI (e.g., dizziness, headaches, insomnia, mood changes) are often monitored through subjective report and are also common in the general population.[1,2] A thorough history and examination is needed to help determine, where possible, when symptoms are secondary to the TBI or are more likely to be from another cause. The severity of TBI does not necessarily correlate with the severity of symptoms or associated

---

The full list of resources and references appears in the digital product found on http://connect.springerpub.com/content/book/978-0-8261-6226-7/part/part01/chapter/ch15

**TABLE 15.1 TRAUMATIC BRAIN INJURY SEVERITY CLASSIFICATION IN ADULTS[3,5]**

|  | GCS | DURATION OF PTA |
|---|---|---|
| Mild | 13–15 | ≤24 hours |
| Moderate | 9–12 | 25 hours–6 days |
| Severe | 3–8 | ≥7 days |

GCS, Glasgow Coma Scale; PTA, post-traumatic amnesia.

impairments. For example, a person with mild TBI may have impairments severely limiting function and a person with severe TBI may eventually have a complete recovery.

## Physical Examination

At the time of TBI, people should be moved to a safe location for evaluation such as a sideline or training room in sport-related concussion.[2] For moderate-to-severe TBI, prehospitalization trauma management should be initiated and not delayed. Restrictions and precautions to minimize secondary injury (e.g., concurrent spine precautions, temperature regulation, avoid alcohol) and safety (e.g., no driving, considerations for avoiding or modifying recreation, work, and caregiving responsibilities) should be started immediately.[2] TBI can impact any and all body systems; on initial clinical evaluation, a complete review of systems and examination including at least screening neurological, psychiatric, and musculoskeletal elements should occur.[2,5] More detailed history and examination are guided by initial findings and symptoms.

Cranial nerve evaluation should include olfactory function.[6] Cranial nerve abnormalities after mild TBI can occur but are rare and should prompt reconsideration of injury severity and possible further assessment (e.g., brain MRI). Abnormal or absent olfactory function should increase the clinician's suspicion for impairments in executive function. Sensory testing with eyes closed allows for less visual interference and testing of both stimulus detection and quality. Examination modification and additional reflexive/brain stem evaluation may be needed in disorders of consciousness (DOC).[7]

TBI can impact motor systems in a variety of ways including strength, coordination, and motor planning. Patients should be screened for active range and strength in upper and lower limbs; coordination in hands and feet; and balance.[2] Vestibular maneuvers may assist evaluation and treatment choice when dizziness is present.

Cognitive function screening is often approached through assessment first of language and basic orientation and then items for cognitive domains including abstraction, attention, executive function, memory, and visuospatial.[2]

## Diagnostic Testing

Advanced imaging is not currently recommended for individual care decisions.[8] Functional neuroimaging may be considered in the clinical evaluation of DOC when there is uncertainty, and the primary clinical question is one of presence or absence of any evidence of awareness. Imaging should still be paired with neurobehavioral observations over time for diagnostic and care planning.[9] Laboratory and other testing should be directed by signs or symptoms and are generally based on the testing recommended for that condition (e.g., labs for electrolyte changes or endocrine function; EEG for concern for seizure).

## Scales and Measures

Clinicians may consider existing tools such as symptom checklists (e.g., neurosymptom inventory, Patient Health Questionnaire 9 [PHQ-9]), clinical screening worksheets (e.g., Montreal Cognitive Assessment [MOCA], SCAT),[2] or outcome measures; examples are linked in the eBook content. Clinicians should understand the psychometrics and target populations of the tools they are utilizing and consider patient's baseline function in considering "normal" and "abnormal" findings.

## Treatment

There is currently no cure for TBI. Medical and rehabilitation treatments are directed at optimizing natural recovery, treating bothersome symptoms, and implementing compensatory strategies.[2] The clinician may prioritize treatment targets based on most bothersome symptoms, the person's individual functional goals, and/or treatable impairments likely to have benefits in multiple functional domains (e.g., agitation, headache, insomnia, mood).

## Medical

Emergency management of TBI is beyond the scope of this chapter, and readers are referred to clinical practice guidelines including those for sports-related concussion and moderate-to-severe TBI.[2,5] A systematic approach is recommended to detect complications and associated impairments (e.g., structured review of systems, systematic approach to history and examination) since the sequela of TBI, including severity and functional impact, vary between individuals.[2,5] Acute management after moderate-to-severe TBI should include seizure prophylaxis for 7 days and enteral nutrition started within 72 hours.[5]

Common complications of TBI include agitation and disruptive behaviors, bladder and bowel dysfunction, delirium, dysphagia, electrolyte disturbances, falls, fatigue, gait/mobility dysfunction, infections, pain, paroxysmal sympathetic hyperactivity, psychological/psychiatric disturbances (including anxiety, depression, and posttraumatic stress disorder [PTSD]), seizures, sleep changes, spasticity, speech and language disorders, substance use, tracheostomy and ventilator management, and venous thromboembolism prevention. These complications including management will be covered in additional chapters. Chronic management should also attend to osteoporosis risk, wound care, and an individualized exercise prescription for all TBI survivors.

Additionally, attention impairments may be treated with stimulant medications (e.g., methylphenidate) or non-stimulants such as amantadine. Subjective or objective impairment in smell or taste should prompt referral to otolaryngology for further evaluation of posttraumatic hyposmia/anosmia, and patients should be counseled for safety regarding fire, natural gas, and food/cooking.[6] Persistent visual signs or symptoms generally warrant additional evaluation by an eye care professional with experience in TBI.

## Rehabilitation

Rehabilitation therapies are commonly indicated after all severities of TBI. Prescriptions for physical therapy, occupational therapy and speech language pathology should be directed based on the patient's impairments, activity limitations, and participation restrictions. Functional vision is often a concurrent target in therapies (e.g., paired with treatments for vestibular dysfunction, balance treatment, reading, pre-road driving evaluation).

Cognitive therapies can assist with TBI-related education, assessment over time, and functional considerations. There is evidence supporting the use of cognitive therapy and training in compensatory strategies and lessening morbidity after TBI, including in the domains of attention, executive function, memory, social communication impairments.[10] Neuropsychological evaluation is a commonly indicated and high-yield tool in assessment and treatment planning after TBI and offers some assistance with expected type and level of cognitive impairments across the severity of TBI.[2]

Rehabilitation counseling (vocational) and services through each state's Division of Vocational Rehabilitation is indicated for patients for futures planning. This includes concerns about return to school or work; counseling regarding applicable benefits and laws (e.g., disability benefits); and/or when counseling specific to work loss is indicated.

Therapeutic recreation is an important referral, especially after moderate-to-severe TBI, to assist with community safety evaluations, adaptive leisure education, transportation, and overall community access and participation.

### Special Considerations for Sports Concussion

After an initial period of relative physical and cognitive rest limited to 24 to 48 hours post-injury, subsymptom threshold physical activity can begin.[2] Studies suggest that early exercise is safe and beneficial for concussion recovery. Exercise tolerance tests can be utilized to help determine recommended intensity of early exercise while symptoms persist. If that is not available, athletes can monitor heart rate to determine their symptom threshold.[11]

Once concussion symptoms resolve completely, the athlete can then continue through the return to play protocol as outlined in Table 15.2.[2] Each step takes a minimum of 24

**TABLE 15.2 PROGRESSING ACTIVITY AND RETURN TO SPORT**

| STEP | AIM | ACTIVITY RECOMMENDATIONS |
|---|---|---|
| 1 | Reintroduction of work/school | Daily activities that do not increase symptoms. |
| 2 | Increase heart rate | Light aerobic exercise such as walking or stationary bike. No resistance training. |
| 3 | Add movement | Running and movement drills. No head impact. Light resistance training. |
| 4 | Increase intensity | Harder training drills including sprinting. Resistance training at normal intensity. |
| 5 | Assess readiness for competition | Normal training with full contact. |
| 6 | Return to sport | Normal game play. |

hours, and the athlete can progress to the next step if they remain asymptomatic. If symptoms occur, they should return to the prior step for at least 24 hours and remain asymptomatic before progressing again. It is also important to discuss a return-to-school and/or work plan.

## Special Considerations for Disorders of Consciousness

Patients with traumatic vegetative state or minimally conscious state (MCS) should receive amantadine between weeks 4 and 16 after injury to optimize functional recovery (starting dose typically 100 mg BID; max 200 mg BID) unless medically contraindicated.[9] Given the uncertainty of experiencing pain and suffering, clinicians should treat pain if a suspected pain generator exists regardless of the level of consciousness.[9] Care for adults with prolonged DOC should include care by, or consultation with, rehabilitation teams with expertise in DOC. It is important to provide counseling regarding what is currently known about the natural history of DOC recovery and the risk/benefit balance of treatments being considered.[9]

# FUNCTIONAL PROGNOSIS AND OUTCOMES

## Mild Traumatic Brain Injury and Sports Concussion

Most athletes recover within a month post-injury with recovery often shorter in adults and on the longer end in children and adolescents.[2] Symptoms that last beyond this expected recovery duration are considered "persistent symptoms" and do not necessarily equate to a persisting brain injury. In cases of persistent symptoms, it is important to evaluate for coexisting physical or psychological conditions and treat them as appropriate. The initial post-injury symptom intensity is the biggest predictor of experiencing prolonged recovery.[2] Migraine headaches, depression, or other mental health conditions are also risk factors for prolonged symptoms.[2]

## Moderate to Severe Traumatic Brain Injury

Trends for worse outcome after TBI include lower GCS, increasing amount of intracerebral blood, bihemispheric edema, older age, fixed pupils, impaired doll's eye sign, eyes do not deviate on caloric testing, decerebrate rigidity, and bilateral brain stem findings on MRI.[12] Threshold values, that define what is statistically unlikely to occur more chronically after TBI, can be helpful given the otherwise wide variability in outcomes after TBI. Clinically helpful threshold values are listed in Box 15.1.[12]

Referral to a multidisciplinary rehab team for prognostic counseling related to DOC is appropriate and should utilize tools such as practice guidelines for DOC.[9] After severe TBI with DOC in adults, progression to MCS within 5 months of injury is associated with more favorable outcomes after DOC. Vegetative state/unresponsive wakefulness syndrome (VS/UWS) more than 12 months after TBI should prompt prognostic conversations around the high likelihood for permanent impairments, long-term assistance, and associated care planning.[9] There is limited information to guide assessment and prognosis for children after traumatic VS/UWS and prolonged DOC.[9]

## Box 15.1

**FUNCTIONAL PROGNOSIS AFTER MODERATE TO SEVERE TRAUMATIC BRAIN INJURY**[12]

- Age greater than 65 years: unlikely to return to work or school/retrain
- Coma less than 2 weeks: unlikely to be dependent in care
- Coma greater than 4 weeks: unlikely to return to work or school
- PTA less than 8 weeks: unlikely to be dependent in care
- PTA greater than 12 weeks: unlikely to return to work or school

## RESOURCES AND REFERENCES

The full list of resources and references appears in the digital product found on http://connect.springerpub.com/content/book/978-0-8261-6226-7/part/part01/chapter/ch15

# Section 2

# MUSCULOSKELETAL MANAGEMENT BY BODY REGION

16

# SHOULDER

AMOS SONG AND NITIN JAIN

## INTRODUCTION

The human shoulder consists of three osseous structures: the scapula, clavicle, and humerus. Within the shoulder, there are two true joints: the humerus attaches to the glenoid fossa of the scapula to create a shallow ball-and-socket joint, the glenohumeral joint, and the clavicle attaches to the acromion of the scapula to form the acromioclavicular joint. The shoulder functions to move the upper extremity through complex, diverse ranges of motion including flexion, extension, abduction, adduction, and external and internal rotation. The lack of bony restraints allows for freedom of motion but makes the shoulder highly prone to both acute and degenerative injury. We will cover in more detail the most common sources of shoulder pain in the text. See Box 16.1 for a more comprehensive differential diagnosis of shoulder pain.

## JOINT PATHOLOGY

### Adhesive Capsulitis

#### Etiology and Pathophysiology

Colloquially known as "frozen shoulder," adhesive capsulitis is most commonly an idiopathic and self-limiting condition. Despite the underlying pathophysiology being

---

The full list of references appears in the digital product found on http://connect.springerpub.com/content/book/978-0-8261-6226-7/part/part02/chapter/ch16

**BOX 16.1**

**DIFFERENTIAL DIAGNOSIS OF SHOULDER PAIN**

**Diagnoses**

**Joint**

Acromioclavicular separation
Adhesive capsulitis
Glenohumeral instability
Labral tear
Scapular dyskinesia
Sternoclavicular separation

**Bone**

Clavicle fracture
Proximal humerus fracture
Scapula fracture

**Tendon**

Biceps tendinopathy
Pectoralis tendinopathy
Rotator cuff tendinopathy

**Nerve**

Axillary neuropathy
Brachial plexopathy
Cervical radiculopathy
Long thoracic neuropathy
Neuralgic amyotrophy
Suprascapular neuropathy
Thoracic outlet syndrome

**Other**

Shoulder impingement syndrome
Snapping scapula syndrome

incompletely understood, it is thought that the glenohumeral capsule becomes thickened, fibrotic, and contracted. The condition is commonly found in female patients and those aged 40 to 60 years. It has been associated with systemic diseases such as diabetes and thyroid dysfunction.[1-3]

## History, Examination, and Diagnostic Testing

Adhesive capsulitis initially presents with insidious onset of diffuse pain for several months. Pain commonly occurs even at rest and is worse at night. This is usually followed by a reduction in shoulder range of motion. On physical examination, a global loss of both active and passive motion is a diagnostic hallmark of adhesive capsulitis. External rotation is usually the plane most affected. X-rays, ultrasound, and MRI may not be diagnostic but can be helpful to rule out other etiologies of shoulder pain.

## Treatment

Physical therapy, with an emphasis on a gradual increase of range of motion, should be initiated once pain is under control. Pain can be managed with non-steroidal anti-inflammatory drugs (NSAIDs), Tylenol, or injections. Glenohumeral joint corticosteroid injections may be most helpful in the early painful stages of the disease process, and there is evidence of improved clinical efficacy with ultrasound guidance. Injections have also been directed at the rotator cuff interval or suprascapular nerve, though based on the literature, there is no clear consensus over the best location to inject patients with adhesive capsulitis. Surgical management, if nonoperative modalities fail, usually involves arthroscopic capsular release and, more rarely, shoulder manipulation under anesthesia.

## Functional Prognosis and Outcomes

Although the condition is self-limiting, prognosis is often prolonged with symptoms persisting up to 2 to 3 years. The natural progression of adhesive capsulitis is commonly divided into four stages: (a) painful stage, which gradually increases, (b) freezing stage, when pain continues to persist and range of motion starts to become restricted, (c) frozen stage, when stiffness becomes the predominant symptom, (d) thawing stage, when pain becomes minimal and range of motion and function begins to improve.

## Basic Order Sets

- ■ X-ray shoulder left/right: Anteroposterior (AP), lateral, axillary, scapular Y-view
- ■ Physical therapy: Begin with low-load gentle stretching followed by strengthening particularly with external rotation and scapular retraction
- ■ Ultrasound-guided glenohumeral joint steroid injection

## Glenohumeral Instability
### Etiology and Pathophysiology

The glenohumeral joint accounts for up to half of all major joint dislocations. The glenohumeral joint is inherently unstable and at risk for dislocation due to the shallow nature of the glenoid fossa where the humeral head articulates. Shoulder instability is most often traumatic. Risk factors for dislocation include a prior history of dislocation and younger age (less than 40 years old).[4-8]

Traumatic shoulder dislocations are most common in the anterior direction by a blow to an abducted and externally rotated arm. Posterior dislocations are less common and usually associated with seizure or electrocutions. Atraumatic shoulder instability can result due to extensive microtrauma (e.g., overhead athlete) or generalized ligamentous laxity (e.g., Ehlers–Danlos syndrome). Associated injuries include labral tears anteroinferiorly (Bankart lesion), an osseous injury on the posterolateral head of the humerus (Hill–Sachs lesion), rotator cuff tears, and axillary nerve injuries.

### History, Examination, and Diagnostic Testing

Patients will present with a subjective sensation of the joint "out of place," often holding onto the affected arm with the contralateral hand, and pain with motion. It is important to elicit prior history and frequency of shoulder joint dislocation. On examination for traumatic instability, inspection is critical to detect obvious deformity of the humeral head. Physical examination maneuvers for atraumatic instability include the sulcus sign, posterior load and shift, and anterior apprehension test that may be provocative. X-rays will be useful in the setting of an acute dislocation, although they may be normal if relocation has already occurred or in cases of instability without dislocation. On x-ray, it is important to evaluate for evidence of an associated Bankart lesion, a Hill–Sachs defect, and glenoid bone loss which may affect treatment options. More advanced imaging such as MRI is rarely needed unless concurrent injuries are suspected.

### Treatment

Treatment of an acute dislocation includes reduction as soon as possible before pain and guarding make this increasingly difficult. A neurovascular check should always be performed before and after reduction. There is no best reduction technique, but the FARES (fast, reliable, and safe) method has been shown to be highly successful. In the FARES method, the patient is supine as the hand is held with the elbow extended and the forearm in neutral rotation. Then, gentle distal traction is applied and the arm is slowly abducted to 120°. While doing so, the patient's arm is vertically oscillated to a depth of around 5 cm, 1 to 2 times per second until reduction occurs. Intra-articular anesthetic injection can be performed if reduction becomes limited due to pain. Radiographic evidence of a successful reduction should be obtained. It remains uncertain whether post-reduction bracing and immobilization improve outcomes. After reduction and with chronic instability, the mainstay of treatment involves physical therapy with focus on strengthening the static and dynamic stabilizers. Surgery is most often indicated for younger patients with traumatic and recurrent dislocations.

### Basic Order Sets

- X-ray shoulder left/right: AP, lateral, axillary, scapular Y-view
- Physical therapy: Regain range of motion followed by scapular stabilization and rotator cuff strengthening exercises.

## Superior Labrum Anterior to Posterior Tear
### Etiology and Pathophysiology

Superior labrum anterior to posterior (SLAP) tears are most often found in overhead athletes (e.g., baseball or volleyball players) or laborers who perform repetitive overhead motions. SLAP tears are thought to occur when the superior labrum separates from the glenoid in a "peel back mechanism" near where the long head of the bicep tendon attaches on the labrum. This injury occurs rarely in isolation and is often associated with rotator cuff and/or biceps tendinopathy.[9–11]

### History, Examination, and Diagnostic Testing

Patients with SLAP tears present variably but often have shoulder pain associated with clicking, locking, or snapping and a decline in sports performance or work function. Physical examination maneuvers do not have strong predictive value, but special tests including O'Brien's and the labral shear may provoke symptoms. When ordering imaging, an MRI arthrogram is considered the gold standard to confirm diagnosis. These results should always be associated with clinical findings, as many individuals begin to develop asymptomatic abnormalities toward middle age.

### Treatment

Physical therapy should be utilized initially to resolve glenohumeral internal rotation deficits (GIRD) and improve scapular stabilizer and rotator cuff strength. NSAIDs, Tylenol, or an ultrasound-guided glenohumeral joint steroid injection can be considered for pain alleviation. Indications for surgery include failure of nonoperative treatment, concomitant presence of significant rotator cuff tear, and large labral tears with significant instability or mechanical symptoms. The best surgical candidates for labral repair are patients under the age of 35.

### Basic Order Sets

- X-ray shoulder left/right: AP, lateral, axillary, scapular Y-view
- MRI arthrogram with contrast: Left/right upper extremity joint, shoulder
- Physical therapy: Regain active/passive range of motion (ROM), posterior capsule mobilization, scapular retraction exercises, rotator cuff strengthening, and proprioceptive neuromuscular rehabilitation exercises.

## Acromioclavicular Joint Sprain and Separation
### Etiology and Pathophysiology

The acromioclavicular (AC) joint is stabilized by three ligaments: (a) AC, (b) coracoclavicular (CC), (c) coracoacromial. Injuries occur most commonly in males aged 20 to 30 years old involved in contact sports. The mechanism of injury usually involves direct trauma to the shoulder or a fall on an outstretched hand.[12-14]

### History, Examination, and Diagnostic Testing

Diagnostic approach should focus on inspection to look for deformities and tenderness to palpation of the AC joint compared to the contralateral side. Special tests include the cross-body adduction test. Plain films should be ordered to confirm the diagnosis and to classify the extent of injury. The Zanca view which involves 15° of cephalic tilt will give the most accurate view of the AC joint. Bilateral films should be performed for comparison to the unaffected shoulder.

### Treatment

AC joint injuries are commonly classified into the Rockwood classification system, which guides treatment options and prognosis. Type I injuries involve sprain of the AC ligament and have no or minimal displacement of clavicle without increase in the CC space. The normal CC space is around 1.1 to 1.3 cm. Type II injuries involve a tear of the AC ligament and are defined as minimal superior displacement of clavicle with a CC space increase of no greater than 25%. Types I and II can be managed nonoperatively using a sling for comfort followed by early range of motion and strengthening exercises in physical therapy. Type III involves a tear of the AC and CC ligaments resulting in superior displacement of the clavicle with a CC space increase of 25% to 100%. Treatment for type III AC joint injuries remains controversial and can be managed either nonoperatively or surgically. Types IV to VI injuries are characterized by varying directions of clavicular displacement and should be treated with surgical repair.

### Basic Order Set

- X-ray shoulder bilateral: True AP view, Zanca view, axillary view
- Physical therapy: Passive and active ROM, scapular stabilization, rotator cuff strengthening

## Scapular Dyskinesis
### Etiology and Pathophysiology

Scapular dyskinesis is the presence of altered scapular positioning and mechanics with movement. The scapula is particularly vulnerable to dyskinesis as it is without significant bony attachments despite the large number of muscles that attach to it. Scapular dyskinesis has been suggested to predispose patients to many different shoulder pathologies. Etiologies for scapula dyskinesis span from muscular imbalance to true neurological injury.[15-17]

### History, Examination, and Diagnostic Testing

Diagnosis of scapular dyskinesis is predominantly based on the physical examination. Inspection for asymmetry with the patient's shirt removed provides the best opportunity to visualize any abnormalities. For this, it is helpful for examiners to locate the inferior angle of the scapulae and place their thumbs there as the patient undergoes shoulder abduction and flexion. Nerve conduction studies (NCS)/electromyography (EMG) can also be helpful in neurogenic causes of scapular dyskinesis. The serratus anterior muscle, which is innervated by the long thoracic nerve, and the trapezius muscle, which is innervated by the spinal accessory nerve, are the two prime movers of the scapula. Medial winging has been classically associated with long thoracic neuropathy and lateral winging with the spinal accessory neuropathy.

### Treatment

Treatment primarily consists of rehabilitation to correct underlying muscular weakness and imbalance.

### Basic Order Sets

- Physical therapy: Shoulder stretching and mobilization, neuromuscular coordination, scapular stabilization, and lower/middle trapezius and serratus anterior strengthening

## BONE PATHOLOGY

### Clavicle Fracture
#### Etiology and Pathophysiology

Clavicle fractures most often occur after a fall on an outstretched hand or direct trauma. The clavicle is divided into thirds: lateral, midshaft, and medial. Most common clavicle fractures occur in the midshaft.[18,19]

#### History, Examination, and Diagnostic Testing

Patients will present with traumatic shoulder pain. On physical examination, it is important to inspect the clavicle and compare it to the unaffected contralateral shoulder to identify deformity including skin tenting. A complete neurovascular examination including at the brachial and radial artery is paramount as neurovascular injury can occur. Bilateral x-rays should be ordered to confirm the diagnosis and assess severity.

#### Treatment

Nonoperative treatment can be tried if there is minimal fracture displacement (<2 cm). This begins with a figure-of-eight sling for up to 2 weeks. Physical therapy should be started as soon as the patient is able to encourage early range of motion. Surgical referral for management is recommended if there is >2 cm displacement, skin tenting, open fracture, neurovascular compromise, or concomitant injury such as a sternoclavicular or glenohumeral joint fracture or AC joint separation.

#### Basic Order Sets

- X-ray shoulder bilateral: Standard AP, Zanca view
- Sling, figure-of-eight brace
- Physical therapy eval and treat: Passive and active range of motion exercises, scapular stabilization, and rotator cuff strengthening exercises

### Proximal Humerus Fracture
#### Etiology and Pathophysiology

Proximal humerus fractures most commonly involve the elderly (>65 years old) female population after a fall or direct trauma.[20]

#### History, Examination, and Diagnostic Testing

Patients often present after trauma with proximal arm pain, swelling, and bruising as well as decreased shoulder ROM. Physical examination should be focused on the presence of obvious deformity and ecchymosis along the proximal arm. A commonly associated condition includes axillary nerve injury which should be evaluated on examination. X-rays will help with diagnosis and clinical decision-making.

#### Treatment

The vast majority of proximal humerus fractures can be treated nonoperatively. Patients can be placed in a figure-of-eight sling for 2 weeks. Physical therapy should start soon thereafter to begin range of motion exercise. Referrals to surgery for management should be made if the fracture is displaced at the surgical neck, anatomic neck, lesser tuberosity, or >5 mm at the greater tuberosity or if there is neurovascular compromise or neurological injury.

### Basic Order Sets

- X-ray shoulder left/right: True AP, glenoid, axillary, scapular Y view
- Sling, figure-of-eight brace
- Physical therapy evaluation and treatment: Passive and active range of motion exercises, scapular stabilization, and rotator cuff strengthening exercises

## TENDON PATHOLOGY

### Rotator Cuff Tendon Tear

### Etiology and Pathophysiology

The rotator cuff is comprised of four rotator cuff tendons: the supraspinatus, infraspinatus, subscapularis, and teres minor. The rotator cuff acts primarily as dynamic stabilizers of the glenohumeral joint. Pathologies involving the rotator cuff occur along a spectrum of disease and may include subacromial bursopathy and impingement, calcific tendinopathy, and a rotator cuff tear. The most common etiology of rotator cuff disease is atraumatic chronic repetitive shoulder movement. Acute injuries occur but are usually limited to the younger patient cohort.[21-24]

### History, Examination, and Diagnostic Testing

On history, patients will report pain and often diminished function of the shoulder with certain motions. There are several physical examination maneuvers and special tests for the rotator cuff. The Jobe test and the full can test have high sensitivity and specificity for supraspinatus injury. The external rotation lag sign and the Hornblower sign have high sensitivity and specificity for infraspinatus and teres minor injury, respectively. The lift-off or bear-hug test can be used to assess the subscapularis. With all of these examination maneuvers, a true positive test is indicated by weakness.

Radiographs may demonstrate proximal migration of the humerus in severe, long-standing rotator cuff tear disease or calcific tendon changes. MRI has been considered the gold standard for rotator cuff diagnosis as it best elicits soft tissues that make up the rotator cuff and characterizes the extent of disease. Emerging evidence has shown that ultrasound can also readily diagnose rotator cuff injuries with similar sensitivity, specificity, and overall accuracy compared to MRI. It should be noted that not all patients with rotator cuff tears on imaging will be symptomatic. Up to 39% of patients with rotator cuff tears are asymptomatic.

### Treatment

There is a lack of evidence to support operative versus nonoperative treatment of rotator cuff tears. Nevertheless, outcomes appear to be similar 1 to 2 years after either nonoperative or operative treatment. Physical therapy is the mainstay of nonoperative treatment and consists of passive range of motion, scapular stabilization, and rotator cuff strengthening exercises. Steroid injections most often performed to the subacromial bursa can be considered for pain control. However, repeat injections are advised against due to negative side effects on tendon health. Orthobiologics, such as prolotherapy, platelet-rich plasma, and stem cells, are currently being investigated for their potential to augment rotator cuff tendon healing or slow progression of disease. Although the use of these biologic adjuvants is increasing, their clinical efficacy remains unclear. Surgery is usually reserved for acute, full-thickness tears. However, other factors to consider include the size and location of the tear as well as patient preference and characteristics. Surgery can also be considered after failure of nonoperative treatment. The greatest risk factor for surgical failure is rotator cuff muscular atrophy due to chronic disease.

## Basic Order Set

- X-ray shoulder left/right: True AP, AP in internal/external rotation, axillary
- Complete joint diagnostic ultrasound: Shoulder left/right
- MRI upper extremity: Shoulder joint left/right without contrast
- Physical therapy: Passive range of motion, scapular stabilization, and rotator cuff strengthening exercises

## NERVE PATHOLOGY

### Acute Brachial Plexus Injury ("Stinger")
### Etiology and Pathophysiology

An acute brachial plexus injury, colloquially known as a "stinger," occurs with trauma to the shoulder or a traction of the arm or shoulder from the neck and trunk. The C5 and C6 nerve roots are most commonly affected during this injury.[25,26]

### History, Examination, and Diagnostic Testing

Diagnosis can be made with a presentation of unilateral numbness and tingling in the upper extremity. Bilateral symptoms must be elicited to rule out a spinal cord injury. A thorough upper extremity neurological and vascular examination should be performed. Milder injuries with transient symptoms do not need further workup. Repeat injuries or those with persistent pain or weakness warrant further workup with imaging as well as a potential NCS/EMG. If obtained, NCS/EMG studies should be delayed 4 to 6 weeks after injury and may show denervation of C5 to C6 muscles including the deltoid, bicep, and brachioradialis while sparing cervical paraspinal muscles.

### Treatment and Prognosis

Treatment is usually nonoperative, consisting of rest, physical therapy, and/or pain management, and most cases are self-limiting. Athletes can return to play when they are asymptomatic without neurological deficit. Early surgical evaluation is warranted in cases of nerve root avulsion or crush-type injury resulting in neurological deficits.

## Thoracic Outlet Syndrome

### Etiology and Pathophysiology

The thoracic outlet is located between the clavicle and first rib with contents including the subclavian artery and vein and the brachial plexus. Thoracic outlet syndrome (TOS) is caused by either a neurogenic or vascular etiology. Neurogenic TOS is caused by compression of the brachial plexus in the thoracic outlet, whereas vascular TOS is due to compression or restriction of blood flow of the subclavian vessels in this same space. Common entities that can cause compression of the thoracic outlet include soft tissue or osseous abnormalities involving either the scalene musculature or cervical first rib. Repetitive shoulder and arm movement has also been reported as a risk factor in some cases.[26,27]

### History, Examination, and Diagnostic Testing

TOS has a highly variable presentation. Patients are usually younger than the age of 40 and present with pain and numbness, tingling, weakness, and vasomotor changes of the upper extremity. Inspection of the affected arm may show cyanotic discoloration in the vasogenic type and Gilliatt-Sumner hand which is characterized by atrophy of the abductor pollicis brevis and hypothenar muscles. Special tests include the Adson's test, which involves palpating for the loss of a radial pulse while extending the patient's arm and turning the head toward the affected side, and Roo's test, which involves provoking symptoms by repeatedly opening and closing the hands with the arms 90° abducted and the elbows 90° flexed. A cervical spine and chest x-ray can show any osseous abnormalities leading to compression. Angiography/venography and NCS/EMG studies are useful in diagnosis of vascular and neurogenic types, respectively.

### Treatment

For treatment, physical therapy should be initiated and involve upper extremity stretching exercises as well as nerve glides. Surgery can be indicated after failure of nonoperative treatment for at least 6 months, especially in cases where there is an obvious soft tissue or osseous compressive etiology.

### Basic Order Sets

- X-ray: Chest x-ray two views, C-spine
- NCS/EMG
- CT angiogram/venogram upper extremity left/right

## REFERENCES

The full list of references appears in the digital product found on http://connect.springerpub.com/content/book/978-0-8261-6226-7/part/part02/chapter/ch16

# ELBOW

PRATHAP JAYARAM, BO SONG, AND TRACEY ISIDRO

## INTRODUCTION

The elbow joint is a series of articulations between the upper and lower arm, consisting of the humeroulnar joint, humeroradial joint, and radioulnar joint. The main function of the elbow is to flex and extend the arm, with its range of motion between 0° of extension and 150° of flexion. The biceps brachii, brachialis, and brachioradialis serve as elbow flexors while the triceps and anconeus serve as elbow extensors. The distal humerus extends to form the medial epicondyle and the lateral epicondyle, the origins for the wrist flexors and extensors, respectively. The medial elbow is stabilized by the ulnar collateral ligament (UCL), and the lateral elbow is stabilized by the radial collateral ligament. Common conditions affecting the elbow joint include joint conditions, bone fractures, common extensor and flexor tendinopathy, distal biceps injuries, ligamentous injuries, and neuropathies which will be covered in the following text. See Box 17.1 for a more comprehensive differential diagnosis of elbow pain.

## JOINT PATHOLOGY

### Elbow Dislocation

### Etiology and Pathophysiology

Elbow dislocations occur at an incidence of about 6 of every 100,000 people and are the most commonly dislocated joint in children and the second most common in adults.[1,2] Posterior dislocation comprises the majority of all elbow dislocations.[1] The understood mechanism is due to be a hyperextension injury, commonly from a fall on an outstretched hand.[1] A true dislocation will affect the lateral UCL first, then the capsule, and then the medial UCL.[1] These forces can also cause associated fractures or cartilaginous damage.[1] Associated orthopedic injuries include radial head/neck fractures, avulsion fractures of the medial/lateral epicondyles, or coronoid fractures.[1] Associated neurovascular injuries include damage to the brachial artery or median nerve.[1]

### History

These injuries always occur with a traumatic mechanism. Males are 2 to 2.5 times more likely to be affected than females.[1] Gymnastics, basketball, football, and wrestling are commonly implicated sports.[1]

---

The full list of references appears in the digital product found on http://connect.springerpub.com/content/book/978-0-8261-6226-7/part/part02/chapter/ch17

## BOX 17.1

### DIFFERENTIAL DIAGNOSIS OF ELBOW PAIN

**Diagnoses**

**Joint**

Elbow dislocation

Olecranon bursitis

**Bone**

Distal humerus fracture

Radial head fracture

Ulna fracture

Olecranon fracture

**Tendon**

Common extensor tendinopathy

Common flexor tendinopathy

Distal biceps tendinopathy

Triceps tendinopathy

**Nerve**

Cubital tunnel syndrome

Radial tunnel syndrome

Pronator syndrome

Musculocutaneous neuropathy

Lateral antebrachial cutaneous neuropathy

## Examination

Obvious deformity along with bruising or swelling can be indicative of a dislocation.[2] A focus on neurovascular status and damage is essential in case acute surgical intervention is necessary.[1] Compartment syndrome is also possible post-injury and should be ruled out, which will present with disproportionate pain with finger and wrist extension.[1]

## Diagnostic Testing

Anteroposterior (AP) and lateral radiographs should be obtained after reduction.[1] CT and MRI are usually more beneficial to evaluate for further injuries or to determine reconstructive planning.[1] However, MRI tends to have limited utility in assessing for chronic instability.[2] Arteriography is recommended for suspicion of arterial injuries.[1]

## Treatment

Reduction should be performed if the injury occurs in the presence of a physician before further workup and radiographs.[1] This is often performed with forearm supination to clear the coronoid under the trochlea while providing longitudinal traction and elbow flexion.[1,2] In this case, an earlier reduction immediately after the injury would be preferable to avoid complication by muscle spasms, swelling, and pain.[1] If not possible, conscious sedation or general anesthesia can be beneficial to accomplish reduction.[1] Multiple attempts should be performed with caution to avoid chondral injury.[1] Surgical indications are for failure to obtain a satisfactory reduction, persistent instability, and suspected intra-articular fragment or neurovascular entrapment.[2] Post-reduction, a 3- to 10-day period of immobilization is recommended followed by rehabilitation to achieve full range of motion.[1]

## Functional Prognosis and Outcomes

Uncomplicated dislocations usually demonstrate good functional recovery.[1] Immobilization >3 weeks is associated with a higher risk of contractures.[1] In general, most patients will report limited extension but will experience improvement up to 6 months.[1] Fifty percent of patients will note long-term discomfort with an average of 15% loss of strength.[1] Other complications include posttraumatic stiffness, heterotopic bone formation (mostly in the medial and lateral collateral ligaments), or neurologic issues including transient paresthesias and nerve palsies.[1] Patients can return to sport once they regain full range of motion without pain.[2]

## Basic Order Sets

Physical therapy (PT) script: Focus early on active range of motion to minimize extension loss. Progress to isokinetic exercises focusing on wrist flexion/extension/supination/pronation and biceps/triceps range of motion and strengthening. No splint is required if the elbow is stable in extension. The extension splint block is gradually decreased for 3 to 6 weeks, after which strengthening exercises are started.

## Olecranon Bursitis
### Etiology and Pathophysiology

Olecranon bursitis develops from an increase of fluid within the posterior elbow bursal cavity.[3,4] Traumatic causes are common, and fractures or penetrating foreign bodies should be ruled out.[3] Chronic bursitis can occur from systematic disorders, prolonged pressure, or multiple acute injuries to the bursa.[4] Septic bursitis can occur from direct inoculation from superficial wounds or from nearby cellulitis; however, hematogenous seeding is rare given the poor blood supply to the bursa.[4]

### History

It is important to differentiate olecranon bursitis from malignancy or neoplasm, which may present with rapid growth, failure of treatment, weight loss, or history of malignancy.[3] A thorough history involving information about trauma is also beneficial. Specifically, a detailed social history including occupation and hobbies can assist in determining the etiology, as manual laborers and athletes are more prone to septic olecranon bursitis.[4]

## Examination

Olecranon bursitis is characterized by a fluid collection along the posterior elbow. Examination should include documenting the size of the bursitis, consistency, erythema, fluctuance, temperature, and any associated lymphadenopathy.[3] Range of motion with pain reproduction should be assessed.[3] In general, elbow range of motion tends to be unaffected in olecranon bursitis.[3] However, if septic arthritis is involved, range of motion can be compromised.[4]

## Diagnostic Testing

Early determination of septic and aseptic causes is critical. The gold standard is with aspiration and gram stain/culture.[3] The most common microorganism involved is *Staphylococcus aureus*.[4] Analysis should also include aspirate and serum white cell, glucose concentration, and protein levels.[3] Basic blood work should consist of a comprehensive blood count, urea levels, electrolytes, glucose levels, and inflammatory markers.[3] Radiographs of the elbow should also be ordered to evaluate for intra-articular causes, osteomyelitis, olecranon spurs, fractures, or foreign bodies.[3] MRI or ultrasound (US) can be considered for better evaluation of infective bursitis.[3]

## Treatment

For noninfective bursitis, initial conservative management includes ice, compression, and anti-inflammatories. Aspiration and steroid injection can be considered, however, present the risk of secondary infection.[3] In the case of noninfective bursitis with accompanying olecranon spur, excision may reduce the risk of recurrence.[3] For infective causes, antibiotics remain the mainstay of treatment, however, with some variability depending on duration and associated treatments.[3] Some practices recommend prolonged oral anticoagulation while others recommend 4 weeks of IV antibiotics depending on the severity of the condition.[3] The option to perform an open incision and drainage is considered for more severe cases.[3] After aspiration however, many studies recommend broad-spectrum antibiotics covering at least *S. aureus*, which comprises >90% of cases.[3]

## Functional Prognosis and Outcomes

Conservative treatments tend to have higher recurrence rates and propensity to become chronic.[4] Corticosteroids have shown symptomatic improvement but can predispose to infection.[4] Operative strategies are considered if conservative treatments are unsuccessful but with complications include impaired wound healing.[4]

## Basic Order Sets

Initial bloodwork including complete blood count (CBC), comprehensive metabolic panel (CMP), urea levels, and inflammatory markers such as C-reactive protein (CRP) and erythrocyte sedimentation rate (ESR) should be ordered first. If infectious etiology is suspected, aspiration/drainage can be considered. Aspirate CBC, glucose, protein, and protein levels should be ordered. Radiographs can be helpful in determining any bony abnormality or presence of septic arthritis.

## BONE PATHOLOGY

### Distal Humerus Fracture

### Etiology and Pathophysiology

Distal humerus fractures are estimated to be 5.7/100,000 per year and comprise one-third of all elbow fractures.[5,6] This fracture most commonly affects males between 12 and 19 and females >90 years old.[5] Traumatic causes predominate in younger patients while elderly patients tend to occur from lower energy forces such as falls.[5,6]

### History

There is almost always a preceding traumatic event prior to injury. An additional detailed history should be obtained to rule out any other coexisting injuries or fractures, which are common.

### Examination

Physical examination should consist of a comprehensive examination around the site of the injury including assessment for erythema, edema, tenderness, and strength. In addition, a neurovascular examination should be performed to rule out any associated nerve or vascular damage.[5]

### Diagnostic Testing

Radiographs, with AP and lateral views are used first line to diagnose distal humerus fractures.[5] CT scans can also be helpful with more complex injuries, for surgical planning, and to rule out other occult fractures.[5]

### Treatment

Nonoperative management can sometimes be an option for nondisplaced fractures with enough stability; however, this option is rarely recommended in younger patients.[5] Surgical fixation is recommended to promote stability and reduce fracture displacement risk.[5,6] Postoperatively it is recommended that immobilization not exceed 3 weeks to promote better functional outcomes.[5]

### Functional Prognosis and Outcomes

Surgical fixation tends to have good outcomes with pain and function, though reduction in elbow range of motion in flexion and extension and strength may be present. Postoperative complications to be aware of include heterotopic ossification, infection, and olecranon nonunion.[5]

### Basic Order Sets

AP and lateral radiographs of the elbow should be ordered to identify the fracture. CT may be beneficial to rule out any other concomitant injuries and help surgical planning.[5] Once a distal humerus fracture is confirmed, referral to an orthopedic surgeon is recommended.

## Radial Head Fracture

### Etiology and Pathophysiology

Radial head fractures usually affect younger active patients and are the most common elbow fractures, consisting of one-third of elbow fractures.[7] These injuries usually occur with falls on outstretched hand or from direct trauma.[7]

### History

A history for suspected radial head fractures should entail mechanism of injury, occupation or sport, medical history, associated symptoms, or history of similar injuries.

### Examination

Palpation of the elbow joint may demonstrate a joint effusion or tenderness at the radial head.[7] The patient may also demonstrate decreased range of motion and pain with all planes of motion mostly in flexion and extension.[7] It is important to differentiate between a mechanical block versus pain-limiting range of motion.[8] A detailed neurovascular examination should be performed to rule out distal nerve damage.[8]

### Diagnostic Testing

AP, lateral, and oblique radiographs should be performed first.[8] These fractures can be subtle, and the only sign may be the presence of a posterior fat pad sign.[8] If the injury is suspected but not seen on initial radiographs, a repeat radiograph in 2 weeks is recommended.[8] CT scan may provide better visualization of radial fractures not seen on initial radiographs and can be beneficial for more complex injuries or to visualize surrounding structures.[8] MRI has not been shown to change treatment plans and prognosis.[8]

### Treatment

Radial head fractures are divided into types I, II, and III injuries.[7] Type I injuries are often nondisplaced and treated with nonoperative measures with early range of motion exercises as tolerated with protected weight-bearing for 6 weeks.[7] Type II injuries are displaced with a mechanical block to motion.[7] There is no universally agreed treatment algorithm for these; nonoperative treatments can be considered for more stable injuries and open reduction internal fixation (ORIF) for more complex injuries.[7] Type III fractures include severely comminuted fractures which usually require the need for radial head excision with or without radial head replacement arthroplasty.[7]

### Functional Prognosis and Outcomes

The most common postsurgical complication of radial head fractures is postoperative stiffness with decreased range of motion, especially in extension.[7] It is also recommended to limit immobilization to less than 3 to 4 weeks to prevent contractures.[7] In general, type I fractures or nondisplaced should regain full range of motion in 1 to 2 weeks while types II and III fractures have more variable outcomes.[7]

## Basic Order Sets

AP, lateral, and oblique radiographs should be ordered of the elbow to help stage the fracture and guide treatment.

## TENDON PATHOLOGY

### Common Extensor Tendinopathy
### Etiology and Pathophysiology

Common extensor tendinopathy of the elbow, also called "lateral epicondylitis" or "tennis elbow," is an overuse phenomenon resulting in chronic symptomatic degeneration of the common wrist extensor tendons at the attachment to the lateral epicondyle.[9,10] It affects approximately 1% to 3% of those between 35 and 54 years old and can be seen with activity that involves repetitive overuse of wrist extension.[9,11] Obesity and smoking are two risk factors.[9,11]

### History

Patients may present with gradual pain along the bony surface of the proximal half of the lateral epicondyle in line with the common extensor mass.[9] Pain may be provoked by wrist movement involving extension and supination.[9]

### Examination

Common on examination, patients will have tenderness to palpation 2 to 5 mm distal and anterior to the lateral epicondyle. Cozen's test most reliably stresses the extensor tendon. To perform the test, the patient holds the elbow extended and the forearm pronated while making a fist and extending the wrist. The patient should hold this position while the examiner applies resistance. Pain at the lateral elbow is considered a positive test. Other tests include Maudsley's test and the chair test.[9] In Maudsley's test, resisted middle finger extension is painful due to selective recruitment for Extensor Carpi Radialis Brevis (ECRB) tendon, whereas in the chair test, the patient is asked to lift a chair in pronation and may present with decreased grip strength.[10] Elbow range of motion is usually intact, but if limited, a concomitant joint pathology should be considered.[9]

### Diagnostic Testing

Diagnosis can be made by clinical assessment alone.[11] If necessary, imaging options include plain radiographs, US, MRI, and nerve conduction studies (NCS)/electromyography (EMG).[11] Plain radiographs can demonstrate cases of calcific tendinosis as well as rule out concomitant bony pathology.[9,10] US and MRI can both show findings of tendinosis and/or tearing.[9,11] While MRI may be beneficial due to reproducibility and ability to visualize intra-articular pathology, US is most ideal to assess structural tendon changes, bone irregularities, calcific deposits, and neovascularization in clinic.[9] NCS/EMG can be utilized to rule out a posterior interosseous nerve (PIN) compressive neuropathy distal to radial head.[9]

### Treatment

Conservative care with activity modification, non-steroidal anti-inflammatory drugs (NSAIDs), PT (see order sets), braces, steroid injections, orthobiologics, and extracorpeal shockwave therapy (ESWT) can be considered first.[9,11] Epicondylar counterforce braces have been particularly popular and work by reducing wrist extensor tension.[9] However, studies have shown no differences between these and placebo braces, and they can even predispose to nerve issues with prolonged use.[9] In the acute phase, NSAIDs can help to decrease inflammation.[9] Steroid injections into the common extensor tendon sheath can be considered for short-term relief, however, may result in no benefit or worse clinical outcomes at 1 year with potential negative side effects on tendon health.[9,12] Platelet-rich plasma (PRP) injections provide a concentrated source of growth factors, which theoretically can enhance tendon healing.[9,11] Growing evidence suggest that PRP injections have long-term benefit on elbow tendinopathy, but there is still much variability among practioners in optimal formulation.[9,12] US-guided tenotomy has also been shown to be effective in treating this condition through stimulating blood flow and has been utilized with other modalities such as PRP with success.[13] Percutaneous ultrasonic tenotomy is another option that works by using thermal energy to emulsify and subsequently debride pathologic tissue.[14] While this has shown efficacy in reducing pain, improving grip strength, and improving quality of life, post-procedure US findings did not show any change in tendon size.[14] Extracorporeal shock wave therapy is another alternative, however, has not been shown to be more effective than other options.[9] Surgery is considered if there is no response to conservative treatment and activity limitation for more than 6 months or in cases of complete tendon rupture.[9,11]

## Functional Prognosis and Outcomes

In general, nonoperative management will improve symptoms 90% of the time even in recalcitrant cases within 12 to 18 months.[9,11] Population studies have shown recurrence rates of 8.5% on average with median time to recurrence around 20 months.[15]

## Basic Order Sets

PT: Focus on stretching and eccentric strengthening of the forearm extensors. Also, include peri-scapular stabilization for the trapezius, serratus anterior, and rotator cuff muscles.[9,11]

## Common Flexor Tendinopathy
### Etiology and Pathophysiology

Common flexor tendinopathy of the elbow, also called "medial epicondylitis" or "golfer's elbow," is the result of overuse activities involving repetitive wrist flexion leading to chronic symptomatic degeneration of these tendons at the attachment to the medial epicondyle.[11] It is less common than lateral elbow tendinopathy, affecting 1% to 6% in those 30 to 50 years old.[11] Throwing athletes like baseball players can be at high risk for this injury due to stress of flexor pronator mass during valgus loading acceleration phase of throwing.[11]

### History

Patients most often present with gradual medial elbow pain. These symptoms are provoked with repetitive wrist flexion and/or forearm pronation.[11]

## Examination

On examination, there may be tenderness over the flexor pronator origin at the medial epicondyle. Symptoms are most often reproduced with resisted pronation or wrist flexion.[11] There can be decreased grip strength.[11] Patients should be assessed for a concurrent ulnar neuropathy.[11]

## Diagnostic Testing

Clinical evaluation is sufficient to confirm a diagnosis in most cases. Additional testing to support this diagnosis includes x-ray, US, MRI, and NCS/EMG. Plain radiographs can show enthesophytes of the flexor pronator origin at the medial epicondyle.[11] US and MRI are beneficial to access for tendinosis as well as tendon tears. NCS/EMG is useful to evaluate for a concurrent ulnar neuropathy at the medial elbow.

## Treatment

Conservative treatment is often successful but can take 6 to 12 months.[11] Activity modification, NSAIDs, and PT are first-line treatments.[11] If there is no improvement, steroid injections into the common flexor/pronator tendon sheath can be considered but have only shown to provide short-term symptomatic relief without long-term disease modification.[11] Additionally, these injections can have negative consequences on tendon and soft tissue health. PRP injections can provide short- and long-term symptomatic relief and have the potential for disease modification; however, more robust studies are needed to demonstrate these results and optimize PRP formulations.[11] Percutaneous ultrasonic tenotomy has shown efficacy in treating this condition.[16] In chronic recalcitrant cases, surgery to debride the common flexor/pronator tendon can be beneficial.[11]

## Functional Prognosis and Outcomes

This condition is relatively self-limiting with resolution in 80% of patients.[17] The literature varies, however, estimates that 5% to 15% will suffer a recurrence.[18] A concomitant ulnar neuropathy with medial elbow tendinopathy has a poorer prognosis.[11]

## Distal Biceps Injury
### Etiology and Pathophysiology

Distal biceps injuries often occur in the dominant arm in men aged 40 to 50 years old.[11] Risk factors include smoking, steroid use, or previous rupture.[11] Ruptures often take place during acute injuries with a large eccentric load with the elbow in 90° of flexion causing tearing of the biceps from the radial tuberosity.[11].

## History

Often, there will be a clear mechanism of injury described as a sharp, sudden, painful pop that improves within several hours followed by a dull ache.[11] Patients will often complain of pain and deformity in the antecubital fossa in maximum eccentric loading along with weakness of elbow flexion and/or supination. This may result in functional difficulties such as turning the doorknob or lifting objects.[11]

## Examination

On inspection, there can be bruising over the medial aspect of the elbow.[19] In a complete rupture, there may be a visible distal biceps retraction known as a "Popeye" deformity.[11] Strength testing of elbow flexion and supination can reproduce symptoms.[11] A Hook test where the examiner flexes the elbow to 90° and fully supinates the forearm, placing the index finger in the lateral antecubital fossa to hook the biceps tendon, can be used to confirm the diagnosis in full-thickness tears.[19]

## Diagnostic Testing

Diagnosis of full-thickness tears is often clinical given the high specificity of the hook test.[19] US or MRI can be used to confirm the diagnosis and identify partial versus complete tears.[19]

## Treatment

Complete distal biceps tendon tears can be managed nonoperatively but may have reduced supination strength or flexion strength.[19] Thus, nonoperative management is reserved for patients with low functional demands or those with significant risk factors for surgery.[19] For appropriate cases, operative treatment is best performed within 1 month of injury.[11] For partial tendon ruptures, activity modifications and PT focusing on elbow flexion and extension are recommended for 3 to 6 months.[11] Surgery can be considered for complete tears or if conservative measures fail.[11]

## Functional Prognosis and Outcomes

Partial and complete tears treated conservatively may have reduced functional outcomes whereas surgery tends to result in full recovery.[11] Studies have estimated 30% to 40% reduction in supination strength and a 20% to 30% reduction in flexion strength in nonoperative treatment.[19] However, complications can occur at a rate of 20% to 45% post-biceps tendon repair depending on the method, including injury to the lateral antebrachial cutaneous nerve resulting in sensory loss.[19,20]

## LIGAMENT PATHOLOGY

### Ulnar Collateral Ligament Injury

### Etiology and Pathophysiology

The UCL has three bundles: anterior oblique, posterior oblique, and transverse ligaments, which function to provide medial elbow joint stability and resist valgus loads.[21] Repetitive tensile stress with high-velocity overhead rotation activity can create microtrauma and weakening of the anterior bundle of the UCL, leading to instability and possible rupture. Approximately 75% of UCL injuries result from contact while 25% are due to throwing injuries.[22] Despite this, throwing injuries tend to be more severe than contact injuries and more likely required surgery.[22] Men's wresting and baseball tend to produce the most number of injuries, at 1.78 per 10,000 and 1.12 per 10,000, respectively.[22]

## History

UCL injury is seen most commonly in athletes who participate in high-velocity overhead rotation activity.[21] Injuries can occur during any acute throwing event or gradually with repetitive activity. The patient will frequently complain of medial elbow pain and instability. Functionally, this may result in a decreased ability to perform overhead activities at full capacity such throwing a baseball at high speed.[21]

## Examination

The patient should be tender to palpation along the medial elbow. Special testing for a UCL injury and subsequent instability includes the Jobe test and milking maneuver. The Jobe test involves flexing the elbow to 25° with gentle stress applied to the medial side of the elbow joint. During the milking maneuver, the patient flexes his or her elbow to 90° and then with the opposite hand passed under the affected arm, pulls the affected thumb in order to stress the medial elbow. A positive test during either of these tests is considered either with pain or laxity.[23]

## Diagnostic Testing

Clinical examination with confirmatory imaging is needed for diagnosis.[21] Plain film radiographs can evaluate for avulsion fractures in acute injury and osseous remodeling in chronic injury at the medial epicondyle.[24] MRI arthrogram has a high sensitivity for detecting abnormalities of UCL.[21] However, athletes may be asymptomatic despite abnormal imaging.[21] MRI without contrast can detect full-thickness tears 100% of the time but can only detect partial tears 14% of the time.[24] US as a dynamic imaging modality is beneficial to diagnose UCL injuries. Not only can US be used statically to evaluate for a ligament partial or full-thickness thickness tear but can assess for gapping of the UCL compared with the contralateral asymptomatic elbow during valgus stress with greater than 1 mm difference being abnormal.[21,24] While US can be utilized as an effective, inexpensive, and safe modality to diagnose UCL injuries, MRI arthrography still has higher specificity and accuracy.[25]

## Treatment

The decision of treatment depends on multiple variables including the location and severity of pathology, activity level and sport, patient goals, and responsiveness to initial nonoperative care.[21] Nonoperative treatment is often tried initially for low-grade partial tears and includes rest, PT, and a brace or splint to prevent valgus stress for 8 to 12 weeks or until pain free.[24] This is followed by progression to a throwing program. Distal UCL injuries have a greater likelihood of failing nonoperative treatment.[21] PRP can also be considered for nonoperative treatment, which has shown good success in improving humeral–ulnar joint space gapping and helping athletes return to a high level of play.[26] For a complete rupture in a patient involved in high-level activity, referral to orthopedic surgery is warranted.[21] UCL reconstruction is the gold standard treatment in this scenario.[21]

## Functional Prognosis and Outcomes

PRP has shown promising results in returning athletes to sport, with some reports indicating up to 88% return to sport an average of 12 weeks post-PRP injection.[26] Regarding therapy alone, some studies have demonstrated up to 94% return to play with this modality; however, special consideration should be made for the degree of injury and comorbid conditions.[22] Postsurgical success allows the athlete to return to the same or higher level of play after procedure >75% of the time. Recovery from UCL reconstruction may take 1 year to 15 months for baseball players without complications.[21]

## Basic Order Sets

There are three phases of UCL rehab: phase 1: 1 to 2 weeks with decreasing pain/swelling, protect against valgus stress, improve ROM, and strengthen the elbow, wrist, hand, and shoulder.[21] Phase 2: 4 weeks to normalize strength and return to sports and begin proprioceptive neuromuscular facilitation with wrist/forearm strengthening.[21] Phase 3: 6 weeks to return to a throwing program. During the nonoperative period, restrict valgus or strain loading for approximately 6 weeks.[21] If asymptomatic, then one can return to a throwing program over an additional 5 to 6 weeks.

## NERVE PATHOLOGY

### Ulnar Neuropathy (Cubital Tunnel Syndrome)
### Etiology and Pathophysiology

Ulnar nerve entrapment at the elbow commonly known as "cubital tunnel syndrome" is the second most common entrapment neuropathy after carpal tunnel syndrome, affecting 24.7 cases per 100,000.[27,28] Entrapment is most common at the elbow at the cubital tunnel and may be due to tumors, ganglion cysts, fractures, osteophytes, accessory musculature, or subluxation of the ulnar nerve over the medial epicondyle with elbow flexion.[27]

### History

It is important to evaluate for repetitive elbow flexion or extension, intensive hand tool use, trauma, and pressure to the elbow.[27] Patients will often complain of decreased sensation or dysesthesias in the fourth and fifth fingers with pain in the proximal medial aspect of the elbow with work-related activities.[27] Also, sometimes individuals complain of weakness with inability to separate the fingers, decreased grip strength, or poor dexterity.[27] A history of neck symptoms should be included to rule out a cervical etiology for the patient's symptoms.

### Examination

Tapping on the ulnar nerve at the elbow (Tinel sign) can sometimes provoke symptoms.[27] Patients may have a positive Froment sign, seen as contraction of the flexor pollicis longus to compensate for a weak adductor pollicis, tested by asking the subject to hold a flat object like a piece of paper between the index finger and the thumb while the examiner tries to pull it out.[27] Patients may also have visibly evident intrinsic hand muscle atrophy especially in the first dorsal interosseous muscles and hypothenar eminence.[27] There may also be an ulnar claw posture with hyperextension of the metacarpophalangeal (MCP) in flexion of the interphalangeal (IP) joints.[27] The ulnar sensory distribution may be impaired to light touch or monofilament.[27] A comprehensive neck examination including Spurling's maneuver should be performed to rule out cervical radiculopathy.[27]

## Diagnostic Testing

Electrodiagnostic studies such as NCS/EMG are the gold standard to diagnose physiological injury of the ulnar nerve.[27] These are also useful to exclude other concurrent conditions such as median neuropathy, peripheral polyneuropathy, or cervical radiculopathy.[27] Other testing includes MRI neurography and US which can provide anatomical information about injury to the ulnar nerve including a potential area of entrapment.[27] US is also particularly beneficial in dynamic evaluation of ulnar nerve subluxation.[29]

## Treatment

Optimal treatment remains unknown at this time. Nonsurgical treatments can be considered initially for patients with early or mild symptoms such as dysesthesias, minimal motor impairment, and normal electrodiagnostic testing. These conservative treatments consist of activity modifications, nighttime splinting, and elbow padding to avoid direct compression.[27] PT exercises including nerve gliding exercises have been shown to be beneficial.[29] Surgery can be considered if there is no improvement with conservative treatment or interference with work and activities of daily living (ADLs).[27] This consists of exploration and/or transposition of the ulnar nerve around the elbow and release of compressive structures if necessary.[27]

## Functional Prognosis and Outcomes

Timing of proper diagnostics is critical for prognosis and return to work.[27] Earlier diagnosis and proper conservative treatment will result in an earlier return to work and function. While some studies have reported up to 90% of patients recover with conservative treatments in 1 to 2 years, the efficacy of which depends greatly on severity of the injury.[30] Those undergoing an ulnar nerve entrapment surgery can return to light-duty work usually within 3 weeks.[27]

## REFERENCES

The full list of references appears in the digital product found on http://connect.springerpub.com/content/book/978-0-8261-6226-7/part/part02/chapter/ch17

# WRIST AND HAND

REBECCA A. DUTTON AND PATRICIA C. SIEGEL

## INTRODUCTION

The wrist and hand consist of several articulations involving the distal radius, distal ulna, carpal, metacarpal, and phalange bones. These articulations are further stabilized and aided in motion by ligaments and tendons throughout the dorsal and volar regions of the wrist and hand. The main functions of the wrist include flexion, extension, radial deviation, and ulnar deviation. The main functions of the hand include finger flexion, extension, abduction, adductions, and thumb opposition. We will cover in more detail the most common sources of wrist and hand pain in the text. See Box 18.1 for a more comprehensive differential diagnosis of wrist and hand pain.

## BONE PATHOLOGY

### Distal Radius Fracture
### Etiology and Pathophysiology

The distal radius is the most common site of fracture in the upper extremity. Peak incidence follows a bimodal distribution, affecting the young and the elderly.[1] Among the elderly, female gender and underlying osteoporosis represent risk factors.[2] Distal radius fractures are often the result of a fall on an outstretched hand but may also arise in the setting of higher energy trauma.

### History, Examination, and Diagnostic Testing

Patients with a distal radius fracture typically present with acute wrist pain and swelling in the setting of trauma.[1] There may be visible deformity if the fracture is displaced and/or angulated. It is important to perform a focused neurovascular examination, with particular attention to distal extremity perfusion, radial and ulnar pulses, as well as median, ulnar, and radial nerve function.[1] Distal radius fractures may be readily confirmed by plain radiographs, which should include anteroposterior, lateral, and oblique views. Plain radiographs are also important to establish radial length, radial inclination, and volar tilt, which often guide subsequent management (Figure 18.1).[1,3] Advanced imaging is generally not necessary for the diagnosis of distal radius fractures in isolation. CT scan can be helpful to evaluate

---

The full list of references appears in the digital product found on http://connect.springerpub.com/content/book/978-0-8261-6226-7/part/part02/chapter/ch18

## Box 18.1

## DIFFERENTIAL DIAGNOSIS OF WRIST AND HAND PAIN

### Bone

Distal radius fracture
Distal ulna fracture
Carpal bone fracture
Metacarpal fracture
Phalange fracture
Kienböck's disease

### Tendon

De Quervain's tenosynovitis
Intersection syndrome (proximal & distal)
Flexor carpi radialis tendinopathy
Extensor carpi ulnar tendinopathy
Dupuytren's Disease
Trigger finger
Jersey finger
Mallet finger

### Ligament

Scapholunate injury
Triangular fibrocartilage complex injury
Thumb ulnar collateral ligament tear
Thumb radial collateral ligament tear

### Nerve

Carpal tunnel syndrome
Ulnar tunnel syndrome
Wartenberg's syndrome

### Other

Ganglion cyst

intra-articular involvement and for surgical planning. MRI should be considered if there is clinical concern for associated soft tissue injuries such as triangular fibrocartilage complex (TFCC) tear or extensor tendon rupture.[1]

## Treatment

The primary goal of management should be restoration of normal anatomic alignment.[3] To this end, extra-articular fractures with minimal displacement generally do not necessitate

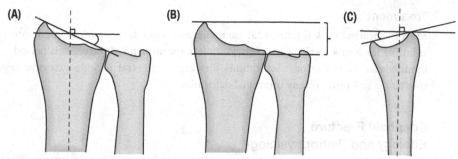

**FIGURE 18.1** Radiographic measures in the evaluation of distal radius fractures. (A) Radial inclination; (B) radial height; (C) volar tilt.

further manipulation and may be managed with immobilization in a short arm cast for 6 to 8 weeks.[3] However, displaced but extra-articular fractures warrant an attempt of closed reduction to restore alignment.[1] Adequate alignment is indicated by less than 5 mm of radial shortening, radial inclination greater than 15°, and volar tilt less than 20°.[1,3] Postreduction, patients should be immobilized in a sugar tong splint, which is maintained for 3 weeks, after which the patient may be transitioned to a short arm cast for an additional 3 to 5 weeks. Plain radiographs should be obtained weekly for the first 3 weeks and at the end of immobilization to ensure maintenance of alignment.[3] Indications for surgical referral include intra-articular, unstable, or inadequately reduced fractures as well as those associated with neurovascular injury. Referral to an occupational therapist may improve range of motion and function following a distal radius fracture.[4]

## Metacarpal Fracture
### Etiology and Pathophysiology

Metacarpal fractures are relatively common, reflecting one of the most frequent injuries of the hand.[5] The highest incidence of metacarpal fractures is observed in young men, 15 to 24 years of age.[6] Such injuries most often occur by way of a direct blow, fall, or crush mechanism. Metacarpal fractures may involve the metacarpal head, metacarpal neck, metacarpal shaft, or metacarpal base. The neck is the weakest segment of the metacarpal and most common site of fracture often a result from punching a wall, a door, or an opponent.[6] A fifth metacarpal is known as a "boxer's fracture."[5] Metacarpal fractures are also frequently sustained through sporting activities such as football, rugby, baseball, hockey, and lacrosse.[5,6]

### History, Examination, and Diagnostic Testing

Patients with metacarpal neck fractures present with acute pain and swelling over the dorsal aspect of the involved distal metacarpal. Malrotation may be indicated by digital overlap or scissoring. Rotational alignment can be readily assessed by having the patient to flex the digits toward the palm. In this position, all fingers should point toward the scaphoid tubercle.[5] Plain radiographs, including anteroposterior, lateral, and oblique views, are useful to confirm diagnosis and evaluate alignment.[6] As a general rule, acceptable angulation is limited to about 10° to 20° for the index and long finger, 30° for the ring finger, and 40° for the small finger.[6]

## Treatment

Most metacarpal neck fractures can be managed nonoperatively with closed reduction and splinting for 3 to 4 weeks. Close observation is recommended during this period to ensure maintenance of reduction.[5] Indications for surgical referral include excessive angulation, shortening (>5 mm), or any rotational deformity.[5]

## Scaphoid Fracture

### Etiology and Pathophysiology

The scaphoid serves as a mechanical bridge between the proximal and distal rows of the carpus. Blood supply to the scaphoid is derived from the radial artery, with the dorsal carpal branch supplying the proximal 70% to 80% of the scaphoid via retrograde blood flow, and the superficial palmar blanch supplying the distal 20% to 30% of the scaphoid. The distinct vascular orientation is noteworthy for increasing the risk of fracture nonunion with distal fractures.[7] The scaphoid represents the most commonly fractured carpal bone, accounting for approximately two-third of carpal fractures.[8] Scaphoid fractures are most commonly the result of a fall on an outstretched, hyperextended wrist.

### History, Examination, and Diagnostic Testing

Patients generally present with radial wrist pain.[8] Tenderness to palpation over the anatomic snuffbox or scaphoid tubercle specifically should raise concern for a scaphoid fracture. Plain radiographs including anteroposterior, lateral, and scaphoid views represent the preliminary study of choice; however, radiographs may be initially negative. Therefore, in clinically suspicious situations, patients should be immobilized and undergo serial radiographs (in 14–21 days) and/or advanced imaging (ultrasound, CT scan, or MRI) to confirm diagnosis.[7,8] In general, MRI is typically favored given a sensitivity and specificity that approaches 100% for the diagnosis of scaphoid fractures as well as the ability to assess surrounding soft tissue structures and the vascular status of the bone.[8]

### Treatment

The need for immediate immobilization in cases of suspected scaphoid fractures cannot be overemphasized. Untreated or undertreated scaphoid fractures are at high risk for nonunion, which has been reported to occur in up to 25% of cases.[8] As aforestated, initially negative radiographs do not exclude a scaphoid fracture. In such scenarios, the patient should be appropriately immobilized in a thumb spica short arm cast until a fracture is definitively confirmed; then management can be directed by the location and stability of the fracture.[7,8] Fracture stability is often defined by the Herbert classification (Table 18.1).[8] Stable and nondisplaced fractures may be managed with cast immobilization. Traditionally, a thumb spica cast has been recommended, although several studies have suggested that inclusion of the thumb is not necessary to promote healing.[9] The application of a long versus short arm cast also remains a matter of controversy. Displaced and unstable fractures necessitate surgical fixation to reduce the risk of malunion and nonunion.[8]

## TABLE 18.1 HERBERT CLASSIFICATION FOR THE STABILITY OF SCAPHOID FRACTURES

| Type A | Stable acute fractures | A1 | Fracture of the scaphoid tubercle |
| | | A2 | Incomplete fracture of the scaphoid waist |
| Type B | Unstable acute fractures | B1 | Distal oblique scaphoid fracture |
| | | B2 | Complete fracture of the scaphoid waist |
| | | B3 | Fracture of the proximal pole of the scaphoid |
| | | B4 | Trans-scaphoid-perilunate fracture dislocation of the carpus |

## Kienböck's Disease

### Etiology and Pathophysiology

Avascular necrosis of the lunate is known as Kienböck's disease. The development of avascular necrosis of the lunate is believed to be multifactorial in nature and likely related at least in part to a combination of mechanical stress and predisposing anatomical factors including variations in vascular supply.[10] Kienböck's disease is observed most commonly in men, between the ages of 20 and 40 years, and is usually unilateral.[10,11]

### History, Examination, and Diagnostic Testing

The diagnosis of Kienböck's disease may be suggested by a history of insidious onset dorsal wrist pain. Pain is often worse with activity. Patients commonly report diminished grip strength.[10] On physical examination, there may be appreciable wrist swelling, as well as tenderness to palpation over the lunate and radiocarpal joint. Diagnosis is confirmed through imaging. Plain radiographs are often sufficient to establish diagnosis and grade the severity of necrosis (Table 18.2).[10] However, MRI may be necessary for diagnosis in early stages of the disease. CT scan, on the other hand, is often used in later stages once lunate collapse has occurred in order to demonstrate the extent of necrosis and lunate fragmentation.[10]

## TABLE 18.2 STAGES OF KIENBÖCK'S DISEASE

| STAGE | IMAGING FINDINGS |
| --- | --- |
| Stage I | No appreciable changes on plain radiographs<br>MRI demonstrates reduced T1 signal within the lunate |
| Stage II | Lunate sclerosis, without significant change in shape |
| Stage IIIa | Lunate collapse, without scaphoid rotation |
| Stage IIIb | Lunate collapse, diminished carpal height, and fixed palmar flexion of the scaphoid |
| Stage IV | Adjacent degenerative changes of the intercarpal joints |

## Treatment

Individuals with early (stage I) Kienböck's disease should be managed with an initial period of immobilization with splinting or casting. However, patients with persistent symptoms or radiographic progression despite immobilization or those with more advanced disease should be referred for surgical evaluation.[10] A decision regarding surgical approach is based on a variety of factors including osseous morphology, cartilage integrity, and lunate vascularity.[11]

## TENDON PATHOLOGY

### De Quervain Tenosynovitis
### Etiology and Pathophysiology

De Quervain tenosynovitis is a condition characterized by tenosynovitis involving the first dorsal extensor compartment of the wrist.[12] The first dorsal extensor compartment is located at the level of the radial styloid and contains the abductor pollicis longus (APL) and extensor pollicis brevis (EPB) tendons.[12] De Quervain tenosynovitis is thought to result from friction or trauma that causes subsequent swelling and thickening of the extensor retinaculum covering the first dorsal compartment. This in turn leads to a narrowed fibro-osseous canal and resisted tendon gliding within the compartment.[13]

De Quervain tenosynovitis is up to three to six times more common in women than men and more often affects individuals in middles age (fourth–sixth decades). It has been especially associated with pregnancy and the postpartum period as well as with activities involving repeated radioulnar deviation, such as hammering, cross-country skiing, racquet sports, golfing, and repetitive lifting. De Quervain tenosynovitis more typically involves the dominant hand.[12]

### History, Examination, and Diagnostic Testing

Diagnosis is often clinical. Patients report dorsal radial-sided wrist pain that tends to be worse when gripping or lifting objects with the wrist in a neutral position. They may also describe swelling about the radial wrist.[13] On physical examination, there is generally focal tenderness to palpation directly over the first dorsal compartment at the radial styloid. Pain may also be exacerbated by resisted thumb movements (particularly extension or abduction) or radial deviation of the wrist.[14] Finklestein test is performed by having the patient grasp their thumb followed by passive ulnar deviation of the hand and wrist. Reproduction of pain with this test is suggestive of de Quervain tenosynovitis.[12] Imaging studies are rarely necessary. However, plain radiographs may have utility to detect contributing bony changes such as bone spurs and also to exclude mimicking diagnoses including basilar arthritis of the thumb, radiocarpal arthritis, or wrist fractures.[13,14] Ultrasound can further support the diagnosis with typical findings of thickening of the extensor retinaculum, distension of fluid within the tendon sheath, and hyperemia within the tendon sheath on color doppler.[15]

### Treatment

Conservative treatment should be tried first. This should include activity modification, ice, and NSAIDs or acetaminophen for pain control.[12] A period of immobilization in a forearm-based thumb spica splint with the wrist in neutral and thumb in 30° of flexion and 30° of abduction is typically recommended.[12] Consideration may be given to an injection targeting the tendon sheath for more severe or recalcitrant symptoms with ultrasound guidance recommended. Surgical referral for first dorsal compartment release may be necessary in severe cases and/or ≥6 months of failed conservative treatment.

Preventative strategies including education, ergonomic or postural correction, and sufficient work breaks have been purported, although there is little evidence currently to support their efficacy.[16]

## Proximal Intersection Syndrome
### Etiology and Pathophysiology

Proximal intersection syndrome refers to tenosynovitis at the site of crossover (or intersection) of the first and second dorsal extensor compartments of the wrist, which occurs approximately 4 to 6 cm proximal to the radial styloid.[14,17] The first dorsal extensor compartment contains the APL and EPB, while the second dorsal extensor compartment contains the extensor carpi radialis longus and brevis tendons. It is believed that repetitive flexion and extension at the wrist can result in friction between the two compartments, ultimately producing an inflammatory response and subsequent tenosynovitis, predominantly involving the second dorsal extensor compartment.[14,17] Individuals engaging in activities that involve repetitive wrist flexion and extension are at greater risk such as rowers, weightlifters, skiers, horseback riders, tennis players, and racquetball players.[17]

### History, Examination, and Diagnostic Testing

On history, patients typically describe dorsal radial-sided wrist and forearm pain with possible swelling over this region. On physical examination, tenderness and localized swelling may be apparent approximately 4 cm proximal to the radial styloid. Pain may be recreated by passive ulnar deviation of the hand or by resisted wrist extension and/or resisted forearm pronation.[17] Imaging with ultrasound may be useful to support the diagnosis and can reveal tendon thickening, fluid within the tendon sheaths as well as peritendinous edema where the first compartment passes over the second.[18] Plain radiographs or advanced imaging such as CT or MRI is indicated primarily to exclude other osseous or soft tissue pathologies.[17]

### Treatment

Initial management should emphasize conservative strategies including activity modification as well as ice, NSAIDs, or acetaminophen for pain control.[14] A course of immobilization in a forearm-based splint in slight wrist extension may be helpful.[14] Should symptoms persist despite these measures, consideration may be given to a corticosteroid injection, targeting the intersection of the first and second dorsal extensor compartments, under ultrasound guidance.[17] Very rarely, in cases refractory to an appropriate course of conservative care, surgical referral for debridement and second dorsal compartment release may be necessary.[14,17] Currently, there are no well-established guidelines for the prevention of intersection syndrome.

## Extensor Carpi Ulnaris Tendinopathy and Subluxation
### Etiology and Pathophysiology

The extensor carpi ulnaris (ECU) assists with wrist extension (particularly when the forearm is supinated) and ulnar deviation and provides both static and dynamic stability to the wrist.[14] The ECU tendon is contained within the sixth dorsal extensor compartment and lies within the groove of the distal ulna and superficial to the TFCC.[14] Injuries of the ECU tenon include tendinopathy, tenosynovitis, and instability. The tendon may be prone to tendinopathy or tenosynovitis in situations of repetitive wrist flexion and extension, especially in supination whereby tension on the retinaculum and subsheath is amplified.[19] Tendon instability or subluxation is the result of frank disruption to the ECU subsheath.[19] ECU injuries reported most commonly in tennis players and golfers.[19]

### History, Examination, and Diagnostic Testing

ECU tendinopathy presents as insidious onset pain over the dorsal ulnar wrist, which may be worse with gripping or heavy activities.[19] ECU subluxation may be preceded by a discrete history of trauma. In addition to ulnar-sided wrist pain, patients may describe a snapping sensation with active wrist movement.[19] On physical examination, there is often focal tenderness to palpation over the ECU tendon. Symptoms (pain and/or snapping) may be reproduced by resisted wrist extension with the forearm in supination.[14] As with most tendinopathies of the wrist, the diagnosis of ECU tendinopathy and/or subluxation is clinical; however, MRI or ultrasound may be considered to confirm diagnosis. Ultrasound has the added value of comparison to the contralateral side in cases of early or subtle tendinopathy as well as dynamic evaluation to assess for tendon instability.[19]

### Treatment

Management should include a trial of conservative measures including activity modification, ice, and NSAIDs or acetaminophen for pain control.[14] A 3- to 4-week course of immobilization in a splint or cast with the wrist in 30° of extension and ulnar deviation may be worthwhile.[19] In addition, a peritendinous injection under ultrasound guidance may have diagnostic and therapeutic value in the management of ECU tendinopathy.[14]

An initial conservative approach is similarly appropriate in cases of ECU subluxation.[19] In the acute setting, tendon reduction followed by immobilization for 6 weeks is suggested. Some advocate use of a long arm cast with the forearm in pronation to promote tendon position within the dorsal ulnar groove, although there is no clear evidence to support one form of immobilization over another.[19,20] Immobilization should be followed by progressive range of motion and strengthening.[19] Surgical referral is appropriate for symptoms of ECU tendinopathy and/or subluxation that are refractory to conservative care.[14,19]

## Dupuytren's Disease
### Etiology and Pathophysiology

The palmar fascia is a triangular structure that covers the underlying hand muscles with extension to the digits. Dupuytren's disease is a condition characterized by progressive fibrosis and thickening of the palmar fascia. Fibroblast infiltration and abnormal collagen deposition lead to the formation of nodules and cords along the fascial bands.[21] This results in contracture and restricted extension of the involved digit(s).

Dupuytren's disease is inherited in an autosomal dominant pattern with variable penetrance. It is observed more frequently in men than women, and incidence increases with age. Additional environmental risk factors include a history of alcohol use, smoking, diabetes mellitus, and manual labor, especially occupations involving vibratory exposure.[21,22] Contractures typically arise at the metacarpophalangeal and proximal interphalangeal joints (PIPJs). The ring finger is the most frequently affected digit.[22]

## History, Examination, and Diagnostic Testing

Patients with Dupuytren's disease will often describe insidious development of painful nodules in the palmar hand, which may be associated with reduced range of motion and impaired daily function.[21] The diagnosis is confirmed by physical examination. In earlier phases of the disease, inspection and palpation may reveal hard nodules within the palmar fascia and puckering of the skin. As the condition progresses, patients may develop contractures at the metacarpophalangeal and PIPJs. This can be readily assessed by Hueston's tabletop test whereby the patient is asked to place the palm of the affected hand on a table and will be unable to fully flatten the fingers.[22] At the time of physical examination, it is also important to evaluate for bilateral involvement as well as ectopic presentations such as Ledderhose disease (plantar fibromatosis), Garrod's pads (dorsal proximal interphalangeal fibromatosis), or Peyronie's disease, as such conditions have been associated with a worse prognosis and higher risk of recurrence.[22] Imaging studies are rarely indicated in the diagnosis of Dupuytren's disease.

## Treatment

A variety of management strategies are available and based on patient preference, disease severity, cost-effectiveness, risk of complications, and concern for recurrence.[22,23] In mild cases, without apparent contracture, stretching and range of motion exercises may be recommended.[22] In addition, minimally invasive procedures such as *Clostridium histolyticum* collagenase (CCH) injection or needle aponeurotomy can play a role in the management of mild-to-moderate disease. CCH injection delivers an enzyme locally to breakdown the collagen and facilitate manual rupture of the cord.[23] CCH injection is more effective in managing metacarpophalangeal joint (MCPJ) over PIPJ contractures and is associated with relatively low risk of complication. Needle aponeurotomy involves needle insertion and disruption to the cord under local anesthesia followed by manual manipulation and rupture.[23] Needle aponeurotomy is similarly more effective in managing MCPJ over PIPJ contractures. CCH injections are more expensive than needle aponeurotomy, may require multiple procedures, and should only be performed on a single cord.[22,23] Potential injection complications include skin damage, digital nerve injury, and tendon rupture. In more advanced disease, surgical fasciotomy should be considered.[22,23] As a general rule, fasciotomy is recommended for any flexion contracture >30° at the MCPJ, flexion contracture >15° at the PIPJ, or significant impairment in hand function and activities of daily living.

## Trigger Finger

### Etiology and Pathophysiology

The flexor digitorum superficialis and flexor digitorum profundus tendons are surrounded by a tendon sheath that is comprised of five annular and three cruciform pulleys. This construct serves to maintain tendon alignment and reduce tendon friction during finger flexion and extension.[24] Stenosing flexor tenosynovitis, or trigger finger, refers to a condition resulting from narrowing of the flexor pulley sheaths, often in combination with hypertrophy and inflammation at the tendon sheath and pulley interface.[25] This results in abnormal flexor tendon gliding and arises most commonly at the first annular (A1) pulley sheath, at the level of the MCPJ.[25] Trigger finger can affect both children and adults. In adults, trigger finger is associated with chronic repetitive use. Other risk factors include diabetes mellitus, thyroid disease, amyloidosis, and rheumatoid arthritis.[25] Peak incidence is between age 40 and 60 years and women are more affected than men. The ring finger is the most commonly involved digit in adults.[25]

### History, Examination, and Diagnostic Testing

Patients with trigger finger classically report pain at the base of the digit as well as clicking, catching, or locking of the affected digit. Patients may report that their finger becomes stuck in a flexed position.[26] Physical examination reveals triggering of the digit with flexion and extension. More advanced cases may present with a nodule at the affected region and a fixed flexion contracture.[24,27] The diagnosis of trigger finger is largely clinical, though ultrasound can have utility and typically reveals thickening of the pulley with sometimes flexor tenosynovitis or tendinosis.[27] Dynamic assessment may further demonstrate abnormal motion of the flexor tendon at the pulley interface.[25]

### Treatment

Earlier or more mild cases of trigger finger are often managed initially with conservative measures including massage, NSAIDs, and nighttime splinting with a metacarpophalangeal blocking splint at 10° to 15°.[24] Other conservative splint options include splinting the metacarpophalangeal joint (MP) in 15° flexion for 6 weeks or limiting the excursion of the flexor digitorum profundus by splinting the distal interphalangeal joint (DIPJ) in extension.[28,29] A ultrasound-guided corticosteroid injection at the tendon sheath and pulley interface can also be helpful for a subset of patients.[24,27] It is worth noting that corticosteroid injections seem to be less effective in those with more chronic (>6 months) or severe symptoms, involvement of multiple digits, and/or a history of diabetes mellitus.[24] Surgical referral for consideration of pulley release should be considered for cases recalcitrant to conservative measures and more severe cases including fixed flexion contractures.[24,27] Ultrasound-guided percutaneous pulley release has also been developed with efficacious and safe results.

## Jersey Finger

### Etiology and Pathophysiology

Jersey finger describes an avulsion injury of the flexor digitorum profundus tendon from its insertion at the base of the distal phalanx.[30,31] The injury is especially common in contact sports, arising as a result of forced extension on a flexed digit, as can occur when the finger becomes caught in a jersey when attempting to grab or tackle an opponent.[30,32] The ring finger is the most commonly involved digit, reflecting up to 75% of cases.[31]

### History, Examination, and Diagnostic Testing

Jersey finger presents with acute pain following the aforementioned mechanism of forced extension on a flexed digit. Tenderness to palpation is particularly pronounced over the volar distal finger, and in some cases, the retracted tendon may be palpated more proximally.[31] At rest, the finger appears slightly extended relative to the surrounding digits. The patient will be unable to actively flex the affected digit at the DIPJ.[31] Plain radiographs are important to evaluate for bony involvement in the form of an avulsion fragment.[30,31] Advanced imaging, either with ultrasound or MRI, can have utility to evaluate the degree of tendon retraction, particularly in more chronic cases.[31]

### Treatment

Jersey finger injuries require a prompt referral to a hand surgeon for operative repair to prevent long-term morbidity.[31,32]

## Mallet Finger
### Etiology and Pathophysiology

Mallet finger refers to an injury resulting from disruption of the terminal extensor tendon near its insertion distal to the DIPJ.[32,33] The injury is common in sports, however, may also arise in the setting of work-related or household activities, such as tucking in a sheet on a bed or from a laceration.[34] The injury is typically caused by direct axial impact to the fingertip when the distal phalanx is in active extension.[32]

### History, Examination, and Diagnostic Testing

Patients can usually recall a clear mechanism for injury, typically characterized by traumatic impaction to the fingertip. On examination, patients will have tenderness and a flexion deformity at the DIPJ, with an inability to actively extend the distal phalanx at the level of the DIPJ.[34] Plain radiographs are important to exclude concomitant avulsion fractures or volar subluxation of the distal phalanx.[33,34]

### Treatment

Nonoperative management, comprised of DIPJ immobilization, is indicated for purely tendinous injuries, nondisplaced injuries, and injuries that involve less the 30% of the articular surface.[32,33] The DIPJ should be immobilized in full extension, generally allowing for free movement at the PIPJ. A variety of splints have been proposed including volar-based Stack splints and cylinder casts with comparable outcomes.[32,33] Splinting should be maintained around the clock, 24 hours per day, for at least 6 to 8 weeks followed by several additional weeks of nighttime splinting.[32,33] Continuous immobilization at the outset is imperative. Should a patient have any disruption in immobilization, it is recommended that the process recommence from the beginning.[33] Referral to a hand surgeon is necessary for all open injuries, as well as any injuries associated with volar subluxation or bony avulsion involving more than 30% of the articular surface.

## LIGAMENT PATHOLOGY

### Scapholunate Ligament Injury

### Etiology and Pathophysiology

The scapholunate (SL) interosseous ligament is an intrinsic ligament of the wrist that bridges the scaphoid and lunate bones. The ligament is comprised of dorsal, proximal, and volar segments, of which the dorsal segment is the most critical to prevent excessive translation between the two bones. Injury to the SL ligament represents an important and common cause of carpal instability.[35] SL ligament injuries can occur acutely, typically in the setting of forced wrist extension and ulnar deviation or a fall on an outstretched hand.[35] However, degenerative processes such as rheumatoid arthritis can also result in chronic SL ligament incompetence.

### History, Examination, and Diagnostic Testing

Patients present with dorsoradial wrist pain and/or swelling. Pain may be exacerbated by activities that load the wrist such as performing a push-up. Additional symptoms may include wrist clicking or reduced grip strength.[35] Physical examination may reveal tenderness to palpation over the anatomic snuffbox or the dorsal SL interval. Watson shift test is performed by applying pressure over the scaphoid tuberosity while deviating the wrist from an ulnar to radial position. Dorsal wrist pain or a palpable clunk represents a positive test and may indicate SL ligament instability.[35] Plain radiographs are important to confirm diagnosis and should include both neutral and stress views. At a minimum, a neutral posterior-anterior (PA) and lateral view should be obtained. Common stress views include PA clenched fist and PA in radial and ulnar deviation. SL ligament injury is indicated by SL interval widening of >3 mm on neutral or stress PA views or an SL angle >70° on the lateral view. Injuries may be categorized radiographically by the Watson classification (Table 18.3).[36] Advanced imaging with ultrasound or MRI may have utility when plain radiographs are unyielding.[35] Diagnostic arthroscopy remains the gold standard for diagnosis.[36]

### Treatment

A trial of nonoperative management may be reasonable for acute, stable SL ligament injuries as well as chronic asymptomatic injuries. This includes 4 to 6 weeks of immobilization

### TABLE 18.3 WATSON CLASSIFICATION OF SCAPHOLUNATE INSTABILITY

| CLASSIFICATION | DEFINITION |
|---|---|
| Predynamic instability | No abnormalities evident on plain radiographs<br>Ligament tear present on advanced imaging or at time of surgery |
| Dynamic instability | Scapholunate widening present on stress radiographs only |
| Static dissociation | Scapholunate widening present on neutral, nonstress radiographs |
| Scapholunate advanced collapse | Scapholunate widening and displaced scaphoid as well as arthritic changes apparent on plain radiographs |

with splinting or casting followed by a progressive rehabilitation program.[35-37] For unstable injuries or those that fail conservative treatment, surgical approach is determined by the severity and chronicity of injury as well as the presence or absence of degenerative changes.[35,36]

## Triangular Fibrocartilage Complex Injury
### Etiology and Pathophysiology

The TFCC is located between the lunate, triquetrum, and ulnar head and is comprised of the triangular fibrocartilage disc, meniscal homologue, dorsal and volar radioulnar ligaments, ulnotriquetral and ulnolunate ligaments, ulnocarpal collateral ligament, and the ECU tendon subsheath.[38] Collectively, the TFCC acts as a stabilizer to the ulnar wrist.[39] Risk factors for injury include activities involving repetitive forced ulnar deviation (as may occur when swinging a bat or club) and positive ulnar variance.[38,39]

### History, Examination, and Diagnostic Testing

Patients typically localize pain to the ulnar aspect of the wrist. The pain may be made worse by activities that load the wrist or pronation/supination activities such as turning a key.[26] On physical examination, pain may be elicited through TFCC compression, by pronating the wrist with ulnar deviation, and axial loading. A positive fovea sign refers to the reproduction of pain with deep palpation over the TFCC.[39] Plain radiographs may be helpful to identify positive ulnar variance, a well-established risk factor for TFCC injury. Radiographs may also reveal an ulnar styloid fracture, which can similarly indicate risk for TFCC injury.[17] Current consensus favors MRI over MR arthrography to further assess the TFCC, although ultimately, wrist arthroscopy reflects the gold standard for the diagnosis of TFCC tears.[39,40]

### Treatment

In the absence of overt instability of the distal radioulnar joint, both acute and chronic TFCC injuries may be managed initially with a conservative approach.[26] Appropriate measures include activity modification and immobilization with a volar wrist splint or short arm cast followed by progressive occupational therapy.[38] Corticosteroid injections to the TFCC or radiocarpal joint are considered in some cases to facilitate pain relief.[26] Referral to a hand surgeon should be considered for cases refractory to the aforementioned strategies.[38]

## Thumb Ulnar Collateral Ligament Tear
### Etiology and Pathophysiology

The MCPJ of the thumb is a diarthrodial joint that functions primarily in flexion and extension and is important in facilitating gripping and pinching motions.[41,42] The UCL is important to uphold lateral stability of the MCPJ which resists radial-directed forces.[42,43] The UCL may be injured as a consequence of chronic repetitive valgus stress (so-called "gamekeeper's thumb") or in the setting of acute hyperabduction or hyperextension of the MCPJ (so-called "skier's thumb").[41,42]

## History, Examination, and Diagnostic Testing

Patients present with acute or insidious onset of pain about the ulnar aspect of the MCPJ. Patients may also report difficulty moving the thumb or weakness and/or instability with grip.[44] Acute cases are typically accompanied by a history of trauma as well as swelling and/or bruising. On physical examination, pain may be reproduced with direct palpation over the ulnar aspect of the MCPJ. A palpable mass in this region is concerning for a Stener lesion (see more in the rest of this section).[41] Stress examination of the MCP should be undertaken to assess ligament integrity. This involves stabilizing the metacarpal while applying a radially directed force to the proximal phalanx in both full extension as well as 30° of flexion, to test both the accessory and proper collateral ligament, respectively.[43] The absence of a firm endpoint or a side-to-side difference of 10° to 15° of laxity is suggestive of a complete injury.[43,44]

Anteroposterior and lateral radiographs are recommended for all patients with a suspected UCL injury. In fact, it is generally suggested that radiographs be obtained prior to undertaking a full physical examination in order to first exclude the presence metacarpal fractures.[41,42] In the context of a UCL injury, plain radiographs may demonstrate MCPJ instability (reflected by radial or volar subluxation of the proximal phalanx) and/or an associated avulsion fracture.[41] Advanced imaging, such as MRI or ultrasound, should be considered to confirm diagnosis and quantify the extent of injury. UCL injuries may be classified as grade I (sprained but intact ligament), grade II (partial-thickness ligament tear), or grade III (full-thickness or complete ligament tear). Grade III injuries may be associated with ligament avulsion, with or without the bony attachment, superficial to the adductor aponeurosis. This is referred to as a Stener lesion and is important to recognize as one indication for surgical referral and repair.[42] Both MRI and ultrasound have demonstrated relatively high sensitivity and specificity in the diagnosis of partial and complete UCL tears. Ultrasound is often more readily available, cost-effective, and allows for dynamic evaluation, however, demonstrates more variable diagnostic accuracy.[41]

## Treatment

As a general rule, grade I and grade II UCL injuries may be managed with a conservative approach focused on early immobilization in a thumb spica cast or splint for 4 to 6 weeks. It has been suggested that the thumb should be immobilized in mild flexion and ulnar deviation at the MCPJ.[44] The interphalangeal joint is typically permitted to move freely in order to limit stiffening.[41,44] After an appropriate course of immobilization, occupational therapy is recommended to first emphasize range of motion, followed by progressive strengthening exercises.[41,44] On average, patients are able to return to full, unrestricted activity about 12 weeks after injury.[41] Grade III injuries and/or the presence of a Stener lesion should be referred to a hand surgeon for surgical repair or reconstruction. Typically, acute injuries (within 3–5 weeks) are considered for ligament repair, while more chronic injuries necessitate ligament reconstruction.[41]

## NERVE PATHOLOGY

### Carpal Tunnel Syndrome
### Etiology and Pathophysiology

The carpal tunnel is formed by the carpal bones and transverse ligament. Important bony landmarks include the scaphoid tubercle and trapezium radially and the hook of the hamate and pisiform ulnarly. The carpal tunnel contains the flexor digitorum superficialis and profundus tendons, the flexor pollicis longus tendon, and the median nerve. Tenosynovitis, hormonal changes, and/or manual activity can yield compression and injury to the median nerve within the carpal tunnel, resulting in so-called "carpal tunnel syndrome."[45]

Carpal tunnel syndrome reflects the most common entrapment neuropathy, affecting up to 1 in 10 individuals.[45,46] In general, carpal tunnel syndrome is considered to be more common in women. Both pregnancy and menopause have been associated with the condition, which has contributed to the notion that hormonal changes may be causative.[45] Other risk factors include hypothyroidism, rheumatoid arthritis, diabetes mellitus, obesity, tobacco smoking, and advancing age.[45,46] While historically implicated in the development of carpal tunnel syndrome, the role of computer use is controversial with recent studies failing to demonstrate a clear association.[45]

### History, Examination, and Diagnostic Testing

The diagnosis of carpal tunnel syndrome is characterized by classic clinical findings of hand paresthesias, pain, and possibly weakness.[45,46] Initially, patients will often report intermittent, nocturnal dysesthesias and paresthesias. Over time, symptoms may become more frequent and occur during waking hours.[45] The distribution of sensory symptoms is expected to involve the radial 3 1/2 digits, although, patients often report more diffuse symptoms in the hand. Moreover, the symptoms can spread proximally to the forearm and upper arm.[45] Over time, individuals may experience frank loss of sensation as well as hand weakness.[45,46] Inspection of the hand may reveal selective atrophy of the thenar eminence in more advanced cases. Physical examination should also include carpal tunnel compression (Durkan's) test. The test is performed by applying direct pressure over the carpal tunnel for 30 seconds. Reproduction of pain or paresthesias represents a positive test.[47] Phalen's test (flexion of the wrist against gravity) and Tinel's test (percussion of the median nerve over the carpal tunnel) are generally less sensitive and specific in the diagnosis of carpal tunnel syndrome.[45]

Confirmatory testing may be undertaken via electrodiagnostic assessment or nerve ultrasonography. Electrodiagnostic evaluation is highly sensitive and provides physiologic data regarding the extent of demyelination and axonal loss. Nerve conduction studies demonstrate prolonged sensory and/or motor latencies, as well as possibly amplitude loss in more severe cases.[48] Electromyography similarly may demonstrate evidence of axonal loss (abnormal spontaneous activity and/or abnormal volitional motor unit morphology), namely of the abductor pollicis brevis, in more severe cases.[48] A grading system, based on the electrodiagnostic findings, has been proposed (Table 18.4) and may be useful to help predict outcome after surgery. However, it is worth noting that the severity of clinical symptoms does not clearly associate with electrophysiologic severity.[48]

**TABLE 18.4 ELECTRODIAGNOSTIC SEVERITY OF CARPAL TUNNEL SYNDROME**

| DIAGNOSTIC SEVERITY | MEDIAN SNAP | MEDIAN CMAP | ELECTROMYOGRAPHY (TO APB) |
|---|---|---|---|
| MILD | Prolonged latency | Normal latency | Normal |
| MODERATE | Prolonged latency | Prolonged latency | Normal |
| SEVERE | Low amplitude/ absent | Low amplitude/ absent | Fibrillation potentials, or Motor unit potential changes |

APB, abductor pollicis brevis; CMAP, compound motor action potential; SNAP, sensory nerve action potential.

Nerve ultrasound may be utilized to provide anatomic data about the median nerve to support the diagnosis of carpal tunnel syndrome.[49,50] Specifically, an increased cross-sectional area (CSA) measured at the carpal tunnel inlet, or level of the pisiform, is consistent with the diagnosis of carpal tunnel syndrome. A cutoff value of 1.0 to 1.2 $cm^2$ is typically used.[49] A CSA difference of >2 mm between the median nerve at the level of the pronator quadratus and carpal tunnel inlet may also have utility in diagnosis.[50] Other supportive sonographic findings may include a loss abrupt flattening of the nerve at the site of compression, loss of the normal fascicular echotexture of the nerve, and hypervascularity in and around the nerve.[50]

## Treatment

Conservative management comprised of activity modification, splinting, and pain management is considered first line for carpal tunnel syndrome in the absence of significant motor deficits. Avoiding repetitive wrist movement and ergonomic modifications to reduce median nerve stress can be helpful.[45]

A neutral or cock-up wrist splint can be prescribed, particularly at night to address nocturnal symptoms.[46] NSAIDs, acetaminophen, or neuropathic medications may be useful adjuvants for pain control.[45,46] An ultrasound-guided median perineural steroid injection and hydrodissection at the carpal tunnel can be both diagnostic and therapeutic. Surgery should be considered in cases refractory to conservative care, more severe cases that involve motor deficits, and in acute traumatic cases (e.g., following open reduction and internal fixation of a distal radius fracture).[45] Surgical decompression is achieved by transection of the transverse carpal ligament. Ultrasound-guided carpal tunnel release has also been developed with efficacious and safe results.

Evidence for effective prevention strategies in carpal tunnel syndrome is generally sparse; however, reducing occupational risk through ergonomic modification has long been purported.[46] Known risk factors include occupations involving forceful repetitive hand and wrist movements, vibration, and/or cold exposure. Given the association between obesity and carpal tunnel syndrome, weight loss, particularly in high-risk workers, has also been recommended for prevention.[46]

## Ulnar Tunnel Syndrome

### Etiology and Pathophysiology

The ulnar tunnel (also known as Guyon's canal) begins at the proximal aspect of the palmar carpal ligament and ends at the aponeurotic arch of the hypothenar muscles, at the level of the hook of the hamate. The boundaries of the tunnel vary along its course but regardless contain the ulnar nerve, ulnar artery, and ulnar vein. Within the tunnel, the ulnar nerve bifurcates into a superficial branch and a deep motor branch. The superficial branch supplies the palmaris brevis and also provides sensation to the hypothenar eminence and ulnar 1 1/2 digits (little finger and ulnar aspect of the ring finger). The deep motor branch innervates the interossei, third and fourth lumbricals, hypothenar muscles (abductor digiti minimi, opponens digiti minimi, and flexor brevis digiti minimi) as well as the adductor pollicis and medial head of the flexor pollicis brevis.[51] Compression of the ulnar nerve at the ulnar tunnel may result from a variety of factors including but not necessarily limited to ganglion cysts, repetitive trauma, ulnar artery thrombosis or aneurysm, hamate fracture, arthritis, palmaris brevis hypertrophy, or fibrous bands.[51]

The incidence of ulnar tunnel syndrome is poorly defined; however, it seems to occur much less frequently than carpal tunnel syndrome or ulnar neuropathy at the elbow. At-risk populations include cyclists, baseball catchers, and those engaging in racquet or club sports such as tennis, golf, and hockey.[51] Occupations that predispose to repetitive wrist trauma, such as hammering, are another risk factor.[51] Finally, wheelchair use has been associated with higher rates of ulnar tunnel syndrome.[52]

### History, Examination, and Diagnostic Testing

Presenting symptoms are determined by the level of compression and involved branches of the ulnar nerve. Clinical presentation may be purely sensory, purely motor, or a combination.[51] Common complaints include ulnar-sided pain, paresthesias, and weakness of the hand intrinsics and finger abduction, ring and small finger flexion, and/or thumb adduction. Typically, sensory symptoms should spare the dorsal ulnar hand, which is supplied by the dorsal ulnar cutaneous nerve proximal to the ulnar tunnel.[51] Physical examination may similarly reveal impaired sensation in the distribution of the superficial branch of the ulnar nerve, including the hypothenar eminence and ulnar 1 1/2 digits, with relative sparing of the dorsal ulnar hand. Tinel's sign over the pisiform of hamate may reproduce symptoms to the ulnar hand. In addition, there may be selective wasting of the hypothenar eminence, interossei, and/or clawing of the ring and little fingers.[51] Functionally, intrinsic hand weakness can be demonstrated by difficulty crossing fingers. Individuals may also demonstrate weakness in grip or pinch. Wartenberg's sign refers to involuntary abduction posturing of the little finger due to unopposed action of the radial-innervated extensor digiti minimi. Froment's sign is assessed by having the patient pinch a piece of paper between the thumb and index finger. A positive Froment's sign is indicated by hyperflexion of the thumb at the interphalangeal joint to compensate for weakness of the ulnar-innervated adductor pollicis.

Imaging studies are useful to identify anatomic causes of ulnar nerve compression at the wrist. Plain radiographs may demonstrate fractures or osteoarthritis, while MRI can identify ganglion cysts, soft tissue masses, aberrant musculature, or vascular lesions.[51] Ultrasound also has an evolving role in demonstrating anatomic causes of compression such as ganglia, while also elucidating findings consistent with nerve compression including increased CSA and loss of normal echotexture.[50,51] Electrodiagnostic studies can provide physiologic data about the injured ulnar nerve and confirm the diagnosis. Nerve conduction studies may demonstrate reduced ulnar sensory responses recording to digit 5, with preservation of dorsal ulnar cutaneous responses. As well, there may be prolonged motor latencies or reduced amplitudes recording to the abductor digiti minimi and/or first dorsal interosseous.[51] Electromyography may also demonstrate evidence of axonal loss (abnormal spontaneous activity and/or abnormal volitional motor unit morphology) involving the abductor digiti minimi and/or first dorsal interosseous.

## Treatment

A trial of nonoperative management is an appropriate, first-line approach in milder cases of ulnar tunnel syndrome without motor deficits. Strategies include activity modification to avoid provocative activities, splinting, and NSAIDs or acetaminophen for pain control.[51] Padded gloves or gel pads may also provide some relief by distributing pressure over the hypothenar eminence. Cyclists should be evaluated for bicycle fit with particular attention to, and possible modification of, handlebar position.[51] Surgical decompression should be considered in recalcitrant or more severe cases (with apparent motor involvement) and in situations involving an organic cause of compression, such as a ganglion cyst.[51]

## REFERENCES

The full list of references appears in the digital product found on http://connect.springerpub.com/content/book/978-0-8261-6226-7/part/part02/chapter/ch18

# HIP AND PELVIS

EUGENE L. PALATULAN, XIAONING YUAN, CAROLINE A. SCHEPKER, AND
CHRISTOPHER J. VISCO

## INTRODUCTION

The hip and pelvis consist of several articulations including the hip, pubic symphysis, and sacroiliac joints. The hip joint consists of an articulation between the acetabulum of the pelvis and the head of the femur. A capsule surrounds the entire joint with hyaline cartilage covering both of these osseous structures. A fibrocartilage labrum is further interposed between the hip joint with attachment to the acetabulum. The hip functions to move the lower extremity through complex, diverse ranges of motion including flexion, extension, abduction, adduction, external, and internal rotation. These motions are aided by several muscle and tendons throughout the anterior, medial, lateral, and posterior hip and pelvis region. The hip is inherently a stable joint but still highly prone to both acute and degenerative injury. We will cover in more detail the most common sources of hip and pelvis pain in the text. See Box 19.1 for a more comprehensive differential diagnosis of hip and pelvis pain.

## JOINT PATHOLOGY

### Labral Tears
### Etiology and Pathophysiology

Labral tears are found across all age groups and commonly in active females, especially those with acetabular dysplasia. The most common location of tears is the anterosuperior labrum. Etiology is multifactorial, including trauma, dysplasia, capsular laxity, osteoarthritis (OA), and femoroacetabular impingement (FAI).[1] Tears can cause pain and intra-articular snapping hip syndrome, though they can also be asymptomatic.

### History, Examination, and Diagnostic Testing

Diagnosis begins with a thorough history and physical examination, including inspection, palpation, and range of motion (ROM). Most patients present with anterior hip and groin pain. Provocative maneuvers include the hip scour and flexion, adduction, and internal rotation (FADIR), an anterior hip impingement test. A 3-Tesla MRI without contrast is now the preferred diagnostic imaging tool, although arthrography was recommended in the past.[1]

The full list of resources and references appears in the digital product found on http://connect .springerpub.com/content/book/978-0-8261-6226-7/part/part02/chapter/ch19

### BOX 19.1

## DIFFERENTIAL DIAGNOSIS OF HIP AND PELVIS PAIN

**Diagnoses**

**Joint**

Avascular necrosis
Hip dislocation
Hip dysplasia
Labral tear
Osteitis pubis
Sacroiliac dysfunction

**Bone**

Acetabular fracture
Femoral neck fracture
Femoroacetabular impingement
Iliac crest contusion
Pelvic fracture

**Tendon**

Adductor tendinopathy
Coxa saltans
Deep gluteal syndrome
Gluteal tendinopathy
Iliopsoas tendinopathy
Proximal hamstring tendinopathy
Proximal quadriceps tendinopathy

**Nerve**

Femoral neuropathy
Meralgia paresthetica
Obturator neuropathy
Pudendal neuropathy
Sciatic neuropathy

## Treatment

Initial treatment includes activity modification, non-steroidal anti-inflammatory drugs (NSAIDs) for pain control, and physical therapy (PT) focusing on core and hip girdle strengthening, lumbopelvic stability, lower extremity flexibility, and soft tissue mobilization for hip flexor and adductor tightness. Ultrasound or fluoroscopically guided intra-articular hip therapeutic injections can aid in pain control, which may include corticosteroid or orthobiologic type procedures. Although the use of orthobiologics is increasing, their clinical efficacy remains unclear. Surgical options include labral debridement versus repair for refractory symptoms with or without correction of bony FAI.

## Functional Prognosis and Outcomes

Functional prognosis and outcomes depend on the presence of comorbid hip conditions such as FAI and patients' functional goals. While most patients will have functional improvements with a nonoperative course, many will also have persistent pain. Patients who are willing to modify their lifestyles or activity are likely to be more satisfied with nonoperative management, particularly if there is mild underlying FAI.[2]

## Avascular Necrosis
### Etiology and Pathophysiology

An estimated 20,000 to 30,000 new cases of avascular necrosis (AVN) arise yearly, ultimately accounting for about 10% of total hip arthroplasty (THAs) performed per year.[3] AVN affects males more than females, age range from 35 to 50 years, and 80% of presenting cases involve both hips. Known risk factors include radiation, trauma, sickle cell disease, alcoholism, smoking, coagulopathies, corticosteroid use, lupus, and viral infections, but pathophysiology is most commonly idiopathic. Intravascular coagulation beginning with intraosseous microcirculation results in venous thrombosis, followed by retrograde arterial occlusion, intraosseous hypertension, and decreased blood flow to the femoral head (FH), which eventually leads to AVN, FH collapse, or chondral fracture. Trauma can sever the medial femoral circumflex blood vessels supplying the FH, causing AVN.

## History, Examination, and Diagnostic Testing

Diagnosis begins with a history assessing risk factors, and physical examination evaluating for an intra-articular pain generator and ROM limitations. Patients may not experience pain as the chief complaint in earlier stages. Radiographs may demonstrate early development of sclerosis and cystic changes within 2 to 6 months. FH asphericity, suggestive of collapse, and joint space narrowing, suggestive of secondary OA, may be detected in later stages. MRI is the gold standard for diagnosis, with 90% to 100% sensitivity and 100% specificity and also can assist in assessing severity.[4]

## Treatment

Nonoperative treatments are limited but include risk factor modification, bisphosphonates, which have shown mixed efficacy,[5] PT, and intra-articular hip injections such as corticosteroids for pain control. Surgical options include core decompression with possible bone grafting (prior to subchondral collapse), rotational osteotomy to offload smaller lesions, and total hip or hemi-arthroplasties for larger lesions or FH collapse.[6]

## Hip Dislocations
### Etiology and Pathophysiology

Hip dislocations are rare without significant trauma. Most commonly, the FH dislocates posteriorly to the acetabulum. A typical traumatic mechanism includes a motor vehicle accident where the knee hits the dashboard with the hip in a flexed, adducted, and medially rotated position.

## History, Examination, and Diagnostic Testing

Upon inspection, the patient presents with the hip oriented in flexion, internal rotation, and adduction. In contrast, the hip is positioned in extension, abduction, and external rotation following anterior hip dislocation. The affected leg will often appear shorter. Patients are typically in severe pain and do not tolerate ROM or strength testing during examination. Diagnostics include AP pelvis radiographs, with special attention in adult patients for acetabular fractures.[7]

## Treatment

Dislocations require emergent reduction, typically under anesthesia, and may require surgery if initial closed reduction attempts are unsuccessful. Other surgical indications include repair of displaced, comminuted fractures, or removal of intra-articular loose bodies.

Following dislocation, non–weight-bearing precautions are maintained for 3 to 4 weeks, followed by 3 weeks of protected weight-bearing. Rehabilitation can begin as early as a few days after reduction. Precautions to adhere to through rehabilitation for posterior dislocations include hip flexion over 90°, hip adduction past midline, and extreme hip internal rotation.

## Functional Prognosis and Outcomes

Prognosis is generally favorable, although complications may include sciatic neuropathy, posttraumatic OA, and AVN.

## Osteitis Pubis
### Etiology and Pathophysiology

Osteitis pubis is a painful degenerative condition affecting the pubic symphysis. While it is most common among athletes and falls within the broader category of core muscle injury (CMI), osteitis pubis may also arise from pelvic trauma, surgery, or pregnancy. Disease pathogenesis is not well understood, but repetitive trauma or microtrauma and overuse are the most likely contributing factors.[8] There is little evidence that the pathology results from true inflammation.

### History, Examination, and Diagnostic Testing

Patients typically report gradual onset of pelvic pain on history, which may radiate into the groin, thigh, or abdomen. History of new training or activity is suggestive. Identifying aggravating factors is essential, such as kicking, twisting, and cutting. Physical examination is notable for tenderness over the pubic symphysis and pain with isometric muscle contraction against the examiner's fist, while lying supine with 90° of hip and knee flexion.

Diagnostics include radiographs, ultrasound, and MRI. Radiographs may be nondiagnostic, but findings include pubic symphysis widening, bone resorption at the pubic symphysis, and osteopenia at the pubic rami. Ultrasound can visualize pubic symphysis widening, while

MRI may demonstrate pubic symphysis joint fluid, periarticular, or subchondral bone marrow edema.

## Treatment

Conservative treatment includes activity modification, ice, NSAIDs, and PT focusing on core, hip girdle, and adductor strength, lower extremity flexibility, and neuromuscular control. Corticosteroid or orthobiologic injections into the pubic symphysis may be considered for pain control, although scant evidence has been published on the efficacy of the latter for osteitis pubis. Patients who fail conservative management may benefit from surgical referral for pubic symphysis debridement, resection, or arthrodesis.

## BONE PATHOLOGY

### Femoroacetabular Impingement
### Etiology and Pathophysiology

FAI arises from abnormal contact between the femur and acetabulum due to bony overgrowth, with three patterns.[9] Cam morphology is characterized by bony overgrowth of the FH, while pincer morphology refers to bony overgrowth extending over the anterosuperior acetabular rim. A third pattern is combined cam and pincer morphology. FAI is common but often asymptomatic in the general population. Activities that require extremes in ROM—such as ballet, gymnastics, and martial arts, or sports with deep flexion and rotation movements (squatting, kicking, pivoting), such as ice hockey—can lead to symptoms. Repetitive abnormal contact of the FH and acetabulum leads to labral degeneration, most commonly anterosuperior, labral separation, chondral delamination, and may predispose to OA.

### History, Examination, and Diagnostic Testing

Patients typically report activity- or position-related groin pain, exacerbated by hip flexion, and mechanical symptoms, although lateral and posterior pain are also reported. End-range flexion and internal rotation are commonly limited. Anterior impingement with a positive FADIR test elicits pain. On radiographs, cam morphology is identified by decreased FH–neck offset ratio <0.15 on elongated femoral neck view or decreased sphericity of the FH on AP view. Pincer morphology is identified grossly or by a lateral center edge angle (CEA) >40° on AP view. CT is useful for assessing associated bony morphology such as coxa vara or acetabular retroversion. MRI without contrast is recommended to evaluate articular cartilage and labral integrity.[10]

### Treatment

Nonoperative management includes PT to improve lumbopelvic stability, neuromuscular control, functional movement patterns, and activity modification to avoid end ROM, repetitive stress, and dynamic overload. NSAIDs or an intra-articular hip CSI can be tried to decrease pain. Surgical options for refractory pain due to FAI alone include arthroscopic osteochondroplasty or FH reshaping. There is currently inconclusive evidence that arthroscopic surgery improves long-term outcomes for FAI versus conservative treatment.

In addition, surgery has not shown to prevent the development of OA seen in association with FAI.

## TENDON PATHOLOGY

### Gluteus Medius Tendinopathy
### Etiology and Pathophysiology

Gluteus medius tendinopathy and tears are primary causes of lateral hip pain, associated with greater trochanteric pain syndrome (GTPS) and bursitis. In a study of patients with lateral hip pain, 88% had MRI findings consistent with gluteal tendinopathy, in contrast to 50% of asymptomatic hips.[11] Symptoms can be triggered by sudden falls, prolonged weight-bearing on one leg during normal or sports activity, overuse, or sports injury. Gluteus medius tears are estimated to affect as many as 25% and 10% of middle-aged women and men, respectively.[12]

### History, Examination, and Diagnostic Testing

The typical patient is a distance runner or woman over 40 years old. Patients may complain of pain localized to the greater trochanter or extension into the lateral thigh or leg. Often, pain is worse when lying on the affected side at night. On palpation, patients have tenderness to palpation directly over the greater trochanter, particularly the posterior fibers of the gluteus medius, which attach to the posterosuperior facet. Flexion, abduction, and external rotation (FABER) reproducing lateral hip pain, hip abduction weakness when tested side-lying, hip external rotation weakness (supine or prone), and positive Ober's test, suggestive of iliotibial band (ITB) tightness, may aid in diagnosis during physical examination. Patients with gluteus medius weakness may present with a trendelenburg gait pattern.

MRI is the most common diagnostic imaging modality for evaluation of tendinopathy and tendon tears. Ultrasound can similarly demonstrate the presence of tendinopathic changes, characterized by hypoechoic tissue changes, tendon thickening, neovascularization with Doppler signal, calcific foci, partial- or full-thickness tears, or bursal fluid.

### Treatment

Treatment includes initial activity modification, ice, ITB rolling, NSAIDs, and acetaminophen for pain control. Rehabilitation focuses on restoration of dynamic and neuromuscular control of the hip girdle, including activation, strengthening, and retraining of the gluteus medius and deep external rotators for dynamic hip stability, core strength and endurance during activity, lumbopelvic control and stability, and progression from isometric to concentric and eccentric strengthening of the gluteal muscles.

Interventional procedures include corticosteroid injection (CSI) to the subgluteus maximus bursa, which is very effective for pain, but repeated corticosteroid exposure can weaken the tendons and predispose to tearing. Ultrasound-guided percutaneous needle tenotomy, with or without orthobiologic injections, and recently, percutaneous ultrasonic tenotomy, are being performed to potentially assist with tendon healing though their clinical efficacy remains unclear. Extracorporeal shock wave therapy (ECSWT) has also demonstrated utility in treatment of GTPS.

Patients with refractory symptoms can be referred for surgical evaluation, ranging from trochanteric bursectomy to gluteus medius tendon repair. Surgical considerations include the etiology and chronicity of disease (acute traumatic vs. chronic degenerative), extent of tendon tearing, with or without retraction, and the patient's functional goals.

## Functional Prognosis and Outcomes

Prognosis is overall favorable, although symptoms may recur if gains from rehabilitation are not maintained and incorporated into the patient's home exercise program (HEP) to prevent future injury.

## Adductor Tendinopathy and Core Muscle Injury (Athletic Pubalgia)
### Etiology and Pathophysiology

Adductor pain is common among athletes, although pathology typically occurs at the enthesis with associated myofascial tightness and muscular pain, rather than true adductor tendinopathy. Groin pain secondary to adductor pathology is common among soccer players (5%–16%) and sports with acceleration/deceleration, sudden changes in direction, trunk rotation, and kicking (football, rugby, ice hockey).

Adductor pain may additionally arise from the abdomen or groin, the pubis (bone or symphysis), and the hip. In athletes reporting chronic adductor-related groin pain, 94% have radiological signs of FAI. CMI encompasses damage to any skeletal muscle between the chest and mid-thigh, including the abdominal wall, adductor, and hip flexor muscles.[13]

Risk factors for adductor tendinopathy in athletes include exaggerated lumbar lordosis with anterior pelvic tilt and imbalance between strong adductor and weak core abdominal wall musculature. Asymmetric core strength may also be implicated with a relatively weak transversalis abdominis.

## History, Examination, and Diagnostic Testing

Patients typically present with groin or medial thigh pain. On examination, tenderness is usually present along the proximal adductors. Pain reproduction occurs with resisted hip adduction. Additional, clinical examination for CMI includes palpation of the abdominal wall (rectus abdominis, rectus diastasis) and pubic symphysis, Valsalva maneuver to evaluate for abdominal wall hernias, and testing for inguinal hernias.

Diagnostics include pelvis and hip radiographs to evaluate for FAI and avulsion injuries, ultrasound to evaluate for tendinopathy, hernias, and transversalis fascia, as well as MRI of the pelvis with an "athletic pubalgia" protocol to better visualize musculature. Pertinent MRI findings for CMI include the presence of fluid between the pubic bone and overlying fibrocartilage plate, and peripubic and bone marrow edema, suggestive of pubic plate detachment.

## Treatment

First-line treatment includes activity modification, ice, NSAIDs, modalities, myofascial work to reduce pain, and rehabilitation focused on core muscle strength, lumbopelvic stability, hip girdle strength, lower extremity flexibility, and eccentric strengthening of involved muscles and tendons. Interventions to consider are CSI for pain control, though repeated injections are advised against due to negative soft tissue side effects. Orthobiologic injections have begun to be utilized for tendinopathy or plate detachments, though their clinical efficacy remains unclear. In refractory cases, operative management can be considered to restore the balance of the rectus abdominis and adductors across the pubic bone by core muscle repair and may include hip arthroscopy for FAI correction.

## Functional Prognosis and Outcomes

Prognosis is overall favorable, with an overall decline in the frequency of athletic groin pain among professional athletes, as injury prevention efforts are on the rise. However, recurrence rates are high even in professional athletes. Amateur athletes have fewer resources or awareness of the underlying condition and associated prevention strategies. Primary and secondary injury prevention is important, by correcting postural dysfunction, lumbar hyperlordosis, anterior pelvic tilt, core abdominal wall weakness, and cross-training to minimize the risk of overtraining.

## Proximal Hamstring Tendinopathy
### Etiology and Pathophysiology

Proximal hamstring tendinopathy can occur either at the origin near the ischial tuberosity or more commonly at the the myotendinous junction. The injury typically arises due to an eccentric hamstring contraction either acutely or with overuse. Common sports for injury include soccer and running. The greatest risk factor is having a previous hamstring injury.[14]

### History, Examination, and Diagnostic Testing

Typical complaints include buttock pain, aggravated by sprinting or accelerating while running, or after prolonged sitting. Pertinent examination findings include localized tenderness and/ or bruising at or near the ischial tuberosity, myotendinous junction, or the muscle depending on the site of pathology. Pain occurs with hamstring stretching or resisted hip extension and knee flexion. Slump test may be equivocal reproducing only local pain but not neural tension. Ultrasound and MRI are both useful for diagnosis of tendinosis and/or tears, although MRI is the more sensitive imaging modality, particularly for myotendinous tears.

### Treatment

Management begins with activity modification, ice, NSAIDs, followed by rehabilitation focusing on soft tissue therapy, lower extremity stretching of the antagonist hip flexors, and progressive eccentric hamstring and core strengthening exercises. ECSWT or ultrasound-guided percutaneous needle tenotomy, with or without orthobiologic injections, can be considered to potentially promote tissue remodeling over CSI, which may only provide temporary pain relief while having negative side effects for soft tissue healing. Surgical tenotomy is an option for cases of tendinosis when conservative measures have failed. In addition, surgical hamstring repair is advised for acute insertional hamstring tears with greater than 2 cm of retraction.[15]

### Functional Prognosis and Outcomes

Hamstring tendinopathy often produces prolonged impairment and a reinjury risk of 12% to 31%.[16] Fortunately, implementation of a Nordic hamstring exercise protocol has shown the ability to halve the rate of proximal hamstring injuries.[17] This type of prevention protocol should be considered for high-risk athletes and sports such as soccer.

## Iliopsoas Tendinopathy

### Etiology and Pathophysiology

Iliopsoas tendinopathy is more common in younger, female patients and typically occurs due to overuse and repetitive movements such as forceful hip flexion. Therefore, hurdlers and jumpers are at the greatest risk of developing symptoms.[18]

### History, Examination, and Diagnostic Testing

On history, pain localizes to the groin but can radiate into the medial thigh. Examination typically reveals tight hip flexors, and pain may be elicited with Stinchfield test. Dynamic testing from FABER to extension, adduction, and internal rotation can elicit snapping of the psoas tendon between the psoas muscle, iliacus muscle, or both (internal snapping hip). Ultrasound is useful to evaluate for tendinopathy and dynamically for internal snapping hip. MRI can additionally be considered for diagnosis as well as assessment of adjacent soft tissues.[19]

### Treatment

Conservative management includes activity modification, NSAIDs or acetaminophen for pain control, and PT. Rehabilitation focuses on eccentric hip flexor strengthening with kinetic chain exercises. Ultrasound-guided CSI into the iliopsoas bursa can be considered for pain control, though repeated injections are advised against due to negative soft tissue side effects. Percutaneous needle tenotomy (PNT), with or without orthobiologic injections, have begun to be utilized for potential tendon healing, though their clinical efficacy remains unclear. Surgery is rarely indicated, but minimally invasive tendon release is available for refractory cases.

## Deep Gluteal Syndrome

### Etiology and Pathophysiology

Deep gluteal syndrome (DGS) is used to describe conditions such as piriformis syndrome that involves buttocks pain along with sciatic nerve compression by focal entrapment or anatomic anomalies in the gluteal space. Common sciatic nerve entrapment sites include at the level of the ischial tuberosity, the obturator internus and gemelli, or piriformis. Anatomic anomalies include a bipartite piriformis (where the sciatic nerve passes through, rather than inferior to the piriformis), variations of the sciatic nerve course, local tumor, or inferior gluteal artery aneurysm. DGS may be associated with FAI and decreased internal rotation resulting in contracture of the deep external rotators and sciatic nerve compression.[20]

### History, Examination, and Diagnostic Testing

History and examination may reveal pain in the posterior gluteal region that radiates down the posterior leg, reproduction of symptoms with FADIR (placing tension across the piriformis), decreased medial hamstring and Achilles reflexes, or loss of strength and sensation in the sciatic nerve distribution. Special tests include the Freiberg (internal rotation of an extended thigh), Pace (resisted hip abduction), and Beatty (active hip abduction in lateral decubitus) maneuvers, which may reproduce buttock pain.[20] MRI and ultrasound are typically unremarkable but may show anatomic anomalies or denervation of sciatic-innervated muscles. Performing electrodiagnostics (EDX) in the FADIR position can transiently prolong the H-reflex and improve sensitivity and specificity for diagnosing piriformis syndrome.[21]

### Treatment

Nonoperative treatments address reversing mechanical causes, such as tight deep external rotators, with PT emphasizing hip mobility and symmetrical neuromuscular control across the pelvis. Activity modification, NSAIDs, muscle relaxants, and dry needling can be considered for pain control. Ultrasound-guided injections with anesthetic or steroids to the piriformis sheath or botulinum toxin injections directly into the piriformis may improve symptoms.[20] Surgical options include piriformis muscle release and external sciatic neurolysis, which are reserved for cases with severe neurological impairment or severe pain refractory to conservative care.

## NERVE PATHOLOGY

### Meralgia Paresthetica
### Etiology and Pathophysiology

Meralgia paresthetica (MP) is caused by compression or damage of the lateral femoral cutaneous nerve (LFCN) of the thigh, which provides sensation to the anterolateral thigh. It can occur in any age group but is most common in those 30 to 50 years old. The etiology is nerve entrapment or injury at the level of the inguinal ligament, due to mechanical forces (tight clothing), rapid weight changes, spine or pelvic surgery, pregnancy, and other conditions with increased intra-abdominal pressure. Diabetes appears to heighten the risk for injury.

### History, Examination, and Diagnostic Testing

MP is typically a clinical diagnosis. Patients present with unilateral anterolateral thigh numbness, paresthesias, pain, or allodynia, although up to 20% of cases are bilateral.[22] Symptoms can be exacerbated by prolonged sitting or deep hip flexion, which may cause nerve compression, or hyperextension of the lumbar spine or hip, which may cause nerve stretch. Tinel's sign may be present at the inguinal ligament and reproduce paresthesias. Physical examination should exclude lumbar or radicular pain etiologies, such as negative dural tension tests. Imaging includes radiographs, CT, or MRI to rule out spinal bony or soft tissue pathology such as vertebral fracture or disc herniation. Ultrasound can be useful to identify nerve compression or an anatomic variant. EDX is often nondiagnostic in mild cases; however, it may reveal a slowed conduction velocity of the LFCN.[22]

### Treatment

Conservative management begins by removing contributing factors, such as educating patients to avoid tight undergarments and belts, prolonged positioning in deep hip flexion or extension, and minimizing rapid weight changes. Treatments include kinesiotaping, acupuncture, transcutaneous electrical nerve stimulation (TENS), low-level laser therapy, manual therapies, and stretching and strengthening exercises. Topical capsaicin or lidocaine, or oral neuropathic pain-modulating medications can be effective in managing dysesthesias.

Ultrasound-guided local anesthetic nerve blocks can be both diagnostic and therapeutic. Following successful nerve block, CSI or nerve hydrodissection can be performed, with the goal of breaking the pain cycle from the afferent contribution to the central nervous system.[23] Patients who fail conservative management may proceed to surgical release of the constricting tissue, neurolysis, or transection with partial excision of the lateral cutaneous nerve of the thigh.

### Functional Prognosis and Outcomes

Prognosis is generally favorable, as the majority of cases self-resolve in 4 to 6 months. MP generally responds well to conservative management, and patients rarely require operative measures.

## Obturator Neuralgia
### Etiology and Pathophysiology

Obturator neuralgia is rare. The most common cause is nerve injury at the adductor compartment due to fascial entrapment as it enters the thigh, but injury can occur due to local hemorrhage, tumor, or surgery. The obturator nerve is usually not injured in isolation but rather as part of a more complex musculoskeletal injury.[24]

### History, Examination, and Diagnostic Testing

Presentation typically includes medial thigh or groin pain, sensory loss, and leg adduction weakness. Examination should focus on thigh sensory and hip adductor strength testing. Radiographs are most helpful to rule out other structural causes, such as intra-articular hip pathology. MRI may demonstrate atrophy or denervation changes of the adductors but can be diagnostically limited in detecting abnormalities of the obturator nerve itself. Ultrasound evaluation of the obturator nerve and adductors may demonstrate focal narrowing ("hourglassing") of the nerve at entrapment site or adductor atrophic changes due to denervation. EDX may demonstrate sensory nerve conduction changes in milder cases or changes in the compound muscle action potential and neuropathic findings on needle examination in severe cases. Local anesthetics nerve blocks can be diagnostic and therapeutic.[24]

### Treatment

Conservative management begins with PT to address hip and lumbar spine mobility and ROM, myofascial release to address focal areas of soft tissue restriction, and gradual introduction of hip and pelvic stabilizer strengthening. Pain can be managed with ultrasound-guided nerve sheath CSI or hydrodissection, neurolytic blockade, or neuromodulation for intractable pain. Surgical decompression can be considered for those with pain and weakness refractory to PT or severe EDX findings.

### Functional Prognosis and Outcomes

A temporal relationship appears to exist between nerve injury and recovery. Those with acute-onset obturator neuralgia respond better to conservative management usually in weeks to months, while those with chronic neuralgia show poorer outcomes.

## Sciatic Neuropathy

### Etiology and Pathophysiology

Sciatic nerve injury can occur due to stretching, compression, or transection anywhere along its course, exiting from the lumbosacral plexus to bifurcating into the common fibular and tibial nerves. Muscles innervated by the common fibular nerve (ankle dorsiflexors, evertors) are more often affected than those innervated by the tibial nerve (knee flexors, ankle plantarflexors, invertors). Causes include trauma, hematoma, malignancy, radiation, pregnancy, and piriformis syndrome. The most common iatrogenic causes occur following THA or injections.[25]

### History, Examination, and Diagnostic Testing

History and examination may reveal radiating pain or numbness in the sciatic nerve distribution (posterior thigh, anterolateral leg and foot), leg muscle weakness and atrophy, foot drop, decreased medial hamstring, or Achilles reflexes. MRI or ultrasound may demonstrate focal narrowing of the nerve at entrapment sites and reveal fibro-fatty atrophy of sciatic-innervated muscles. EDX are key in confirming the diagnosis and severity of sciatic neuropathy.

### Treatment

Cases are generally managed conservatively. PT may relieve mechanical restrictions in the hip, spine, and pelvis that may contribute to symptoms. Desensitization techniques can be helpful, including TENS. Soft tissue mobilization and myofascial release can promote mobility and ROM. An active program centered around strengthening the dynamic stabilizers of the hip, spine, and pelvis will optimize nerve positioning and mobility and prevent repeat injury. In rare and refractory cases, sciatic neuroplasty can be performed if there is a localized area of injury.

### Functional Prognosis and Outcomes

Prognosis is variable, depending on the extent of injury on EDX. However, iatrogenic sciatic nerve palsy following THA has shown poor recovery, with only 35% to 40% likelihood of complete functional recovery to preoperative strength.[26]

### Basic Order Sets

---

#### Hip radiographs[27]

Order an anteroposterior (AP) pelvis radiograph with lateral and false-profile views

- AP pelvis: to assess for pincer morphology, acetabular morphology, calculate lateral center-edge angle (CEA)
  - Recommend supine radiographs with 15° of anteversion (feet internally rotated by 15°)
- Lateral views: to assess for cam morphology, FH sphericity
  - 45° or 90° Dunn, cross-table lateral, or frog-leg lateral views
- False-profile view: to assess for acetabular morphology, calculate anterior CEA

---

## MRI of the hip

Typically order without contrast; request proton density sequences
- Wide field of view: including both hips to assess symmetry
- Sagittal view: to assess for cartilage, labral, psoas, and hamstring pathology
- Coronal view: to assess the labrum, capsule, gluteus medius and minimus, adductors, pubic symphysis
- Axial view: to assess the hip flexors, gluteal muscles, adductor muscles, and pubic symphysis for core muscle injuries

## CT scans with three-dimensional reconstruction

Order to assess hip morphology, cam morphology, acetabular dysplasia, femoral and acetabular version

## PT prescription

Diagnosis: femoroacetabular impingement
One to two times/week for up to 12 sessions
Core and hip girdle strengthening, including hip abductors, deep external rotators
Lumbopelvic stabilization, assess pelvic tilt
Lower extremity flexibility, hamstring, and quadriceps stretching
Neuromuscular retraining
Single leg exercises and balance
Progress to functional activities, multidimensional and multiplanar exercises, plyometrics
Manual therapies, modalities as needed
Teach HEP
Precautions: avoid exercise at end-range ROM

## PT prescription

Diagnosis: gluteus medius tendinopathy
One to two times/week for up to 12 sessions
Core and hip girdle strengthening, including hip abductors, deep external rotators
Progress to eccentric strengthening of the gluteal muscles
Lumbopelvic stabilization
Lower extremity flexibility, ITB stretching
Neuromuscular retraining
Single leg exercises and balance
Progress to functional activities, multidimensional and multiplanar exercises, plyometrics
Manual therapies, modalities as needed
Teach HEP
Precautions: none

**PT prescription**

Diagnosis: adductor tendinopathy

One to two times/week for up to 12 sessions

Core and hip girdle strengthening, lumbopelvic stabilization

Progress to eccentric strengthening of the adductor muscles

Lower extremity flexibility

Neuromuscular retraining

Single leg exercises and balance

Progress to functional activities, multidimensional and multiplanar exercises, plyometrics

Manual therapies, modalities as needed

Teach HEP

Precautions: none

---

**PT prescription**

Diagnosis: proximal hamstring tendinopathy

One to two times/week for up to 12 sessions

Core and hip girdle strengthening

Progress to eccentric strengthening of the hamstring muscles

Lumbopelvic stabilization, assess pelvic tilt

Lower extremity flexibility

Neuromuscular retraining

Single leg exercises and balance

Progress to functional activities, multidimensional and multiplanar exercises, plyometrics

Manual therapies, modalities as needed

Teach HEP

Precautions: none

---

**PT prescription**

Diagnosis: iliopsoas tendinopathy

One to two times/week for up to 12 sessions

Core and hip girdle strengthening

Progress to eccentric strengthening of the hip flexor muscles

Lumbopelvic stabilization, assess pelvic tilt

Lower extremity flexibility

Neuromuscular retraining

Single leg exercises and balance

Progress to functional activities, multidimensional and multiplanar exercises, plyometrics

Manual therapies, modalities as needed

Teach HEP

Precautions: none

## PT prescription

Diagnosis: sciatic neuropathy

One to two times/week for up to 12 sessions

Core and hip girdle strengthening

Lumbopelvic stabilization

Lower extremity flexibility

Neuromuscular retraining

Nerve mobilization techniques

Gait and balance training, evaluate for assistive device as needed

Progress to functional activities

Manual therapies, myofascial release, modalities as needed

Teach HEP

Precautions: none

## RESOURCES AND REFERENCES

The full list of resources and references appears in the digital product found on http://connect .springerpub.com/content/book/978-0-8261-6226-7/part/part02/chapter/ch19

# KNEE AND LOWER LEG

ALEXANDER LLOYD, ISAIAH LEVY, ALLISON BEAN, AND KENTARO ONISHI

## INTRODUCTION

The knee consists of four osseous structures: the femur, tibia, fibula, and patella. The knee joint is comprised of three separate articulations involving the medial and lateral femorotibial joints and the patellofemoral joint. A capsule surrounds the entire joint with a synovial lining. Hyaline cartilage covers the osseous articulations with meniscus interposed between the medial and lateral femorotibial joints. The knee joint is further stabilized intra-articular by the anterior and posterior cruciate ligaments and extra-articular by the medial and lateral collateral ligaments. Flexion and extension are the primary motions of the knee with internal and external rotation as secondary motions. The lower leg is comprised of four compartments (anterior, lateral, superficial posterior, and deep posterior) with each containing separate muscle and neurovascular structures that are susceptible to injury. We will cover in more detail the most common sources of knee and lower leg pain in the text. See Box 20.1 for a more comprehensive differential diagnosis of knee pain.

## KNEE INJURIES

### Joint Pathology
### Medial and Lateral Meniscus Injuries

*Etiology and Pathophysiology*

The menisci are crescent-shaped fibrocartilaginous tissues that absorb shock and distribute load in the knee. Traumatic injuries are most commonly seen in the younger population and a result of rotational stresses when the knee is flexed and the foot is planted. Common sports for this to occur are football and soccer. Degenerative menisci are most commonly seen in the older population, which may become painful in the absence of trauma and often associated with osteoarthritis (OA).

*History, Examination, and Diagnostic Testing*

Classic presentation includes knee pain with weight-bearing activity. Mechanical symptoms such as swelling, catching, and locking may be present. Typical physical examination findings include joint line tenderness. An effusion and decreased knee range of motion may or may not be present. For special testing, McMurray's, Thessaly's, or Apley's test may be used to

---

The full list of references appears in the digital product found on http://connect.springerpub.com/content/book/978-0-8261-6226-7/part/part02/chapter/ch20

## BOX 20.1

### DIFFERENTIAL DIAGNOSIS OF KNEE PAIN

**Diagnoses**

**Joint**

Knee dislocation
Meniscal injury
Patella dislocation
Patellofemoral syndrome
Plica
Tibia-fibula instability

**Bone**

Femoral condyle fracture
Fibula fracture
Osteochondritis dissecans
Patella fracture
Tibial plateau fracture

**Tendon**

Hamstring tendinopathy
Patellar tendinopathy
Quadriceps tendinopathy

**Ligament**

Anterior cruciate ligament sprain or tear
Lateral collateral ligament sprain or tear
Medial collateral ligament sprain or tear
Medial patellofemoral ligament sprain or tear
Posterior cruciate ligament sprain or tear
Posterolateral corner injury

**Nerve**

Fibular neuropathy (common, deep, and superficial)
Saphenous neuropathy
Tibial neuropathy

**Other**

Baker cyst
Fat pad impingement
Infrapatellar bursopathy (superficial and deep)
IT band syndrome
Pes anserine bursopathy
Pre-patellar bursopathy

identify meniscal injury. Weight-bearing radiographs can be considered to evaluate for underlying osseous abnormalities such as OA. MRI is the most sensitive imaging modality to detect a meniscal injury. MRI can also help to characterize the tear pattern which helps direct further management. However, MRI findings must be interpreted cautiously over the age of 45 as asymptotic meniscal tears are common.

## Treatment

In the absence of mechanical symptoms, initial management should focus on pain relief, with PRICE (protection, rest, ice, compression, elevation), or acetaminophen. Adjunctive non-steroidal anti-inflammatory drugs (NSAIDs) can be used but should be avoided as long-term therapy due to possible side effects and detrimental impacts on tissue healing. A physical therapy program should also be initiated for improvement of mechanical symptoms as well as pain.[1] An intra-articular knee joint steroid injection can be considered for pain control, though this does not alter the disease course. Repeat injections are advised against due to negative side effects on joint health. Hyaluronic acid injections can be considered as an alternative. Orthobiologics, such as platelet-rich plasma and stem cells, are currently being investigated for their potential to aid meniscus healing. Although the use of these biologic adjuvants is increasing, their clinical efficacy remains unclear. Arthroscopic surgery may be considered in patients with persistent pain over 3 months or mechanical symptoms such as locking. Surgery typically depends on the type of tear and can include debridement, partial meniscectomy, or meniscal repair and should be followed by a robust rehabilitation program. Surgical outcomes are better for younger patients with isolated tears rather than older patients with degenerative tears.[2]

## Basic Order Set

Physical therapy prescription:
- Diagnosis: Medial or lateral meniscus tear
- Frequency and duration: Two to three times per week for 6 weeks
- Protocol: Improve strength of knee stabilizers, including hip girdle, quadriceps, and hamstrings. Balance and proprioceptive training. Modalities as appropriate. Transition to home exercise program.
- Precautions: Avoid painful loading and ROM

# Patellofemoral Pain Syndrome

## Etiology and Pathophysiology

Patellofemoral pain syndrome (PFPS), also known as runner's knee, is believed to result from patellar maltracking most often caused by increased valgus forces at the knee due to muscular imbalance between the vastus medialis and vastus lateralis (Figure 20.1). PFPS is more common in females than males, presumably because of the greater baseline valgus at the knee.[3] Foot disorders such as rear-foot eversion or pes planovalgus can contribute to PFPS due to altered biomechanics that change the forces through the knee (Figure 20.1).

## History, Examination, and Diagnostic Testing

PFPS is defined as pain around or behind the patella, which is aggravated by at least one activity that load the patellofemoral joint during weight-bearing on a flexed knee (jumping,

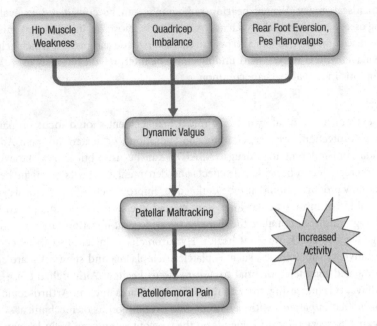

**FIGURE 20.1** Common biomechanical risk factors and causes for Patellofemoral Pain Syndrome.[4]

running, squatting, and climbing stairs). Physical examination findings suggestive of PFPS include pain with palpation over the patellar facets and a positive patellar grind test. Dynamic valgus is often seen during a single-leg squat. Radiographs are rarely needed to confirm the diagnosis but can assist in evaluation of predisposing biomechanical malalignments. MRI can be considered in recalcitrant cases to identify structural joint or soft tissue abnormalities.

### Treatment

Physical therapy is first-line treatment for PFPS and should focus on strengthening the muscles surrounding the knee and hip specifically the quadriceps and hip abductors and rotators, respectively. NSAIDs can be used for pain relief in the short term. Taping or bracing to limit lateral patellar movement may also be helpful.[4] For patients with foot abnormalities, orthoses may improve lower limb kinematics but should be utilized in conjunction with physical therapy.[5] While rarely necessary, surgery may be considered for patients with PFPS who have structural joint abnormalities such as cartilage defects or significant patellar subluxation and who have not responded to appropriate conservative management.

### Basic Order Set

Physical therapy prescription:

- Diagnosis: PFPS
- Frequency and duration: One to three times per week for 4 to 6 weeks
- Protocol: Improve strength in hip and knee stabilizers, progress to single-leg exercises, taping and modalities as indicated
- Precautions: None

## Tendon Pathology
### Patellar Tendinopathy

*Etiology and Pathophysiology*

Patellar tendinopathy, also known as "jumper's knee," is a common condition affecting athletes and young, active adults. It is frequent in sports such as volleyball and basketball that involves repetitive knee flexion and extension. Like other tendinopathies, it is believed to be a chronic overload injury to the tendon initially resulting in reactive inflammation followed by inadequate repair and subsequent degeneration.[6]

*History, Examination, and Diagnostic Testing*

Patients present with anterior knee pain inferior to the patella exacerbated by activities such as jumping, squatting, and stair climbing. Physical examination typically reveals tenderness at the inferior pole of the patella and pain with resisted knee extension and single-leg squat. Diagnosis of this condition is largely clinical, though ultrasound or MRI can be helpful to confirm the diagnosis and assess severity. It should be noted, however, that asymptomatic individuals may have tendinopathic changes on ultrasound and appropriate clinical correlation is essential.[7]

*Treatment*

Standard treatment consists of initial activity modification with progressive tendon loading and muscle strengthening. Underlying weakness and kinetic chain abnormalities should be addressed. Steroid injections are not advised, because they may lead to worse outcomes and potential tendon rupture.[8] New conservative treatment options that are being studied include extracorporeal shockwave therapy, platelet-rich plasma injections, ultrasound-guided tendon scraping, and percutaneous ultrasonic tenotomy.[9] If nonsurgical management fails, surgical referral may be warranted.

*Basic Order Set*

Physical therapy script (patellar tendinopathy):
- Diagnosis: Patellar tendinopathy
- Frequency and duration: Two to three times per week for 4 to 6 weeks
- Protocol: Please start with isometric exercises loading the patellar tendon and progress to isotonic lower extremity exercises emphasizing the eccentric phase of loading. Progress to heavy concentric exercises and energy-storing exercises such as plyometrics before moving to activity-specific exercises.
- Precautions: Progress based on pain with level no higher than 5/10.

## Ligament Pathology
### Lateral Collateral Ligament Sprain/Tear

*Etiology and Pathophysiology*

The LCL originates on the lateral epicondyle of the femur and inserts onto the anterior and lateral aspect of the fibula. It resists tibial external rotation and varus deformation. It is commonly injured with a blow to the medial side resulting in varus stress to the knee or with hyperextension.

### History, Examination, and Diagnostic Testing

Patients will typically present with lateral-sided knee pain and instability. On physical examination, there will be tenderness and swelling along the course of the LCL along with increased varus laxity. Injuries are graded according to the amount of tibial translation with varus stress (Table 20.1). Due to anatomic proximity, the posterolateral corner of the knee should also be assessed with a dial test if an LCL injury is suspected. Musculoskeletal ultrasound and MRI can both be used to evaluate and grade LCL injury as well as concurrent ligament or meniscal injuries (Table 20.1).

### Treatment

Isolated grades I and II injuries can be managed conservatively by utilizing PRICE and a hinged brace for 3 to 6 weeks. Physical therapy focusing on hip and knee strengthening and proprioception can be initiated after approximately 3 weeks. Surgical evaluation should be considered for grade III injuries, particularly when other ligamentous or meniscal injuries are present. However, some studies have shown that athletes with isolated grade III LCL tears can be managed successfully nonoperatively.[10]

### Basic Order Set

Physical therapy prescription:

- Diagnosis: Grade I/II LCL injury
- Frequency and duration: Two to three times per week for 4 to 6 weeks
- Protocol: Continued hinged bracing for 3 to 6 weeks with no restriction in flexion/extension; progressive open and closed kinetic chain strengthening exercises targeting hamstrings, quadriceps, and gluteal musculature; proprioceptive exercises
- Precautions: Avoid varus and external rotational stresses

## Medial Collateral Ligament Sprain and Tear

### Etiology and Pathophysiology

The medial collateral ligament (MCL) originates on the posterior aspect of the medial femoral epicondyle and inserts onto the medial condyle and to the body of the tibia. It resists tibial internal rotation and valgus knee deformation. Injury typically occurs with excessive valgus stress either by a direct blow to the lateral knee or with rapid direction change.

**TABLE 20.1 GRADING LATERAL COLLATERAL LIGAMENT INJURIES**

| BASED ON PHYSICAL EXAMINATION | | BASED ON MUSCULOSKELETAL ULTRASOUND OR MRI | |
|---|---|---|---|
| Grade | Degree of laxity | Grade | MRI findings |
| Grade I | <5 mm | Grade I | Subcutaneous fluid around ligament, no tearing |
| Grade II | 5–10 mm | Grade II | Partial tearing |
| Grade III | >10 mm, instability | Grade III | Complete tearing |

## History, Examination, and Diagnostic Testing

Patients typically describe sudden onset of medial knee pain and instability. Laxity on physical examination can be assessed by applying a valgus force to the knee in 30° of flexion and is graded based on the amount of tibial translation (Table 20.2). Of note, the anterior cruciate ligament (ACL) and medial meniscus can also be concomitantly injured and should be thoroughly evaluated. While MCL injury can typically be diagnosed clinically, patients with suspected multiligament injury should undergo MRI. Ultrasound can also be utilized to characterize the grade of the medial collateral ligament (MCL) injury (Table 20.2).

## Treatment

For isolated Grades I and II tears, nonsurgical treatments can be trialed with a hinged brace to limit valgus motion. Once pain has subsided, a physical therapy program focusing on strengthening of the quadriceps and hamstrings should be implemented.[11] For athletes, return to competition is permitted once full range of motion is pain-free, there is no instability on examination, and strength is comparable to the uninjured side. For Grade III injuries, nonoperative management is an option, but patients may have residual laxity that can predispose to reinjury. In cases where either there is chronic pain, instability, or additional associated ligamentous injury, surgical consultation and repair should be considered.[12] For isolated MCL injuries, 75% of patients return to preinjury activity levels within 3 months, and over 85% have normal knee function and strength after 4 years.[13]

## Basic Order Set

Physical therapy prescription:
- Diagnosis: Grade I/II LCL injury
- Frequency and duration: Two to three times per week for 4 to 6 weeks
- Protocol: Continue hinged bracing for 4 to 6 weeks; strengthening of hamstrings, quadriceps, and gluteal musculature; proprioceptive training
- Precautions: Avoid valgus and adduction stress

## Anterior Cruciate Ligament Sprain and Tear

### Etiology and Pathophysiology

The ACL originates from the posteromedial aspect of the lateral femoral condyle and

## TABLE 20.2 GRADING MEDIAL COLLATERAL LIGAMENT INJURIES

| BASED ON PHYSICAL EXAMINATION | | BASED ON MUSCULOSKELETAL ULTRASOUND OR MRI | |
|---|---|---|---|
| Grade | Degree of laxity | Grade | Imaging findings |
| Grade I | <5 mm | Grade I | Subcutaneous fluid around ligament, no tearing |
| Grade II | 5–10 mm | Grade II | More tearing of superficial fibers, preservation of deeper fibers |
| Grade III | >10 mm, instability | Grade III | Complete tearing of both superficial and deep fibers |

inserts into the intercondylar notch of the anterior tibia. It resists anterior motion and tibial external rotation. It is the most commonly injured knee ligament with over 100,000 injuries per year.[14] Injury generally occurs with excessive external rotation of the femur on a fixed tibia or a direct blow causing knee hyperextension or valgus. High school soccer and basketball athletes are at the highest risk of ACL injury, and female athletes have a higher risk compared to men.[15]

### History, Examination, and Diagnostic Testing

Patients often describe a "pop" at the time of the injury, followed by acute swelling and knee instability. While weight-bearing may be tolerated, pain is often elicited by squatting or pivoting. Special physical examination maneuvers including Lachman, anterior drawer, and pivot shift tests are useful for clinical diagnosis of ACL injury. Importantly, care should be taken to ensure a tibial sag from a PCL injury is not present since this may mimic a positive anterior drawer. Diagnosis can be confirmed with MRI. Common associated injuries that should also be evaluated for include meniscal injury, MCL injury, bone contusion, and a Segond fracture.

### Treatment

Treatment can be either operative or nonoperative depending on the severity of the injury and the patient's functional goals. Patients with concomitant injury of other structures, such as the meniscus or other ligaments, typically require ACL repair for adequate stability. Younger and more active patients are likely to undergo ACL repair due to higher activity and lifestyle demands. Preoperative rehabilitation to normalize range of motion and increase muscular strength and dynamic stabilization can facilitate postoperative recovery. Postoperative rehabilitation follows a formal progression, initially focusing on closed kinetic chain exercises and progressing to open kinetic chain exercises. The immediate postoperative phase (1–7 days postop) should focus on restoring full knee range of motion and quadriceps control. The second phase (2–4 weeks postop) should focus on normalizing proprioception and active knee ROM with strengthening exercises. The third phase (4–10 weeks postop) should focus on improving muscular endurance and enhancing proprioception. The last phase (10–16 weeks postop) should focus on increasing power and progressive return to play.[16] Preventive programs for ACL injury have been developed focusing on neuromuscular control of the knee joint with success.[17]

### Basic Order Sets

Imaging:
- MRI of the knee without contrast including coronal oblique views

Physical therapy prescription:
- Diagnosis: ACL tear
- Frequency and duration: One to two times per week for 12 to 16 weeks
- Protocol:
  - Acute ACL tear without operative repair or plan to return to high-level sports: Implement post-op ACL protocol without ROM restrictions; ROM and strengthening of the knee stabilizers with secondary focus on hip and ankle stability; progressive lower extremity proprioception and neuromuscular control to high-level single-leg balance

❑ Acute ACL tear with plans to return to sport at high level: Multiphasic exercises with progression from passive knee extension to quadricep strengthening followed by proprioception and endurance to power and sport-specific drills
■ Precautions: Avoid knee hyperextension

## Posterior Cruciate Ligament Sprain and Tear

### Etiology and Pathophysiology

The posterior cruciate ligament (PCL) originates from the posterior intercondylar tibia and attaches to the medial femoral condyle, preventing posterior motion and internal rotation of the tibia. Classic mechanisms of injury include motor vehicle accidents with the tibia striking the dashboard.

### History, Examination, and Diagnostic Testing

In contrast to ACL injuries, a "pop" is rarely reported. Physical examination can reveal tenderness of the popliteal fossa and effusion. Positive posterior drawer test is suggestive of PCL injury, while the dial test can be used to assess for both PCL and posterolateral corner injuries. MRI should be obtained to further evaluate the PCL and possible concomitant injuries.

### Treatment

Patients with limited symptoms and minimal posterior tibial translation can be managed nonoperatively. Rehabilitation progression is described in Table 20.3.[18] If the patient has significant tibial translation or severe pain with instability, repair may be necessary.

### Basic Order Set

Physical therapy prescription:
■ Diagnosis: PCL tear (no-operative management)
■ Frequency and duration: One to two times per week for 12 to 16 weeks
■ Protocol: Maintain knee ROM while progressing to proprioception and strengthening exercises; begin with open chain and progress to closed-chained and sport-specific exercises
■ Precautions: Avoid knee hyperextension

## Medial Patellofemoral Ligament Sprain and Tear

### Etiology and Pathophysiology

The patella is the largest sesamoid bone and is stabilized by the bony constraints of the trochlear groove of the femur, muscles of the quadriceps, patellar tendon, and medial and lateral retinacula/ligaments. Instability can result from disturbances in bony and reticular/ligamentous anatomy or poor quadriceps activation that alters the dynamic stability of the patella. Trochlear dysplasia, where the femoral trochlea is abnormally flat or prominent, is common in individuals with patellar instability.[19] Patella alta may result in inadequate bony contact and abnormal patellar tracking.[19] Women are at increased risk of patellar subluxation and dislocation likely due to increased Q angle.[20] Lateral subluxation/dislocation of the patella due to disruption of the medial patellofemoral ligament (MPFL) is believed to be the most

**TABLE 20.3 PCL LIGAMENT REHABILITATION**

| PHASE | DURATION POST INJURY | FOCUS |
|---|---|---|
| Protective phase | Weeks 1–6 | • Knee range of motion<br>• Progressive strengthening of quadriceps and proximal hips<br>• Avoid knee hyperextension |
| Transitional phase | Weeks 6–12 | • Proprioception and strengthening of lower extremities |
| Functional phase | Weeks 12–16 | • Light exercise, such as slow jogging<br>• Closed-chained exercises |
| Return to play | >16 weeks | • Resume sport-specific exercises with emphasis placed on neuromuscular control to prevent reinjury |

PCL, posterior cruciate ligament.

common injury leading to patellar dislocation. A sprain or tear of the MPFL may occur as a result of a laterally directed blow to the medial patella or with strong quadriceps contraction while the knee is in a flexed and valgus position with a relatively internally rotated femur.

### History, Examination, and Diagnostic Testing

Patients typically present with an acute episode of anteromedial knee pain often with patella subluxation or dislocation. On physical examination, swelling is often present, and tissue defect in the area between medial patella and medial femoral condyle may be palpable. A positive patellar apprehension test at 30° of knee flexion is characteristic. Patellar grind and apprehension tests are generally positive. Patellar tilt may also be asymmetric reflecting underlying medial ligamentous laxity or lateral ligamentous tightness. Lateral translation of the patella with knee extension, also known as the "J sign," may also be seen. Lateral and Merchant view radiographs are most helpful for diagnosis and can reveal patella alta and abnormal patella angulation. Ultrasound and MRI allow for assessment of the degree of MPFL disruption, though MRI can also demonstrate osteochondral involvement.[19]

### Treatment

Initial management of patellar dislocation involves reduction by application of lateral pressure while simultaneously extending the knee.[20] Immobilization should be maintained for 2 to 3 weeks, followed by physical therapy. Recurrence is common, and the patient may report a sense of instability or buckling. Physical therapy for patellar instability should emphasize quadriceps strengthening and activation to maintain dynamic stability of the patella with gradual return to activity.[20] Taping or bracing can be trialed to enhance patellar stability. If symptoms persist, surgical referral is recommended for MPFL repair or reconstruction.

### Basic Order Sets

Imaging:
- XR of the knee including anteroposterior (AP), lateral and Merchant views
- MRI of the knee (if significant intra-articular pathology is suspected)

■ Ultrasound of the anterior knee evaluating the retinacula/ligamentous structures of the patella

Physical therapy prescription:

■ Diagnosis: Patellar instability in context of patellar subluxation/dislocation
■ Frequency and duration: One to two times per week for 4 to 6 weeks
■ Protocol: Strengthening and coordinated activation of dynamic stabilizers, particularly quadriceps; progress to functional movements and single-leg exercises; use taping and bracing to enhance patellar stability as needed
■ Precautions: None

## Nerve Pathology
### Fibular Neuropathy

*Etiology and Pathophysiology*

The common fibular nerve is vulnerable to trauma or compression at the fibular neck where the nerve is most superficial. Extrinsic etiologies include leg crossing, lower extremity casts, or tight-fitting orthoses. Intrinsic etiologies include tibiofibular joint cysts, fibular fracture, or a knee dislocation. Traction injury can occur in individuals with multiple ankle inversion injuries or those with significant *genu varum*.[21]

*History, Examination, and Diagnostic Testing*

The initial symptom of common fibular nerve injury is often dorsiflexion and eversion weakness. In more severe cases, frank foot drop may occur, resulting in a steppage gait. Complaints of pain, paresthesias, or burning sensation over the lateral lower leg and dorsum of the foot are also frequent.[21] If common fibular neuropathy is suspected clinically, intrinsic etiologies should be ruled out using musculoskeletal ultrasound or MRI. In addition, these imaging modalities can provide anatomic information about the health of the nerve and aid in localizing the injury. A nerve conduction study and electromyography (NCS/EMG) can further confirm the diagnosis, classify the severity of the nerve injury, and rule out other peripheral nerve conditions. NCS/EMG should not be performed until 3 weeks post injury as this is when initial abnormal activity may be seen.

*Treatment*

Treatment depends on the etiology. Compressive neuropathies usually improve once the source is localized and compression is alleviated. Physical therapy can aid recovery of function and provide compensatory strategies. Neuropathic pain-modulation medications can be considered for pain control. Ultrasound-guided hydro-release/dissection of the common fibular nerve has been trialed by some practitioners, but no published literature exists at this time. Surgical intervention should be considered if nonoperative measures have failed, if symptoms are progressive, or if there is a defined lesion such as a fracture, laceration, or mass lesion compressing the nerve. In chronic cases, if weakness and foot drop persist, an ankle brace or ankle foot orthosis (AFO) can be used. Recovery is dependent on nerve injury severity.[21]

## Other Pathology

### Iliotibial Band Syndrome

#### Etiology and Pathophysiology

The iliotibial band (ITB) is a lateral thickening of the tensor fascia lata in the thigh that passes over the lateral femoral condyle and attaches to Gerdy's tubercle on the anterolateral aspect of the tibia as well as distal lateral femur. It is generally thought to be due to compression over the lateral aspect of the knee related to ITB overload rather than abnormal movement or friction due to ITB tightness. Potential contributing factors include weak hip abductors, varus knee alignment, and excessive foot pronation often in the setting of increased exercise volume or intensity.[22]

#### History, Examination, and Diagnostic Testing

ITB syndrome typically presents as pain in the lateral aspect of the distal femur and is often exacerbated by walking or running downhill. Physical examination is typically notable for tenderness over the lateral femoral condyle and Gerdy's tubercle. Ober's test is often positive. Noble's compression is also used and is more specific than sensitive. Imaging studies such as radiographs, musculoskeletal ultrasound, and MRI are not typically necessary but can help to rule out other lateral knee pathology.

#### Treatment

Treatment should initially focus on load reduction and stretching, with gradual reintroduction of nonprovocative activities.[23] Physical therapy should be prescribed with emphasis on hip and knee stabilization with progression to single-leg exercises and plyometrics.

#### Basic Order Set

Physical therapy script:
- Diagnosis: ITB syndrome
- Frequency and duration: One to two times per week for 4 to 6 weeks
- Protocol: Stretching of the tensor fascia latae and gluteus medius; initial focus on hip abductor strengthening and neuromuscular coordination; start with uphill treadmill walking to reintroduce activity; progress to slow split squats with heavy loads and eventually to plyometrics
- Precautions: None

### Prepatellar Bursopathy

#### Etiology and Pathophysiology

The prepatellar bursa lies superficial to the patella and assists with smooth patellar movement during knee flexion and extension. Prepatellar bursopathy, also known as housemaid's knee, may develop acutely due to trauma, infection, or gout or due to chronic direct pressure over the patella.[24]

#### History, Examination, and Diagnostic Testing

Patients with acute bursopathy (or "bursitis") present with tenderness directly over the patella, swelling, and erythema. Chronic bursopathy is typically non-tender and non-erythematous with a globular mass over the patella. Diagnosis is clinical but can be confirmed with musculoskeletal ultrasound or MRI if required. Additional workup is targeted at determining an etiology for the bursopathy which should include obtaining basic vital signs, serology, and a bursa fluid sample for analysis.

## Treatment

Treatment depends on the etiology. In most acute cases the bursa can be aspirated with careful adherence to aseptic technique, though fluid re-accumulation can occur. Bursopathy related to an infectious etiology should empirically be treated with antibiotics until a causative organism is confirmed. Bursopathy secondary to a crystal pathology should be treated with usual care for crystal-associated diseases. Noninfectious bursitis can be treated additionally with a corticosteroid injection to reduce inflammation and pain.[24] Chronic bursopathy is usually managed with activity modification with no need for aspiration.[24]

## Basic Order Sets

Serology:
- Complete blood count (CBC) with differential
- Serum uric acid
- Blood cultures if concern for sepsis

Bursal fluid analysis:
- White blood cell count (WBC)
- Gram stain
- Culture
- Crystal evaluation

# Pes Anserine Bursopathy

## Etiology and Pathophysiology

The pes anserine bursa is located between the proximal medial tibia and the confluence of the semitendinosus, gracilis, and sartorius tendons. Some experts have suggested that "pes anserine bursopathy" may actually be a tendinopathy rather than secondary to bursa inflammation. It is often associated with underlying OA.[25]

## History, Examination, and Diagnostic Testing

Patients typically present with pain at the insertion of the pes anserine tendons distal to the medial knee joint line. Physical examination reveals tenderness at this location and potential swelling. Plain radiographs can be useful to evaluate for OA or proximal tibial bone injury. Ultrasound or MRI may show swelling near pes anserine tendons, but these are frequently absent and, therefore, not necessary.

## Treatment

Treatment options include activity modification, icing, NSAIDs, and physical therapy focused on stretching and strengthening of the medial hamstrings and quadriceps. Bursal injections of corticosteroids under ultrasound guidance can be considered for recalcitrant symptoms.[26]

## LOWER LEG INJURIES

### Acute Compartment Syndrome
### Etiology and Pathophysiology

Acute compartment syndrome (ACS) typically occurs as a result of severe traumatic injury. The highest risk is seen with compound or open fractures due to bleeding and limited compartment expansion capacity.[27] Increased compartment pressures lead to compression of the vasculature, causing tissue ischemia and eventual necrosis. It is important to note that open fractures do not release a compartment and ACS can still occur.

### History, Examination, and Diagnostic Testing

The classic findings in ACS are the five Ps: pain out of proportion to appearance, pallor, pulselessness, paresthesias, and paralysis. However, these are often found in the late stages of ACS and may signal irreversible damage.[27] Their absence does not rule out ACS. In this scenario, the leg may appear swollen and tense and is often painful with passive muscle stretch. Sensory and motor nerve compression can result in paresthesias and weakness. ACS is a clinical diagnosis that does not require imaging. Intracompartmental pressure greater than 15 mmHg is generally used for diagnosis based on the modified Pedowitz criteria; however, there are no established values determining the need for acute surgical decompression and should not delay this treatment.[27]

### Treatment

When identified, ACS requires emergent surgical referral for compartment release with open fasciotomy as ischemic duration directly correlates with long-term morbidity. Recovery after fasciotomy is often slow and may be complicated by infection or need for skin grafting. Return to activity is heavily dependent on severity of neurovascular injury. There is no standardized postoperative physical therapy regimen specific to ACS.

### Chronic Exertional Compartment Syndrome
### Etiology and Pathophysiology

Chronic exertional compartment syndrome (CECS) is a painful leg condition that can affect both athletes and sedentary individuals. Muscle swelling of up to 20% can occur during exercise as a result of fluid shift and vascular congestion, while the relatively stiff fascia is unable to accommodate the increase in volume, leading to increased compartment pressure.[28] While the cause of pain is presumed to be related to ischemia, increased pressure on other structures (nerves, connective tissues, muscles, and periosteum) may also contribute.[28]

### History, Examination, and Diagnostic Testing

Clarifying the location, timing, precipitating factors, and training regimen help differentiate CECS from medial tibial stress syndrome (MTSS) and stress fracture. CECS typically presents with leg pain during exertion of a specific length, intensity, or duration. Pain progressively worsens and can shift from a dull, aching fullness to sharp pain. As the syndrome progresses, symptoms may be triggered with simple activities like walking. Muscle weakness in the affected compartment and paresthesias may also occur. The compartment may feel firm and tender following activity. Symptoms generally improve with rest. Diagnosis of CECS is most commonly made using the Pedowitz criteria with compartment pressures greater than 15, 30, and 20 mmHg at rest, 1 minute postexertion, and 5 minutes postexertion, respectively.[29] Exertional MRI protocols have also been described to make the diagnosis of anterior compartment CECS.[28]

## Treatment

Activity modification is at the core of conservative management with initial avoidance of aggravating activity followed by gradual reintroduction.[30] Ice, NSAIDs, massage, stretching, shoe modification, and alteration of gait mechanics may also be trialed, but failure rates are high. Chemodenervation to decrease compartment muscle activation has shown some success.[30] Open or endoscopic surgical fasciotomy is the definitive treatment and has success rates of over 80% for anterior and lateral compartments.[31] More recently, experimental ultrasound-guided fascial release has been described for anterior and lateral compartments.[32] Rehabilitation following surgical fasciotomy generally begins with passive range of motion for the first several days after surgery followed by progressive walking over a period of approximately 4 weeks. Gentle aerobic exercise with slow progression of sport-specific activity may be started 6 weeks postoperatively provided symptoms do not recur.

## Basic Order Sets

Physical therapy prescription (preoperative conservative management):
- Diagnosis: CECS
- Frequency and duration: One to two times per week for 3 to 4 weeks
- Protocol: Gradual reintroduction of physical activity. If unable to tolerate, evaluate gait mechanics and retrain as indicated.
- Precautions: Stop activity if symptoms recur.

Physical therapy prescription (postoperative)*:
- Diagnosis: Status post-compartment decompression for CECS
- Frequency and duration: Two to three times per week for 8 to 12 weeks
- Protocol: Gradually restore ROM with concomitant scar tissue massage and desensitization; advance to progressive strengthening, balance, and proprioception exercises; once general strength is adequate, progress to activity-specific movements
- Precautions: Monitor and control any postactivity swelling, avoid eccentric exercises initially, avoid friction over scar tissue

## Gastrocnemius Strain
### Etiology and Pathophysiology

Gastrocnemius strain ("tennis leg") is a common injury in the athletic population. Injury typically occurs with rapid acceleration/deceleration during knee extension and ankle dorsiflexion, when the muscle is in its more elongated position.[33] Risk of gastrocnemius strain may be higher with inadequate warmup or when fatigued.[33] The medial head is more commonly injured than the lateral head.

**TABLE 20.4 GRADING OF GASTROCNEMIUS STRAINS[35]**

| GRADE | SYMPTOMS | SIGNS | PATHOLOGY | RADIOLOGY |
|---|---|---|---|---|
| 1/mild | Pain with activity, able to continue | Mild localized pain, minimal loss of strength/ROM | <10% muscle fiber disruption | Edema on MRI, <5% muscle fiber involvement |
| 2/moderate | Pain with activity, unable to continue | Significant localized pain, loss of strength/ROM | 10%–50% muscle fiber disruption | Abnormal myotendinous junction, edema, and hemorrhage |
| 3/severe | Immediate severe pain with disability, unable to continue any activity | Loss of muscle function, palpable defect/mass | 50%–100% muscle fiber disruption | Complete disruption of muscle, extensive edema/hemorrhage, retraction |

## History, Examination, and Diagnostic Testing

Patients typically present with acute posterior leg pain described as the sensation of being kicked or hit in the leg. Swelling and ecchymosis may occur and can mimic Achilles tendon injury. MRI or ultrasound can be used to make a definitive diagnosis and determine the degree of injury (Table 20.4).

## Treatment

Initial treatment consists of PRICE. Immobilization is rarely required but may be indicated in severe strains.[34] Physical therapy should be initiated to restrengthen the gastrocnemius/soleus complex and provide sport-specific instructions on movement patterns to prevent recurrence.[34] Gradual return to activity is guided by pain. While data is limited, most individuals return to preinjury activities within 4 to 7 weeks.

## Medial Tibial Stress Syndrome
### Etiology and Pathophysiology

MTSS, commonly known as "shin splints," is a frequent cause of activity-induced athletic leg pain, typically occurring along the posteromedial border of the tibia. The etiology of MTSS is incompletely understood, but the most popular theory suggests that pain is the result of a periosteal stress reaction secondary to tension at the insertion of the tibialis posterior, soleus, or flexor digitorum longus tendons onto the tibia.[36]

## History, Examination, and Diagnostic Testing

Patients typically present with tenderness over the lower third of the posteromedial border of the tibia. Swelling or palpable periosteal reaction may occur. Unlike stress fractures, night pain and percussive pain are not typically present in MTSS, and the pain is generally more diffuse. Stress fracture pain also remains constant during activity, while MTSS may initially subside during early activity. In contrast to CECS, pain in MTSS may not resolve rapidly upon activity cessation. MTSS is a clinical diagnosis; however, imaging with MRI may be helpful in differentiating MTSS from a stress fracture.

## Treatment

Conservative management is generally successful, although precise protocols have not been studied. Rest and activity modification are initiated first. Addressing gait mechanics, knee and ankle strength, and flexibility with physical therapy is typically beneficial.[37] Modalities such as massage, acupuncture, electrotherapy, and extracorporeal shockwave therapy have shown limited success in reducing symptoms.[37] Shoe orthotics may be helpful in preventing recurrence.[37] Return to activity should be gradual and occur in a stepwise pain-free fashion.

## Basic Order Set

Physical therapy prescription:
- Diagnosis: MTSS
- Frequency and duration: One to two times per week for 4 weeks
- Protocol: Evaluate biomechanics and assess overall lower extremity strength; include strengthening of knee and ankle stabilizers with secondary focus on hip stabilization; modalities PRN for symptom relief; gradually progress to activity-specific movements
- Precautions: None

## REFERENCES

The full list of references appears in the digital product found on http://connect.springerpub.com/content/book/978-0-8261-6226-7/part/part02/chapter/ch20

# ANKLE AND FOOT

SHERRY IGBINIGIE, BRIAN MUGLESTON, MATT LACOURSE, AND MARK HARRAST

## INTRODUCTION

Ankle and foot injuries are some of the most common sports injuries. Ankle injuries alone account for 10% to 30% of all sports injuries.[1] One study on National Football League (NFL) players found that 53.2% of players had a history of ankle injury.[2] Another study found that 31% of running injuries involved the ankle or foot.[3] This chapter will review the anatomy, biomechanics, and common injuries of the ankle and foot. We will cover in more detail the most common sources of ankle and foot pain in the text. See Table 21.1 for a more comprehensive differential diagnosis of ankle and foot pain.

**TABLE 21.1 DIFFERENTIAL DIAGNOSIS OF ANKLE AND FOOT PAIN BY PAIN LOCATION**

| REGION | DIAGNOSES |
|---|---|
| Lateral ankle pain | **Bone**<br>Distal fibula fracture<br>Talus fracture and osteochondral injury<br><br>**Tendon**<br>Peroneal tendinopathy<br>Peroneal tendon subluxation<br><br>**Ligament**<br>Lateral ankle sprain<br>Syndesmosis/AITFL sprain<br><br>**Nerve**<br>Radiculopathy—S1<br>CRPS<br><br>**Other**<br>Anterolateral impingement syndrome<br>Sinus tarsi syndrome |

*(continued)*

The full list of references appears in the digital product found on http://connect.springerpub.com/content/book/978-0-8261-6226-7/part/part02/chapter/ch21

**TABLE 21.1 DIFFERENTIAL DIAGNOSIS OF ANKLE AND FOOT PAIN BY PAIN LOCATION (continued)**

| REGION | DIAGNOSES |
|---|---|
| Medial ankle pain | **Bone**<br>Distal tibia (medial malleolar) fracture<br>Talus fracture and osteochondral injury<br><br>**Tendon**<br>Tibialis posterior tendinopathy<br>Flexor hallucis longus tendinopathy<br><br>**Ligament**<br>Medial ankle sprain<br><br>**Nerve**<br>Tarsal tunnel syndrome<br>Radiculopathy—L4–5<br>CRPS<br><br>**Other**<br>Medial impingement syndrome |
| Anterior ankle pain | **Bone**<br>Talus fracture and osteochondral injury<br><br>**Tendon**<br>Tibialis anterior tendinopathy<br><br>**Ligament**<br>Syndesmosis/AITFL sprain<br><br>**Nerve**<br>Radiculopathy—L4–5<br>Anterior tarsal tunnel syndrome<br>Superficial peroneal neuropathy<br>CRPS<br><br>**Other**<br>Anterior impingement syndrome<br>Anterolateral impingement syndrome |
| Posterior ankle pain | **Bone**<br>Os trigonum fracture<br><br>**Tendon**<br>Achilles tendinopathy<br>Plantaris tendinopathy<br><br>**Nerve**<br>Radiculopathy—S1<br>Sural neuropathy<br>CRPS<br><br>**Other**<br>Posterior impingement syndrome<br>Retrocalcaneal bursitis<br>Haglund's syndrome<br>Accessory soleus |

(continued)

**TABLE 21.1 DIFFERENTIAL DIAGNOSIS OF ANKLE AND FOOT PAIN BY PAIN LOCATION** (*continued*)

| REGION | DIAGNOSES |
|---|---|
| Hindfoot pain | **Bone**<br>Calcaneal fracture<br><br>**Ligament**<br>Plantar fasciopathy<br><br>**Nerve**<br>Radiculopathy—S1<br>Tarsal tunnel syndrome<br>Inferior calcaneal nerve entrapment<br>Medial calcaneal nerve entrapment<br>CRPS<br><br>**Other**<br>Fat pad contusion and/or syndrome |
| Midfoot pain | **Bone**<br>Tarsal fractures (navicular, cuboid, and cuneiform)<br>Cuboid syndrome<br>Tarsal coalition<br>Os naviculare injury<br><br>**Tendon**<br>Extensor digitorum tendinopathy<br>Tibialis posterior tendinopathy<br>Peroneal tendinopathy<br>Abductor hallucis strain<br><br>**Ligament**<br>Mid-tarsal joint sprain<br>Plantar fascia strain<br>Lisfranc injury<br>Bifurcate ligament injuries (calcaneonavicular and calcaneocuboid ligament)<br><br>**Nerve**<br>Superficial peroneal neuropathy<br>Radiculopathy—L5–S1<br>Tarsal tunnel syndrome<br>Medial plantar nerve entrapment<br>Inferior calcaneal nerve entrapment<br>Anterior tarsal tunnel syndrome (deep peroneal nerve entrapment)<br>CRPS |
| Forefoot pain | **Bone**<br>Fifth metatarsal injury: Jones fracture, pseudo–Jones fracture<br>Metatarsalgia<br>Metatarsal fracture<br>Hallux valgus<br>Hallux limitus<br>Hammer toe<br>Sesamoid injuries: fracture, sesamoiditis, bipartite |

(continued)

**TABLE 21.1 DIFFERENTIAL DIAGNOSIS OF ANKLE AND FOOT PAIN BY PAIN LOCATION (continued)**

| REGION | DIAGNOSES |
|---|---|
| Forefoot pain | **Tendon**<br>Flexor hallucis longus tendinopathy<br>Extensor hallucis tendinopathy<br>Abductor hallucis tendinopathy<br><br>**Ligament**<br>"Turf toe"—first[t] MTP joint sprain<br><br>**Nerve**<br>Superficial peroneal neuropathy<br>Morton's neuroma<br>Radiculopathy—L5–S1<br>Tarsal tunnel syndrome<br>Anterior tarsal tunnel syndrome (deep peroneal nerve entrapment)<br>Joplin's neuritis<br>CRPS<br><br>**Other**<br>Synovitis/capsulitis of the MTP joints<br>Synovitis of the metatarsal–cuneiform joint<br>Subungual hematoma<br>Subungual exocytosis<br>Corns and calluses<br>Onycocryptosis<br>Plantar wart |

AITFL, anterior inferior tibiofibular ligament; CRPS, complex regional pain syndrome; MTP, metatarsophalangeal.

## ANATOMY AND BIOMECHANICS

The ankle is a three-joint complex consisting of the talocrural (tibiotalar), distal tibiofibular, and subtalar (talocalcaneal) joints. The talocrural joint is a hinged synovial joint with primarily sagittal plane motion of dorsiflexion and plantarflexion, though there is some degree of rotation and abduction/adduction at this joint. The distal tibiofibular articulation is a fibrous joint, or syndesmosis. The primary motion of the subtalar joint is inversion/eversion. The terms pronation and supination are triplanar motions at the talocrural joint, subtalar joint, and forefoot. Pronation is dorsiflexion, subtalar eversion, and forefoot abduction. Supination is plantarflexion, subtalar inversion, and forefoot adduction.

During ambulation, there is significant stress across the foot and ankle given the large amount of force placed on a small surface area.[4] Derangements in biomechanical stress affecting the lower limb often result in injury to the ankle and foot. Rehabilitation for the majority of ankle and foot injuries typically begins with reduction in pain followed by restoration of range of motion, neuromuscular reeducation and strengthening (including the foot intrinsic musculature or "foot core"), proprioception/balance, functional exercises, and return-to-sport activities.

## ANKLE

### Bone Pathology
### Traumatic Distal Fibular Fractures

#### Etiology and Pathophysiology

Distal fibular fractures are typically caused by a direct blow to the lateral leg or an ankle inversion injury resulting in disruption of the lateral ligaments causing the talus to contact, then fracture, the distal fibula.

#### Diagnostic Approach

Distal fibular fractures present with swelling, tenderness, and possible deformity at the lateral malleolus or slightly more proximal. Patient may have a positive dorsiflexion external rotation test. Ottawa ankle rules (Table 21.2) apply. Ankle radiographs (see the following "Basic Order Set(s)") can confirm the diagnosis.

#### Treatment

Weber type A fractures are usually stable and can be treated with a walking boot and weight-bearing as tolerated (WBAT) for 6 to 8 weeks. Weber type B fractures may be stable and treated similarly to Weber A but can be associated with instability and may require open reduction internal fixation (ORIF). Type C fractures are commonly unstable requiring ORIF. Typically, with this type of injury, the presence of a medial ankle lesion (deltoid ligament disruption or bimalleolar fracture) or >2 mm talus–fibula interval is an indication for surgery. See Table 21.3 and Figure 21.1 for details on Weber classification. Follow-up radiographs should be obtained to ensure proper healing.

#### TABLE 21.2 OTTAWA ANKLE RULES

*Ankle or foot radiographs are required if one or more of the following is present:*

| ANKLE | FOOT |
|---|---|
| • Tenderness to palpation over the distal 6 cm of posterior edge of the fibula or tibia or the tip of the lateral or medial malleolus<br>• Unable to take four steps immediately following the injury and in the ED | • Tenderness to palpation over the navicular or over the base of the fifth metatarsal<br>• Complaints of pain in the midfoot<br>• Unable to take four steps immediately following the injury and in ED |

#### TABLE 21.3 WEBER CLASSIFICATION

| | |
|---|---|
| Weber type A | Avulsion-type fractures of the distal fibula below the level of the ankle mortise. |
| Weber type B | Fracture of the distal fibula at the level of the ankle mortise. |
| Weber type C | Fracture of the distal fibula above the level of the ankle mortise. |

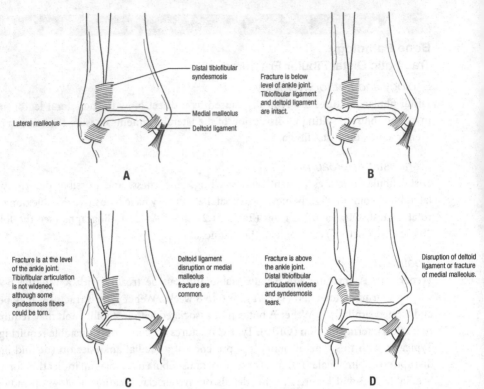

**FIGURE 21.1** Weber classification: (A) normal, (B) Weber A, (C) Weber B, (D) Weber C.

## Functional Prognosis and Outcomes

Overall, fibular fractures have a good prognosis regardless of type if properly treated. The most common complication from an ankle fracture is posttraumatic arthritis, which is most commonly seen in bimalleolar and trimalleolar fractures.[4] Nonunion is uncommon.

## Basic Order Set(s)

Weight-bearing ankle x-ray with anteroposterior (AP), mortise, and lateral views +/− oblique views. Consider external rotation stress views if concerned for a concurrent deltoid ligament injury.

## Ligament Pathology

### Lateral Ankle Sprain

#### Etiology and Pathophysiology

Ankle sprains account for 14% to 21% of sports injuries and 85% of all ankle injuries and also carry the highest rate of reinjury.[5] Lateral ankle sprains result from inversion forces on a plantarflexed foot and occur in a predictable sequence, with the anterior talofibular ligament (ATFL) commonly being the first and only ligament injured followed by the calcaneal fibular ligament (CFL).

## Diagnostic Approach

Patients present with pain, swelling, and ecchymosis at the lateral ankle, along with difficulty weight-bearing. Examiners should inquire about a history of prior lateral ankle sprains, as patients who have had multiple events have a greater risk for reinjury. Common tests include the anterior drawer and talar tilt to evaluate for ATFL and CFL integrity, respectively. The squeeze test can evaluate for concomitant syndesmotic injury. The Ottawa Ankle Rules are used to determine the need for radiographs. (See Table 21.2). This is primarily a clinical diagnosis. However, MRI, to evaluate for concurrent injuries other than solely a lateral ligamentous sprain, may be considered if recovery is longer than expected (>4–6 weeks) with minimal improvement or general failure of conservative management.

## Treatment

Initial injuries are treated with the RICE (rest-ice-compression-elevation) protocol until patients are able to ambulate with normal gait. Time-limited protected weight-bearing with use of a walking boot, aircast, or other ankle orthosis can be helpful for pain and swelling management as well as to expedite a more normal gait and thus lessen stress on other structures due to antalgia. Early mobilization within the first week should be encouraged when possible. Surgical intervention has not been shown to result in better outcomes, though considerations should be made on an individual basis for severe injuries.[6] Surgical intervention (lateral ligament reconstruction) is generally only considered after failure of conservative management and persistent instability. Physical therapy (PT) should be included for all injuries, which helps to restore ankle range of motion (ROM), proprioception, and balance for return to sport and to prevent subsequent injury.

## Functional Prognosis and Outcomes

Approximately one third of injured individuals experience long-term, residual symptoms, and thus, appropriate treatment of an acute lateral ankle sprain is paramount.[7] Positive prognostic factors include early weight-bearing, milder severity, and younger age.

## Basic Order Set(s)

Generally, no imaging is needed unless Ottawa Ankle Rules apply. If so, order weight-bearing ankle XR with AP, lateral, oblique, and mortise views to rule out syndesmotic injury or fracture. PT ordered should follow a progressive protocol of restoration of full ankle range of motion, active ankle muscle strengthening, proprioceptive retraining, and functional exercises.

# Syndesmosis and Anterior Inferior Tibiofibular Ligament Sprain

## Etiology and Pathophysiology

Syndesmosis sprains result when an eversion force is applied to a dorsiflexed ankle, which commonly occur during contact sports that combine high-intensity cutting and jumping movements, such as in football and soccer.

### Diagnostic Approach

Patients present with diffuse pain, which is more prominent along the anterolateral ankle, and have difficulty weight-bearing. Examiners should inspect the joint for swelling, as well as palpate the ligaments for tenderness. The squeeze test evaluates for syndesmotic injury, and the external rotation test evaluates for AITFL injury. Weight-bearing radiographs are typically performed to evaluate the presence of fracture or tibiofibular diastasis. MRI can be performed to grade injury severity, as well as to identify concurrent injuries.

### Treatment

Treatment depends on the severity of the injury. Lower grade injuries, characterized by a partial tear of the AITFL with no tibiofibular diastasis, can be treated conservatively with the RICE protocol along with 2 to 4 weeks of immobilization in a walking boot with WBAT. Higher grade injuries, which involve a complete tear of the AITFL and resultant ankle instability, require surgery.

### Functional Prognosis and Outcomes

Syndesmotic injuries are associated with the worst prognosis of ankle ligament injuries, with recovery nearly four times longer than those for lateral ankle sprains, typically taking 6 to 8 weeks.[8]

### Basic Order Set(s)

Weight-bearing ankle XRs (AP, lateral, and mortise views) to evaluate for fracture or tibiofibular diastasis. MRI of the ankle can be obtained to grade injury severity and identify concurrent injuries.

## Tendon Pathology
## Achilles Tendinopathy

### Etiology and Pathophysiology

Achilles tendinopathy is most prevalent in middle-aged male patients and in those who participate in running sports, especially if training errors occur. Tendinopathy is classified by duration, such as acute or chronic (>6 weeks), or location, which can be insertional (within 2 cm of tendon insertion) or midsubstance (2–6 cm proximal to tendon insertion), with the latter being more common.

### Diagnostic Approach

Patients report posterior heel pain that is worse in the morning and at the beginning of exercise. Diagnosis is made primarily by clinical assessment (pain/tenderness at the site, swelling, erythema, warmth, and thickening or a palpable nodule). Although not always needed, radiographs can identify insertional calcifications, a characteristic of insertional tendinopathy, as well as a prominent calcaneal tuberosity (Haglund's deformity), which is a cause of Haglund's syndrome (insertional Achilles tendinopathy with a retrocalcaneal bursitis at the site of a Haglund's bump). MRI or ultrasound (US) can confirm the diagnosis and gauge severity, especially when symptoms do not respond to conservative measures.

### Treatment

Treatment depends on severity and consists of activity modification, ice, a heel lift to offload the calf–Achilles complex, immobilization with a walking boot for severe symptoms, and PT. PT focuses on eccentric strengthening exercises, stretching, myofascial work, and evaluating the entire kinetic chain of the lower limb for any biomechanical deficits that may contribute to symptoms. Eccentric exercises are more beneficial for the treatment of midsubstance over insertional tendinopathy.[9] Nitro patches are commonly used in conjunction with eccentric strengthening, but patients should be counseled that this medication can frequently cause headache as a side effect. For chronic Achilles tendinopathy that has failed conservative treatment, US-guided procedures (platelet-rich plasma [PRP] injection, needle tenotomy, percutaneous tendon scraping, and/or tenotomy), and extracorporeal shockwave therapy (ESWT) are commonly considered prior to surgical debridement.

### Functional Prognosis and Outcomes

Approximately 20% of patients have symptoms at least 6 months following initial injury.[9] There is low risk of progression to Achilles tendon rupture with one study showing only 4% of individuals with Achilles tendinopathy progressed to frank rupture.[10]

### Basic Order Set(s)

Weight-bearing foot or ankle (AP and lateral views) radiographs are considered to evaluate for a bony source of posterior heel pain or evaluate for a Haglund's deformity that may contribute to insertional Achilles tendinopathy. For midportion Achilles tendinopathy, PT ordered should follow an eccentric strengthening protocol.

## Achilles Rupture

### Etiology and Pathophysiology

Achilles tendon rupture typically occurs in the watershed zone where there is decreased blood supply, located 2 to 6 cm above the insertion site. It is more commonly seen in males than females with a peak age of 30 to 40 years old. Risk factors include obesity, use of fluoroquinolones, corticosteroid exposure, or anabolic steroid use.

### Diagnostic Approach

Patients presents with sudden, sharp posterior ankle pain +/– a notable "pop," with a sensation often described as "someone hit me in the back of the leg." Patients will have difficulty bearing weight on the affected leg. Physical examination reveals bruising and edema over the area with a palpable defect. Thompson test is positive which is a lack of plantarflexion when the calf muscle is squeezed. US imaging or MRI can confirm the diagnosis.

### Treatment

Nonoperative treatment includes 2 weeks of non-weight-bearing (NWB) followed by WBAT in a walking boot with a 20-degree heel wedge that is progressively decreased over 8 to 12 weeks. Rehabilitation is initiated once the patient transitions to weight-bearing. Surgical repair is recommended in young and active patients.

### Functional Prognosis and Outcomes

Overall, the risk of rerupture is low, but surgical repair reduces the risk of rerupture and allows for a quicker return to activity compared to nonsurgical treatment.

### Basic Order Set(s)

MRI or US of the ankle to confirm the diagnosis.

## Peroneal Tendinopathy

### Etiology and Pathophysiology

The peroneal tendons assist with ankle eversion and plantarflexion. Injuries more often occur in patients with a cavovarus hindfoot alignment, as well as during activities that place excessive pronation and eversion stress on the peroneal tendons, such as running on sloped or uneven surfaces.

### Diagnostic Approach

Patients present with posterolateral ankle pain and dysfunction that can be difficult to distinguish from lateral ankle ligament injuries. Examination reveals tenderness posterior to the lateral malleolus and sometimes a palpable nodule. Tendon subluxation due to tearing of the superior peroneal retinaculum can occur, with patients demonstrating a positive Kleiger test (pain with knee flexed and passive ankle external rotation) on examination. US and MRI are used in recalcitrant cases to confirm the characteristics of tendinopathy or the presence of subluxation or split tears. Imaging can reveal fluid within the peroneal tendon sheath, though this finding is nonspecific and can be seen in asymptomatic individuals.

### Treatment

Treatment for tendinopathy is RICE and eccentric strengthening exercises. Orthoses with lateral heel wedging can be prescribed to off-load the peroneal tendons. US-guided peroneal tendon sheath injections are considered for pain control in refractory cases. Subluxation is treated with immobilization (casting or boot), NWB × 2 weeks, followed by progressive WB over the next 4 weeks, and if it fails, surgical treatment is considered.

### Functional Prognosis and Outcomes

Acute tendinopathy responds well to conservative therapy, though subluxation typically requires surgical evaluation due to the risk of chronic instability and recurrent subluxation.

## Tibialis Posterior Tendinopathy

### Etiology and Pathophysiology

The tibialis posterior acts as a powerful inverter and plantarflexor of the foot, as well as a dynamic stabilizer of the medial longitudinal arch. Injuries occur from overuse and rapid increases in activity.

## Diagnostic Approach

On examination, patients display posteromedial ankle pain, excessive pronation of the foot, and difficulty performing consecutive heel raises. Pes planus and the "too many toes" sign can be seen in later stages of tendon dysfunction. While imaging is generally not necessary, US and MRI are used in recalcitrant cases to confirm the characteristics of tendinopathy or the presence of a tear. Imaging can reveal fluid within the tibialis posterior tendon sheath, though this finding is nonspecific and can be seen in asymptomatic individuals.

## Treatment

Treatment for tendinopathy is RICE and eccentric strengthening exercises. Arch support with medial heel wedges can off-load the tendon. Severe cases may require several weeks of immobilization with a walking boot. US-guided tibialis posterior tendon sheath injections can be considered for pain control in refractory cases. If basic conservative management fails, surgical debridement can be considered.

## Functional Prognosis and Outcomes

Patients with early stages of tendon dysfunction respond well to conservative management.

# Nerve Pathology
## Tarsal Tunnel Syndrome
### Etiology and Pathophysiology

Tarsal tunnel syndrome (TTS) is the result of posterior tibial nerve compression within the tarsal tunnel that is formed by the overlying flexor retinaculum that extends from the medial malleolus to the medial calcaneus. Compression of the tibial nerve may be idiopathic, due to a tenosynovitis, stretch injury from excessive pronation, trauma, or external compression from a variety of sources, including ganglion cysts.

### Diagnostic Approach

TTS typically presents with medial ankle pain and/or paresthesias along the plantar surface of the foot that are worse at night. Symptoms are worsened with activity. Chronic cases may have atrophy of the foot intrinsic muscles, but permanent neurologic injury is rare. A Tinel's sign at the area of entrapment may be positive. Stressing the area with forceful active pronation or by sustained passive eversion can elicit pain. Neurologic examination should rule out competing diagnoses, such as peripheral polyneuropathy or radiculopathy. In challenging cases, electrodiagnostic studies can be helpful. MRI and US imaging may rule out an anatomic lesion but are rarely necessary.

### Treatment

TTS is treated conservatively with rest (including a walking boot for severe symptoms), foot orthoses to limit excessive pronation, and correcting biomechanical deficits with ankle rehabilitation (including Achilles stretching and proprioceptive training) and foot core strengthening (to improve medial longitudinal arch support and lessen excessive pronation). US-guided injections and surgical release are reserved for recalcitrant cases.

*Functional Prognosis and Outcomes*

There is a high perioperative complication rate for individuals who undergo surgery. Favorable surgical outcomes include a positive Tinel's sign or the presence of a space-occupying lesion.

## Other
## Ankle Impingement Syndromes

*Etiology and Pathophysiology*

*Anterior impingement* is caused by entrapment of bony or soft tissue between the talus and tibia during dorsiflexion and is seen more commonly in soccer players and other kicking athletes or those who perform repetitive extreme ankle ranges of motion. *Anterolateral impingement* is commonly seen after repeated lateral ankle sprains and is related to scarring of the soft tissues and synovial hypertrophy. *Posterior impingement* is bony entrapment of the posterior talus by the posterior aspect of the distal tibia at terminal plantarflexion commonly seen in ballet dancers, gymnasts, and footballers. This may be related to an enlarged posterior talus process or os trigonum.

*Diagnostic Approach*

Symptoms occur at the site of impingement. Anterior and anterolateral impingement worsen with ankle dorsiflexion, including deep squatting and lunges (both physical examination and provocative maneuvers). Posterior impingement worsens with ankle plantarflexion (downhill running or walking and wearing high-heeled shoes). Passive plantarflexion is the posterior impingement test. Ankle radiographs can demonstrate osteophytes along the neck of the talus and anterior rim of the tibia to suggest anterior impingement or an os trigonum/enlarged posterior talus process to suggest posterior impingement.

*Treatment*

Initial treatment is conservative with activity modification limiting impingement, a walking boot for more severe symptoms, and PT, including manual mobilization techniques at the foot and/or ankle. US-guided corticosteroid injections at the site of impingement may help with symptom relief. Surgical debridement or resection in bony impingement may be considered for those who fail conservative care.

*Functional Prognosis and Outcomes*

Conservative management is generally satisfactory. Sixty-one percent of those moving onto surgery for posterior impingement are dancers that require a high level of activity.[11] The majority of patients are able to return to their previous level of activity following surgery.

*Basic Order Set(s)*

Ankle XR: weight-bearing AP, mortise, lateral views in extension and flexion. PT: focus on ankle stability and proprioception exercises, stretching exercises, pain modalities as needed, home exercise program.

## FOOT

### Bone Pathology
### Metatarsalgia

#### Etiology and Pathophysiology

The synovium of the metatarsal phalangeal joint becomes inflamed following chronic pressure due to overpronation, hammer toes, high arches, or a shortening of the first metatarsal (Morton's foot) resulting in excessive weight-bearing on the second metatarsophalangeal (MTP) joint most frequently.

#### Diagnostic Approach

Patients present with pain and tenderness over the plantar aspect of the metatarsal heads that worsens with toe dorsiflexion and ambulation. Calluses may be present over the affected joints. X-ray imaging of the foot may demonstrate a "V" sign, or separation of the toes, which may be a sign of joint synovitis.

#### Treatment

Conservative management is standard. A metatarsal pad/bar or other orthosis to off-load pressure on the affected joint is a first-line measure. A corticosteroid injection may be appropriate if the patient fails more conservative treatment. Although surgical metatarsal osteotomies can be performed if the patient has no relief from other measures, evidence shows this procedure has a high failure rate.[12]

### Fifth Metatarsal Fracture (Jones and Pseudo–Jones Fracture)

#### Etiology and Pathophysiology

A Jones fracture occurs in the proximal fifth metatarsal at the level of the articulation between the fourth and fifth metatarsals (metaphyseal–diaphyseal junction). A pseudo–Jones fracture, which is more common, is a fifth metatarsal fracture proximal to that articulation, often a result of avulsion where the peroneus brevis tendon inserts at the proximal tubercle. Both fractures generally occur with ankle inversion or forefoot adduction forces ,respectively.

#### Diagnostic Approach

Patients classically present with lateral foot pain at the fifth metatarsal base. Both fractures are typically visible on radiographs and can be classified by zone, which is important to distinguish as treatment differs.

#### Treatment

Jones fractures are treated surgically with screw fixation for better outcomes and faster return to play. Pseudo–Jones fractures are treated nonoperatively in a walking boot or short-leg walking cast WBAT for 2 to 3 weeks unless the fracture is largely displaced (>2–3 mm) or extends through the articular surface.

#### Functional Prognosis and Outcomes

Jones fractures occur at a vascular watershed area leading to a high risk of nonunion. Surgical revision may be necessary in these cases. Screw failure is not common. In all cases of fifth metatarsal fractures, radiologic evidence of healing is an appropriate safety measure before a return to sport. One study showed that all patients with a type of pseudo–Jones fractures returned to preinjury functional status by 1 year with 20% return to play (RTP) at 3 months and 85% by 6 months.[13]

## Ligament Pathology
## Plantar Fasciopathy

### Etiology and Pathophysiology

True plantar fasciopathy occurs at the medial tuberosity of the calcaneus. It is the most common cause of heel pain and typically seen in patients with high BMI and long hours of standing but also in distance runners.

### Diagnostic Approach

A common presentation includes insidious onset of inferior and medial heel pain, often worse with the first steps in the morning or immediately following a period of inactivity. Physical examination is notable for tenderness at the medial tuberosity of the calcaneous and pain with dorsiflexion of the first toe. Radiographs are not indicated as calcaneal spurs are commonly seen in the asymptomatic population. US and MRI can characterize the degree of pathology of the plantar fascia (thickening, tears) as well as rule out other diagnoses.

### Treatment

Initial management consists of activity modification, weight loss if appropriate, heal pads or cups for comfort, night splints that hold the foot in dorsiflexion (thus putting the plantar fascia on stretch), foot orthoses or low-dye taping to support the arch of the foot and lessen stress on the plantar fascia, stretching of the fascia, gastrocnemius and soleus, and friction massage with ice or other trademarked devices (e.g., Graston technique). If basic conservative management fails, interventional procedures to consider include ESWT, US-guided steroid injection for short-term pain relief, US-guided PRP injection, and potentially US-guided or surgical plantar fasciotomy if the patient has failed all other treatment options. A randomized controlled study showed that PRP injections significantly reduced pain and increased function better than corticosteroid injections at 12 months.[14] Additionally, steroids have known negative soft tissue side effects.

### Functional Prognosis and Outcomes

Up to 80% of patients undergoing plantar fasciopathy will experience full resolution of the condition within 12 months regardless of treatment.

## First Metatarsophalangeal Joint Sprain ("Turf Toe")

### Etiology and Pathophysiology

This injury involves hyperextension to the first MTP joint causing damage to the plantar plate, joint capsule, and ligaments. This commonly occurs in athletes, especially those who play on rigid surfaces like turf (soccer and American football players). It is categorized as grade I (mild), grade II (partial ligament tear and plantar capsule disruption), and grade III (complete ligamentous tear and plantar capsule disruption). Risk factors include playing on artificial turf, pes planus, and limited ankle dorsiflexion range.

### Diagnostic Approach

Patients present with pain while weight-bearing that worsens with first toe movement. Pertinent examination findings include swelling, ecchymosis, and tenderness with palpation of the first MTP joint. Radiographs are typically not helpful but can rule out a fracture, including an accompanying plantar plate avulsion fracture of the MTP joint capsule. US and MRI can confirm the diagnosis and grade the injury.

### Treatment

Treatment typically includes RICE and taping of the great toe and forefoot to provide stabilization of the MTP joint. Limiting first toe dorsiflexion is the goal of initial treatment and thus transitioning from the postoperative shoe to a running shoe with a carbon fiber insert and Morton's extension is typical for the running athlete. Avoidance of weight-bearing for 48 to 72 hours post-injury followed by WBAT in a postoperative shoe can be done for severe injuries.

### Functional Prognosis and Outcomes

Athletes with a grade I injury can return to play as tolerated. Grade II injury requires at least 2 weeks of rest prior to return to play, and grade III injuries typically necessitate 6 to 10 weeks of recovery. Recovery can be complicated by the development of hallux rigidus.

### Basic Order Set(s)

X-rays for suspected plantar plate avulsion fracture: AP and lateral views of foot with great toe in forced dorsiflexion.

## Nerve Pathology

## Inferior Calcaneal Nerve (Baxter's Nerve) Entrapment

### Etiology and Pathophysiology

Baxter's neuropathy involves entrapment of the first branch of the lateral plantar nerve, typically the inferior calcaneal nerve; however, the medial calcaneal nerve may be less often involved. The nerve can be entrapped at various sites but most frequently occurs between the fascia planes of the abductor hallucis muscle and the quadratus plantae or at the medial calcalaneal tuberosity due to enthesophytes. Poorly fitting footwear and overpronation are common causes of compression.

### Diagnostic Approach

This condition can often be erroneously diagnosed as plantar fasciopathy. Patients typically participate in a repetitive activity such as running and complain of heel pain and paresthesias from the medial plantar surface of the heel to the medial arch of foot. A nerve conduction study and electromyography (NCS/EMG) NCS/EMG, though technically challenging, may demonstrate abnormalities involving the abductor digiti minimi muscle in chronic cases. MRI and US imaging may help to visualize the nerve, as well as possible areas of entrapment.

### Treatment

Initial management includes activity modification, properly fitting footwear, and shoe orthoses. If conservative care fails, rare interventions to consider include US-guided steroid injection, US-guided radiofrequency ablation, or a surgical nerve release.

## Morton's (Interdigital) Neuroma

### Etiology and Pathophysiology

Compression of the interdigital nerve, typically in the second or third webspaces, occurs from impingement under the intermetatarsal ligament, MTP joint synovitis, or tight-fitting (narrow toe box) or high-heeled shoes.

### Diagnostic Approach

Symptoms consist of plantar forefoot pain and paresthesias radiating to the affected toes. Signs include a positive compression test (pain at the site with squeezing the metatarsal heads together) and Mulder's sign (a palpable click with the compression test). US can visualize the neuroma. Electrodiagnostic studies can evaluate for more proximal neuropathies as the source of symptoms but cannot rule in an interdigital neuroma. An interdigital block with local anesthetic can help confirm the diagnosis.

### Treatment

Initial treatment involves ensuring appropriate footwear (cushioned, wide toe box, low heel), a metatarsal pad, and potentially a steroid injection from a dorsal approach. Surgical neuroma resection is reserved for recalcitrant symptoms.

### Functional Prognosis and Outcomes

Conservative treatment with an orthosis or a steroid injection improved symptoms in 48% and 85% of individuals, respectively.[15,16] Surgical removal of the neuroma and nerve is associated with an 80% to 90% cure rate, with recurrences being rare.[17]

## REFERENCES

The full list of references appears in the digital product found on http://connect.springerpub.com/content/book/978-0-8261-6226-7/part/part02/chapter/ch21

# SPINE—AXIAL PAIN

RUDY GARZA, JENNIFER LEET, TYLER CLARK, MEGAN THOMSON, AND AMEET NAGPAL

## INTRODUCTION

Axial pain refers to localized low back, middle back, or neck pain without radiation to the extremities. This condition can present as a challenge to providers. Treatments have provided mixed results often because the underlying pathology is either not accurately identified or is not completely understood. When evaluating a patient with axial pain, there are overarching concepts and steps that can be applied to help with the diagnosis and treatment plan, as outlined here.

## EVALUATION

As part of the initial evaluation, it is important to differentiate between a benign and nefarious etiology. Red flag symptoms (fever, chills, night sweats, unexplained weight loss, bowel/bladder/sexual dysfunction) can suggest a progressive or nefarious etiology. The prevalence of pathology varies with age, with discogenic pain being most common in patients between 20 and 50 years of age, and degenerative processes (e.g., spondylosis, osteoporotic fractures) more likely in elderly patients.[1] Nefarious conditions such as cancer and infection account for only a small prevalence but do increase in prevalence with increasing age.[2]

### Differential for Axial Pain

- In a study by DePalma et al., the prevalence of causes of chronic axial pain was identified after the diagnosis was verified in patients. Pertinent to their presenting symptoms and examination, each patient underwent diagnostic procedures, such as discography, dual diagnostic facet joint blocks, intra-articular sacroiliac joint (SIJ) injections, vertebral augmentation, and anesthetic blocks, in the areas of interest. The prevalence of each pathology was stratified according to age.[2]
  - ❑ Intervertebral disc (IVD) (42%)—internal disc disruption, most common in younger patients with varying etiologies
  - ❑ Zygapophyseal ("z") joint process (31%)—localized paramedian pain, prevalence increases with age, much more common in those over 50
  - ❑ SIJ (18%)—buttock and/or posterior superior iliac spine (PSIS) pain, prevalence is also much higher in patients greater than 50 years of age

The full list of references appears in the digital product found on http://connect.springerpub.com/content/book/978-0-8261-6226-7/part/part02/chapter/ch22

❑ Vertebral insufficiency fracture (2.9%)—more common in older population, with or without spine tenderness
❑ Other sources of back pain cited in the study accounted for the remaining 6% of patients with chronic back pain, including pelvic insufficiency fractures and Baastrup's disease; these causes of back pain are not discussed further in this chapter
■ Other spinal conditions[1]
❑ Studies on prevalence of etiologies of back pain also include neoplasia (0.7%), inflammatory arthritis (0.3%), and infection (0.01%)

## History and Physical

History should focus on the mechanism of injury and/or symptoms. Clinicians should be cognizant of "red flag" symptoms that may be indicative of a nefarious etiology. Any prior trauma or symptom should be noted as well as past treatment successes and failures. An assessment of social and psychologic factors (e.g., depression, smoking status) may yield information that can also affect the treatment plan.

As part of the initial evaluation, a thorough neurologic examination should be performed, including evaluating for weakness and reflex changes. Several special maneuvers can be helpful and will be discussed in subsequent sections.

## Workup

Even though plain-film radiographs are used first line, findings often do not help to establish a diagnosis for acute axial pain. Advanced imaging such as MRI of the spine has a high rate of degenerative findings in asymptomatic persons. In studies of asymptomatic adults, nearly two-thirds of the patients had nonspecific, abnormal findings on lumbar spine MRI evaluation.[3] Therefore, imaging should be used in carefully selected patients and interpreted with appropriate clinical correlation. Because most cases of acute back pain resolve with conservative treatment, immediate imaging is rarely indicated before 4 to 6 weeks unless radicular symptoms, neurologic deficits, or red flag symptoms are present. If clinical suspicion is sufficiently high, it may be necessary to proceed directly to advanced imaging.

## CONSERVATIVE THERAPY

For most acute and even chronic episodes of axial pain, the simplest treatments stem from lifestyle and activity modifications. Avoidance of activities that place strain on the spine (excessive extension or flexion) is an early option. Previously published studies have dealt with various therapeutic modalities of axial pain, but the evidence of their efficacy is highly inconclusive.[4] The McKenzie therapy protocol seems to be an effective technique, but long-term randomized controlled trials are still lacking. The McKenzie method of lower back pain treatment is explained by the principle that exercises that encourage disc centralization should be promoted, and exercises that encourage disc peripheralization should be avoided.[5] Across all studies in a systematic review by Namnaqani et al., a significant improvement in pain level was seen in the McKenzie group at 2 to 3 months compared to the manual therapy (MT) group. At 6 months, significant improvements in the disability index were reported by two trials in the McKenzie group compared to the MT group. At 12 months, there were no significant differences in measurements of low back pain, but three studies reported that the McKenzie method group had a better disability level than the MT group. In patients with chronic low back pain, many pain measures showed that the McKenzie method is a successful treatment to decrease pain in the short term, while the disability measures determined that the McKenzie method is better in enhancing function in the long term.[5]

## MEDICATION MANAGEMENT

Generally, one should maximize medications that have the least adverse effects for each patient, taking into account patient comorbidities, dosing, and likelihood of adherence. Chronic pain often shares biochemical and neurohormonal pathophysiology with sleep and mood disturbances; therefore, medications that can address multiple complaints can be considered.

1. Non-steroidal anti-inflammatory drugs (NSAIDs): Various randomized controlled trials have shown that NSAIDs are more effective than placebo in decreasing pain intensity and slightly more effective than placebo regarding disability scores. However, the level of evidence is low, and the degree of change is noted to be minimal. Additionally, no evidence supports statistically significant differences in efficacy between different NSAID types, including selective versus nonselective NSAIDs.[6] Providers must also take into account the risks of these medications including potential gastrointestinal, cardiac, and renal side effects.

2. Paracetamol (acetaminophen): Traditionally paracetamol is considered a first-line analgesic for treating acute low back or axial pain; however, no high-quality evidence supports this recommendation.[7]

3. Muscle relaxers: A short course (<4 days) of cyclobenzaprine or methocarbamol has shown some effectiveness in acute low back pain (not chronic).

4. Antidepressants: SNRIs and tricyclic amines (TCAs) have neuropathic analgesic properties. Duloxetine is Food and Drug Administration (FDA) approved for chronic musculoskeletal pain including osteoarthritis of the back.

5. Gabapentinoids (pregabalin and gabapentin): This class of drugs has demonstrated benefit for neuropathic pain conditions but not for nonspecific chronic low back pain. Prescribers should be aware of emerging evidence of gabapentinoid abuse and misuse, especially among those with a history of opioid abuse.[8]

6. Opioids: After thorough evaluation, consideration of alternative treatments, review of current medications, and discussions of risks, a short course of opioids may be indicated for acute pain. It is important to use the lowest effective dose that provides pain relief (as reflected by improved function) for a limited period of time.[9] The prevalence of psychological distress, unhealthy lifestyles, and healthcare utilization has been shown to increase incrementally with duration of opioid use. The extended prescription of opioids (>8 weeks) for the treatment of chronic pain has questionable benefits for individual patients and presents substantial public health risks.[6] The risks of overdose and addiction from this prescribing practice—both among patients with chronic pain and the public at large—increase with higher doses (>60 MME/day), longer duration of prescribing, and perhaps the use of long-acting opioids.

## PROCEDURES

Image-guided interventions can be used for both diagnostic and therapeutic purposes. Patients who are significantly debilitated or unable to fully participate in physical therapy (PT) and rehabilitation due to limitations posed by pain should be considered for intervention. Interventions used based on diagnosis will be discussed in further detail.

## INDICATIONS FOR REFERRAL

Any patient with axial pain with additional signs of cauda equina syndrome (lower extremity weakness, bowel and/or bladder dysfunction, saddle anesthesia, hyporeflexia) or myelopathy (extremity weakness, bowel and/or bladder dysfunction, impaired ambulation, hyperreflexia, upper motor neuron signs) warrants immediate, emergent referral to a spine surgeon or emergency room.

## PROGNOSIS AND OUTCOMES

Most patients with nonspecific low back pain recover within 4 to 6 weeks, and 80% to 90% improve within 3 months regardless of treatment modality. After an episode of nonspecific low back pain, 20% to 44% of patients have a recurrence within 1 year, and up to 85% have a recurrence during their lifetime.[10] Less than half of patients disabled for longer than 6 months return to work and nearly 0% after 2 years.[11]

## DIFFERENTIAL DIAGNOSES

### Degenerative Disease

### Zygapophyseal (Facet) Joint Syndrome

*Etiology and Pathophysiology*

Spondylosis is an age-related condition that affects the joints and discs of the spine as a result of "wear and tear" of the soft tissue, cartilage, and bones. Degeneration of the intervertebral discs (IVDs) can place increased stress on the z-joints. Chronic inflammation of the articulating synovial z-joints can lead to degradation of articular surfaces, capsular laxity, subluxation, and hypertrophy.[11,12] Prevalence studies of z-joint-mediated pain are flawed due to the lack of standardization in diagnosis, but studies have estimated cervical z-joints to account for 36% to 60% of chronic neck pain, thoracic z-joints in 34% to 48% of chronic mid to upper back pain, and lumbar z-joints in 15% to 45% of chronic low back pain.[3,13] There is a significantly higher prevalence of z-joint arthritis in those older than 45 years of age.[12] The C6–7 and C5–6 levels are most commonly affected, likely because these levels experience the most flexion and extension.[3] Thoracic spondylosis is less studied compared to the cervical and lumbar regions; however, it is estimated that degenerative changes are found most commonly at T11–12 and T1–2.[3] Lumbar spondylosis most commonly affects the L5–S1 and L4–5 levels.[3,12]

Z-joint arthropathy can also be a result of trauma such as whiplash injury, which can produce a variety of associated painful injuries, one being z-joint capsular stretch and inflammation.

## Presentation and Physical Examination

History and physical examination have limited diagnostic validity in identifying z-joints as the source of pain.[14] Symptoms can be unilateral or bilateral and can mimic other common sources of back pain such as sacroiliac joint pain and radiculopathy; however, there should not be any neurological deficits.

The cervical z-joint syndrome is defined as axial neck pain rarely radiating past the shoulders, pain elicited with pressure over z-joints, and pain and limited motion with extension and rotation.[15] Pain from thoracic z-joints can cause upper or mid-back pain that may refer into the chest wall.[3] Features suggestive of lumbar z-joint syndrome include low back pain that typically radiates to the buttock, hip, groin, and thighs and usually remains proximal to the knee. Pain may be provoked with palpation, standing or sitting positions, lumbar extension, or rotation, following stress, exercise, or after periods of inactivity.[14]

## Diagnosis

Plain radiographs are not sensitive for detection of mild osteoarthritis of the z-joints but can detect severe cases of z-joint arthrosis. MRI is often the imaging modality of choice for adequately assessing the z-joints as well as evaluating for most other spinal pathology. Bone scan/SPECT can be utilized to determine active z-joint inflammation. It is important to reiterate that degenerative spinal changes on imaging do not correlate to clinical symptoms of axial pain. Cervical and lumbar z-joint arthritis have been observed to be present in approximately one third of asymptomatic patients.[12,14]

Dual diagnostic comparative medial branch blocks (MBBs) of the corresponding z-joint are the accepted and validated criterion standard for diagnosing z-joint–mediated pain.[3,15]

## Treatment

Initially analgesia and modification of aggravating activities/positions should be emphasized. Modalities such as superficial cryotherapy or heat and soft tissue mobilization/massage may be beneficial. Use of cervical collars or lumbar support braces should generally be avoided as it can further weaken key postural muscles with prolonged use. After pain reduces, the patient should begin a restorative PT program.

Example PT orders:

- Cervical: Static–dynamic cervico-scapulothoracic strengthening, endurance, and flexibility exercises to include biofeedback, posture reeducation, and sustained natural apophyseal glides. Teach home exercise program and mindfulness exercises.[16]
- Lumbar: Stretching of hip flexors, hamstrings, quadratus lumborum, paraspinals, gluteals; core and lower extremity strengthening, aerobic exercise, patient education,[11] biofeedback, postural training, and improve gait mechanics.

Interventional techniques for z-joint pain, such as intra-articular injections and MBB and neurolysis, are often pursued if symptoms persist for over 3 months. There is level II evidence for long-term effectiveness of radiofrequency neurotomy in the lumbar and cervical levels as well as for z-joint nerve blocks in all spinal segments.[13] Intra-articular z-joint steroid injections have been shown to have a low response rate, unless active capsular inflammation is present.[12]

A referral to surgery is rarely required, as there is no strong evidence that supports surgery as an effective treatment for z-joint-mediated pain.[14]

## Discogenic and Intervertebral Disc Disease

### Etiology and Pathophysiology

IVDs are made up of the cartilaginous end plates, the nucleus pulposus (NP), and the annulus fibrosis (AF) and allow for flexibility and absorption of compressive loads. IVDs are largely avascular and receive nutrients through a diffusion gradient. Normal age-related changes of the IVD involve loss of proteoglycan content, progressive decline in disc nutrient supply through decreased blood supply, and changes in the extracellular matrix composition. Ultimately, these changes may lead to dehydration, altered structure, and metabolism.[17] Internal disc disruption refers to structural disorganization within the disc, often from fissures within the AF, which can lead to disc bulge, herniation (protrusion, extrusion, sequestration, migration), and/or discogenic pain.[3,11,18] Modic changes refer to end-plate abnormalities seen on imaging. IVDs are innervated anteriorly from the sympathetic trunks, laterally from the vertebral nerve, and posteriorly from the sinuvertebral nerves.[19] The exact mechanism of pain from disc degeneration without radiculitis or myelopathy is controversial and not well defined, though it is also thought to be mediated in part by chemical nociception through the release of inflammatory substances and an ingrowth of nociceptive receptors.[3,11,19]

Cervical discogenic pain without disc herniation or spondylosis is believed to account for 16% to 44% of chronic neck pain cases.[19] Thoracic discs have been shown to elicit pain and cause chronic upper back and mid-back pain; however, prevalence of discogenic pain in the thoracic level has not been well studied.[3] Prevalence of lumbar discogenic pain is estimated to be 26% to 42% in those with chronic low back pain without radicular symptoms.[3,20]

### Presentation and Physical Examination

Presentation of discogenic pain is classically axial (as opposed to predominately radicular pain from an acutely herniated disc) and somatic in nature but can mimic and/or coexist with radicular pain.[3] Discogenic pain can be described as band-like or poorly localized, deep, aching pain exacerbated by extension (though dependent on where the disc is degenerated) and Valsalva maneuvers (sneeze, cough, defecation, etc.). There should be no neurological deficits on examination and neural tension signs (i.e., straight leg raise, seated slumped root test, etc.) should be negative.

### Diagnosis

Radiographic and MRI evidence of disc abnormalities exist in asymptomatic people and do not accurately diagnose the discs as the source of pain. The lack of a correlation between the presence of gross tissue pathology and pain presents a conundrum in establishing a criterion standard for discogenic pain.[3] A systematic review by Malik et al. found a paucity of reliable data for the diagnosis and treatment of presumptively painful IVDs due to the use of diverse nomenclature and diagnostic and treatment approaches across studies.[21]

Provocation discography attempts to correlate distorted IVD architecture to symptomatology; however, controversy exists about its clinical usefulness and the risk of accelerating disc degeneration, therefore, it is now rarely utilized.[21,22] In summary, discogenic pain is often diagnosed based on history, physical examination, and exclusion of other common causes of axial pain.

### Treatment

The evidence for the treatment of discogenic pain is riddled with the same issues found in diagnosis.[21] Discogenic pain is often difficult to treat due to the lack of evidence, poor healing potential, and limited blood supply of IVDs.

PT should be centered around extension-biased strengthening programs.

A lumbar program should include strengthening of the core and lower abdominal muscles, integrating the pelvis, and stretching the hip flexors. A cervical program should include strengthening muscles responsible for normal cervical alignment, lengthening hypertonic muscles and shortened fascia, providing postural reeducation, and restoring scapulothoracic mechanics.

Interventional techniques include intradiscal electrothermal annuloplasty, intradiscal steroids, caudal epidural steroid injections, biacuplasty, spinal cord stimulation, and other intradiscal injections (platelet-rich plasma, methylene blue, or bone marrow concentrate). All of these have insufficient evidence to support their use.[22,23]

Surgical treatment is rarely indicated for axial discogenic pain. Studies have shown no correlation of fusion outcomes with positive discography findings. Surgical intervention is much more effective in improving radicular pain rather than axial pain.[3,24]

## Vertebral Body Compression Fracture

### Etiology and Pathophysiology

There are more than 1.4 million cases of vertebral compression fracture (VCF) worldwide, comprising half of all osteoporotic fractures in the United States. VCFs are likely the result of minimal trauma and typically occur in the mid-thoracic or thoracolumbar transition zone of the spine.[25]

### Presentation and Physical Examination

Vertebral fractures are directly correlated with increasing age and incidence of osteoporosis. They most commonly occur among Caucasian women and are less common among men and women of African American or Asian ethnicity. Many fractures may develop insidiously, and chronic compression fractures are commonly detected incidentally on chest x-rays. When symptomatic, patients complain of sudden-onset severe, focal back pain that may radiate anteriorly. Patients may have severe spinal pain worse with sitting up, standing, or ambulating. VCF pain is typically localized to the spine but may radiate to the flank or abdomen. If lower limb radicular pain is described, further workup should look for spinal cord compression or cauda equina syndrome. Patients may describe progressively decreased mobility and pulmonary function.

On physical examination, inspect for a kyphotic posture. Palpate for midline spinal or paraspinal tenderness near the area of interest, pain with spine motion, or pain with direct spinal percussion. Assess neurologic status, including upper motor or lower motor neuron signs.

### Diagnosis

In instances of vertebral fractures, radiographs can be helpful to establish a diagnosis. Any loss of height more than 20% of the vertebra, presence of end-plate deformities, and/or altered appearance of the vertebra should be considered a fracture and assessed further. The age of the fracture should also be assessed to determine whether the present fracture is responsible for current symptoms of the patient. On conventional radiographs, it is often difficult to determine the age of the fracture unless prior radiographs are available for comparison. If there is cortical disruption or impaction of the trabeculae, then the diagnosis of acute fracture is obvious. In the absence of these features, the fracture is generally considered to be chronic. However, many times, such a clear-cut differentiation is not possible.[26] MRI and nuclear scan can help in such cases, as lack of edema on MRI and lack of radiotracer uptake on a bone scan indicate an old fracture.[27.]

### Treatment

Acute compression fractures may be treated with analgesics such as acetaminophen, NSAIDs, calcitonin, and opioids in severe cases. Researchers hypothesize that NSAIDs may slow the rate of bone healing, but this is controversial.[28] Calcitonin can be prescribed for a duration of 4 weeks and appears to be effective for pain relief and osteoporosis treatment; it is indicated for patients presenting with evidence of spontaneous vertebral fracture on imaging and evidence that inciting event or start of symptoms occurred within the past 5 days.[29]

Physical therapists focus to improve paraspinal muscle strength and proprioception to limit further fractures, improve posture, and ambulation.[25] Instructions to the therapist should include any spine motion limitations to prevent progression of fracture or bony compromise (tailored to the patient's specific injury).

Bracing has been shown to improve vertebral alignment and limit axial loading on fractured vertebrae, improving muscle strength, posture, quality of life, and ability to complete activities of daily living (ADLs). Limitations of bracing include increased pain, skin breakdown, deconditioning, weakness with prolonged use, and impaired ability to complete ADLs depending on their prior level of function. A practitioner must be selective in deciding which patient is most appropriate for bracing. Thoracolumbar orthoses for thoracic or lumbar fractures include Jewitt, cruciform anterior spinal hyperextension, and Taylor braces. Lumbosacral orthoses may be used to treat upper lumbar fractures (L1–3) but are contraindicated in lower lumbar (L4–S1) fractures as these braces can increase movement of the affected vertebrae.[25]

It is important to note that spontaneous VCFs warrant further workup for osteoporosis, including a dual x-ray absorptiometry (DEXA) scan and laboratory studies including vitamin D 25-OH and calcium levels. Depending on these results, a referral to an endocrinologist may be warranted for evaluation and management.

Indications for vertebral augmentation procedures include patients with acute or subacute fracture with pain in the area of the fracture that increases with axial loading. The fracture must not be completely collapsed (i.e., vertebra plana), and the fracture must not involve the posterior wall of the vertebra which will increase the risk of cement extrusion. Kyphoplasty is indicated for patients with osteoporotic VCF who are neurologically intact with progressive symptoms unresponsive to conservative therapy (oral analgesics, therapy). Kyphoplasty has been shown to improve vertebral body height and correct spinal angle of kyphosis. Vertebroplasty comes with some controversy as prior studies have shown no benefit compared to sham procedure. However, recent research has shown improved mortality with both vertebroplasty and kyphoplasty.[30]

Indications for emergent open surgical decompression include symptoms of neurologic compromise, unstable fractures, or vertebral fragment retropulsion into the spinal canal.

### Prognosis and Outcomes

Although genetic predisposition and age of puberty onset play a significant role, a multitude of lifestyle and environmental factors increase the risk of developing osteoporosis. These include lack of exercise and low body mass index, insufficient dietary calcium, low vitamin D production, glucocorticoid medication, smoking, and excessive alcohol intake. The presence of one vertebral fracture confers a 5 to 12.6 times risk of subsequent vertebral fractures. At the same time, with advances in early detection and treatment of osteoporosis, early initiation of bisphosphonates and selective estrogen receptor modulators can reduce the risk of vertebral and other insufficiency fractures by 40% to 65% and mitigate the subsequent morbidity and mortality associated with them.[31]

## Infectious
## Vertebral Osteomyelitis and Discitis

### Etiology and Pathophysiology

Vertebral osteomyelitis and discitis occur as a result of blood-borne infection from other sites, including urinary tract infections, indwelling catheters, skin infections, and injection sites for intravenous (IV) drugs.[32]

### Presentation and Physical Examination

Presentation typically consists of fever and spine tenderness with percussion. Patients with possible vertebral osteomyelitis and discitis should be questioned on their history of infection and drug use.

### Diagnosis

An MRI with contrast should be ordered and blood cultures should be obtained prior to antibiotic treatment. Initial laboratory studies include complete blood count (CBC), erythrocyte sedimentation rate (ESR), and C-reactive protein (CRP).

### Treatment

Treatment of vertebral osteomyelitis should begin with empiric antimicrobial therapy once infection is suspected. In the case of an unstable patient (i.e., sepsis, severe neurologic symptoms), broad-spectrum antibiotics should be initiated while cultures are pending. Therapy duration will depend on the location and extent of infection but will likely continue for 6 weeks. Therapy duration increases to 3 months if due to *Brucella* spp.

Image-guided aspiration biopsy is only recommended when cultures and previous tests do not yield a diagnosis, yet vertebral osteomyelitis is highly suspected.

Surgical intervention is recommended in patients with progressive neurologic deficits, deformity, or spinal instability. Should a patient have severe, recurrent bloodstream infections, surgical debridement is indicated.

### Prognosis and Outcomes

Patients' response to antimicrobial therapy and the likelihood of treatment failure can be tracked using clinical status of the patient, systemic inflammatory markers, and imaging. Vertebral osteomyelitis patients with a 50% reduction in ESR after 4 weeks will rarely develop treatment failure.

## Mechanical Back Pain

## Sacroiliac Joint Dysfunction and Sacroiliitis and Posterior Sacroiliac Complex Pain

### Etiology and Pathophysiology

The SIJ is a diarthrodial joint that is about 1 to 2 mm wide and lined with hyaline cartilage and stabilized by posterior sacroiliac ligaments. It allows for the transmission of forces from the lower limbs to the axial skeleton and vice versa. Pain is thought to arise from the SIJ itself as well as the extra-articular ligaments. Of those with clinically suspected SIJ pain, 13% to 30% have a positive anesthetic response to diagnostic injections into the joint.[33] Minimal data exist regarding the contribution from extra-articular ligamentous pain. SIJ pain also occurs in the setting of sacroiliitis related to ankylosing spondylitis.

### Presentation and Physical Examination

SIJ pain is often nonspecific; 94% of patients present with buttock pain, 72% with lower lumbar pain, and 14% with groin pain, but 50% present with associated lower limb pain and 14% described pain reaching the feet.[34] Patients are more likely to experience unilateral pain as compared to bilateral pain in a 4:1 ratio. Pregnancy can predispose to SIJ pain, with possible mechanisms including increased lordosis, increased joint laxity due to relaxin hormone release, and increased abdominal weight. Multiple special tests exist for the SIJ, including Faber's, Gillet's, Gaenslen's, SI compression, and sacral thrust maneuvers. Prior studies attempted to establish a single maneuver or combination of multiple maneuvers to aid in the accurate diagnosis of SIJ dysfunction; however, the data were inconsistent in favor of any certain approach. Recent literature has been consistent in demonstrating that when compared to diagnostic SIJ anesthetic blocks, physical examination maneuvers, whether a single maneuver or multiple, add very little to the accurate diagnosis of SIJ dysfunction.[35]

### Diagnosis

There is little correlation between SIJ pain and imaging findings, but imaging may be helpful to rule out sacroiliitis. The current reference standard to diagnose SIJ pain is an injection of anesthetic into the SIJ with fluoroscopic guidance. However, this does not take into account posterior ligamentous causes of pain.

### Treatment

Initial treatment may include activity modification, ice, heat, and analgesics. PT is often used to help improve either mobility or stabilization. MT including mobilization and manipulation can assist with SIJ dysfunction.[33]

If there is minimal improvement with conservative treatment, intra-articular SIJ injection with anesthetic and steroid is often tried first which can be diagnostic and therapeutic. Fluoroscopy guidance provides improved intra-articular accuracy, although ultrasound-guided injections can still be efficacious likely due to the extra-articular ligamentous component of sacroiliac pain. Another extra-articular source that has been targeted is the dorsal innervation to the SIJ which arises from the L5 dorsal ramus and the S1–3 lateral branches. Multisite, multidepth lateral branch blocks were developed to compensate for the complex regional anatomy that limits the effectiveness of single-site, single-depth lateral branch injection. A study by Dreyfuss et al. established a physiologic analgesic effect of 70% using a multisite multidepth approach to the sacroiliac posterior ligament complex.[36] Lateral sacral branch blocks with subsequent radiofrequency ablation (RFA) may assist with further pain relief in select patients who do not respond to intra-articular injections. Available studies show pain relief in 32% to 89% of SIJ posterior ligament complex pain with sacral lateral branch RFA, but more research is needed in this area.[37]

SIJ arthrodesis is a surgical approach only indicated in patients with acute fracture and severe instability. Even then, arthrodesis for SIJ pain remains very controversial with several studies showing incomplete relief of pain.[33]

## REFERENCES

The full list of references appears in the digital product found on http://connect.springerpub.com/content/book/978-0-8261-6226-7/part/part02/chapter/ch22

# SPINE—RADICULAR PAIN

ANTHONY KENRICK, JOHN CHAN, LYNDLY TAMURA, MANOJ MOHAN, KEVIN BARRETTE, AND JOSH LEVIN

## INTRODUCTION

Radicular pain is defined as neurologic dysfunction that is attributed to mechanical compression or chemical irritation of a spinal nerve root. The clinical presentation may include sensory symptoms (numbness and tingling), motor deficits (weakness), and pain radiating down the limb in the respective nerve root distribution. While the term radiculopathy is often used for this type of pain, in the absence of a neurologic deficit or electrodiagnostic abnormality, a more accurate term is "radicular pain."

## PREVALENCE, PATHOPHYSIOLOGY, AND PROGNOSIS

### Prevalence

A population-based analysis in Rochester, Minnesota, reported an annual incidence of cervical radicular pain of 107.3 per 100,000 for men and 63.5 per 100,000 for women with a peak at 50 to 54 years of age.[1] Precise prevalence rates of lumbar radicular pain have not been clearly delineated in the literature but are typically cited at 2% to 5% in men and 3% to 5% in women with an approximate incidence of 2.2% to 8% overall.[2]

### Pathophysiology

Mechanical compression can cause nerve root dysfunction. An intraoperative study noted a reduction in intra-radicular blood flow and a decrease in nerve root mobility caused by herniated discs in patients undergoing discectomy surgery for radicular pain.[3] While mechanical compression clearly contributes to some nerve root dysfunction, inflammation can also play a key role in the pathogenesis of radicular pain. Nerve roots in pig models that were exposed to autogenous nucleus pulposus (without compression) displayed a pro-inflammatory response and subsequent nerve cell damage.[4] Additionally, the prevalence of asymptomatic mechanical nerve compression as evidenced by neural foraminal narrowing as demonstrated on MRI suggests that mechanical compression does not always result in radicular pain. Common causes of nerve root dysfunction secondary to compression

The full list of resources and references appears in the digital product found on http://connect.springerpub.com/content/book/978-0-8261-6226-7/part/part02/chapter/ch23

or inflammation include disc herniations in the young population and spondylosis and stenosis in the older population. Other atypical etiologies of radicular pain include infection, cancer, epidural lipomatosis, and facet synovial cysts.

### Prognosis—Cervical Radicular Pain

A systematic review concluded that for cervical radicular pain, most improvement occurs in the first 4 to 6 months, and that 83% of patients recovered completely within 2 to 3 years.[5] Further studies are needed to accurately demarcate the timeline of recovery from cervical radicular pain depending on the underlying pathology.

### Prognosis—Lumbar Radicular Pain

The natural history of lumbar radicular pain secondary to disc herniation is typically favorable. Approximately 40% of patients treated nonoperatively reported significant improvement in pain within 6 weeks, with 90% demonstrating relief at long-term follow-up.[6] While disability from lumbar radicular pain caused by a disc herniation can be significant, typically only 1% to 10% of patients proceed to surgery in the acute phase.[7] Of patients who fail conservative management and undergo an epidural steroid injection, 75% of patients reported >50% pain reduction at 6 months.[8] However, about 75% had recurrent pain and 50% went on to have surgery after 5- to 9-year follow-up. Unfortunately, successful treatments, including early surgery, did not change the natural history, highlighting the fact that this tends to be a recurrent problem for a large number of patients.[9]

## DIAGNOSTIC EVALUATION

### History

Radicular pain is a clinical diagnosis. Classically, radicular pain involves pain referring from the spine down a limb concordant to the affected nerve root. While the symptoms may follow a specific anatomic pattern and the practitioner should attempt to delineate the location of the symptoms, there is growing evidence that radicular pain patterns do not always match the expected location of symptoms.[10] Correlation between the history, physical examination, and imaging is therefore necessary to diagnose the specific affected level. Using the region of spine involvement as a guide, history should also evaluate for red flag symptoms (fever, chills, night sweats, unexplained weight loss, bowel/bladder/sexual dysfunction) that suggest a progressive or nefarious etiology.

### Physical Examination

Examination of the patient with radicular pain includes traditional musculoskeletal assessment with focused attention on strength, reflexes, evaluation for upper motor neuron signs, sensation, and special tests. With regard to strength testing, practitioners should closely evaluate for true, non–pain-inhibited weakness, which can lead to significant functional deficits. Specific myotomal tests have been used which are based on the American Spinal Cord Injury Association (ASIA) impairment scale for spinal cord injury, which includes testing hip flexors for L2, knee extensors for L3, ankle dorsiflexors for L4, great toe extension for L5, and ankle plantarflexors for S1.[11] Due to difficulty in accurately assessing ankle plantarflexion strength manually, full strength in this muscle group should be defined as the ability to perform at least 10 unipedal calf raises. In the cervical myotomes, elbow flexion strength can be assessed for C5, wrist extension for C6, triceps for C7, finger flexors for C8, and finger abductors for T1. Reflexes associated with specific spinal levels include biceps for C5, brachioradialis for C6, triceps for C7, knee jerk for L3 and L4, medial hamstring for L5, and ankle jerk for S1. Hyporeflexia could suggest a radiculopathy, while hyperreflexia would be more suggestive of central nervous system pathology such as myelopathy. Other upper motor neuron signs which could be suggestive of central nervous system pathology include clonus, Hoffman's sign, and Babinski sign. With regard to sensory testing, diminished sensation in a dermatomal distribution may also be suggestive of radiculopathy, though it should be noted that there can be significant dermatomal overlap between adjacent spinal levels. Special tests for radicular pain include the Spurling's test in the cervical spine, and dural tension signs in the lumbar spine such as the straight leg raise, seated slump, and femoral stretch. The Spurling test, which is used to evaluate for cervical radicular pain, has been shown to have low sensitivity (30%) and high specificity (93%), making it more useful as a confirmatory study as opposed to a screening tool.[12] Similarly, the straight leg raise is used to evaluate for lumbar radicular pain, with measured sensitivities and specificities from 52% to 84% to 78% to 89%,[13] while the seated slump test may be more sensitive (84%) with similar specificity (83%).[14] The femoral nerve stretch test has been shown to have a very high sensitivity of up to 100% and a specificity of 78% in the evaluation of upper lumbar radicular pain.[13]

## Imaging

The decision about whether to obtain imaging is a complex topic that depends on a number of variables including but not limited to the severity and duration of the symptoms, the presence of neurologic deficits (particularly a progressive neurologic deficit), or red flag signs. A full discussion regarding imaging indications is beyond the scope of this chapter. Plain film, two-view anteroposterior (AP) and lateral radiographs can be useful as a first-line screen for some osseous etiologies of radicular pain. Flexion/extension films could be considered in select cases when a dynamic spondylolisthesis is suspected. CT is often used in the evaluation of trauma or acute symptoms; however, it is limited in its ability to fully evaluate the discs and other soft tissues. This, in conjunction with the radiation exposure associated with CT imaging, limits its utility in the assessment of radicular pain. MRI allows for better visualization of discs, nerve roots, and the spinal canal and is therefore the typically preferred imaging study in the evaluation for radicular pain. That being said, up to 90% of asymptomatic adults have disc pathology on MRI[15] with rates of abnormalities increasing with age. Age-specific prevalence estimates for disk degeneration are 37% at age 20, 52% at age 30, 68% at age 40, 80% at age 50, 88% at age 60, 93% at age 70, and 96% at age 80.[16] Specifically, disk bulges, protrusions, and annular fissures follow a similar pattern, while disk extrusions are rare in the asymptomatic population, with most studies reporting prevalence rates of <2%.[17] Imaging findings, therefore, must be correlated with a patient's clinical presentation.

## Electrodiagnostic Testing

Electrodiagnostic testing can be a useful diagnostic utility in some cases of radiculopathy.[18] Sensory nerve conduction studies are usually normal as the pathology is proximal to the dorsal root ganglia, thereby leaving the connection between the cell body and its distal axons intact. Motor nerve conduction studies may be abnormal, but only if the affected nerve root innervates the muscle that the specific nerve conduction test is evaluating (typically C8/T1 in the upper limb and L5/S1 in the lower limb) and the motor axons are affected. In order to diagnose radiculopathy on electromyography (EMG), abnormalities should be demonstrated in at least two muscles that receive innervation from the same nerve root but different peripheral nerves. If there is axon loss, the study may show abnormal spontaneous activity (positive sharp waves and fibrillation potentials) beginning at approximately 3 weeks after the onset of symptoms in the muscles innervated by that nerve root. If reinnervation occurs, polyphasic motor unit action potentials can be seen in the subacute to chronic phase, followed by large amplitude, long-duration motor unit action potentials. The testing of paraspinal muscles can increase sensitivity as they are the most proximal muscles affected in radiculopathy but should be used cautiously as they can yield a false-positive result in asymptomatic individuals. Electrodiagnostic studies have several significant limitations, most notably that they should not be considered as a diagnostic evaluation of pain. Instead, they are diagnostic studies of nerve function. If radicular pathology is purely demyelinating or if it only affects sensory fibers, the electrodiagnostic study is expected to be normal.

## Noninterventional Treatment

Noninterventional treatments, which can be divided into pharmacological and non-pharmacological categories, are often the first line in management of radicular pain in the absence of red flag symptoms. However, there is a paucity of high-quality data to direct noninterventional treatments, and the literature surrounding conservative management is confounded with the heterogeneity of underlying patient etiologies. Because of this, performing stratification based on categorical data between responders and nonresponders may be beneficial in determining if subsets of patients may respond to treatment. Many medications and treatment modalities might not otherwise reach a minimal clinically important difference, and it is important to consider this additional critical appraisal to not overlook potentially beneficial interventions for appropriately selected patients.

## Pharmacological Management

Non-steroidal anti-inflammatory drugs (NSAIDs) are among the most commonly prescribed medications for those with radicular pain. Evidence supporting this practice, however, is lacking. A comprehensive systematic review of noninvasive treatments for low back pain found that NSAIDs were no more effective than placebo in improving radicular low back pain.[19] A Cochrane review from 2016 found that NSAIDs are more effective in "overall improvement" when compared to placebo; however, the quality of these studies was found to be low.[20] The evidence in the cervical spine is also limited. It is therefore prudent for practitioners to do a risk benefit calculation for the patient prior to prescribing these medications, considering the potential of gastrointestinal and vascular complications, including heart attack and stroke, posed by NSAID use.[21]

Anticonvulsants are another class of medications frequently used in the treatment of radicular pain; however, the data on this class is also limited. Chou et al. found inconsistent evidence on the effects of gabapentin, topiramate, and pregabalin on improving radicular pain.[19] This review found that low-dose gabapentin (1,200 mg/day) was no different than placebo in improving pain, but a higher dose (3,600 mg/day) resulted in greater improvement in radicular pain at rest versus placebo. Two trials involving topiramate showed improvement in radicular pain when compared to placebo. Pregabalin alone demonstrated no benefit over placebo, but pregabalin plus celecoxib was associated with lower pain scores versus celecoxib alone. However, the effect size from all of the anticonvulsant medications was small and below minimum clinically important differences (MCID) calling into question their efficacy.

Systemic corticosteroids are also commonly administered for radicular pain despite mounting evidence against their efficacy. Several large trials have consistently demonstrated no difference in pain when comparing treatment with systemic steroids and placebo, and systemic steroids are associated with a significantly increased risk for adverse events.[22] Although one small study on cervical radicular pain has reported short-term pain reduction with a short course of high-dose oral prednisolone,[23] the clinical significance of this response is unclear, as there was no patient follow-up beyond 10 days, and additional studies have not replicated these results.

Opioid analgesics are often considered for radicular pain, but a systematic review has demonstrated neither improvement in pain nor positive patient-perceived global effect with opioid use.[24] Considering the high risk for adverse events, dependency, and abuse associated with opioids, there are few cases where the optimal management strategy for radicular pain involves opioid analgesia.

Other commonly prescribed analgesics, including acetaminophen, antidepressants, and muscle relaxants, also lack evidence to suggest efficacy in treating radicular pain.[19]

## Nonpharmacological Intervention

Physical therapy is the most common type of non-pharmacological conservative management prescribed for radicular pain. Chou et al. evaluated two fair-quality trials that supported back-specific physical therapy over sham therapy or usual care in patients with lumbar radicular pain. They found that education plus physical therapy correlated with functional improvements when compared to usual care, but that these effects were small[19] and like medications, failed to reach the MCID. For patients with cervical radicular pain, most studies have found that physical therapy does not change the natural course of the disease, although there may be moderate short-term benefit in neck pain.[25] While a short course of focused physical therapy is a low-risk option for those with radicular symptoms, its effects beyond natural history are questionable, and monetary costs are high. See sample physical therapy prescription in supplementary material.

There is evidence, however, to suggest that a subset of patients who experience a centralization phenomenon with back and radicular pain may benefit from physical therapy. Centralization describes a clinically induced abolition of midline pain or distal-to-proximal change in location of pain derived from mechanical movements and positions. McKenzie originally described the operational categorization of patients into a centralization group, a partial reduction group, and a noncentralization group.[26] Studies have since suggested that using a physiotherapy regimen based on the McKenzie method of physical manipulation in a centralizing group can reduce healthcare utilization and improve pain compared to standard therapy.[27,28] However, similar to the studies discussed earlier, this literature also suffers from diagnostic heterogeneity.

An important yet commonly forgotten eschewed treatment for radicular pain is the tincture of time. Given the known favorable natural history of the disease process, and the risks, side effects, costs, and limited effectiveness of the currently available conservative treatment options, this readily available, safe, and cost-free treatment could be considered and counseled for appropriate patients.

## Interventional Treatments for Radicular Pain

When symptoms are refractory to conservative interventions, or when there are clinical characteristics to suggest that an individual would likely have a positive response to invasive treatment, epidural steroid injections may be a reasonable option. Early studies were designed without image guidance, without control groups, and implemented undefined or invalid outcome measures, which limited clinical applicability. It was not until recently that high-quality data became available, informing the use of epidural interventions for radicular pain and advancing the practice of spine interventions.

## Lumbar Interventions

Steroid can be introduced into the epidural space in one of several ways, including transforaminal, interlaminar, and caudal injections, each named for their respective anatomic approach. Of these, the transforaminal approach has the greatest evidence for clinically significant symptomatic relief,[29] which suggests that the targeted injection of steroid around an affected nerve root diminishes the local inflammatory processes associated with disc herniation.[17,18] This is in contrast to those individuals who experience radicular pain from spondylosis, stenosis, or large disc herniations which may have associated mechanical stress altering the structure of the nerve root itself. In these cases, there may be some pain relief from epidural steroids due to downregulation of local inflammation, but it is less likely to provide a robust response.[30]

In appropriately selected patients who experience radicular pain from intervertebral disc herniation with MRI characteristics of low-grade nerve compression, pain relief from epidural steroid injection can be very significant. In a randomized controlled study by Ghahreman et al., 76% of patients who met these criteria had at least 50% relief of pain after fluoroscopy-guided transforaminal epidural steroid injections at 1 month post-intervention. Some had relief of symptoms for up to 6 months, and a minority experienced pain relief as far as 12 months. These results correspond to a single injection and do not include the possible benefit of repeated or rescue injections.[31] Independent systematic reviews have similarly demonstrated that transforaminal epidural steroid injection is an effective means of controlling radicular pain.[29,32]

Beyond pain relief, lumbar transforaminal epidural steroid injections appear to effectively restore function, reduce healthcare utilization, reduce sick days from work, and, in some cases, lead to surgery avoidance.[29,31,33] These results are demonstrated in large systematic reviews on the treatment of acute and chronic radicular pain from disc herniations.[29] This illustrates that in a well-selected patient population with lumbar radicular pain, epidural steroid injections serve as a practical treatment that can provide significant relief of pain and restoration of function.

## Lumbar Complications

Lumbar transforaminal epidural steroid injections practiced by current guidelines are generally safe with few severe complications. Patients undergoing the procedure are counseled on risks including exacerbation of pain, reaction to steroid, bleeding, infection, and damage to the underlying soft tissues and structures including the spinal nerves.[34] Both mild and severe complications are infrequent, with a study of over 26,000 consecutive procedures demonstrating that fewer than 2% of procedures resulted in any complications, with vasovagal reaction being the most frequently cited adverse event, and fewer than 0.1% of interventions resulted in the transfer of a patient to a higher level of care for complications including allergic reaction, chest pain, and symptomatic hypertension.[35]

However, in rare circumstances, severe neurologic compromise has been reported following lumbar and sacral transforaminal injection of steroids. Most reported cases occurred when particulate steroid was used, and neurologic insult was thought to have been the result of inadvertent arterial injection with embolization in terminal branches of arteries supplying the spinal cord. This is exemplified by case series of individuals who developed paraplegia from spinal cord infarct after receiving transforaminal epidural injections of particulate steroid-like betamethasone and methylprednisolone.[36,37] Because of this, performing injections with depot preparations of methylprednisolone, triamcinolone, and betamethasone should not be considered as first-line treatment.[38] Non-particulate steroid preparations are instead preferred and have been shown to be equally as effective as particulate steroids in pain and subsequent surgical rate reduction.[8,39] Additionally, injections should be performed with an adequate volume of contrast medium under continuous imaging to ensure no vascular uptake, with the field of view including the proximal spinal canal so that arterial uptake may be detected.[34]

## Cervical Interventions

Less data is available to inform the management of cervical radicular pain. Treatment tends to mirror the paradigm for lumbar radicular pain, with conservative management preceding cervical epidural injections. Engel et al. performed a systematic review of 16 primary publications and determined that 50% of patients with painful cervical radicular pain experience about 50% pain relief at 4 weeks after cervical transforaminal injection of epidural steroid.[40] Beyond this, the effects of cervical epidural steroid injection on function, healthcare utilization, and surgery avoidance have not yet been fully evaluated. Although less robust, the data suggests that in select patients with cervical radicular pain, an epidural steroid injection may provide at least temporary pain relief and postpone or avoid surgical intervention. In these cases, no comparative outcome studies have been reported for transforaminal and interlaminar approaches.

## Cervical Complications

When compared to lumbar transforaminal epidural steroid injections, cervical interventions similarly have risk for mild, transient complications such as increased pain and vasovagal reaction.[41] Cervical epidural injections, however, have an increased risk of catastrophic complications. Documented complications have included tetraparesis, stroke, epidural hematoma, arachnoiditis, abscess, spinal anesthesia, direct spinal cord trauma, and even death.[41,42]

It is worth noting that these complications are differentially distributed between cervical transforaminal and interlaminar approaches for cervical epidural access. Stroke and spinal cord infarct are greater risks following cervical transforaminal epidural steroid injections, as major arterial branches reside close to the path of the needle in the posterior neuroforamen, and the vertebral artery is present within the neuroforamina above C6.[41] Even with adequate visualization, inadvertent vascular access in cervical transforaminal epidural injections is common, with one study documenting intravascular needle placement in nearly 33% of 121 fluoroscopically guided procedures (although the large majority are venous).[43] The use of nonparticulate steroid in cervical injections is therefore again recommended to mitigate the risk of embolic infarct.[38]

In the case of interlaminar injections, aberrant needle placement within the thecal sac or within the spinal cord itself can lead to spinal anesthesia or direct spinal cord trauma.[41] Additionally, despite appropriate technique, development of an epidural hematoma post-injection could cause a myelopathy and progressive neurologic sequelae.[44-46] Given the proximity of the spinal cord to the roof of the vertebral canal in the cervical spine, and the paucity of posterior epidural fat in the proximal cervical spine, interlaminar injections are typically recommended to be performed at the C7-T1, or sometimes the C6-7 level. This should only be done after confirming an adequate amount of posterior epidural fat on the patient's imaging studies.[36,38] Though these are rare, potentially devastating complications exist with both the transforaminal and the interlaminar approaches.[47]

## When to Refer to Surgery

When patients present with cervical or lumbar radicular pain, it is important to be able to recognize if there are concerning features on history, examination, and imaging that would warrant surgical evaluation. Red flag symptoms, as previously described, should prompt the need for imaging and potential surgical evaluation. Neurologic deficits on examination, such as progressive neuromuscular weakness, new hyperreflexia, hyporeflexia, or areflexia, unmasking of primitive reflexes, gait dysfunction, progressive sensory dysfunction, and bowel and/or bladder dysfunction may warrant further investigation with imaging and surgical evaluation in the appropriate clinical context.[48,49] As with nonoperative treatments, surgical efficacy for the treatment of radicular pain is confounded by the heterogeneity of underlying patient etiologies, and a full discussion regarding surgical treatment options is beyond the scope of this chapter.

## RESOURCES AND REFERENCES

The full list of resources and references appears in the digital product found on http://connect .springerpub.com/content/book/978-0-8261-6226-7/part/part02/chapter/ch23

# OSTEOARTHRITIS

RYAN NUSSBAUM, CHAD HANAOKA, AND PRAKASH JAYABALAN

## INTRODUCTION

Osteoarthritis (OA) is associated with older age, female sex, obesity, and prior history of joint injury. It is a leading cause of disability worldwide with symptomatic OA affecting approximately one in eight Americans.[1] OA is a clinical diagnosis based on joint pain, stiffness, and functional limitations that hinder activities of daily living. Imaging such as plain radiographs can be helpful in confirming the diagnosis and staging the radiographic severity of OA. Common OA features on plain radiographs include joint space narrowing, osteophytes, subchondral bone sclerosis, and bone cysts.[1] The primary goals in managing the disease are to relieve pain, optimize function, and improve quality of life.[2]

Although abundant evidence exists for a wide variety of treatments, the vast majority have been investigated and directed toward knee OA.[3] The extent to which recommendations for knee OA can be extrapolated to other joints may be dependent on the joint affected, safety profile of the treatment, and the patient's individual circumstance. The objective of this chapter is to provide a broad overview of primary and secondary interventions available for the practitioner managing OA.

## DEVELOPING AN OVERALL TREATMENT STRATEGY

The Osteoarthritis Research Society International (OARSI) has recommended a universal treatment algorithm for any type of OA to most effectively address a patient's needs (see Figure 24.1 for a modified version of their algorithm[3]). Individuals undergo an initial assessment that evaluates the location of their OA disease, comorbidities (e.g., gastrointestinal, cardiovascular, frailty and widespread pain, and depression), clinical and functional status, and emotional and environmental factors. Based on this information, one or more primary treatments should be selected. Primary treatment options have the highest quality of supporting evidence. Post-intervention reassessment is crucial to determine if both the patient and clinician agree that the current treatment plan is effective. If deemed insufficient, potential barriers to adherence should be evaluated thoroughly before using secondary interventions to achieve a more acceptable state. If the patient continues to demonstrate minimal improvement, consider reassessing the diagnosis and having a specific conversation about the patient's goals. As a

---

The full list of references appears in the digital product found on http://connect.springerpub.com/content/book/978-0-8261-6226-7/part/part02/chapter/ch24

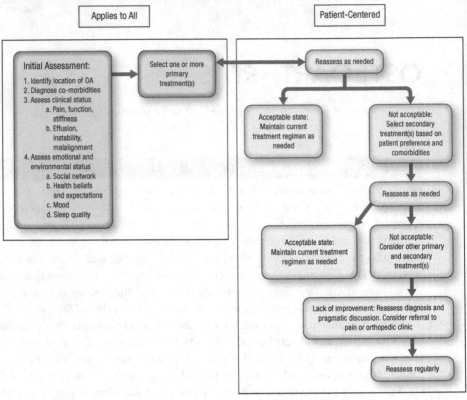

**FIGURE 24.1** Framework for the management of osteoarthritis.

last resort, referral to a pain clinic or orthopedic surgery may be warranted for potential joint replacement.[3] An example order set for diagnosis and treatment of knee OA is provided at the end of the chapter.

## PRIMARY INTERVENTIONS

### Osteoarthritis Education

Essential to the treatment plan for the patient is a conversation educating the patient about their condition. Patients should have basic knowledge about the etiology, course of disease, and treatment options. With this information, they will have a better understanding about outcomes and will be more engaged with their treatment plan.

### Physical Activity
### The Benefits of Physical Activity

There is significant evidence for the benefits of physical activity in the management of OA. Current U.S. guidelines for physical activity in adults with chronic conditions recommend at least 30 minutes of moderate-intensity exercise 5 days a week or 75 minutes a week of vigorous-intensity activity.[4] However, the adoption of physical activity in patients with OA has been inconsistent due to patient concerns regarding exacerbation of pain and potential worsening of the structural joint disease.[5] This leads to variable adherence to exercise programs in the long term and difficulty in promoting behavioral change.[6] The types of exercise programs with the strongest support in the current literature include land based, mind–body, and aquatic training as discussed in more detail in the following.[3]

## Prescribing Exercise

The ultimate goal for any exercise prescription is to optimize physical fitness while minimizing the generation of symptoms. The initial step involves determining the patient's specific activity goals, including the amount of exercise they engage in during a week and the specifics about their current workout plan (e.g., type of activity:aerobic, resistance, and leisure; plyometrics, free weights, and number of repetitions). It is also important to evaluate the patient's impairments, strength, range of motion, estimated aerobic fitness, and balance before providing specific recommendations. Formulating the exercise prescription should also be done by prioritizing patient preferences and interests as this provides the greatest likelihood of adherence.

Patient's questions and concerns should be addressed early in the treatment plan. Typical concerns include experiencing pain with joint loading during the exercise. Based on studies in individuals with knee OA, patients should know that experiencing pain during load-bearing exercise is likely normal as long as their pain is not lasting more than 2 hours after the activity has been completed.[7] Further, there is minimal evidence supporting that physical activity will worsen structural degeneration of the knee joint.[8] These findings can be applied to other joints impacted by OA, though all have not been clearly studied.

## Land-Based Programs

Aerobic and resistance training are strongly supported as exercises that substantially improve pain, function, and quality of life in patients with OA.[3,8] Prior studies of land-based exercise demonstrated the benefits of 20 to 60 minutes of exercise 2 to 3 days a week. In these trials, aerobic exercise typically involved either walking programs or cycling classes. Resistance training was comprised of varying sets of Theraband, free weight, or weighted cuff exercises at a 10-repetition maximum.[8]

A randomized controlled trial (RCT) of individuals with knee OA studied the efficacy of a 12-week instructor-led stationary cycling program in 37 subjects. The group-based program was specifically modified to minimize the weight-bearing load on the knee joint to refrain from aggravating symptoms of OA, such as pedaling at maximum resistance or in the standing position. Subjects attended a minimum of two classes per week, starting off at 40 minutes and gradually progressed to 60 minutes of exercise by the end of the program. Each session was comprised of a low-intensity warm-up followed by alternating higher cadence pedaling or hill climbing and a brief stretching period. Subjects were instructed to achieve levels of vigorous-intensity exercise at 70% to 75% of their maximum heart rate.[9] Significant improvements in knee pain, function, stiffness, and activities of daily living were found at completion of the program.

Another study investigated the impact of 8 weeks of high resistance, low resistance, and no exercise on 102 subjects with knee OA and observed similar improvements in both high- and low-resistance groups with the added benefits of muscle strengthening. Subjects performed unilateral exercises on a leg press machine three times per week for approximately 40 minutes. The authors described high-intensity exercise as requiring "an extra amount of time (duration or frequency) or resistance (strength or effort)." In line with this definition, high-resistance training was designated by calculating 60% of the subject's one-repetition maximum, and low-resistance strengthening was classified as 10% of the one-repetition maximum. Repetitions and sets were adjusted accordingly to achieve similar total outputs of training under both conditions. While the resistance training groups significantly improved function when compared to the nonexercise control group, there were no significant differences between the high- and low-intensity exercise groups at the end of 8 weeks.[10]

## Step Counts

Personal electronic devices have grown in popularity and provide a way to monitor a patient's physical activity. This can help quantify the effectiveness of an intervention to promote activity in individuals with OA, specifically lower-extremity OA. Walking is the most common form of exercise and has shown benefits to improve pain and functional limitations in patients with knee OA. Walking, compared to the interventions mentioned earlier, may be the most cost-effective and requires the least amount of resources. The American College of Sports Medicine has endorsed at least 7,000 steps per day to maintain cardiorespiratory, musculoskeletal, and neuromotor fitness.[7] A reasonable approach for a step count intervention can begin with a goal of 6,000 steps a day and increase that amount by 1,000 steps every 1 or 2 days while using experience of pain to determine the target step goal.[7]

## Mind–Body and Aquatic Training

Tai chi and yoga have displayed benefits for OA with little to no risk of adverse effects. An RCT for knee OA involving 40 subjects incorporated a 12-week instructor-led tai chi course that met two times a week for 60 minutes. The intervention was comprised of sessions in self-care, tai chi movements and principles, breathing techniques, and relaxation. Additional modifications were implemented to limit the stress placed on knee joints, such as the removal of movements that required flexion beyond 90°. Improvements in pain, function, psychological well-being, and quality of life were observed in the intervention group at 12 weeks. Additional improvements in self-efficacy and depression were also observed at 24 and 48 weeks.[11]

Aquatic therapy provides physiological benefits by partially off-loading the force experienced at the joints and facilitates joint mobilization. A study involving 152 subjects investigated the efficacy of tai chi and aquatic training to treat symptomatic hip or knee OA. The 12-week programs involved specially designed exercises that occurred over 1 hour of training twice a week with professionally trained instructors. Tai chi was offered in a modified format of the Sun style. The aqua therapy protocol included cardio, mobility, balance, and strengthening exercises performed in waist-high water, such as walking (forward, backward, laterally), pool-side stabilized exercises (hip abduction/adduction, lateral lunges, squats, etc.), seated leg lifts, deep water noodle movements (scissors, cycling, knees to chest, etc.), free-standing joint circles, and pool stair climbing (among others). Substantial improvements in pain and function were observed in both groups at 12 and 24 weeks.[12]

## Weight Loss

In overweight and obese patients, weight loss is another strongly supported treatment for OA. A recent RCT by Messier et al.[13] involving an 18-month interventional program for diet and/ or exercise investigated how varying levels of weight loss altered symptoms of knee OA and the biochemical composition of the knee joint. Of note, this study involved a closely monitored diet prescription that incorporated two meal replacement shakes per day with a weekly recipe plan for third meals of 500 to 750 kcal that were high in vegetable count and low in fat. The caloric distribution was designed to achieve a breakdown of 15% to 20% protein, <30% fat, and 45% to 60% carbohydrates. Nutrition and behavioral educational sessions were administered multiple times per week. Exercise protocols involved sessions with certified trainers with 30 minutes of aerobic training, 20 minutes of strength training, and a 10-minute cool down three times per week. The study found that the diet and diet plus exercise groups lost significantly more weight than the exercise group, highlighting the effectiveness of diet regulation for weight loss. Greater weight loss also resulted in superior clinical and functional outcomes of knee OA, including statistically significant improvements in pain, function, physical quality of life, inflammatory marker levels, and joint compressive forces. Thus, if done safely without surgical or pharmacological interventions, weight loss can provide clinically significant improvements in pain and enhance function in overweight and obese patients with knee OA.

## SECONDARY INTERVENTIONS

### Pharmacologic Treatments
### General Approach

Medications may be considered when primary interventions do not suffice for managing pain and preserving function. When choosing a medication, factors to consider are the patient's comorbidities, including conditions related to the gastrointestinal system, cardiovascular system, frailty, widespread pain, and depression which may limit prescription options.[3] Additionally, topical agents should be considered before oral agents in order to reduce the chances of systemic organ toxicity.

### Topical Agents

#### Topical Non-Steroidal Anti-Inflammatory Drugs

Non-steroidal anti-inflammatory drugs (NSAIDs) reduce inflammation by inhibiting cyclooxygenase (COX), which thereby reduces prostaglandin and thromboxane synthesis. Diclofenac gel is the most strongly supported topical therapy for musculoskeletal joint pain.[14] Evidence has shown that patients benefit from this medication particularly when the joint is superficial in relation to the skin, that is, knee and hand.[3,15] Deeper joints, such as the hip and shoulder, tend to show less benefits. Patients should not apply topical NSAIDs to broken, inflamed, or infected skin, and it is important to note that diclofenac gel can elevate liver enzymes.

#### Capsaicin Cream

Capsaicin theoretically desensitizes and degenerates cutaneous nociceptive neurons; additionally, substance P depletion is thought to reduce pain transmission to the central nervous system (CNS). Though OARSI guidelines recommended against capsaicin due to poor quality evidence, there have been many placebo-controlled trials showing its benefit.[3,14] Similar to other topical medications, capsaicin cream should not be applied to damaged, broken, or irritated skin. A burning sensation at the site of application is a common issue experienced by patients.

## Oral Agents

### Acetaminophen

Acetaminophen analgesic mechanism of action is unknown, but there is evidence to support that it is more effective than placebo at reducing pain from OA. However, the most recent OARSI recommendations state that acetaminophen shows little to no efficacy in the treatment of OA. Patients taking daily dosages of 3 to 4 g on a long-term basis should have their liver enzymes monitored.

### Non-Steroidal Anti-Inflammatory Drugs

Nonselective NSAIDs and COX-2 inhibitors have both demonstrated significant reductions in OA-related pain. While NSAID selection is determined based on a patient's comorbidities, individuals with no comorbidities may be prescribed any type of NSAID. Patients with gastrointestinal disease should take COX-2 inhibitors only. Any patient with a history of cardiovascular disease or frailty should refrain from taking NSAIDs due to the risk of myocardial infarction. In general, NSAIDs should be administered at the lowest effective dose possible and for the shortest period of time and potentially with a proton-pump inhibitor for gastric protection.[3] Individuals with kidney disease should not take NSAIDs due to risk of worsening renal function.[14]

### Opiates

Opiates display mild benefits for relieving symptoms of OA.[3] However, the complications of chemical dependence, constipation, respiratory depression, and sedation make the class of medication a very suboptimal selection. Tramadol is a class of opiate medication that has been shown in the literature to result in small positive effects for OA pain management. The drug acts as a weak mu opioid receptor agonist with serotonergic effects. The American College of Rheumatology (ACR) presents a conditional recommendation for the use of tramadol in knee OA when administered in combination with oral NSAIDs and topical pain relievers.[14] In general, opiates should be prescribed extremely sparingly for OA pain management, particularly with older individuals who are more susceptible to sedation.

### Duloxetine

Duloxetine inhibits the reuptake inhibition of norepinephrine and serotonin in the CNS. There is mild evidence that supports its use to improve pain in patients with combinations of knee OA and/or widespread pain with depression.[3]

## Intra-Articular Injections

Intra-articular (IA) corticosteroid injections (CSIs) and hyaluronic acid (HA) have been widely accepted as treatment options for knee OA when a patient is unresponsive to noninterventional treatments. CSIs exhibit anti-inflammatory properties that may alleviate pain in individuals with OA. However, repeated administration of CSIs must be approached with caution. A recent study by McAlindon et al.,[16] in which 40 mg of triamcinolone acetonide was injected into the knee joint every 3 months for 2 years for knee OA, found that CSIs resulted in significantly greater cartilage volume loss and no significant reduction in pain when compared to placebo.

HA is a fundamental component of synovial fluid that forms a shock-absorbing lubricant to protect articular cartilage, which can lead to reductions in pain and improved function. They have shown to be of particular benefit in younger individuals with milder symptoms and structural disease. While an abundance of evidence exists for the benefits of these injections, the effects of CSIs and HA injections have also been shown to gradually attenuate in the long term.[17] Thus, these injections should be used only when necessary to alleviate symptoms.[15]

## Psychosocial Interventions

Psychosocial interventions show moderate evidence, regardless of a patient's psychological history, to improve pain and function in individuals with knee OA. Keefe et al.[18] demonstrated in an RCT that a 12-week intervention combining spouse-assisted coping skills training with exercise improved strength, physical fitness, pain coping, and self-efficacy compared to either intervention alone. A study by Bennell et al.[19] found that a 12-week physical therapy program incorporating both pain coping skills training and exercise resulted in statistically significant improvements in function at 32 weeks post-treatment compared to the standalone interventions. When treating patients experiencing OA and associated pain and depression, cognitive behavioral therapy may be considered as part of a multidisciplinary pain management program.[3]

## Dietary Supplements

Dietary supplements are alternative therapeutic agents with purported benefits to relieve clinical symptoms of OA. While growing in popularity, these nutritional supplements still lack conclusive, high-quality evidence in spite of some promising outcomes and a higher safety profile than traditionally prescribed NSAIDs.

### Glucosamine and Chondroitin Sulfate

Glucosamine and chondroitin sulfate are naturally occurring compounds in the human body with anti-inflammatory properties. They are classified as symptomatic slow-acting drugs (SYSADOAs) and disease-modifying OA drugs (DMOADs) that theoretically supply building blocks for the synthesis of proteoglycans, a fundamental component of articular cartilage. They have also been shown to inhibit the production of proteolytic enzymes and are believed to promote HA synthesis in the synovium. Studies have shown the efficacy of glucosamine and chondroitin sulfate at maximum dosages of 1,500 mg/day over durations of 2 months to 2 years. However, due to the heterogeneity of design and outcome measures across studies, it is currently unclear whether glucosamine and chondroitin sulfate can be administered safely for the long-term treatment of osteoarthritic symptoms. While individual administration of each supplement was shown to be beneficial, prescribing both simultaneously is not recommended due to a lack of evidence for significant benefits.

A recent meta-analysis of 30 RCTs found that glucosamine showed statistically significant improvements in stiffness while chondroitin sulfate resulted in significant improvements in pain and function. The study also compared the number of adverse events that occurred in interventional and placebo groups as a safety measure and found no significant differences between the groups. Another analysis of 29 trials found that glucosamine and chondroitin sulfate individually resulted in statistically significant decreases in pain but no change in function. However, both of these meta-analyses found that the combination of the two agents did not result in any significant added benefit.[2,20]

## Turmeric

Turmeric is an agent with anti-inflammatory effects. Its primary component, curcuminoid, has been shown to modulate pro-inflammatory cytokines by promoting antiapoptotic activity in addition to its antioxidant properties. Current evidence indicates that turmeric can cause significant improvements in pain and function but may have equal or less of an effect compared to ibuprofen (and potentially other NSAIDs). Safe dosage recommendations are currently under question, with several studies indicating that a maximum of 1,200 mg/day for up to 4 months would minimize the potential of adverse effects. Curcuminoids display a poor bioavailability with evidence of extremely low amounts measured in serum and tissues following oral administration, but caution must be exhibited in prescribing higher dosages as limited evidence indicates that excessively high doses of turmeric may lead to an iron deficiency. However, similar to the aforementioned agents, turmeric at moderate dosages has been demonstrated to show no significant differences in adverse events compared to placebo medications or ibuprofen.[21,22]

## Gait Aids and Orthoses

Gait aids and orthoses play a vital role in improving function for individuals with OA. Patients with advanced or severe symptoms of hip or knee OA may need a cane (that should be used on the contralateral side to symptoms) or walker.[3] Commonly used treatments for knee OA include taping, knee sleeves, and off-loading braces. There is mild evidence that taping the patella with a medial pull improves short-term patellofemoral knee pain and is well tolerated in patients with OA. Although a specific type has not yet been identified, knee sleeves have been shown to be well tolerated and provide modest short-term improvements. Off-loading braces for medial femorotibial OA has also shown mild evidence to reduce pain and function, but it is often not well tolerated due to discomfort and poor fit at the joint.

Shoe insoles have been suggested to be of benefit by the ACR, including lateral wedge insoles for medial OA and medial wedge insoles for lateral femorotibial involvement. Insoles for hip OA have not been well-studied.[23] For OA of the carpometacarpal OA, the European League Against Rheumatism (EULAR) and ACR recommend thumb splinting to immobilize the carpometacarpal joint. No specific design (rigid/semirigid) has been shown to be superior, but it has been recommended that the splint be worn at night.

## Modalities

Modalities cover a broad range of accessible treatment options with mild evidence that patients may be interested in. Therapeutic ultrasound for 10 to 15 minutes demonstrates modest benefits with minimal risk in knee OA, but the limited evidence is inconsistent.[14] Cold packs applied for no more than 20 minutes can decrease swelling and pain over time in knee OA. Ice massage has also been shown to improve knee range of motion, function, and strength following 20 minutes of use. Conversely, heat application for 20 minutes did not display benefits for knee OA.[24]

## OUTCOME MEASURES TO CONSIDER

With each treatment plan, evaluating progress is essential to optimize outcomes. Patient responses can provide insights that may change the treatment plan to focus on areas of greatest need or impairment. There are multiple validated patient-reported outcome measures to consider for use in a clinical setting. The Western Ontario and McMaster Universities (WOMAC) OA index can be used to assess the functional status of patients with knee or hip OA. The Knee Injury and Osteoarthritis Outcome Score (KOOS) can evaluate clinical symptoms of knee OA, while the Hip Disability and Osteoarthritis Outcome Score (HOOS) measures clinical symptoms of hip OA.[1] Additionally, the Disabilities of the Arm, Shoulder, and Hand (DASH) Questionnaire can be used in the treatment of various types of upper-extremity OA.[25]

## FUTURE INTERVENTIONS

Future agents and treatment modalities with limited evidence that require further investigation and more high-quality evidence before they can be recommended include, but are not limited to, the following[3]:

- Massage
- Mobilization
- Manipulation
- Thermotherapy
- Taping interventions
- Electromagnetic therapies
- Laser therapy
- Genicular nerve block therapy (i.e., radiofrequency ablation)
- IA platelet-rich plasma (PRP)
- IA stem cell therapy
- Fibroblast growth factor-18, dextrose prolotherapy
- DMOADs (i.e., methotrexate)
- Long-acting IA extended-release corticosteroid (i.e., FX006)
- Anti-nerve growth factor (anti-NGF) and nutraceuticals

## BASIC ORDER SET

## Osteoarthritis Management Order Set

| DIAGNOSIS | |
|---|---|
| CLINICAL | Joint pain, stiffness, and functional impairments hindering daily living |
| RADIOGRAPHIC | *X-ray three view:* anterior–posterior, lateral, and sunrise views<br>*Diagnostic criteria:* joint space narrowing, osteophytes, subchondral sclerosis, bone cysts |
| **PRIMARY TREATMENTS** | |
| PHYSICAL ACTIVITY | *Exercise guideline:* 150 minutes of moderate-intensity exercise or 75 minutes of vigorous exercise per week.<br>*Intervention options should be based on patient preference and include:*<br>• Land-based—aerobic and resistance training<br>• Step count—aim for 7,000 steps per day<br>• Taichi and yoga<br>• Aquatic therapy<br>*Weight loss:*<br>For patients who are overweight or obese, focusing on both diet and exercise is most beneficial for symptom management. |
| **SECONDARY TREATMENTS** | |
| MEDICATIONS | *Must consider the patient's comorbidities involving the gastrointestinal system, cardiovascular system, frailty, widespread pain, and depression.*<br>*Topical agents (preferred due to lowest systemic side-effect profile):*<br>• Topical NSAIDs<br>• Capsaicin cream<br>*Oral agents:*<br>• Acetaminophen—caution in use with liver pathology<br>• NSAIDs—avoid use with history of cardiovascular disease or kidney disease and use COX-2 inhibitor for history of gastrointestinal disease.<br>• Tramadol—prophylactically treat constipation and use cautiously with older adults<br>• Duloxetine—consider with history of depression |
| INTRA-ARTICULAR INJECTIONS | *Can utilize an injection when no benefit is seen with earlier treatments.*<br>• Corticosteroid injection<br>• Hyaluronic acid injection |
| PSYCHOSOCIAL INTERVENTIONS | • Regardless of psychological history, patients benefit from interventions combining coping skills training and exercise. |
| DIETARY SUPPLEMENTS | • Glucosamine and chondroitin sulfate<br>• Turmeric |

(continued)

## Osteoarthritis Management Order Set (*continued*)

| | |
|---|---|
| GAIT AIDS AND ORTHOSES | • Cane or walker<br>• Knee taping with medial pull on the patella<br>• Off-loading braces for medial femorotibial OA<br>• Lateral wedge insoles for medial femorotibial OA<br>• Medial wedge insoles for lateral femorotibial OA |
| MODALITIES | • Therapeutic ultrasound for 10- to 15-minute duration<br>• Cold packs daily for 20-minute duration<br>• Ice massage daily for 20-minute duration |

NSAIDs, non-steroidal anti-inflammatory drugs; OA, osteoarthritis.

## REFERENCES

The full list of references appears in the digital product found on http://connect.springerpub.com/content/book/978-0-8261-6226-7/part/part02/chapter/ch24

# STRESS FRACTURES

STEPHANIE R. DOUGLAS AND ADAM S. TENFORDE

## INTRODUCTION

Bone stress injuries (BSIs) represent failure of the bone in the setting of repetitive stresses that exceed the ability of the bone to remodel. Stress fractures represent the advanced stage of injury with the presence of fracture line seen on imaging along with clinical symptoms to confirm true injury. Bone is constantly in dynamic balance between resorption and new bone formation. In the setting of mechanical strain, increased intensity or duration of loading leads to microscopic injury and initiation of a healing response. Unrecognized stress fractures may progress to complete fracture if untreated. Many general practitioners are likely to encounter patients with BSI at some point in their practice, and this chapter describes the epidemiology and risk factors associated with BSI along with general principles for their evaluation and management. Though insufficiency fractures are a subgroup of stress fractures, this injury type will be discussed in further detail in the osteoporosis/metabolic bone disease chapter.

## EPIDEMIOLOGY

Given the role of repetitive loading on the development of BSI, athletes and military recruits are the populations most commonly affected. Data suggest that around 8% to 52% of runners have a history of BSI, and college athletes in the United States experience stress fractures at a rate of 5.70 per 100,000 athletic exposures over 10 years.[1,2] Runners and gymnasts are thought to be at highest risk due to the repetitive nature of the sport and the significant loads placed on bone.[1] Prospective studies of U.S. military recruits show a stress fracture incidence of 3.3% to 8.5%.[2] BSIs occur at greater frequency in young adults, possibly due to higher rates of participation in competitive sports or strenuous activity. A large majority of BSI affect the lower extremities, with 38% occurring in the metatarsals, 22% in the tibia, and 12% involving the pelvis in a population of college athletes.[1] As expected, site of injury varies by sport. While data in populations with disability, including adaptive sport athletes, is limited, overuse or traumatic injuries to bone should also be considered within physiatry practice. One report in para-athletes identified 9.2% with history of BSI attributed to sport, and half of all athletes reported history of fracture.[3]

---

The full list of references appears in the digital product found on http://connect.springerpub.com/content/book/978-0-8261-6226-7/part/part02/chapter/ch25

## RISK FACTORS

### Biological

Risk for injury may be affected by a number of biological factors that either cause or correlate with reduced bone strength or resilience. History of fracture is a robust predictor of future bone injury, and females with a history of fracture have been found to have a six-fold increase in risk of fracture.[4,5] Female sex confers elevated risk of BSI. In a sample of collegiate athletes, the relative risk of stress fracture in females across sex-comparable sports was 2.06 elevated risk compared to male athletes.[1] Female Athlete Triad (Triad) risk factors include low energy availability with or without disordered eating, menstrual dysfunction, and low bone mineral density (BMD).[6] A positive correlation between the number of triad risk factors and BSI risk has been observed in female athletes.[7] The concept of triad has been expanded to Relative Energy Deficiency in Sport (RED-S), which describes the multiple health and performance impairments from low energy availability state in both female and male athletes, including athletes with disability.[8]

Nutritional deficiencies, including low energy availability, are risk factors for suboptimal bone health in all patients. Low BMD is a risk factor for BSI in females and delayed bone healing in males.[5,9] Calcium and vitamin D play an important role in bone health.[5,10-15] Certain medications confer increased bone injury risk as a result of their effect on BMD, cell turnover, or effect on gastrointestinal absorption of nutrients. Examples of offending medications include contraceptives, other hormonal medications, antacids, anticonvulsants, and antidepressants (see online supplemental material for a full list of these medications).[5,10,16] Genetic loci both with and without a well-understood role in bone biology are known to modulate fracture risk.[17] Medical conditions such as systemic inflammatory diseases and endocrine abnormalities may affect bone health or healing and may lead to increased risk of BSI.

### Biomechanical

Biomechanical intrinsic risk factors for BSI vary by location, but a number of commonalities are seen across anatomical sites. Leg length discrepancy can lead to asymmetric loading along the entire kinetic chain and does not have to be large in magnitude (usually exceeding 0.5–1 cm) to have clinical significance in the setting of repetitive activities such as running.[18-21] Consideration for a partial lift in the shoe of the affected limb can be trialed to see if this helps improve mechanics. Variability in bone microarchitecture in healthy individuals may affect BSI risk, with reduced trabecular number and thickness seen in soldiers with tibial BSI.[22] Other anatomic factors such as bone diameter and geometry have been shown to affect rates of bone injury.[23-25] Muscle weakness and fatigue may lead to greater transmission of force to bone and increase injury risk; for example, smaller calf girth and pes planus (an indicator of foot weakness) are associated with tibial and metatarsal BSI, respectively.[21,26] Muscle tightness and dynamic loading patterns likewise affect the forces seen by bone and the consequent risk of bone injury.[18,27-30]

Extrinsic factors related to training (load, progression, and surface), equipment, and footwear may affect the risk of bone injury associated with exercise. Specifically, chronic overload or abrupt changes in training volume or intensity place people at elevated risk for BSI.[4,31] Changes in footwear or equipment may lead to altered biomechanics and changes in patterns of bone loading, leading to the possibility of stress injury.[31-33]

## EVALUATION

### History

Patients with BSI classically describe focal pain, often of insidious onset, which increases with activity. Over time, symptoms may be provoked with less activity and can progress to pain at rest. Patients occasionally present with abrupt onset of increased pain on top of milder symptoms if fracture occurs at the site of a chronically stressed area.

A thorough exercise history should be obtained, including any recent change in volume or intensity of training. History of fracture places the patient at higher risk of bone injury, and prior orthopedic injuries may provide clues to areas of weakness or biomechanical deficits.[4,5] Suspicion for BSI should prompt assessment of nutritional status, including calcium and vitamin D intake, dietary restrictions, symptoms of malabsorption, and current or prior history of disordered eating. In female patients, clinicians should inquire about menstrual irregularities. Personal or family history of low BMD, rheumatologic disease, endocrine conditions (such as thyroid disease), or orthopedic issues should be assessed. Medications affecting bone health should be noted, including corticosteroids, hormonal contraceptives, estrogen, and progesterone, as well as antacids, anticonvulsants, and antidepressants.[5,10,16] Patients should be asked about tobacco use as it may affect time to bone healing. The patient's activity and occupation should be determined as it may influence treatment planning.

### Physical Examination

Patients with BSI often exhibit focal bony tenderness on examination, along with pain with direct and indirect percussion. Swelling or subtle bruising may be present in advanced cases.[25,34] Reproduction of index pain with single-leg hop test is sensitive for lower extremity BSI, though care should be taken to avoid worsening of advanced or high-risk injuries.[35] The fulcrum test can help identify injury to long bones such as the humerus or femoral shaft and is performed by placing one hand beneath the location of pain and applying pressure to the end of the bone to generate stress on the suspected injury site.[36] Axial loading of the affected bone may also cause pain. Neurovascular status should be assessed, though compromise is rare.

Various special examination maneuvers may be helpful in diagnosing BSI of specific locations. In the presence of sacral or pelvic BSI, sacroiliac provocative testing using the thigh thrust or Flexion ABduction and External Rotation (FABER) maneuver may cause pain, as may pelvic distraction or compression. Stress injuries of the femoral neck or lesser trochanter may be aggravated by hip internal rotation, and femoral acetabular impingement with a positive Flexion ADduction and Internal Rotation (FADIR) maneuver is a common finding in patients with these injuries.[37] Iliopsoas tendinopathy as indicated by a positive Stinchfield's test is often seen in conjunction with lesser trochanter injuries.[38] The presence of pain with calcaneal squeeze test can help distinguish calcaneal stress injuries from retrocalcaneal bursitis or plantar fasciitis. In the upper extremity, muscle strength testing may provoke pain in patients with a stress injury of the humeral shaft.

The patient should be examined for findings suggestive of ligament injury or tendinopathy, which may provide an alternate explanation for the presenting symptoms. Examination can also reveal predisposing factors for injury. The clinician should assess for limb-length discrepancy, genu varus or valgus limb alignment, pes cavus or planus foot, joint range of motion, and muscle strength and flexibility of the affected anatomical region. Weakness, instability, or balance deficits may be evident on gait analysis in patients with lower extremity BSI. Stigmata of anorexia or bulimia nervosa such as lanugo or Russell's sign may be present in patients with a history of disordered eating. Rash or abnormal joint examination may provide evidence of underlying rheumatologic or systemic inflammatory disease.

## Imaging

Clinical evaluation may be sufficient to diagnose a portion of injuries, particularly low-risk BSI. Imaging is an important adjunct for injuries at anatomical locations that could suggest high risk for nonhealing or in patients desiring a rapid return to sport or with occupational demands. Plain radiographs may show periosteal elevation, cortical lucency or thickening, and sclerosis. However, x-rays have poor sensitivity for detecting early BSI as the radiographic features lag behind clinical symptoms by up to 2 to 3 weeks.[39-41] Once commonly used, bone scans have fallen out of favor for diagnosis of BSI due to their low specificity. MRI is both sensitive and specific for diagnosing BSI and provides useful prognostic information (Table 25.1).[9,42] In lower-grade injuries, periosteal or bone marrow edema can be seen. Grade 4 injury, referred to as stress fracture, is defined by the presence of a fracture line on T2 or T1 images (Figure 25.1). Severity of injury as assessed by MRI may correlate with expected healing time.[9,42] Ultrasound is gaining in popularity as a low-cost imaging modality with good sensitivity and specificity for diagnosis of metatarsal stress fractures and possible utility as a screening tool for BSI at other sites.[43,44]

## MANAGEMENT

### General Principles

Activity modification and a period of immobilization are the mainstays of treatment of BSI, along with addressing modifiable risk factors. During healing, activity should remain pain free, and reintroduction of bone loading should be gradual. Return to full activity should follow a stepwise symptom-free protocol. Specific recommendations by site of injury are outlined next. Ice and acetaminophen can be used for pain control, if needed. Non-steroidal anti-inflammatory drugs (NSAIDs) should be avoided due to a possible detrimental effect

**TABLE 25.1 MRI GRADING SYSTEM FOR BONE STRESS INJURY[9,42]**

| INJURY GRADE | MRI FINDINGS |
|---|---|
| Grade 1 | Mild periosteal or marrow edema on T2 and T1 normal |
| Grade 2 | Moderate periosteal or marrow edema on T2 and T1 normal |
| Grade 3 | Severe periosteal and marrow edema on T2 and T1 |
| Grade 4 | Severe periosteal and marrow edema on T2 and T1, plus presence of fracture line |

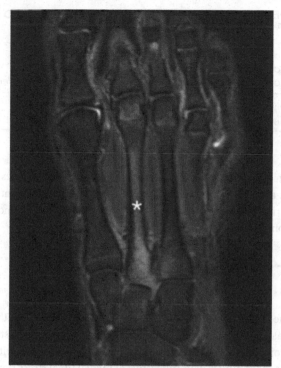

**FIGURE 25.1** MRI with long axis Short-TI Inversion Recovery (STIR) showing marrow edema of the left second metatarsal (indicated by asterisk) consistent with grade 3 bone stress injury.

on bone healing.[45,46] Patients should be counseled on smoking cessation as tobacco use is associated with delayed bone healing.[47] Physical therapy is helpful in addressing biomechanical contributors to injury such as core muscle weakness or instability and mobilizing tissues after a period of restricted activity. Patients with a history of multiple lower-extremity BSI may benefit from formal gait evaluation. Education on training techniques, training progressions, and recovery may help prevent future injury.

Given the important role of nutrition on bone health, patients with BSI should be advised to ensure adequate intake of calcium and vitamin D as well as macronutrients. Due to the high prevalence of vitamin D deficiency, patients with BSI should be screened by checking 25-OH vitamin D levels and provided with supplementation if indicated (Table 25.2). If low energy availability is suspected, referral for nutrition assessment by a registered dietician with a sports nutrition background is appropriate. A multidisciplinary treatment team may be required in certain cases, such as presence of eating disorder.[8,49]

Clinicians should consider screening for low BMD using dual-energy x-ray absorptiometry (DXA) for patients with recurrent or poorly healing BSI, amenorrhea, family history of low BMD, history of disordered eating, or other predisposing conditions such as malabsorption syndromes, systemic inflammatory illness, or chronic use of glucocorticoids or other medications affecting bone health. Laboratory evaluation for biological contributors to injury

**TABLE 25.2 RECOMMENDED DAILY INTAKE OF CALCIUM AND VITAMIN D BY INSTITUTE OF MEDICINE[48]**

| Calcium | 1,300 mg daily for ages 9 to 18<br>1,000 mg daily for women ages 19 to 50, men ages 19 to 70<br>1,200 mg daily for women ages 51 and older, men ages 71 and older |
|---------|---|
| Vitamin D | 600 IU daily up to age 70<br>800 IU daily for ages 71 and older |

may also be indicated. Referral to an endocrinologist with experience with athletes and/or familiarity with triad/RED-S may be more appropriate for patients with recurrent injury, significant hormonal irregularities, or low BMD. Patients with lower BMD may demonstrate slower healing and benefit from a more gradual return to activity.[9]

## Recommendations by Location
## Low-Risk Injuries
### Medial Tibia

The distal tibia is among the most common locations for BSI, and injuries of this area generally respond well to conservative management. Most injuries occur in the distal third of the tibia along the posteromedial aspect of the bone. Focal pain associated with bone injury may be preceded by the more diffuse pain suggestive of medial tibial stress syndrome. Recovery time is typically from 3 to 12 weeks, but full return to sport may take up to 20 weeks in high-risk athletes.[42] During this time, patients should avoid painful activities. A short period of stabilization in an air cast or walking boot may be required to achieve pain-free ambulation.

### Fibula

Fibular stress injuries typically exhibit rapid healing over a period of 3 to 6 weeks followed by a gradual return to activity when asymptomatic.[50] Non–weight-bearing status or rigid immobilization are rarely required, except in cases with slight displacement or those associated with injury to the common peroneal nerve. Proximal injuries may require a more conservative timeline due to the increased biomechanical forces at that location.

### Metatarsal Shaft

BSIs of metatarsal shafts two to five carry a good prognosis for uncomplicated healing. Low-grade injuries can often be treated with a firm-soled shoe with metatarsal pad, though some injuries may require immobilization in a walking boot to achieve pain-free ambulation.[50] Clinical follow-up should identify healing based on pain-free examination, with repeat radiographs considered at 4 to 6 weeks for high-grade injuries or concern for poor healing based on clinical symptoms. Patients may begin to resume normal activities at around 6 to 8 weeks when signs of healing are evident on radiographs and clinical examination, with goal to advance activity as long as pain free. Operative intervention is indicated for rare cases where there is displacement of the fracture or symptomatic nonunion.[51]

## Moderate-Risk Injuries

### Sacrum and Pelvis

Sacral and pelvic BSIs often present as high-grade injury In some patients, crutches may be required in order to achieve pain-free ambulation but can be discontinued when walking is nonpainful. Time to return to full activity ranges from 12 weeks to 20+ weeks depending on location and biological risk factors.[9,52]

### Femoral Shaft

The proximal posteromedial cortex of the femur is the most common location due to the combined effects of muscle activity at the insertion of the adductor brevis and origin of the vastus medialis.[53] Because of the severe consequences of a complete fracture, patients with suspected injury to the femoral shaft should be made non–weight-bearing until BSI has been ruled out. With advanced-grade injury, patients should remain non–weight-bearing with crutches for at least 3 weeks followed by 3 weeks of weight-bearing ambulation and subsequent reincorporation of progressively increasing levels of activity over several weeks.[54] These injuries usually respond to conservative treatment if no cortical break or displacement is present, allowing a return to full activity in 8 to 12 weeks.[50]

## High-Risk Injuries

### Femoral Neck and Lesser Trochanter

Patients with dynamic femoral anteversion, genu valgum, confusion assessment method (CAM) deformity, or leg length discrepancy are at higher risk for BSI of the femoral neck.[19,37] Injuries of the femoral neck are considered high risk due to the risk of disruption of the tenuous blood supply to the femoral neck and the potential for serious complications associated with nonunion. Patients should be non–weight-bearing until BSI is ruled out. Tension-side (superolateral) fractures require a surgical consultation with a trauma surgeon given risk for nonunion or development of complications including avascular necrosis. If managed nonoperatively, tension-sided injuries typically require 1 to 2 weeks of bed rest if no widening of the fracture is seen on serial imaging, followed by use of crutches for 4 to 8 weeks.[55] Weekly radiographs should be obtained for the first 4 to 6 weeks and then bimonthly until 12 weeks to confirm that no displacement has occurred. Compression-side (inferomedial) fractures can be managed with crutches and strict non–weight-bearing status for 6 weeks, with consideration for repeat imaging and examination to confirm healing prior to advancing to weight-bearing status. Lesser trochanter fractures can progress to involve the femoral neck and are managed with similar precaution of non–weight-bearing for 6 weeks.[38] Healing is expected in 2 to 3 months. Early consultation with an orthopedic surgeon is recommended for tension-side injuries or if bony healing is not evident on repeat radiographs. Low-impact cross-training is permitted when patients are pain free on examination and demonstrate radiographic evidence of cortical bridging.

### Anterior Tibial Cortex

Injuries of the anterior tibial cortex make up only 5% of tibial BSI. In contrast to BSI of the medial tibia, injuries of the anterior cortex are considered high risk as they occur on the tension side of the tibia and are subject to increased forces interfering with healing. In the presence of fracture, the "dreaded black line" may be seen on plain radiographs (Figure 25.2). Injuries should be treated with initial non–weight-bearing with crutches for 6 weeks minimum and gradual increase in weight-bearing and progression back into sport pain free. Repeat radiographs should be obtained before allowing progressive weight-bearing. BSI of the anterior tibial cortex complicated by nonunion may require surgical fixation with an intramedullary rod to achieve stability and allow healing to occur.

### Second Metatarsal Base

BSIs of the second metatarsal base are distinct from other metatarsal injuries due to their high rate of nonunion, particularly if the fracture extends into the Lisfranc joint.[40,56] They most commonly occur in ballet dancers due to repetitive extreme plantar flexion. Morton's toe is a risk factor because of the resulting increased forces through the second ray of the foot.[25,57] Due to the high risk of complications, injuries in this area should be treated with a minimum of 4 weeks of immobilization. The patient should be carefully examined and repeat radiographs obtained to confirm bone healing before weaning from a boot. Custom orthosis with a metatarsal pad beneath the second metatarsal may reduce the risk of future injury.

### Proximal Fifth Metatarsal

Known as a Jones fracture, stress fractures of the proximal fifth metatarsal are at risk for delayed healing and nonunion because of the relative avascularity of the bone distal to the tuberosity. Initial treatment in a CAM walking boot can be considered, but studies suggest that patients may have better outcomes and faster return to sport with surgical treatment, typically with intramedullary screw fixation and bone grafting.[58,59] Management without

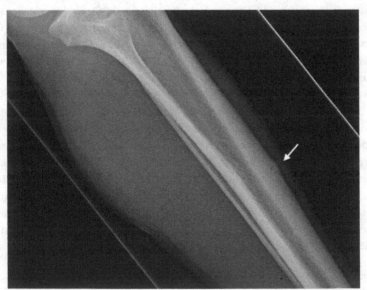

**FIGURE 25.2** Plain radiograph showing "dreaded black line" characteristic of tibial stress fracture.

surgery requires both walking boot and crutches for 6 weeks to maintain non–weight-bearing status, followed by weaning from crutches and boot and formal physical therapy. With surgical treatment, return to activity is possible beginning as early as 12 weeks.

## Tarsal Navicular

Navicular stress injuries make up 10% to 30% of stress fractures and are most common in runners.[60] Risk of injury and delayed healing are increased due to the relatively avascular zone in the central navicular due to the watershed blood supply. Unlike management of BSI at other locations, partial weight-bearing is inadequate for healing of navicular stress fractures due to the high risk of nonunion.[61] Type 1 injuries that are limited to the dorsal cortex are most likely to respond to conservative treatment.[62] Strict non–weight-bearing status for at least 6 weeks should be implemented initially, with immobilization in a CAM boot to prevent passive plantar flexion. Type 2 injuries extending into the navicular body warrant surgical referral but can be given an initial trial of nonoperative treatment with similar boot and non–weight-bearing restrictions. Type 3 injuries extending into the plantar cortex are at highest risk for nonunion when treated conservatively. Studies suggest improved outcomes for high-grade injuries treated surgically. Surgical referral may also be appropriate if diagnosis is delayed more than 3 months from symptom onset; however, patients may respond to 8 weeks of immobilization and non–weight-bearing status even following a delay in diagnosis. CTs should be obtained to assess the healing response in the setting of chronic injury or if patients are not asymptomatic after 10 to 12 weeks of conservative treatment.

## REFERENCES

The full list of references appears in the digital product found on http://connect.springerpub.com/content/book/978-0-8261-6226-7/part/part02/chapter/ch25

# PEDIATRIC INJURIES

SHERRY IGBINIGIE AND BRIAN J. KRABAK

## INTRODUCTION

Youth physical activity is helpful in combating obesity and promoting a healthy lifestyle. Children are becoming active and specializing in sports at younger ages than in the past. This has led to an increase in pediatric musculoskeletal injuries. It is important for clinicians to understand musculoskeletal injuries in the skeletally immature population as their presentation and treatment may differ compared to adults.

## OSTEOCHONDRAL DEFECTS

### Etiology and Pathophysiology

Osteochondritis dissecans or osteochondral defects (OCD) are the formation of a fragment of separated subchondral bone and cartilage. The etiology of this condition remains unclear. However, bones and cartilage are their weakest during periods of rapid growth, likely increasing their susceptibility to injury with repetitive trauma and/or vascular insult.[1-3]

### Diagnosis

The patient typically presents with gradual vague joint pain that worsens with activity. Their symptoms may also proceed following a traumatic event. Patients can have mechanical symptoms such as catching, locking, clicking ,or popping if the bony fragment is partially or fully detached. If found at the ankle, they may have a chronic history of ankle instability or laxity. Joint swelling may be present. The knee is the most frequent site of OCD in youth, followed by the ankle. Knee OCDs are typically found at the lateral aspect of the medial femoral epicondyle. These defects are best viewed on the tunnel view of knee radiographs (Figure 26.1—OCD knee). Lesions in the ankle typically involve the talar dome, mostly in the medial aspect. Standard weight-bearing plain films often help to identify the lesion. MRI is the gold standard for diagnosis as well as helping to stage the osteochondral lesion at all sites.[4]

### Treatment

The treatment of OCD is determined by the stage, size, location, and patient age. Overall, healing is more successful in the skeletally immature population.[5,6] Stable lesions (Stages 1 and 2) can be treated nonoperatively for 3 to 6 months with a period of immobilization (6–18

The full list of references appears in the digital product found on http://connect.springerpub.com/content/book/978-0-8261-6226-7/part/part02/chapter/ch26

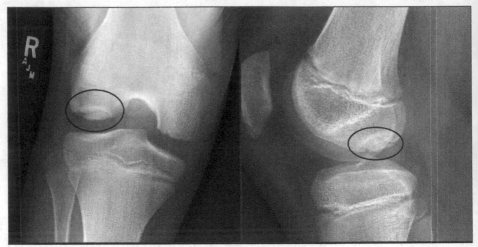

**FIGURE 26.1** Tunnel view of knee osteochondral defect.

*Source:* Reprinted by permission from Mugleston BJ, Krabak BJ. Caring for and counseling the youth runner. In: Harrast M, ed. *Clinical Care of the Runner*. Elsevier; 2020.

weeks) and/or non–weight-bearing followed by physical therapy.[1,7] The role of orthobiologics in treatment of this condition lacks high-level evidence and remains inconclusive at this time. Surgical management is reserved for stage 3 and 4 lesions. Proper treatment of these lesions is imperative as there is a high risk of osteoarthritis development in adulthood if inappropriately managed.

### Basic Order Sets

- X-rays of the knee: Weight-bearing anteroposterior (AP) view, tunnel view (most important), sunrise view, and lateral.
- X-rays of the ankle: Weight-bearing AP view, mortise view, and lateral.

## ACUTE FRACTURES

### Salter–Harris Classification

i.   Type I: Fracture through the physis only
ii.  Type 2: Fracture through the physis and the metaphysis (most common)
iii. Type 3: Fracture through the physis and epiphysis
iv.  Type 4: Fracture through the metaphysis and epiphysis
v.   Type 5: Crush injury to the physis

### Etiology and Pathophysiology

The etiology of acute fractures is typically traumatic, but poor underlying bone mineralization should also be considered. Epiphyseal fractures are most common in the distal radius but are often seen in other bones.

## Diagnosis

The patient often presents with pain and swelling at the site of the fracture usually after a traumatic event. Radiographs will help determine the presence and type of fracture and the need for reduction (open/closed) (Figure 26.2—x-ray Salter–Harris 2). It is important to note that Salter–Harris type 5 fractures may be missed on radiographs. If there is high suspicion of fracture and radiographs are negative, advanced imaging should be ordered such as CT scan or MRI.

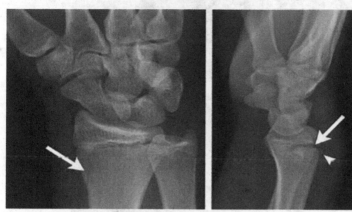

**FIGURE 26.2** X-ray of Salter–Harris type 2 fracture.

## Treatment

Treatment is generally with cast immobilization for 6 to 8 weeks depending on the rate of healing. However, if the fracture involves the joint or articular surface (types 3–5), then anatomic reduction is required. Growth disruption is not common in type 1 and type 2 fractures. There is a high risk of growth disruption in Salter–Harris type 5 fractures. The exact timing for return to activity may differ per individual and fracture type. Generally, advancement in activity is determined per patient's reported level of function and tolerance. After appropriate bone healing has been demonstrated on imaging, the patient should focus on functional mobility and strength, followed by activity-related exercises and ultimately return to sport. Generally, advancement in activity is determined per patient's reported level of function and tolerance.

## Apophysitis
### Etiology and Pathophysiology

Apophysitis is a common overuse injury seen in the skeletally immature. As children grow, the length of long bones increases faster than that of muscles and tendons, which places strain on the tendon at its insertion site on the apophysis.[2] The apophysis is the secondary ossification center where tendons attach to the bone. Repetitive stress to this area leads to irritation and injury to the apophysis.

## Diagnosis

Youth typically present with pain at the site of the apophysis that is worse with activity and better with rest. On physical examination, there is tenderness to palpation over the site of injury and pain reproduced with passive stretch of the involved tendon or activation of the attached muscle group. Radiographs of the area can be helpful to rule out an avulsion fracture (Figure 26.3—anterior inferior iliac spine [AIIS] avulsion fracture).

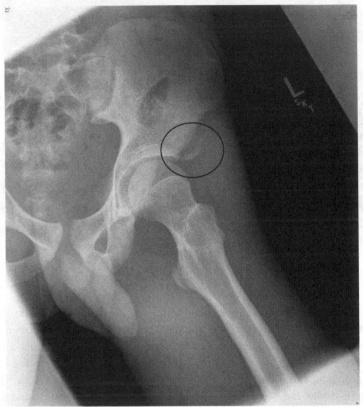

**FIGURE 26.3** X-ray of AIIS avulsion fracture.

*Source*: Reprinted by permission from Krabak BJ, Snitily B, Milani CJ. Running injuries during adolescence and childhood. *Phys Med Rehabil Clin N Am*. 2016;27(1):179–202.

## Treatment

Most injuries respond well to conservative management with a focus on rest, ice, pain medication (anti-inflammatories), activity modification, orthosis, correction of poor biomechanics, and training errors with therapy. Surgical intervention is rarely required with these types of injuries unless significant avulsion displacement or nonunion.

See Table 26.1 for specific types of common apophyseal injuries and their presentations.

## TABLE 26.1 COMMON APOPHYSEAL INJURIES AND PRESENTATION

| NAME | LOCATION | PRESENTING SYMPTOMS |
|---|---|---|
| LITTLE LEAGUE SHOULDER | Head of the humerus at the insertion of the rotator cuff | Presents with shoulder pain, particularly with throwing. Patient may have tenderness to palpation of the proximal shoulder. |
| LITTLE LEAGUE ELBOW | Medial epicondyle at the humeral origin of the ulnar collateral ligament | Presents with medial elbow pain, especially while throwing. Patient may have tenderness to palpation over the medial epicondyle. |
| ASIS) APOPHYSEAL INJURY OR AVULSION | Origin of the Sartorius and tensor fascia lata muscles at the ASIS | Presents with insidious or acute (if an avulsion) pain in the area of the ASIS and anterior thigh that can be associated with history of a "pop" sensation, localized swelling, tenderness, and bruising. May lead to compression of the lateral femoral cutaneous nerve resulting in meralgia paresthetica. |
| AIIS APOPHYSEAL INJURY OR AVULSION | Origin of the rectus femoris muscle at the AIIS | Presents with insidious or acute (if an avulsion) pain in the area of the AIIS and anterior thigh that can be associated with history of a "pop" sensation, localized swelling, tenderness, and bruising. |
| SINDING-LARSEN–JOHANSSON LESION | Patellar tendon origin at the inferior pole of the patella | Presents with insidious onset of pain of the anterior knee located at the base of the patella that is worse with high-impact activity, such as jumping and running. |
| OSGOOD–SCHLATTER LESION | Patellar tendon insertion at the tibial tuberosity | Presents with an insidious onset of anterior knee pain located at the tibial tuberosity that is worse with high-impact activity, such as jumping or running. There is often an associated palpable mass at the area of pain. |
| SEVER'S DISEASE | Achilles tendon insertion | Presents with an insidious onset of heel pain that is worse with direct compression. Symptoms often are bilateral and rarely associated with swelling. |
| ISELIN'S DISEASE | Base of the fifth metatarsal at the insertion of the fibularis brevis and tertius tendons | Presents with lateral foot pain that is worse with weight-bearing activity and wearing shoes as well as tenderness to palpation at the base of the fifth metatarsal. |

AIIS, anterior inferior iliac spine; ASIS, anterior superior iliac spine.

## Slipped Capital Femoral Epiphysis
### Etiology and Pathophysiology

Slipped capital femoral epiphysis (SCFE) is a Salter–Harris type 1 fracture that is strongly associated with obesity.

### Diagnosis

The child commonly presents with a limp, ipsilateral groin, thigh, or knee pain. This is typically seen in obese males, ages 11 to 13, and may be associated with endocrine disorders.[8] On physical examination, there is a loss of internal rotation of the hip when flexed. Radiographs of the hip (AP and frog-leg views) demonstrate posterolateral displacement of the epiphysis (abnormal Klein's line) and/or widening of the physis (Figure 26.4—x-ray SCFE). Up to 30% to 40% of cases are bilateral.

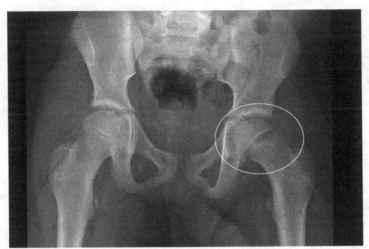

**FIGURE 26.4** X-ray of slipped capital femoral epiphysis.

### Treatment

The child is immediately placed in non–weight-bearing status and referred to orthopedics for surgical stabilization.

### Basic Order Set(s)

X-ray hip: AP and frog-leg lateral views

## Perthes Disease (Legg-Calve-Perthes Disease)
### Etiology and Pathophysiology

Perthes disease is osteonecrosis of the femoral epiphysis. Its etiology is unknown but is commonly thought to be related to repetitive microtrauma.[9] Another study suggests a possible systemic etiology.[10]

## Diagnosis

The child typically presents similarly to SCFE but is mostly seen in boys aged 4 to 8 years old. On physical examination, there is limited hip abduction. Radiographs (AP, frog-leg views) (Figure 26.5—Legg-Calve-Perthes) show sclerosis and fragmentation of the femoral head and a positive "crescent" sign. MRI of the hip can also be obtained for both diagnosis and prognosis especially in the early and late stages.[11]

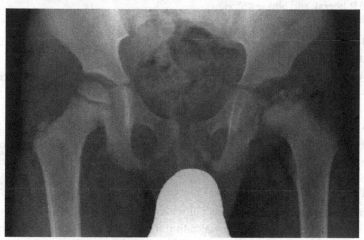

**FIGURE 26.5** X-ray of Legg-Calve-Perthes disease.

*Source*: Courtesy of Dr. J. Lengerke.

## Treatment

The patient is placed in crutches or a walker to decrease femoral head deformation that may occur with weight-bearing. An abduction brace may also be used. Physical therapy helps to maintain range of motion of the hip. Prognosis is better for children less than 10 years old as the development of osteoarthritis is more common in those above the age of 10 years.

## Basic Order Set(s)

X-ray hip: AP and frog-leg lateral views

## Kohler's Disease
### Etiology and Pathophysiology

Kohler's lesion is osteonecrosis of the navicular thought to be due to abnormal strain on the navicular resulting in decreased blood flow to the avascular zone in the central one-third portion.

## Diagnosis

The child typically presents with a limp and pain in the medial aspect of the arch of the foot. On physical examination, there is tenderness to palpation over the medial navicular. Radiographs of the foot demonstrate sclerosis, collapse, and fragmentation of the navicular.

## Treatment

Kohler's disease is treated conservatively. The child is placed in a walking boot or short-leg cast for a period of 4 to 6 weeks. Non-steroidal anti-inflammatory drugs (NSAIDs) can be given for pain management.

## Basic Order Set(s)

X-ray foot: AP, lateral, and blique 45° views

## Freiberg's Disease
## Etiology and Pathophysiology

Freiberg's lesion is osteonecrosis of the second or third metatarsal heads. Its etiology is unclear and likely multifactorial.[12]

## Diagnosis

This presents with pain and tenderness over the metatarsal head. It is more commonly seen in adolescent females. Radiographs of the foot demonstrate flattening of the metatarsal head.

## Treatment

Conservative management is often successful when diagnosed early. This includes relative rest and the use of orthotics (i.e., metatarsal cutout, rocker bottom). Chronic lesions may be treated with surgical debridement and loose body removal if present.

## Basic Order Set(s)

X-ray foot: AP, lateral, and oblique 45° views

## Blount's Disease
## Etiology and Pathophysiology

Blount's disease is osteonecrosis of the medial tibial epiphysis with an unclear etiology but thought to be associated with obesity.

## Diagnosis

The patient presents with bowing of the legs (genu varus) and a lateral thrust when ambulating. This is often seen in tall, obese adolescents. Most lesions are unilateral. Radiographs demonstrate a "beaking", thickening of the proximal medial tibia and a metaphyseal–diaphyseal angle less than 80°.

## Treatment

Typical treatment is weight loss, but bracing may be effective in the infantile form of Blount's disease before the age of 4.[13] If conservative treatment is ineffective, then an osteotomy may be performed.

## Basic Order Set(s)

X-rays tibia-fibula (bilateral): Standing long-cassette AP and lateral views

## Scheuermann's Disease

### Etiology and Pathophysiology

Scheuermann's disease is focal osteonecrosis of the superior and inferior endplates of the thoracic vertebral body, likely due to repetitive stress on weaker growing bone.[14] This condition may be associated with genetic factors.

### Diagnosis

It is commonly seen in male adolescents that present with mid-back pain, barrel chest, and poor posture. On physical examination, there is rigid kyphosis. Radiographs of the spine demonstrate irregular endplates with Schmorl's nodes, kyphosis =/> 45°, and three adjacent thoracic vertebral bodies with at least 5° of anterior wedging.

### Treatment

This is mostly treated nonsurgically with physical therapy (posture and extension exercises) and bracing, except for individuals with severe deformity who require surgery.

### Basic Order Set(s)

X-ray thoracic spine: AP and lateral views

## Spondylolysis

### Etiology and Pathophysiology

Pars defects (spondylolysis) are an overuse injury due to repetitive stress to the bone that can result in a stress reaction or fracture most commonly at the L4 or L5 level. If spondylolysis occurs bilaterally, spondylolisthesis may occur.

### Diagnosis

This is typically seen in adolescent athletes whose activities involve repetitive lumbar hyperextension and is the most common cause of low back pain in this population. The patient presents with low back pain that is worse with extension, physical activity, and lying prone. On physical examination, often there is pain with range of motion greatest in extension, increased lumbar lordosis, hamstring tightness, core weakness, and a positive Stork test. Radiographs (standing AP, lateral, flex/ext, oblique views) may show bony defects at the level of injury (Figure 26.6—Spondylolysis), but these may also be negative. If radiographs are negative, advanced imaging should be ordered to confirm the diagnosis. Which imaging should be ordered is controversial.[15] Bone scan with SPECT is the most sensitive and may show changes as early as 1 week after symptom onset. However, it is nonspecific and may be positive with other etiologies such as infection, arthritis, or malignancy. SPECT may be followed by a CT scan with thin slices focused at the L4 and L5 levels for better visualization of a bony defect and staging. Both SPECT and CT scan have significant levels of radiation exposure, making MRI a desirable option, especially in the pediatric athlete. Advantages of MRI are the lack of radiation exposure and the ability to visualize early bone stress reaction and evaluate concurrent lumbar etiologies, though the reliability of MRI in diagnosing pars defects is not well-defined at this time.

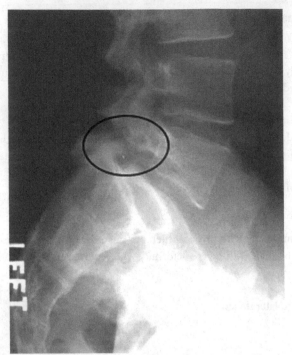

**FIGURE 26.6** X-ray depicting lumbar spondylolysis.

## Treatment

Most lesions are treated nonoperatively with relative rest, bracing, and physical therapy. For most clinicians, relative rest is for at least a period of 3 months as one study showed healing in greater than 90% of acute cases at 3 months.[16] Bracing remains controversial and may not affect clinical outcomes. Surgical intervention is used when there are neurologic deficits, instability, or symptoms that persist greater than 6 months with conservative management.

## Basic Order Set(s)

X-ray lumbar spine: AP, lateral, and oblique views; may add flexion and extension views if concerned about spondylolisthesis

## Juvenile Rheumatoid Arthritis (Still's Disease)
### Etiology and Pathophysiology

Still's disease is an autoimmune, rheumatologic disorder with an unknown etiology.

## Diagnosis

The child usually presents with persistent, intermittent knee effusions associated with warmth and decreased range of motion lasting more than 6 weeks. This may occur in other joints as well. The child may also complain of morning stiffness. There may be a family history of rheumatoid arthritis. Radiographs are often normal but may show periarticular osteopenia.[17]

Serological testing may demonstrate elevated erythrocyte sedimentation rate (ESR), C-reactive protein (CRP), or anemia which is associated with active arthritis. Rheumatoid factor (RF) and antinuclear antibody (ANA) should also be tested, but negative results do not exclude the diagnosis.[17] Arthrocentesis should be performed and sent for lab studies to rule out infection.

### Treatment

This is typically treated conservatively by restricting use of the joint in its inflamed state. NSAIDs may be taken to help with pain and swelling. In some cases, disease-modifying antirheumatic drugs (DMARDS) are started. Referral to a rheumatologist is imperative for further evaluation and management.

## REFERENCES

The full list of references appears in the digital product found on http://connect.springerpub.com/content/book/978-0-8261-6226-7/part/part02/chapter/ch26

# Section 3

# PHYSICAL MEDICINE AND REHABILITATION MANAGEMENT BY PROBLEM

## 27

# ANXIETY

DAVID ROTHMAN, AMY STAROSTA, AND JESSE FANN

## CORE DEFINITIONS

Anxiety in the face of uncertain and potentially threatening situations, whether the threat is physical or psychological, can be adaptive and functional, as it allows for increased attention, vigilance, and threat detection.[1] As such, anxiety related to major life changes, physical injury, and uncertain treatment and recovery can be a normative and understandable reaction.

In addition to the psychological components, anxiety is usually accompanied by physiological responses, which can include increased heart rate, increased blood pressure, feelings of muscle tension, feeling hot or increased sweating, shortness of breath, chest tightness, or dizziness. While some anxiety may be normative and helpful for patients in times of increased change, excessive or disproportionate anxiety is less functional and may start to cause impairment in function and distress for the patient.

The *Diagnostic and Statistical Manual of Mental Disorders*[2] (*DSM-5*) states that anxiety disorders are characterized by "excessive fear and anxiety and behavioral disturbances." This definition focuses on concerns surrounding future threats, either real or perceived. According to the *DSM-5*, anxiety disorders comprise autonomic arousal and avoidance behaviors to decrease the reaction associated with the feared stimulus. The topic of the feared stimulus is the predominant distinction between the disorders.

---

The full list of references appears in the digital product found on http://connect.springerpub.com/content/book/978-0-8261-6226-7/part/part03/chapter/ch27

## ETIOLOGY AND PATHOPHYSIOLOGY

Rehabilitation populations experience many unknown challenges not only in the early stages of their rehabilitation but throughout their life. These patients often deal with significant stress, such as after receiving a new diagnosis, or adjusting to functional change, or managing chronic medical issues.

Both subclinical and clinical levels of anxiety symptoms are common in rehabilitation populations. Anxiety disorders are prevalent among individuals with traumatic brain injury (TBI). Posttraumatic stress, generalized anxiety disorder (GAD), obsessive–compulsive disorder, and panic disorder are the most common among individuals with a history of TBI.[3] For individuals with spinal cord injury (SCI),[4] 45% report symptoms of anxiety, with a lower incidence of clinically significant anxiety (27%–32%). In association with clinical levels of anxiety, among individuals with SCI, GAD and panic disorder were found in 5% of the population, while only 2.5% were found to have agoraphobia.[4] In individuals who sustained a stroke, over a 12-month period, pooled prevalence of overall anxiety disorders was 29.3%.[5] Additionally, prevalence of anxiety disorders among individuals undergoing amputation ranges from 25.4% to 57%.[6] These rates are noteworthy as among individuals enrolled in inpatient rehabilitation programs, multiple studies have highlighted worse outcomes for patients experiencing anxiety.[7]

## DIAGNOSTIC APPROACH

### Screening Tools

Two anxiety screening tools that have been validated within medical settings are the Generalized Anxiety Disorder-7[8] (GAD-7) item measure and the Hospital Anxiety and Depression Scale (HADS)—Anxiety.[9] The GAD-7 was designed to be a brief screening measure to diagnose and assess the severity of GAD. While the measure was specifically designed for GAD, it is common practice to use this measure to assess for an individual's symptoms of anxiety, especially in healthcare settings. The GAD-7 assesses physiological sensations, psychomotor agitation, irritability, future-focused anxiety, and worry and is useful as a screener for individuals experiencing anxiety symptoms and disorders.[10] While the GAD-7 has well-established psychometrics for diagnosis of GAD, the GAD-7 is less specific when attempting to diagnose other anxiety disorders.

Unlike the GAD-7, the HADS focuses less specifically on the criteria for a specific disorder and rather assesses for anxiety as an overall construct. The HADS anxiety subscale includes items focused on general physiological distress, future-oriented fear, worrying, and feelings of panic. The HADS anxiety subscale will identify individuals experiencing anxiety symptoms but require a referral to a psychology provider for further assessment of their specific anxiety disorder. In doing so, individuals can work with providers to identify a strong treatment plan to decrease their experience of anxiety, specific to their circumstance.

### Adjustment Disorder With Anxiety

Adjustment disorders occur in association with an identifiable stressor or set of specific stressors, which in the context of rehabilitation populations is usually a new diagnosis or injury. Moreover, they are limited to 6 months following the specific stressor. In contrast,

**TABLE 27.1 EXAMPLES OF PATIENTS EXPERIENCING ANXIETY WITH NEW SPINAL CORD INJURY**

| | ADJUSTMENT DISORDER WITH ANXIETY | SOCIAL ANXIETY |
|---|---|---|
| START OF SYMPTOMS | Following SCI | Predating SCI |
| SPECIFIC WORRIES | Anxiety about bowel/bladder program, fear about going outside due to SCI-based limitations, fear of negative social evaluation because of their SCI | Fear of social interactions, where the SCI may or may not be component |

SCI, spinal cord injury.

individuals experiencing anxiety disorders do not have to experience a specific stressor or set of stressors that lead to their anxiety. Instead, their anxiety occurs without a direct link to their injury or diagnosis and occurs chronically (see Table 27.1).

Note that when an individual's anxiety relates directly to their SCI, both in topic and temporality, adjustment disorder is a more appropriate diagnosis. It is expected that this anxiety would decrease over time as the individual with a new SCI becomes acclimated to their new normative routines, interactions with others, and functional challenges. In contrast, the individual with an anxiety disorder reports symptoms that predate the SCI. These symptoms are likely compounded by the new SCI, but the new injury is not the primary driving force behind their social anxiety. Thus, when considering the continuum of anxiety disorders as compared to adjustment disorders, time and link back to a discrete stressor are important to consider. Although many physical medicine and rehabilitation (PM&R) providers meet with individuals who meet criteria for both adjustment disorders and anxiety disorders, a referral to a psychologist when uncertainty or significant distress exists should be strongly considered.

## Panic Disorder

When working with individuals in either an inpatient or outpatient rehabilitation setting, providers may encounter individuals who experience panic attacks. In general, the prevalence of panic attacks ranges from 2.1% to 27.4% depending on the country of origin.[11] Panic attacks and disorder are more common among a variety of medical populations.[12] A panic attack is when an individual experiences a significant increase in fear and/or physical discomfort which surges within minutes including 4 of 13 symptoms (as in Box 27.1).

Not all individuals who experience a panic attack meet criteria for panic disorder. Rather, in order to be diagnosed with panic disorder, individuals must present with at least a month of (a) concern about having another panic attack or fear of what the panic attack means, (b) maladaptive behavior change related to the panic attack, (c) the panic which is not associated with a medical condition. Within a rehabilitation population, panic attacks can be challenging as many of the associated symptoms can also be a signal of medical concerns. For example, shortness of breath and tachycardia can be associated with a panic attack or can be an indication of a cardiac event. Increased blood pressure and sweating can be related to anxiety or autonomic dysreflexia. Additionally, panic attacks can occur in isolation or can be related to medical symptoms.

> ## BOX 27.1
>
> ### SYMPTOMS OF PANIC ATTACK
> An abrupt surge of intense fear of discomfort that reaches a peak within minutes and during which time four (or more) of the following symptoms occur.
> 1) Palpitations, pounding heart, or accelerated heart rate
> 2) Sweating
> 3) Trembling or shaking
> 4) Sensations of shortness of breath or smothering
> 5) Feelings of choking
> 6) Chest pain or discomfort
> 7) Nausea or abdominal distress
> 8) Feeling dizzy, unsteady, light-headed or faint
> 9) Chills or heat sensations
> 10) Paranesthesia's
> 11) Derealization or depersonalization
> 12) Fear of losing control or "going crazy"
> 13) Fear of dying

Individuals could misinterpret normal symptoms associated with their medical condition as dangerous or threatening, resulting in a panic attack. Unfortunately, increased anxiety and panic may also contribute to worsening of medical symptoms, resulting in a bidirectional relationship between physical symptoms of anxiety and comorbid medical conditions.[12]

When PM&R providers identify that a patient is experiencing a panic attack or panic disorder, there may be a role for brief intervention. Specifically, if they are experiencing changes in respiration, cardiac, or gastrointestinal functioning, education about how these symptoms can increase panic symptoms may be useful for patients and providers alike. Should individuals continue to express concern or experience panic attacks, a referral for cognitive behavioral therapy for panic attacks should be considered. Behavioral interventions have been found to be effective in the treatment panic attacks, especially exposure-based techniques.[13]

## TREATMENT

### Psychotherapy
Anxiety disorders have been found to be responsive to psychotherapeutic interventions, with research regularly finding a medium to large effect on symptom reduction.[13,14] Moreover, there are multiple effective psychotherapeutic interventions to treat anxiety disorders, including cognitive behavioral therapies, and mindfulness-based interventions.[13,14] Of note, cognitive behavioral therapies are more effective at treating fear-based symptoms associated with anxiety disorders, while mindfulness-based strategies were more efficacious in treating internalizing anxious distress.

When considering information to provide patients about anxiety disorders associated with rehabilitation diagnoses, resources can be found in a variety of locations. One good resource that can be applied to variety of individuals is the Model Systems Knowledge Translation Center (https://msktc.org). Each of the model system websites has handouts focused either on anxiety explicitly or emotional distress following these injuries. These handouts are useful as they help patients and families understand symptoms, self-help techniques, and discussion of when to seek help/who to seek help from.

## Pharmacologic Interventions

Benzodiazepines act quickly and are occasionally necessary for short-term treatment for acute anxiety, particularly in the first few weeks of rehabilitation or when a patient's anxiety is so extreme that they cannot focus or function. However, benzodiazepines are not recommended for long-term use, particularly among individuals with acquired brain injury who are more susceptible to their potential adverse effects. If benzodiazepines are needed, they should be used initially at lower doses because of their propensity to exacerbate or cause cognitive and motor impairment and sedation. The high prevalence of substance use disorders in patients with TBI adds to the risk of benzodiazepines and may preclude their use in some patients. Periodic attempts at tapering are recommended as adjunctive therapies (e.g., selective serotonin reuptake inhibitors [SSRIs], psychotherapy) take hold. If available, assistance with dosage monitoring from a caregiver can help prevent inadvertent overuse and allow for monitoring of side effects.

SSRIs, serotonin norepinephrine reuptake inhibitors (SNRIs), and tricyclic antidepressants (TCAs) may have efficacy for anxiety in the rehabilitation setting, particularly when there is co-morbid depression.[15] SSRIs and SNRIs have also been found to be effective in decreasing mood lability and compulsions after brain injury, although these effects may take several weeks. Because the initial activating effects of serotonergic agents may be particularly problematic for anxious individuals, which can in turn lead to nonadherence or early discontinuation, these medications should be started at 50% or 25% of the usual starting dosage. However, as with treatment for depression, higher dosages may be needed to achieve maximum therapeutic effect.

Valproic acid, gabapentin, and pregabalin may be of benefit for anxiety, especially in patients with concomitant mood lability or seizures. Buspirone is another option for generalized anxiety symptoms and is generally well tolerated. Antipsychotics should not be used as first-line treatments for anxiety or posttraumatic stress disorder (PTSD) and should be reserved for patients with psychotic symptoms. When these agents are indicated, quetiapine and olanzapine may be the most useful for anxiety and sleep.

## SPECIAL CONSIDERATIONS

### Anxiety and Ventilator Weaning

Anxiety is very common among patients requiring mechanical ventilation. Prolonged anxiety and distress may predispose patients to more long-term negative psychological outcomes.[16] From a patient's perspective, psychological challenges weaning from the ventilator include fear of not being able to breathe, feeling out of control, and changes in self.[17] Physiological manifestations of anxiety such as tachycardia, shallow breathing, or hypertension can decrease an individual's ability to wean from the ventilator.[16] There is limited research on managing anxiety during ventilator weaning. Anecdotally, providing clear information to the patient and family, using a structured weaning schedule that helps the patient know what to expect, and preplanning effective coping strategies such as distraction, mindfulness, or pleasant activities have all been associated with positive outcomes.

## Pain and Anxiety

Not only does anxiety cause psychological distress, it can also impact an individual's report of pain.[18] Interactions between anxiety and pain have been shown to worsen outcomes post-surgery, medication needs, and reports of acute pain severity.[19] There are numerous proposed mechanisms including "fear-avoidance" behaviors and similar neural network activation in anxiety and pain.[18] Fear avoidance behaviors are those which lead to decreased participation in movement or actives, leading to deconditioning.[18] Within the context of rehabilitation populations, both anxiety, pain, and their co-occurrence are common clinical phenomena.

Nonpharmacologic pain interventions have been found to improve outcomes across multiple populations.[20] Therefore, individuals who are experiencing significant acute pain or chronic pain may benefit from a psychology referral, especially when significant pain-related anxiety (cognitions or behaviors) is present to help promote recovery and participation with therapies.

## REFERENCES

The full list of references appears in the digital product found on http://connect.springerpub.com/content/book/978-0-8261-6226-7/part/part03/chapter/ch27

# AGITATION AND DISRUPTIVE BEHAVIORS

LESLEY ABRAHAM AND CHERRY JUNN

## CORE DEFINITIONS

According to the International Psychogeriatric Association, agitation is defined broadly as (a) occurring in patients with a cognitive impairment or dementia syndrome; (b) exhibiting behavior consistent with emotional distress; (c) manifesting excessive motor activity, verbal aggression, or physical aggression; and (d) evidencing behaviors that cause excess disability and are not solely attributable to another disorder (psychiatric, medical, or substance related).[1]

Agitation that occurs after a traumatic brain injury (TBI) can be defined as a subtype of delirium unique to survivors of a TBI in which the survivor is in the state of posttraumatic amnesia and there is excess of behaviors that include some combination of aggression, akathisia, disinhibition, and/or emotional lability.[2]

## ETIOLOGY AND PATHOPHYSIOLOGY

The pathophysiology of agitation is not completely understood. Certain anatomical regions such as the frontal and temporal lobes, amygdala, and hippocampus have been implicated.[3] Cognitive impairment that limits one's ability to understand events, neurochemical imbalance, and external factors may also contribute.[3,4] It has been reported that up to 70% of patients with TBIs and up to 98% of patients with dementia may experience agitation.[4,5]

## DIAGNOSTIC APPROACH

It is important to obtain detailed information from the patient, family, and hospital staff to better characterize the type and severity of symptoms. It is also important to perform a thorough physical examination and workup to assess for causes of agitation including infection; inadequately controlled pain; abnormal sleep–wake cycle; overstimulation; presence of restraints, lines, and tubes; sundowning; alcohol/drug withdrawal; seizures; hydrocephalus after TBI; electrolyte abnormality; recent medication change; and endocrine dysfunction after TBI.

There are several tools that may be utilized to evaluate and monitor agitation.

---

The full list of resources and references appears in the digital product found on http://connect.springerpub.com/content/book/978-0-8261-6226-7/part/part03/chapter/ch28

## Agitated Behavior Scale

The Agitated Behavior Scale is a well-validated tool that assesses 14 types of behavioral disturbances within three categories: aggression, disinhibition, and lability. It is most useful when serially administered under similar circumstances (e.g., by nursing at the end of a night shift).[6]

## Overt Aggression Scale

Useful for rating aggressive events, it is divided into four categories: verbal aggression, physical aggression against objects, physical aggression against self, and physical aggression against others. There is also a modified version for use in neurorehabilitation (Overt Aggression Scale-Modified for Neurorehabilitation [OAS-MNR]).[7]

## Neuropsychiatric Inventory

This is a valid and reliable tool to assess the frequency and severity of 10 behavioral disturbances: delusions, hallucinations, dysphoria, anxiety, agitation/aggression, euphoria, disinhibition, irritability/lability, apathy, and aberrant motor activity.[8]

## TREATMENT

Treatment should first involve behavioral and environmental modifications with pharmacotherapy if needed. Behavioral and environmental modifications include adequately treating pain; establishing a proper sleep–wake cycle; minimizing lines, tubes, and restraints, decreasing overstimulation; and maintaining consistency.

There are several classes of medications that may be used in the treatment of agitation, although there is no clear expert consensus. Therefore, the treatment should be individualized based on the type and severity of agitation and patient comorbidities. The following is a list of commonly used medications, starting doses, and adverse effects.

Beta-blockers have the greatest evidence for use in agitation.[9] They are also useful in akathisia. Lipophilic beta-blockers should be chosen as they cross the blood–brain barrier. Common agents may include propranolol 10 mg BID/TID (up to 420 mg/day) or pindolol 5 mg BID (up to 30 mg/day; has less effect on heart rate and blood pressure). Adverse effects include low blood pressure, bradycardia, fatigue, and bronchospasm in asthmatics.

There have been several studies that suggest improvement in agitation with anticonvulsants/mood stabilizers.[10–12] They require routine lab monitoring due to potential side effects. These may include the following:

1. Valproic acid 250 mg daily (often extended release [ER]). Adverse effects may include hepatotoxic, thrombocytopenia, teratogenic, rash, gastrointestinal (GI) upset, fatigue, weight gain
2. Carbamazepine 100 to 150 mg BID. Adverse effects may include aplastic anemia, hyponatremia (SIADH), hepatic impairment, teratogenic, renal failure, fatigue, dizziness

Antidepressants such as selective serotonin reuptake inhibitors (SSRIs) and tricyclic antidepressants (TCAs) may be useful if depression, anxiety, and/or mood lability are present.[10,13] They can also be titrated up as needed. Common SSRI agents and doses include fluoxetine 20 mg daily, sertraline 25 mg daily, or citalopram 10 mg daily. Adverse effects of SSRIs include erectile dysfunction, hyponatremia, fatigue, or nausea. Use of fluoxetine with clopidogrel should be avoided due to interaction. TCAs such as amitriptyline 25 mg should be used at bedtime due to somnolence. Other adverse effects of TCAs include arrhythmia, anticholinergic effects, or delirium.

Several studies have evaluated the use of neurostimulants. Agents to consider include methylphenidate 5 mg BID (8 a.m., noon) or amantadine 100 mg BID (8 a.m., noon—maximum 400 mg/day). Adverse effects of methylphenidate include tachycardia, anxiety, decreased appetite, or hypertension. In an initial trial, amantadine was found to reduce irritability when compared to placebo. A subsequent multisite study did not find increased benefit.[14] Hallucinations, cardiac arrhythmia, lower seizure threshold, and livedo reticularis are potential side effects of amantadine. Amantadine is also contraindicated in end-stage renal disease (ESRD) (CrCl <15 mL/min).

Several studies suggest that antipsychotics may decrease agitation. However, animal studies also demonstrate that antipsychotic medications, especially typical antipsychotics, may impair cognitive function, prolong posttraumatic amnesia, and impair neuro recovery after brain injury.[15] Alternatives in this class include quetiapine 12.5 to 25 mg HS or BID, olanzapine 2.5 mg daily—intramuscular and oral dissolving formulations, or risperidone 0.5 mg HS or BID. Adverse effects may include corrected QT interval (QTc) prolongation, metabolic syndrome, extrapyramidal side effects, and neuroleptic malignant syndrome.

Benzodiazepines may increase confusion, cause paradoxical agitation, and delay recovery.[3,16] Adverse effects include sedation and dependence/addiction potential. Their use should be reserved for emergent situations. Options include lorazepam 1 mg IM/IV, lorazepam PO 1 mg (shorter half-life), or diazepam PO 2 mg (longer half-life).

## FUNCTIONAL PROGNOSIS AND OUTCOMES

Agitation and disruptive behaviors may cause distress for patients, friends and family members, and hospital staff. It may also disrupt care, pose risk to others, limit progress in rehabilitation, and prolong recovery.[3,5]

## BASIC ORDER SETS

- Regulate sleep–wake cycle—may trial sleep medication at bedtime.
- Minimize noise, overstimulation, restraints/lines/tubes.
- Perform infectious workup (chest x-ray, urinalysis/urine culture, complete blood count, other pertinent studies).
- Evaluate for electrolyte abnormality (basic metabolic panel).
- Evaluate for drug/alcohol withdrawal.
- Consider evaluating for hydrocephalus if TBI, seizures, and endocrine abnormality.

## RESOURCES AND REFERENCES

The full list of resources and references appears in the digital product found on http://connect.springerpub.com/content/book/978-0-8261-6226-7/part/part03/chapter/ch28

# AUTONOMIC DYSREFLEXIA

AUDREY S. LEUNG AND DEBORAH A. CRANE

## CORE DEFINITIONS

Autonomic dysreflexia (AD) is a disorder of the autonomic nervous system seen in individuals with spinal cord injury (SCI) at or above the sixth thoracic level (T6). It is defined by acute episodic hypertensive events caused by unmodulated sympathetic reflexes below the level of injury triggered by a noxious stimulus. Other terms that have been used for this condition include autonomic hyperreflexia, paroxysmal hypertension, paroxysmal neurogenic hypertension, autonomic spasticity, sympathetic hyperreflexia, and neurovegetative syndrome.

## ETIOLOGY AND PATHOPHYSIOLOGY

Individuals with SCI at T6 or above are generally at risk of developing AD, although cases with injuries as low as T10 have been reported. When a noxious visceral or somatic stimulus occurs below the level of injury, sensory nerves below the level of injury transmit impulses to the spinal cord, which then ascend via the spinothalamic and posterior columns. Sympathetic neurons in the interomediolateral gray matter of the spinal cord are stimulated by these impulses and at levels T6 through L2 provide sympathetic innervation to the splanchnic vascular bed, leading to vasoconstriction. In SCI, descending supraspinal inhibitory impulses are blocked at the level of injury. Therefore, in injuries at T6 and above, there is relatively unopposed sympathetic outflow to the splanchnic vascular bed, which receives approximately 25% of the body's cardiac output and ultimately results in an elevation in blood pressure. This can lead to potentially life-threatening hypertension, which can have severe consequences such as hypertensive encephalopathy, stroke, cardiac arrest, seizure, and death.[1]

AD can occur in either nontraumatic or traumatic cases of SCI. Not all individuals with SCI at or above the T6 level develop AD, with the prevalence reported anywhere between 48% and 91%.[2-4] The majority of cases first occur 3 to 6 months after injury,[3] with only 5.7% of individuals presenting with AD within the first month of injury.[5]

## DIAGNOSTIC APPROACH

The magnitude of hypertension required to be considered AD varies across studies, but current clinical practice guidelines set by the Consortium for Spinal Cord Medicine state that

---

The full list of resources and references appears in the digital product found on http://connect
.springerpub.com/content/book/978-0-8261-6226-7/part/part03/chapter/ch29

systolic blood pressure (SBP) of 20 to 40 mmHg above baseline may be a sign of AD in adults. In the pediatric population, greater than 15 to 20 mmHg above baseline for adolescents and greater than 15 mmHg above baseline in children may signify AD. In addition to elevated blood pressure, individuals may also experience concurrent symptoms such as headache, sweating, flushing of skin above the injury level, piloerection, nasal congestion, blurred vision, and anxiety. Although AD has classically been associated with bradycardia due to the baroreflex system attempting to counteract the increase in blood pressure by increasing vagal parasympathetic output to the heart, several studies have reported tachycardia being either equally as common or more common than bradycardia.[3,6,7] Some individuals may have minimal or no symptoms despite elevations in blood pressure (silent AD).

## TREATMENT

Initial measures to treat AD include immediately sitting the individual up if they are lying down, loosening any clothing or constrictive devices, and identification and removal of the noxious stimulus. The most common cause of AD is bladder distension followed by bowel impaction. If an indwelling urinary catheter is not in place, the individual should be catheterized, and lidocaine jelly should be placed into the urethra prior to the insertion of the catheter if possible to prevent exacerbating the AD. If the patient has an indwelling catheter, the system should be checked for kinks or obstructions and for correct placement. If there is blockage within the catheter, irrigation of the bladder via the indwelling catheter with 10 to 15 mL of fluid such as normal saline should be done. If the catheter is still not draining, then the catheter should be removed and replaced. If symptoms of AD persist, fecal impaction should be suspected next, followed by any other source of noxious stimulus (i.e., infection, skin wounds, renal stones).

There are no studies demonstrating the exact point at which elevated blood pressure becomes dangerous or which agents are the most optimal in treating AD. The Consortium for Spinal Cord Medicine suggests that treatment of SBPs at or greater than 150 mmHg in adults, 140 mmHg in adolescents, 130 mmHg in children 6 to 12 years old, and 120 mmHg in infants and children under 5 years old should be considered.[8] Antihypertensive agents used should have a short onset and duration to prevent uncontrollable drop in blood pressure. Nifedipine and nitrates are most commonly used, although use of other oral drugs such as hydralazine, mecamylamine, diazoxide, and phenoxybenzamine has also been reported. Intravenous drip of sodium nitroprusside for rapid titration of blood pressure can be used in closely monitored settings. If 2% nitroglycerin ointment is used, it should be applied to the skin above the level of injury. Consideration should be taken for individuals using phosphodiesterase (PDE) type 5 inhibitors (i.e., sildenafil), as concurrent use of nitrate medications to treat AD can result in a precipitous drop in blood pressure. Therefore, alternative short-acting antihypertensive agents are recommended such as prazosin or captopril. Given that blood pressure can fluctuate rapidly in patients with AD, it is also important to monitor blood pressure every 2 to 5 minutes for resolution or exacerbation of hypertension once the noxious stimulus is removed and/or if pharmacological treatment is used.

Once the individual with SCI is stabilized, the cause of the AD episode should be discussed with the individual and other caregivers, as well as education provided on how to minimize risks of triggering another AD episode. A written guide or alert can be downloaded and provided to the patient (link provided under Patient Education Resources available online for this chapter) and can be particularly helpful in individuals with limited cognition or verbal skills.

## FUNCTIONAL PROGNOSIS AND OUTCOMES

It is imperative that one identify and promptly treat AD appropriately because untreated AD can lead to further disability or death. Hemorrhagic strokes, retinal hemorrhages, seizures, and cardiac arrhythmias are potential sequelae of untreated AD and can ultimately lead to death.

## BASIC ORDER SETS

For signs/symptoms of AD, or if SBP >150 or SBP >40 mmHg above baseline, check pulse, respiratory rate, and blood pressure every 5 minutes.

Initiate AD orders if patient has the following: flushing, gooseflesh above level of spinal injury, onset of severe headache, blurry vision, nasal congestion, profuse sweating above the level of spinal injury, SBP >150, or SBP >40 mmHg above baseline.

- Transfer patient to bed.
- Loosen any tight or constrictive clothing.
- Elevate head of bed to at least 45°.
- Lower foot of bed.
- Reposition patient.
- Examine skin for irritation.

### Urinary Catheter

- Insert Foley to gravity. Premedicate with lidocaine topical 2% jelly in sufficient quantity for transurethral lubrication 2 minutes prior to insertion.
- Irrigate with 15 mL normal saline at body temperature and withdraw. Inspect Foley for kinds or other obstructions.
- If Foley catheter is not draining, remove and replace with new catheter of same size. Premedicate with lidocaine topical 2% jelly in sufficient quantity for transurethral lubrication 2 minutes prior to replacing.

### Digital Rectal Stimulation

- Premedicate with lidocaine topical 2% jelly of sufficient quantity for rectal lubrication 2 minutes prior to digital rectal stimulation. Proceed with fecal disimpaction PRN.
- If blood pressure (BP) increases or heart rate decreases with rectal stimulation/disimpaction, then stop. Instill generous amount of lidocaine topical 2% jelly into rectum and recheck for the presence of stool in 20 minutes.

### Medications

- Lidocaine topical 2% gel
  - One application, topical, on call, PRN for transurethral lubrication 2 minutes prior to Foley catheter placement or replacement

❏ Application, topical, on call, PRN for lubrication 2 minutes prior to digital rectal stimulation or disimpaction
■ Nitroglycerin 2% transdermal ointment 1 inch topical, q8h, PRN. Apply to chest or forehead above level of spinal injury for SBP >150. May repeat × 1 after 10 minutes if ineffective. Remove ointment if SBP <130.
■ Hydralazine 10 mg, IV, on call, PRN. For continued SBP >150, 10 minutes after application of 2 inches of nitroglycerin ointment, may repeat × 1 in 10 minutes if ineffective.

## RESOURCES AND REFERENCES

The full list of resources and references appears in the digital product found on http://connect .springerpub.com/content/book/978-0-8261-6226-7/part/part03/chapter/ch29

# BLADDER

PHILIPPINES G. CABAHUG, JUNGHOON CHOI, ALBERT C. RECIO, AND CRISTINA L. SADOWSKY

## CORE DEFINITION

Neurogenic bladder is bladder dysfunction, either flaccid or spastic, caused by central or peripheral neurologic damage. Symptoms include, but are not limited to, urinary urgency and/or incontinence, retention, and dysuria.

## ETIOLOGY AND PATHOPHYSIOLOGY

Neurogenic bladder can be categorized by the location of the injury.[1–4] Its presentation varies depending on the classification.

### Suprapontine (Upper Motor Neuron)

Suprapontine neurogenic bladder is caused by brain damage (e.g., stroke, traumatic brain injury, multiple sclerosis, Alzheimer's dementia). It leads to detrusor overactivity without detrusor sphincter dyssynergia (DSD) due to impairment of cerebral regulation and inhibition. Typically, suprapontine lesions do not lead to increased post-void residual (PVR) volume.

### Suprasacral (Upper Motor Neuron)

Suprasacral neurogenic bladder is associated with injuries below the pons and above the sacral micturition center including most traumatic and nontraumatic spinal cord injury (SCI). It results in a spastic bladder (detrusor hyperreflexia) and sphincter. This results in the following:

- High bladder pressures with frequent and low-volume urination
- High PVR volume (greater than 50–150 mL)
- DSD, co-contraction of the bladder, and sphincter, which leads to high bladder pressure
- Bladder hypertrophy with diminished bladder compliance if not well controlled

### Infrasacral (Lower Motor Neuron)

Infrasacral neurogenic bladder involves injuries of the peripheral nerves at or below the sacral micturition center including cauda equina syndrome and diabetes mellitus. This results in the following:

- Hypotonic detrusor and normal or hypotonic sphincter
- Overflow incontinence from urinary retention or incontinence from decreased sphincter tone

---

The full list of resources and references appears in the digital product found on http://connect.springerpub.com/content/book/978-0-8261-6226-7/part/part03/chapter/ch30

- Continuous incontinence that may require use of condom catheters (males) or indwelling catheters (females)

## DIAGNOSTIC APPROACH

Neurogenic bladder should be suspected if patients have symptoms that are consistent with upper motor neuron (UMN) and/or lower motor neuron (LMN) bladder dysfunction, as described previously.[2-4]

### History

Discuss ability/inability to void, frequency, and volume of urination; urinary urgency; urinary incontinence; bladder sensation; and frequency of urinary tract infection (UTI).

### Physical Examination

Evaluate mental status, sensation, reflexes, anal sphincter tone, and ability to contract voluntarily.

### Laboratory Studies

Appropriate studies may include urinalysis, urine culture, and a basic metabolic panel (BMP) to assess for baseline kidney and bladder function and to rule out acute infection or kidney damage. The recommended frequency of laboratory and imaging studies is detailed in Table 30.1.[1,3]

### Imaging Studies
### Renal/Bladder Ultrasound

This is used to evaluate kidney and bladder anatomy and function and is useful to rule out complications such as hydronephrosis or urinary retention by measuring PVR. PVR volume of <50 mL is considered normal; >50 mL increases potential for UTI, although <100 mL is usually acceptable. It is recommended to catheterize for ultrasound (US)-detected PVR volumes >100 mL (when checked with US). It can also be measured directly using post-void catheterization.

### Cystoscopy

Cystoscopy is used to evaluate the anatomy of the bladder and urethra using a hollow camera tube. It may identify stones, bladder tumor, and cystitis.

### Voiding Cystourethrogram

This assesses bladder neck and urethral function during filling and voiding phases using contrast and x-ray/US. It is used to diagnose vesicoureteral reflux (VUR) or urethral obstruction.

## TABLE 30.1 RECOMMENDED TESTING SCHEDULE FOR PATIENTS WITH NEUROGENIC BLADDER

| TEST | INDICATION/REASON |
|------|-------------------|
| Urinalysis and urine culture | 6 months or yearly but often not routinely checked |
| Urine culture | Whenever symptomatic to monitor for infection |
| Renal/bladder ultrasound | Yearly to evaluate bladder function and rule out hydronephrosis or other kidney abnormalities |
| BMP | Yearly check to evaluate kidney functions |
| Cystoscopy | Every 2 years for patients with indwelling catheters |

BMP, basic metabolic panel.

### Cystometry (Urodynamics Study)

This is a comprehensive test to evaluate for neurogenic bladder. Refer to Chapter 65 for more details.

## SPECIAL CONSIDERATIONS

### Spinal Shock

Acutely after SCI, temporary areflexia/hyporeflexia and autonomic dysfunction occur regardless of type of injury (UMN or LMN).[1,3,5] Bladder dysfunction is described in four phases, with progression from areflexia to hyperreflexia. Reflexes begin to return within 24 hours. Spinal shock-related bladder dysfunction may last days or months after SCI with typical duration of 4 to 12 weeks post injury.

### Vesicoureteral Reflux

This refers to the backflow of urine from the bladder into the ureter.[1,5] VUR is typically caused by bladder wall hypertrophy and loss of the vesicoureteral angle, leading to malfunction of the valve mechanism of the submucosal ureter against the detrusor muscle. If severe or untreated, it can lead to hydronephrosis. High PVRs (100 cc or higher) with elevated intravesical pressure have been associated with VUR.

## TREATMENT

The main goal of treatment is to preserve kidney and bladder function while preventing/minimizing medical complications and undesired voiding in social setting.[1,3,4]

### Nonpharmacological
### Behavioral Strategies

Voiding diaries, timed voiding, and caffeine regulation are strategies that support voiding routines.

### Triggered Reflex Voiding (Crede or Valsalva Maneuvers)

Use for patients with LMN injuries or those who had sphincterotomy, where there is less risk for elevated pressure/reflux. It is not recommended for UMN neurogenic bladder due to risk of further elevating bladder pressures.

### Intermittent Catheterization Programs

This is the preferred method of treating neurogenic bladder dysfunction and is associated with decreased complications (e.g., UTI) when compared to indwelling catheters. It should only be used in patients who have a minimum bladder capacity of 200 mL. In a typical program, intermittent catheterization (IC) should be performed every 4 to 6 hours for a target output volume not to exceed 400 to 500 mL (depending on bladder capacity and patient size). Fluid intake should be adjusted to meet target output (usually restricted to 2–2.5 L/day). Patients with urethral pathology (e.g., false passages or strictures) should not use IC.

### Condom Catheters

They are generally not recommended but occasionally used during nighttime or during prolonged activity when IC is not realistic to achieve socially acceptable continence.

### Indwelling Catheters

This is an alternative for patients unable or unwilling to perform IC as it has been associated with complications such as bladder stones, prostatitis, epididymitis, transitional cell and squamous cell carcinoma of the bladder, and higher risk of UTIs.

### Pharmacological

Pharmacological interventions are widely used and may include medications to decrease detrusor tone/spasms and increase bladder capacity (Table 30.2),[6,7] decrease urethral outflow resistance (Table 30.3), or combination therapy for complex deficits. Prolonged use of anticholinergic medications is associated with increased risk for dementia in older patients; thus, use of beta-3 agonists (e.g., mirabegron) may be considered to reduce risk.

### Procedures and Surgical Interventions

### Botulinum Toxin Injections

These are a common treatment method for neurogenic bladder. Injection may be done at the bladder (for hyperactivity) or at the external sphincter (external sphincter injection not recommended for women as it frequently leads to incontinence).[4,8,9] Dosage varies between 100 and 300 units, divided into several areas of the bladder. They usually need to be repeated every 3 to 9 months.

### Surgery

Surgical interventions are used when nonsurgical interventions are ineffective or contraindicated.[1,3,4]

Suprapubic catheters are placed by inserting a catheter through the lower abdomen into the bladder. They are indicated for patients who have difficulty performing IC due to urethral

**TABLE 30.2 MEDICATIONS TO DECREASE DETRUSOR TONE/SPASM AND INCREASE BLADDER CAPACITY (ANTICHOLINERGICS)**

| | INITIAL DOSAGE | MAXIMUM DOSAGE | SIDE EFFECTS |
|---|---|---|---|
| Oxybutynin IR | 5 mg BID | 5 mg QID | Dry mouth, dry/blurry eyes, urinary retention, constipation |
| Tolterodine IR | 1 mg BID | 2 mg BID | |
| Darifenacin | 7.5 mg daily | 15 mg daily | More constipation |
| Solifenacin | 5 mg daily | 10 mg daily | More constipation |
| Trospium | 20 mg BID | 60 mg daily[a] | Dry mouth, constipation |
| Oxybutynin ER | 5 mg daily | 30 mg daily | Side effects less than IR |
| Tolterodine ER | 2 mg daily | 8 mg daily | |
| Mirabegron[b] | 25 mg daily | 50 mg daily | HR and BP increase, less anticholinergic side effects than other medications earlier. |

Dose adjustment may be required for renal or hepatic impairments.

[a]Extended release formulation.

[b]Not anticholinergic but a beta-3 agonist.

BP, blood pressure; ER, extended release; HR, heart rate; IR, immediate release.

**TABLE 30.3 MEDICATIONS TO DECREASE URETHRAL OUTFLOW RESISTANCE (ALPHA ADRENERGIC ANTAGONISTS)**

| | INITIAL DOSAGE | MAXIMUM DOSAGE | SIDE EFFECTS |
|---|---|---|---|
| Terazosin | 2 mg daily | 10 mg daily | Dizziness and postural hypotension |
| Doxazosin | 2 mg daily | 8 mg daily | |
| Tamsulosin | 0.4 mg daily | 0.8 mg daily | Ejaculatory problems |

abnormalities (i.e., stricture, fistula, enlarged prostate) or hand dexterity and perineal skin breakdown due to urine leakage. They are usually placed after comprehensive evaluation and diagnostic testing.

A Mitrofanoff appendicovesicostomy is performed by creating a channel from the bladder to the umbilicus (most commonly) using the patient's appendix (or part of small bowel if the patient does not have an appendix). This makes catheterization easier for the patients as the abdomen is easier to access.

Bladder augmentation is typically done by attaching a portion of the small bowel to the bladder to increase bladder volume. This procedure has become much rarer with the advent of botulinum toxin injections.

Other surgical or procedural interventions used for the management of neurogenic bladder include transurethral sphincterotomy (TURS), urethral stent, posterior sacral rhizotomy with electrical stimulation, urinary diversion, sacral neuromodulation, and posterior tibial nerve stimulation.

## FUNCTIONAL PROGNOSIS AND OUTCOMES

Patients with neurogenic bladder are expected to require lifelong treatment.[1] Complications from neurogenic bladder, such as kidney failure, used to be the number one cause of death for SCI patients. Appropriate care for neurogenic bladder significantly decreases morbidity and mortality.

## RESOURCES AND REFERENCES

The full list of resources and references appears in the digital product found on http://connect .springerpub.com/content/book/978-0-8261-6226-7/part/part03/chapter/ch30

# BOWEL

PHILIPPINES G. CABAHUG, CRISTINA L. SADOWSKY, AND ALBERT C. RECIO

## CORE DEFINITION

Neurogenic bowel is the impairment of gastrointestinal (GI) and anorectal function arising from a lesion, injury, or disease of the nervous system.[1,2] This can result in severe constipation, fecal incontinence, or both.

## ETIOLOGY AND PATHOPHYSIOLOGY

Neurogenic bowel is seen in patients with neurologic disease or dysfunction such as spinal cord injury (SCI), multiple sclerosis (MS), stroke, Parkinson's disease (PD), myelomeningocele (MMC), and cerebral palsy (CP), among others.[2]

The level and extent of the lesion or injury to the nervous system determines the pattern of presentation and symptoms of neurogenic bowel in neurologic disease.

When the spinal cord is involved, neurogenic bowel can be classified as supraconal or conus/cauda equina.

### Supraconal (Above Conus Medullaris)

Injuries at or above the 12th thoracic vertebra (T12) present as an upper motor neuron (UMN) or reflexic (spastic) bowel, resulting in impaired sensation and voluntary control. The autonomic reflex arcs between the cord and sigmoid colon/anorectum remain intact. Colonic and anal sphincter tone is increased. Colonic transit time is slowed. Persons with UMN bowel present with constipation and stool retention. Reflex uncontrolled evacuation may still occur.[1,3,4]

### Within the Conus or at the Level of Cauda Equina

Injuries at or below the first lumbar vertebra (L1) present as a lower motor neuron (LMN) or areflexic (flaccid) bowel. The autonomic reflex arcs between the spinal cord, colon, and anal rectum are damaged, with loss of reflex activity of the sigmoid and anorectum. Colonic transit time is slowed and the external anal sphincter (EAS) is atonic; thus, persons with LMN bowel can present with both constipation and high risk of fecal incontinence.[1,3,4]

Constipation is a frequent presentation in other neurological conditions such as stroke, CP, and PD. In stroke, impaired cortical inhibition, urge to defecate, and anal sphincter con-

The full list of resources and references appears in the digital product found on http://connect.springerpub.com/content/book/978-0-8261-6226-7/part/part03/chapter/ch31

trol combined with problems in communication, cognition, and mobility can lead to constipation and fecal incontinence.

## DIAGNOSTIC APPROACH

### History

Premorbid bowel function, current bowel symptoms and bowel program, diet, fluid intake, medications, premorbid or current GI or sphincter dysfunction, surgical procedures, and other comorbidities that can affect bowel function should be discussed (see Table 31.1).[1,3,4]

Patients can have atypical presentation due to impairments in sensation or function. SCI patients with fecal impaction can present only with nausea and early satiety. Diarrhea may be due to overflow incontinence and not related to infection or food intake. Autonomic dysreflexia (AD) is a frequent presentation in individuals with neurologic injury at T6 level and above.

**TABLE 31.1 NEUROGENIC BOWEL CLINICAL HISTORY[1,4]**

| | | |
|---|---|---|
| Premorbid bowel function | Review bowel frequency, any bowel symptoms prior to injury/disease | |
| Current bowel function | Sensory: Can the patient tell if rectum is full and/or needs to evacuate? Motor: Is there voluntary control of anal sphincter? | |
| Bowel symptoms | Constipation<br>Fecal incontinence<br>Flatus incontinence<br>Bowel urgency<br>Unplanned evacuations (bowel accidents) | Abdominal pain<br>Bloating, abdominal distention<br>Nausea<br>Early satiety<br>Rectal bleeding<br>Autonomic dysreflexia |
| Frequency of bowel movement | Ideally not less than two times per week | |
| Average time spent toileting | Ideally less than 1 hour (includes transferring to the toilet/commode till end of defecation and transfer away from toilet). If done in bed, then it is the time required from beginning to end of bowel management. | |
| Stool consistency | Bristol Stool Form Score to describe consistency | |
| Defecation method | Valsalva maneuver/straining<br>Digital anorectal stimulation<br>Digital evacuation | Enemas<br>Transanal irrigation system<br>Colostomy |
| Diet and fluid intake | Assess frequency and content of meals<br>Assess fiber and fluid intake<br>Take note of any allergies or food intolerance<br>Take note of any conditions that can interfere with adequate food or fluid intake (cognitive deficits, dysphagia) | |

(continued)

## TABLE 31.1 NEUROGENIC BOWEL CLINICAL HISTORY[1,4] (continued)

| Medical history | GI or anorectal sphincter dysfunction<br>Functional GI disorders (e.g., irritable bowel syndrome)<br>Obstetric: Anal sphincter dysfunction following childbirth<br>Pelvic organ prolapse<br>Hemorrhoids, anal fissures<br>GI surgical procedures |
|---|---|
| Medication review | Use of stool softeners, laxatives, or antidiarrheal medications<br>Bladder anticholinergics (e.g., oxybutynin), opiates, NSAIDs, antispasticity meds, antibiotics, etc., can worsen bowel dysfunction symptoms |
| Functional and cognitive history | UE strength, fine motor skills, transfers, balance, walking, communication, cognitive impairment<br>In SCI: Physical functioning, equipment, and caregiver support needed are dependent on level of injury |
| Environmental factors | Use of assistive device/equipment, toilet accessibility, availability of caregiver support |

GI, gastrointestinal; NSAIDs, non-steroidal anti-inflammatory drugs; SCI, spinal cord injury; UE, upper extremity.

## Physical Examination
### Abdominal Assessment

Include inspection for distention, auscultation for presence of bowel sounds, percussion for widespread tympany (suggestive of flatus retention), and palpation for tenderness, masses (e.g., hernia), or hard stool along the course of the colon.[1,4,5]

### Rectal Examination

Examine the anal orifice for pathology (anal fissures, hemorrhoids, etc.). The digital rectal examination provides information about sensation of deep anal pressure, anal tone, voluntary anal contraction, and presence of masses such as hemorrhoids or stool in the rectal vault.

### Neurologic Examination

Check for anocutaneous (EAS contraction in response to perianal skin stimulation by touch or pin prick) and bulbocavernosus (EAS contraction in response to pinching the glans penis or pressing the clitoris) reflexes. The presence of these reflexes is suggestive of areflexic bowel.

### Functional Assessment

Evaluate upper limb strength and hand function, spasticity, sitting tolerance, balance, transfers, walking, sensation and risk of skin breakdown, and level of activity. Assess the ability to learn and to direct care. Consider environmental factors (need for assistive devices, home adaptations for accessibility) and availability of caregiver support.[4]

## Assessment Tools
### Bristol Stool Form Scale

A validated seven-point scale of stool form that can be used to guide the bowel regimen.[5] Used to describe stool form.

## Neurogenic Bowel Dysfunction Score

Used to assess bowel symptoms. Consists of 10 questions, with scores ranging from 0 to 47. A score of 14 or more is consistent with severe dysfunction.[5] This has been validated in adults with SCI and children/adolescents with spina bifida.[5-7] It has been used in MS.[5]

## The International Spinal Cord Injury Bowel Function Basic Data Set

A standardized format for collecting and reporting a minimal amount of information on bowel function in clinical practice and research. The revised version includes the neurogenic bowel dysfunction score to allow its use among children with SCI.[8]

## Laboratory and Imaging Studies
## Abdominal X-Ray

Obtain a plain film of the abdomen to assess degree of fecal loading or colonic dilatation if patient presents with increased constipation or abdominal distention or if overflow incontinence is suspected.[1,2,4,5]

## Stool Examination

Evaluate fecal leukocytes, *Clostridium difficile* toxin, ova and parasites, or other enteropathogens in cases of unexplained diarrhea.

## CT Scan or MRI of the Abdomen

If "red flag" symptoms are present, that is, blood loss, weight loss, or worsening of a previously stable bowel program. Consider in females with progressive symptoms when there is concern for ovarian cancer.

## Fecal Occult Blood Test

Should be performed every 2 years in individuals 50 years of age with a negative family history for colorectal cancer as part of colon cancer screening. False positive results may occur if hemorrhoids are present.

## Endoscopy (Rectosigmoidoscopy, Anoscopy, Colonoscopy)

Consider these tests if cancer or structural abnormalities are suspected.

## TREATMENT

The primary goals of managing neurogenic bowel are to (a) provide a predictable, effective, and efficient way to evacuate the bowels and (b) prevent fecal incontinence and evacuation problems and minimize other GI complications.[1]

## Acute and Subacute

Regular physical examination should be performed to identify any changes in anal tone, sensation, and presence of feces in rectum. Daily digital removal of stool is recommended if feces are present in the rectum. In SCI, the spinal cord will be areflexic acutely due to spinal shock. Once out of spinal shock, the initial bowel program should be established based on the underlying pathology (i.e., reflexic vs. areflexic bowel).[1] The bowel program should be reevaluated upon commencing rehabilitation, modifying with changes in physical function, level of consciousness, oral intake, progression to independent self-care, and so forth.[4]

## Chronic

Annual evaluation of bowel program efficacy is recommended, with modifications done as needed. Screening for colorectal cancer is the same as in the general population, as per guidelines.[4]

An individualized bowel care program should consider the following: pattern of neurogenic bowel dysfunction (reflexic vs. areflexic bowel); patient's physical and cognitive function; patient's goals and societal obligations; availability of caregiver support; and environmental barriers (Table 31.2).[1,4] Detailed clinical guidelines are available.[1,4] An interprofessional team approach (physicians/advance practice providers, nurses, occupational therapists, mobility specialists, dieticians, social workers) is important to optimize the bowel program.[6]

## TABLE 31.2 DESIGNING THE INITIAL BOWEL CARE PROGRAM[1,4]

| CORE COMPONENTS | COMMENTS |
|---|---|
| Optimize fiber and fluid intake to achieve desired stool consistency:<br>- Reflexic bowel: Bristol Stool Scale 4 (smooth, soft like sausage)<br>- Areflexic bowel: Bristol Stool Scale 3 (like sausage with cracks on surface) | Fiber: Start with 15 g of fiber daily and gradually increase.[b] |
| | Fluid: Goal of 1.5–2 liters per day; or urine of pale straw color. May need to increase catheterization with increased fluid intake |
| Establish bowel care schedule to develop predictable response and avoid colorectal overdistention | Frequency: Should be done on same time of day, depending on physiologic and lifestyle needs<br>• Reflexic bowel: Daily or every other day<br>• Areflexic bowel: Daily or twice daily |
| | Duration: ≤60 minutes |
| Defecation method | Mechanical methods:<br>• Reflexic bowel: Digital anorectal stimulation (use of finger to trigger rectal contractions and anal relaxation)<br>May be used with suppository to trigger defecation<br>• Areflexic bowel: Digital evacuation (finger used to remove stool in rectum)<br>Note: Rectal stimulation may trigger AD in SCI patients with lesions at T6 and above |

(continued)

**TABLE 31.2 DESIGNING THE INITIAL BOWEL CARE PROGRAM[1,4] (continued)**

| CORE COMPONENTS | COMMENTS |
|---|---|
| Defecation method | Chemical rectal agents: Used in reflexic bowel. Not effective in areflexic bowel.<br>• Suppositories: Shorter bowel care time, time to flatus and defecation period is seen with PGB bisacodyl than HVB bisacodyl. Use glycerin suppository in those who cannot tolerate bisacodyl or are transitioning from bisacodyl to digital stimulation.<br>• Enemas: Small-volume enemas (5 mL) containing docusate can trigger defecation; available with benzocaine for those who get AD with rectal stimulation |
| | Assistive techniques: Abdominal massage, Valsalva maneuver, deep breathing, ingestion of warm fluids may be helpful.<br>• Caution with Valsalva maneuver in those with cardiac issues, hypertension, hemorrhoids. Empty bladder before doing Valsalva as this can lead to vesicoureteral reflux |
| Nutrition | Food and/or fluid intake 30 minutes prior to bowel care to facilitate gastrocolic reflex<br>Do not skip meals<br>Note diuretic/stimulant food/fluids (alcohol, caffeine, prunes, pure fruit juice sorbitol sweetener) |
| Medications | For constipation: Stool softeners, laxatives if initial management not optimum<br>For diarrhea: Consider loperamide<br>Review medications for side effects, drug interactions that can exacerbate bowel symptoms |
| Equipment and assistive devices | Coordinate with OT and nursing |
| Education and training of patient and caregiver | Discuss anatomy, defecation process, and effect of SCI on bowel function; goals of bowel program, techniques, interventions; and recognition, prevention, and treatment of complications |
| Periodic evaluation of effectiveness of bowel care program | Evaluate for constipation, unplanned and/or prolonged evacuations, or presence of other GI symptoms and complaints<br>Check for adherence to program, identify barriers.<br>Evaluate after 3–5 cycles of bowel care after each revision, making one change at a time. |

AD, autonomic dysreflexia; GI, gastrointestinal; HVB, hydrogenated vegetable oil-based; OT, occupational therapy; PGB, polyethylene glycol-based; SCI, spinal cord injury.

## Pharmacologic Intervention
### Stool Softeners (Docusate Sodium, Docusate Calcium)

Use if soft, formed stool is desired. They increase water content in the stool by decreasing colonic reabsorption of water. Adequate fluid intake is required.[1,3,4]

### Bulk Forming Agents (Psyllium, Calcium Polycarbophil, Methylcellulose)

These absorb water in the stool, causing luminal distention, and stimulate colonic peristalsis. Adequate fluid intake is required.

### Peristaltic-Stimulating Agents (Senna)

Stimulation of myenteric plexus leads to colonic peristalsis. Give 6 to 12 hours prior to bowel program. Long-term use can cause melanosis coli (benign staining of colon) and atonic bowel (decreased responsiveness over time).

### Bowel Contact Irritants (Bisacodyl)

Irritation of colonic mucosa stimulates peristalsis. Oral form is used if with problems with bowel program. May lead to fecal incontinence.

### Saline (Magnesium Citrate, Milk of Magnesia) and Hyperosmolar (Lactulose, Percutaneous Endoscopic Gastrostomy [PEG]) Laxative Agents

Stimulates colonic motility by drawing fluid into colon. PEG does not cause electrolyte abnormalities and is safe for chronic use.

### Promotility Agents (Prucalopride)

Improve colonic transit time by promoting high-amplitude propagation contractions. Prucalopride is a 5-hydoxytryptamine receptor agonist with no cardiac toxicity.

### Transanal Irrigation

Facilitates bowel evacuation by introducing water into the colon and rectum via a single-use catheter or cone. Transanal irrigation (TAI) use resulted in lower rates of stoma surgery, urinary tract infections (UTIs), fecal incontinence, and improved quality of life (QOL).[9-11]

### Alternative Methods

Anorectal biofeedback has been used in patients with incomplete SCI, MMC, and MS.[3,12] Sacral anterior root stimulation involves stimulator and lead implantation over the S2 to S4 anterior nerve roots via laminectomy, resulting in increased colonic activity, defecation frequency, and decreased constipation. Sacral nerve stimulation is less invasive, with electrode placement via sacral foramen between S2 and S4.[3]

Other surgical options include antegrade continence enema (ACE) and colostomy. ACE is more common in children with spina bifida, though it has been used in adults.[13] Colostomy is used in cases of intractable bowel complications or to divert stool from sacral wounds. Colostomy is associated with reduced bowel time, decreased fecal incontinence, decrease laxative use, and improved QOL.[14,15]

## FUNCTIONAL PROGNOSIS AND OUTCOMES

Complications of neurogenic bowel include hemorrhoids, fecal impaction, abdominal pain, rectal bleeding and prolapse, UTIs, skin breakdown, anal fissures, and AD (in SCI patients). Hospital admissions due to complications of fecal impaction, constipation, megacolon, or volvulus occur more than twice as often compared to individuals without neurologic disease. In patients with SCI, symptoms of abdominal pain and discomfort can persist even years after initial injury.[3] In a study of individuals aging with SCI over a period of 19 years, constipation worsened while fecal incontinence improved.[16] Though strategies for daily bowel management remained stable, more people increased oral laxatives or chose to have a stoma. Neurogenic bowel can have a negative impact on the QOL, social integration, and personal independence.[2,4]

## BASIC ORDER SETS

### Reflexic (Upper Motor Neuron) Bowel

Medications[1,4,17]:

Docusate 100 mg PO TID

Senna 8.6 mg/tab two tabs HS

Bisacodyl 10 mg rectal suppository daily (during bowel program)

Polyethylene gycol 17 g daily PRN constipation

Lidocaine gel 2% rectally with digital stimulation

Note that clinical bowel care guidelines recommend the use of anesthetic lubricants (e.g., 2% lidocaine) in patients with reflexic (UMN) bowels at risk for AD. However, in a recent study on the use of 2% lidocaine during *at-home* bowel care versus placebo, it was found that use of lidocaine lubricants prolonged time of bowel care, worsened AD, and increased incidence of cardiac abnormalities.[18]

Nursing:

Perform bowel program daily/every other day (same time).

Position patient in left side ying. Remove any stool in rectum. Perform digital stimulation for 15 to 20 seconds. Insert suppository in rectum. Wait 5 to 15 minutes for suppository to work. Repeat digital stimulation to ensure rectum is empty 5 to 10 minutes after stool is passed.

### Areflexic (Lower Motor Neuron) Bowel

Medications[1,4,17]:

Psyllium one packet orally BID

Docusate 100 mg daily if hard stool or no bowel movement for 2 days

PEG 3350 17 g oral once daily PRN for constipation or no bowel movement for 2 days

Nursing:

Perform bowel program daily (same time)

Position patient in left side lying or bedside commode/toilet if able to transfer. Empty bladder prior to bowel program. Perform digital evacuation of feces until rectum is empty. Digitally check after 5 to 10 minutes to ensure rectum is empty.

## RESOURCES AND REFERENCES

The full list of resources and references appears in the digital product found on http://connect .springerpub.com/content/book/978-0-8261-6226-7/part/part03/chapter/ch31

# DELIRIUM

ASHLEY M. EAVES AND AMY K. UNWIN

## CORE DEFINITION

Delirium is defined as an acute, acquired disorder of attention and cognition. It is common, costly, significantly impacts function and quality of life, and increases mortality risk for older adults. As a result, it is important to recognize, treat, and prevent delirium.[1-3]

## ETIOLOGY AND PATHOPHYSIOLOGY

The pathophysiology of delirium is not well understood. Evidence supports various pathways including chronic stress, inflammation and neurotoxicity from hypoxia, ischemia, metabolic derangements, shock, and/or sepsis. This may lead to neuronal injury and alterations in neurotransmission from anticholinergic deficiency and dopaminergic excess, as well as activation of microglia and astrocytes, apoptosis, free radical, glutamate, and nitric oxide production.[1,4,5]

The incidence of delirium during hospital admission is as high as 61% after hip fracture, with rates of 53% after general surgeries, and up to 30% in all inpatients. It is found in 60% to 80% of ICU patients who have been on mechanical ventilation and up to 50% of those in the ICU without the need for mechanical ventilation. Those on hospice services have a 29% prevalence rate, and end-of-life prevalence can be as high as 83%. Community dwellers over 85 years of age have a 14% prevalence rate, and at hospital admission or presentation to the emergency department, patients have up to 30% prevalence rates. Long-term care or post-acute care facilities see up to a 60% delirium rate. About 10% of patients screened positive for delirium at inpatient rehabilitation facility admission, and the incidence in inpatient reha-bilitation facilities (IRFs) is 10% to 16% overall. One study found that delirium was present in about 3% of stroke survivors that were admitted to an inpatient rehabilitation unit. Some studies have also shown that right brain strokes have double the risk of delirium compared to strokes in the left brain.[2,6,7]

Although there is not much data on the racial prevalence of delirium, a study at a universi-ty-affiliated, safety-net hospital found that African American race does not confer increased risk of ICU-associated delirium, and African American patients aged 18 to 49 years old de-veloped delirium in the ICU at lower rates than their Caucasian counterparts, regardless of gender.[8] However, based on information from the National Nursing Home Survey in 2004,

---

The full list of resources and references appears in the digital product found on http://connect .springerpub.com/content/book/978-0-8261-6226-7/part/part03/chapter/ch32

physical restraints including trunk restraints, bed rails, and side rails were more commonly used for black nursing home patients than whites, and therefore, clinicians should be mindful of this data when caring for delirious patients.[9]

## Significance and Functional Consequences

It was originally thought that the majority of patients with delirium fully recover regardless of treatment. However, new studies have shown that delirium is associated with impairments in long-term cognitive function and may take months or even years to resolve. Delirium has been found to be present at rates up to 41% at 12 months post-discharge, although it was unclear if this was persistent or recurrent delirium.[5,10] Patients with delirium at inpatient rehabilitation facilities had stays that were 6 days longer than patients without delirium.[11]

Prognostic implications of delirium include hospital-acquired complications such as falls and pressure wounds, longer hospital stays, higher readmission rates, and increased healthcare costs. Hospitalized patients 65 years and older with delirium are at three times increased risk of both institutionalization and functional decline.[12] Mortality rates within 1 year of delirium in hospitalized patients can be as high as 40%, especially when associated with malignancy or severe medical illness.[6]

Premorbid delirium carries a three- to sixfold risk of dementia, and coexisting delirium and dementia lead to double the rates of mortality at 12 months post discharge from a post-acute care rehabilitation facility.[4,11] However, delirium is a marker of brain vulnerability and mediates noxious injuries. Delirium may unmask preexisting dementia or lead to permanent cognitive deficits and eventual dementia. It is not clear if delirium and dementia are on the same continuum or mutually exclusive pathologies.[1,3,4,10]

## DIAGNOSTIC APPROACH

### Risks Factors and Screening

Predisposing factors are chronic conditions that increase patient vulnerability to delirium. Precipitating factors are acute events that initiate delirium. If a patient has multiple predisposing factors, they often require fewer precipitating events to cause delirium.

### Predisposing Factors

Comorbidities include alcoholism; chronic pain; terminal illness; history of baseline lung, liver, kidney, heart, or brain disease; history of stroke or transient ischemic attack (TIA), and Parkinson's disease.

Demographic factors include age >65 years old, male sex, and infants or young children with fevers.

With specific regard to geriatric patients, common predisposing conditions include dementia or preexisting cognitive impairment, depression, elder abuse, falls, history of delirium, malnutrition, polypharmacy, pressure ulcers, and functional and sensory impairments.

### Precipitating Factors

Acute insults include cardiac or cerebral ischemia, dehydration and electrolyte disturbances, high BUN:creatinine ratio, fracture, hypoxia, infection or sepsis, intoxication or withdrawal from substances, metabolic derangement, new psychoactive, sedative or hypnotic medication, prescribed or over-the-counter medications, polypharmacy, poor nutrition, severe illness, shock, major surgery or anesthesia, uncontrolled pain, prolonged time to ambulation following hip fracture, trauma or urgent hospital admission, coma, and urinary or stool retention.

Environmental exposures include ICU stay or extended hospitalization, mechanical ventilation, sleep deprivation or sleep–wake cycle disturbances, tethers such as catheters and intravenous (IVs), and physical restraints.[1,2,4,7]

## Diagnostic Criteria

There are no definitive laboratory tests, biomarkers, imaging methods, or other objective diagnostic tools to confirm the diagnosis of delirium, aside from a provider's clinical history, examination, and assessment of the patient.[2,3]

The definition of delirium based on *DSM-5* criteria includes the following:

1. Disturbance in attention (ability to direct, focus, shift, and sustain attention) and awareness (orientation to the environment).
2. Disturbance develops acutely (hours or days) and the severity fluctuates throughout the day.
3. At least one additional cognitive disturbance (memory/learning, disorientation—most commonly time and place, language, visuospatial ability, perception).
4. These disturbances are not better explained by another condition and do not occur in conjunction with severely reduced level of arousal (coma).
5. Evidence based on history, physical examination, labs, or imaging that this disturbance is a direct physiologic consequence of a medical condition, intoxication, or withdrawal of a medication side effect, substance, toxin, or multiple etiologies.[6]

Acute delirium lasts for a few hours to days, while persistent delirium can last for weeks, months, or even years. Delirium can be described as hyperactive, hypoactive, or mixed level of activity. Hypoactive and mixed delirium are often more difficult to recognize, resulting in frequent underdiagnosis. Additional descriptive features include behavioral and emotional disturbances, and changes in these features may occur more frequently at night or when other stimulation and environmental cues are absent.[1-3,6,13]

## History

It is important to determine the patient's baseline mental status and the timing of their mental status change, including events surrounding the onset of the mental status change such as medication initiation, physical symptoms, falls, or trauma. The approach to the evaluation and diagnosis of delirium is summarized in Table 32.1. A thorough medication history is crucial, including scheduled and as-needed prescriptions, over-the-counter medications, supplement substances not prescribed, and details about dosages and administration times. The prescription drugs commonly associated with delirium are summarized in Table 32.2. Inquiring about sensory deprivation and performing a pain assessment is also helpful. Much of the history will likely need to be supplemented from family members, friends, caregivers, and those familiar with the patient, and a chart review is likely helpful if the patient has been

**TABLE 32.1 APPROACH TO THE EVALUATION AND DIAGNOSIS OF DELIRIUM[1,3]**

| 1 | Define baseline mental status |
|---|---|
| 2 | Evaluate current mental status and cognition |
| 3 | Perform careful physical and neurologic examination |
| 4 | Assess delirium risk with validated instrument for delirium/another condition that may present similarly (acute psychosis, dementia, depression, mania) |
| 5 | Institute delirium prevention and treatment measures, starting with nonpharmacologic strategies |
| 6 | Identify and treat underlying precipitating factors for delirium |
| 7 | Measure delirium severity for changes and response to interventions |

**TABLE 32.2 COMMON MEDICATIONS ASSOCIATED WITH DELIRIUM[2,6,7]**

| CLASS | EXAMPLES |
|---|---|
| Anticholinergic | Tricyclic antidepressants—amitriptyline, doxepin, imipramine |
| Antiemetics | Promethazine |
| Anticonvulsants | Primidone, phenobarbital, phenytoin |
| Antihistamines | Cyproheptadine, diphenhydramine, hydroxyzine, H2-receptor antagonists (cimetidine, ranitidine) |
| Antimuscarinics | Oxybutynin, tolterodine |
| Antiparkinsonian | Levodopa, benztropine, trihexyphenidyl |
| Antispasmodics | Scopolamine |
| Antiarrhythmics | Disopyramide, quinidine |
| Barbiturates | Lorazepam, midazolam |
| Benzodiazepines | Long acting > short acting |
| Corticosteroids | Prednisone |
| Dihydropyridines | Nifedipine |
| Dopamine agonists | Bromocriptine |
| Hypnotics | Zolpidem |
| Opioids | Meperidine |
| Skeletal muscle relaxants | Cyclobenzaprine, tizanidine |

previously hospitalized. Past medical history can help give insight into predisposing factors, including mental health conditions. Details about substance use, changes in employment, stressful life events, and family history are all useful as well.[2,3]

## Physical Examination

This should include vital signs, a general medical examination, including heart, lungs, and abdomen. Perform a neurologic examination for any focal neurologic deficits, and a cognitive and mental status examination, focusing on testing for attention if unable to complete the entire examination. Conduct a skin check for bruises, wounds, abscesses, and/or evidence of intravenous (IV) drug use.

## Screening Tests

Another important tool for diagnosing delirium in a quick, clinical context is the Confusion Assessment Method (CAM).[14] Delirium diagnosis via the CAM is based on four cardinal features:

1. Acute mental status changes with fluctuating course
2. Inattention
3. Disorganized thinking
4. Altered level of consciousness

A positive diagnosis via the CAM assessment requires features 1 or 2, plus features 3 or 4, to be present.[14] The CAM continues to be one of the most widely used assessment tools in the world and takes 5 minutes on average to administer. The CAM has demonstrated high sensitivity (94%), high specificity (93%), and good interrater reliability.

## Laboratory Studies, Imaging, and Procedures

Table 32.3 summarizes the potential laboratory studies and tests to be ordered to elucidate the underlying cause of delirium.

**TABLE 32.3 LABORATORY STUDIES AND TESTS TO EVALUATE FOR UNDERLYING CAUSE OF DELIRIUM[2,3,7]**

| LABS AND TEST ORDERS | POSSIBLE ETIOLOGY TO EVALUATE |
| --- | --- |
| CBC W/ DIFF<br>BLOOD CULTURES, ESR, CRP<br>LACTIC ACID | Severe anemia/rapid blood loss<br>Infection—sepsis, wounds, HIV, syphilis |
| DUPLEX U/S<br>CT-PE PROTOCOL | Thrombus or embolus |
| SERUM ELECTROLYTES<br>MAGNESIUM, PHOSPHORUS | Electrolyte disorders (i.e., hyper- and hyponatremia)<br>Acidosis, alkalosis<br>Urine-specific gravity, serum osmoles |
| BUN, CREATININE | Dehydration<br>Renal failure<br>Uremic encephalopathy |

*(continued)*

**TABLE 32.3 LABORATORY STUDIES AND TESTS TO EVALUATE FOR UNDERLYING CAUSE OF DELIRIUM[2,3,7] (*continued*)**

| LABS AND TEST ORDERS | POSSIBLE ETIOLOGY TO EVALUATE |
|---|---|
| GLUCOSE | Hypoglycemia<br>Severe hyperglycemia, DKA<br>Hyperosmolar state, HHNS |
| ALBUMIN, PREALBUMIN | Malnutrition, social isolation |
| LIPASE, AMYLASE, TAGS | Pancreatitis |
| LFTS, INR, AMMONIA | Liver failure w/ hepatic encephalopathy |
| UA, CULTURE<br>BLADDER ULTRASOUND | Urinary tract infection<br>Urinary retention |
| ABDOMINAL X-RAY | Renal stones<br>Constipation |
| PELVIC ULTRASOUND OR CT ABD/PELVIS | Gynecologic or obstetric issues |
| CXR, O₂ SATS<br>SPUTUM CULTURES/TRACHEAL ASPIRATES | Pneumonia<br>Congestive heart failure<br>Hemoglobin variants |
| ECG, TROPONIN<br>VITALS—BP, HR | Myocardial infarction<br>Arrhythmia<br>End-organ damage due to hypertension |
| ABG | Hypercarbia in chronic obstructive pulmonary disease |
| DRUG/TOXIN LEVELS | Medication side effect or toxicity<br>(may happen at "normal" serum levels, change with renal function, etc.) |
| BLOOD/URINE TOXICOLOGY SCREEN | Ingestion (more common in younger patients)<br>Recreational drugs and alcohol intoxication or withdrawal<br>(EtOH, barbiturates, sedative hypnotics)<br>Heavy metals—lead, manganese, mercury |
| CEREBRAL IMAGING—CT, MRI<br>PT, PTT, INR | Stroke or hemorrhage<br>Brain mass, metastasis with a known cancer history<br>Sequelae of TBI, HIE, such as DAI<br>Herniation<br>Abscess<br>Hydrocephalus<br>Subdural hematoma<br>Vasculitis |
| LUMBAR PUNCTURE WITH CSF ANALYSIS (S/P NEUROIMAGING) | Meningitis<br>Increased intracranial pressure<br>Encephalitis<br>Syphilis |
| EEG | Seizure or postictal state |

(*continued*)

**TABLE 32.3 LABORATORY STUDIES AND TESTS TO EVALUATE FOR UNDERLYING CAUSE OF DELIRIUM[2,3,7] (continued)**

| LABS AND TEST ORDERS | POSSIBLE ETIOLOGY TO EVALUATE |
|---|---|
| TSH, FREE T4<br>ACTH, CORTISOL STIM<br>PTH, CA | Hypo/hyperthyroidism, myxedema<br>Hyper/hypoadrenocorticism<br>Hyperparathyroidism |
| VITALS—TEMPERATURE<br>CK | Hypo- or hypothermia—environmental<br>Neuroleptic malignant syndrome<br>Serotonin syndrome |
| VITAMIN LEVELS | Vitamin B12/nitrous oxide<br>Folic acid<br>Niacin<br>Thiamine<br>Vitamin D<br>Zinc |

ABD, abdominal; ABG, arterial blood gas; ACTH, adenocorticotropic hormone; BP, blood pressure; BUN, blood urea nitrogen; CA, calcium; CBC, complete blood count; CK, creatine kinase; CRP, C-reactive protein; CSF, cerebrospinal fluid; CXR, chest x-ray; DAI, diffuse axonal injury; DKA, diabetic ketoacidosis; ESR, erythrocyte sedimentation rate; EtOH, ethyl alcohol; HHNS, hyperglycemic hyperosmolar nonketotic syndrome; HIE, hypoxic ischemic encephalopathy; HR, heart rate; INR, international normalized ratio; LFTs, liver function tests; PT, prothrombin time; PTH, parathyroid hormone; PTT, partial thromboplastin time; TAGS, triglycerides; TBI, traumatic brain injury; TSH, thyroid stimulating hormone; UA, urinalysis.

## Differential Diagnosis

Dementia, depression, and psychosis may commonly mimic delirium. Table 32.4 contrasts the features of delirium, dementia, and depression. Agitation, delusions, hallucinations, and language disturbances associated with delirium may be confused for bipolar or depressive disorders with psychotic features, brief psychotic disorder, schizophrenia, or schizophreniform disorder. Delirium also has some overlapping features of posttraumatic amnesia (PTA) following a traumatic brain injury (TBI). There are also stroke syndromes that may mimic delirium.

**TABLE 32.4 FEATURES OF DELIRIUM COMPARED TO ALTERNATIVE DIAGNOSES[1,3,4,6]**

| | DELIRIUM | DEMENTIA | DEPRESSION |
|---|---|---|---|
| Acute onset | +<br>(hours–days) | −<br>(months–years) | +/− |
| Inattention | + | −/+ if severe dementia | +/− |
| Altered consciousness | + (fluctuates) | −/+ if severe dementia | − |
| Disorganized thinking | + | +/− | + |
| Altered psychomotor activity | + | +/− | +/− |
| Duration | Days–years | Months–years | Days–years |

Atypical presentation may be due to malingering or factitious disorder, if all other etiologies are ruled out. It can be difficult to distinguish between delirium, dementia, delirium superimposed on dementia, and another preexisting neurocognitive disorder (NCD) such as Alzheimer's disease. Altered level of consciousness and acute onset are more unique to delirium and less common with NCDs. If in doubt, it is best to manage the patient for delirium initially.

## TREATMENT

Treatment of delirium should aim to correct the underlying disease and remove precipitating factors when possible (e.g., medications).

In non-ICU hospitalized patients 65 years and older, implementing nonpharmacologic prevention and intervention strategies has been shown to be cost effective, reduces the risk of delirium in the hospital by 53%, shortens length of stay, and reduces the risk of falls by 62% (Box 32.1).[2,3,7,15]

### Pharmacologic Management for the Agitated Patient

There is minimal evidence that pharmacologic therapy for delirium is beneficial to patients and should be reserved for when there are safety risks to the patient or healthcare workers. Pharmacotherapy with antipsychotics and benzodiazepines has not been associated with improved outcomes.[3,16] It should be noted that minimal studies evaluated functional outcomes; the populations studied were homogenous, and very few studies taking place in rehabilitation units and nursing home settings have been included in systematic reviews or meta-analyses.[16] There is modest evidence for the association of pharmacotherapy with increased rates of institutionalization, higher delirium symptoms scores, and worse survival.[3]

---

**BOX 32.1**

**NONPHARMACOLOGIC INTERVENTIONS FOR THE MANAGEMENT OF DELIRIUM**

1. Implement good sleep hygiene
2. Minimize physical restraints
3. Mobilize early – ambulation, range of motion, therapy involvement, make assistive devices available
4. Re-orient and familiarize the patient with calendars, clocks, phone, lighting, and minimize room changes
5. Make introductions, explain your role, facilitate visits by family and friends, provide consistent staff/caregivers
6. Offer cognitively stimulating activities for the patient
7. Minimize tubes, lines, drains, catheterization
8. Optimize sensory input: glasses, hearing aids, dentures, impacted ear wax
9. Encourage PO intake for maintenance of fluids, nutrition, and ensure adequate oxygen
10. Make call light available
11. Ensure healthcare providers are educated in delirium management

**TABLE 32.5 MEDICATIONS THAT MAY BE USED FOR AGITATION ASSOCIATED WITH DELIRIUM[1-3,17]**

| MEDICATION | DOSE | BENEFITS | SIDE EFFECTS |
|---|---|---|---|
| Haloperidol | 0.25, 0.5, or 1 mg PO q4h; may repeat Q20–30 minutes if needed for agitation, do not exceed 3–5 mg/day | -Nonsedating<br>-Few hemodynamic effects | -EPS, increased with >3 mg/day<br>-Torsades de pointes increased with IV form, so use in monitored settings only<br>-Worse cognitive recovery after TBI |
| Lorazepam | Three times a day as needed | -For sedative and EtOH withdrawal, neuroleptic malignant syndrome history | -Paradoxic excitation—more respiratory depression than haloperidol |
| Olanzapine | 2.5, 5, or 10 mg PO, IV, or IM daily as needed | -Fewer EPS than Haldol | -More sedating than haloperidol |
| Quetiapine | 12.5, 25, or 50 mg PO BID as needed. | -Fewer EPS than haloperidol | -Most sedating atypical antipsychotic<br>-Hypotension |
| Risperidone | 0.25–1 mg PO or IV q4–12h as needed | -Nonsedating<br>-Few hemodynamic effects | -Slightly fewer EPS than haloperidol |

EPS, extrapyramidal side effects; EtOH, ethyl alcohol; IM, intramuscular; IV, intravenous; TBI, traumatic brain injury.

Providers should start with the lowest possible dose of medication, utilize the lowest effective dose for the shortest duration possible (typically <2 days), and then taper as possible (Table 32.5). Haloperidol is often considered first line due to fewer hemodynamic effects and less sedation compared to other agents. However, haloperidol impairs cognitive recovery in TBI, so it should be used with caution, or providers may consider an alternative agent such as quetiapine or risperidone instead. Benzodiazepines should be avoided unless specifically used for alcohol or benzodiazepine withdrawal. Clinicians should avoid using drugs to treat hypoactive delirium.

## RESOURCES AND REFERENCES

The full list of resources and references appears in the digital product found on http://connect.springerpub.com/content/book/978-0-8261-6226-7/part/part03/chapter/ch32

# DEPRESSION

DAVID ROTHMAN, AMY STAROSTA, AND JESSE FANN

## CORE DEFINITIONS

According to the *Diagnostic and Statistical Manual for Psychiatric Disorders (DSM-5)*[1] depression is the "presence of sad, empty, or irritable mood accompanied by somatic and cognitive concerns that significantly affect an individual's capacity to function."[1] In order to meet criteria for a major depressive disorder (MDD), an individual must experience five of the following nine symptoms for more than half of the days over a 2-week period:

- Depressed mood (sad, empty, hopeless)*
- Decreased interest or pleasure in activities*
- Five percent weight loss or gain without intent
- Insomnia/hypersomnia
- Increased/decreased motor agitation (as noted by others)
- Fatigue or loss of energy
- Feelings of worthlessness or guilt out of proportion to the situation
- Decreased concentration or decisiveness
- Thoughts of death or suicidal ideation
    - ❏ Cause significant impairment in functioning (social, occupational, other domains)
    - ❏ Not due to substance use disorder (SUD) or medical condition
    - ❏ Not better explained by other depressive disorder and no presence of mania

The cardinal features of MDD (*) are depressed mood and decreased interest or pleasure in activities. The presence of one of these symptoms is required for diagnosis.

## ETIOLOGY AND PATHOPHYSIOLOGY

Depression is common in rehabilitation populations. Patients with traumatic brain injury (TBI),[2] spinal cord injury (SCI),[3] and stroke[4] all present with increased rates of depressed mood. While depression may be more common among rehabilitation populations, it is by no means ubiquitous. Among those patients who reported clinical levels of depressed mood at one time point, three major trajectories were identified: persistent, recovery, and delayed.[2] Similar patterns are also noted among individuals with SCI[3] and individuals involved in traumatic events, independent of diagnosis.[5] In chronic conditions (i.e., multiple

---

The full list of resources and references appears in the digital product found on http://connect.springerpub.com/content/book/978-0-8261-6226-7/part/part03/chapter/ch33

sclerosis [MS]), there is less variability, with a tendency for individuals to remain consistent in their reports of depression, across three trajectories: low (subclinical: 63.8%), moderate (above clinical threshold: 26.2%), and high (10%). Therefore, among individuals in PM&R populations, depression is a common occurrence, and many individuals experience clinical levels of distress over time.

## DIAGNOSTIC APPROACH

### Screening

Given that depression is present at higher rates in PM&R populations and may develop at different time points during the rehabilitation process, it is critical to conduct repeated assessment of individuals over time. Common "red flags" or indications that depression assessment is needed include decreased hygiene, low social participation, decreased participation in care, and expression of a belief/feeling that they feel hopeless or helpless. In addition to clinical interview, there are multiple measures to assess symptoms of depression used across the literature. These tools can be used in response to concerning symptoms or as broad screeners.

One of the most widely used and validated measures in healthcare settings to assess for depression is the Patient Health Questionnaire 9 (PHQ-9).[6] There is strong support for the PHQ-9's use as a screening tool across multiple populations, including rehabilitation. Furthermore, the PHQ-9 has the benefit of serving as an initial screening tool for suicidal ideation via item 9. The use of a PHQ-9 cutoff of 10 provides an acceptable balance of sensitivity and specificity for depression.[7] Additionally, the PHQ-9 is sensitive to change in symptoms and can be used repeatedly to measure clinically significant change based on an increase or decrease of five points.

The second measure often used across a variety of studies and clinical settings is the Hospital Anxiety and Depression Scale (HADS).[8] This measure assesses both anxiety and depression across hospitalized patients. Unlike the PHQ-9, the HADS does not include the somatic symptoms associated with depression and instead is focused on the anhedonia symptoms associated with depression. The HADS focuses on the past week, allowing for more frequent assessment and measurement of change and has demonstrated stability across multiple assessments.[9] One theorized strength of the HADS is that by removing the somatic symptoms, the interference of physical health conditions will be limited; however, there does not seem to be strong support for this concept in research and practice. Thus, when selecting between the PHQ-9 and the HADS, factors including time (e.g., 1 week) and combined assessment of anxiety and depression simultaneously may be useful in selection. Furthermore, assessment of suicidal ideation is not contained on the HADS.

When working with older populations, providers may consider using the Geriatric Depression Scale (GDS).[10] Unlike other measures noted earlier, which use a severity scale (i.e., 0–3, with higher scores connoting increased severity), the GDS focuses on a Yes/No format for responses. For the purposes of the current screening measures, the GDS-15 is the most common and well-supported version of the GDS.[10]

## Clinical Presentation

Patients in rehabilitation settings will likely experience a range of reactions throughout their life. Primary factors to consider in determining appropriate diagnosis to consider are: (a) Is the distress excessive? (b) Where does the depressed mood result from? and (c) time since the stressor (see Table 33.1).

It is important to note that not all sadness is MDD. From a diagnostic perspective in order to meet criteria for MDD, symptoms must interfere with daily functioning or be out of proportion to what would be expected based on the circumstances. Many people may experience normative, proportionate sadness that does not significantly impact their daily functioning.

Some patients may experience mood concerns following a traumatic event, possibly related to their injury. While it is important to consider acute/posttraumatic stress (see Chapter 46), for patients who experience depressed mood following a trauma, a more appropriate diagnosis may be adjustment disorder with depressed mood. In order to meet criteria for adjustment disorder with depressed mood, the following criterion must be met:

- Symptoms of depression begin within 3 months of the stressor.
- Symptoms of depression relate directly to the stressor.
- Reaction must be out of proportion to the stresses and cause direct impact to normal functioning.

Patients experiencing adjustment disorder with depressed mood may present with many of the same symptoms as MDD; however, symptoms directly relate back to the stressor. People are resilient and often symptoms related to adjustment disorder decrease over time.

### Depression and Aphasia

One common experience for providers working in rehabilitation settings is assessing patients who are unable to or have limited ability to communicate. As most depression assessments rely on patients' ability to report their symptoms, it can be challenging to evaluate depression in patients with communication impairments. However, it is critical to assess depression among those with communication difficulties as this subgroup experiences higher rates of depression and lower rates of treatment. The Stroke Aphasic Depression Questionnaire[11] is a

## TABLE 33.1 COMPARISON OF FACTORS IMPLICATED IN ADJUSTMENT TO INJURY

| FACTOR | NORMAL ADJUSTMENT | ADJUSTMENT DISORDER WITH DEPRESSED MOOD | MAJOR DEPRESSIVE DISORDER |
|---|---|---|---|
| Distress | Low/med/high | Med/high | Med/high |
| Stressor | Related to injury | Related to injury | Multiple factors including injury and external factors |
| Time | Immediate | 1 month post to 6 months following an acute stressor (longer if stressor is ongoing) | Period of 6 months with clinically significant distress following event |

measure developed to evaluate individuals with aphasia who may be experiencing depressed mood. This measure focuses on behavioral ratings of individuals rather than relying on self-report and can be found online.

## Safety Concerns

In addition to increased rates of depression, there is an elevated risk of suicide attempts and death by suicide for patients with TBI,[12] SCI,[13] and stroke. Furthermore, chronic pain, a common symptom among PM&R populations, has been found to be associated with increased suicidal ideation and attempts. Many patients struggling with suicidal ideation and depression do not have access to appropriate mental healthcare, and medical providers are often the last point of contact for patients before a suicide attempt. Some providers have expressed concerns that discussing suicide with distressed patients may induce suicidal thoughts; however, there is no evidence to suggest that asking about suicide increases distress or suicidal ideation. Instead, reviews of the existing literature suggest that acknowledging and talking about suicide may actually reduce distress and suicidal ideation.[14] Therefore, it is crucial that all providers who screen for depression also ask patients about thoughts of suicide.

Providers should ask patient in a direct, nonjudgmental manner, using language such as "Are you thinking of killing yourself?" "Are you thinking of suicide?" or "Have you had thoughts about taking your own life?" For patients endorsing suicidal thoughts, intent, or plan, mental health provider should be consulted for further assessment and management. There are excellent resources available for clinics that would like to develop more systematic approaches to assessing and managing suicide risk for their patients, such as the Suicide Prevention Toolkit for Primary Care Practices. This resource is included online.

## TREATMENT

### Psychotherapeutic Interventions

The primary psychotherapeutic approaches at this time include (a) Cognitive behavioral therapy for depression, (b) mindfulness-based techniques, and (c) acceptance and commitment therapy for depression. All three interventions can be implemented in both inpatient and outpatient settings and have been found to be effective in reducing symptoms of depression, even when implemented in brief formats.[15]

*Cognitive behavioral therapy:* Focuses on identifying maladaptive cognitions (i.e., I cannot live with my injury). Providers work with the patient to identify logical challenges and modify maladaptive cognitions, decrease emotional reaction to maladaptive cognitions, and focus on increased behavioral activation and participation in pleasurable activities.

*Mindfulness-based techniques:* Focuses on increasing an individual's present attention versus past negative thoughts or future worries. It seeks to help individuals enjoy current abilities and focus on present capabilities while working to decrease suffering. Techniques often include meditation or visual imagery.

*Acceptance and commitment therapy:* Helps patients increase their acceptance of their current situation via mindfulness-based techniques. Providers work with patients to increase their focus on personal values while focusing on increasing participation in valued activities and continued work on acceptance of the distress that may result in new challenges.

## Pharmacological Interventions

Selective serotonin reuptake inhibitors (SSRIs, such as citalopram or sertraline) or serotonin norepinephrine reuptake inhibitor (SNRI, such as venlafaxine extended release or duloxetine) is usually the first-line antidepressant for patients in the PM&R setting due to favorable side-effect profiles.[16–18] In rehabilitation populations, these agents should be started at about half of their usual starting dose and titrated slowly. Dosages should be titrated to normal therapeutic doses when tolerated. SNRIs have the added potential benefit of decreasing neuropathic pain. Serotonin-induced restlessness sometimes can be mistaken for TBI-related agitation. In some patients with acquired brain injury, serotonergic agents may produce or exacerbate apathy, which can be mistaken for increased depression. SSRI use has been associated with an increased risk of hemorrhagic complications and increased risk of falls in the elderly, so caution is warranted when considering their use in this population.

Bupropion may help with fatigue but is associated with an increased risk of seizures, a particular concern following severe TBI or stroke. Mirtazapine may be considered in patients with comorbid anxiety, insomnia, or anorexia. While studies using tricyclic antidepressants (TCAs) have suggested efficacy, potential for side effects such as sedation and orthostatic hypotension limits their safety in vulnerable populations. Among TCAs, nortriptyline or desipramine may cause the fewest side effects and may also be helpful for neuropathic pain. Because of the potentially problematic properties of monoamine oxidase inhibitors (MAOIs), they should be used with extreme caution if at all.

Methylphenidate, a psychostimulant, has antidepressant effects and may concurrently enhance arousal, cognitive processing speed, fatigue, and participation in rehabilitation.[19] Long-term use is not recommended due to potential for misuse. Ketamine and newer antidepressants such as vilazodone, levomilnacipran, and vortioxetine have not yet been systematically studied in rehabilitation patients with depression.

## FUNCTIONAL PROGNOSIS AND OUTCOMES

Among individuals enrolled in inpatient rehabilitation programs, multiple studies have highlighted worse outcomes for patients experiencing depression than those without depression both while hospitalized and post discharge.[20] These findings include multiple outcome variables, including poorer scores on functional independence measures, increased length of stay, lower self-reported quality of life, and reduced social participation. Moreover, there seems to be a bidirectional relationship between these variables, such that depression predicts poorer physical outcomes, and worse physical outcomes are associated with increased depression; therefore, early intervention for the management of depression is likely to improve outcomes across multiple domains.[20]

## RESOURCES AND REFERENCES

The full list of resources and references appears in the digital product found on http://connect
.springerpub.com/content/book/978-0-8261-6226-7/part/part03/chapter/ch33

# DERMATOLOGIC RASHES OF REHABILITATION

EVAN SWEREN, RONALD J. SWEREN, JENNIFER M. ZUMSTEG, AND LUIS GARZA

## ACTINIC KERATOSIS

### Core Definitions

Actinic keratosis (AK) is an atypical keratinocyte proliferation secondary to photodamage, occurring in areas subjected to prolonged sun exposure, such as the face, neck, and arms. Prevalence increases with age. Individuals with lighter skin colors (Fitzpatrick types I and II) are more at risk. A small percentage of AKs may progress to squamous cell carcinoma (SCC), which can become invasive. AKs are considered "premalignant" and require treatment, especially in immunocompromised individuals.[1,2]

### Etiology and Pathophysiology

Chronic sun exposure (work and leisure) and tanning (outdoor and tanning bed use) are the primary causative agents. UVB (285–315 nm) and UVA (315–400 nm) penetrate the epidermis and dermis, respectively, damaging DNA, initiating inflammatory and free radical cascades, and deregulating skin tissue homeostasis.

### Diagnostic Approach

AKs present as scaly, keratotic, erythematous, tan/gray plaques or papules on the scalp, ears, face, lips (actinic cheilitis), trunk, back, and extremities. They are often small (<5 mm), asymptomatic, and appear in multiples, though larger (1–2 cm) AKs also occur. Most commonly, complaints include itching or ill-defined prickling in the affected area, and bleeding may result from scratching or frictional irritation, though not in great quantities. Larger ones may be confused with SCC, requiring a biopsy to differentiate.

### Treatment

Numerous treatment options exist, including monitoring very small pinpoint lesions. The most common treatments include cryosurgery with liquid nitrogen and 5 fluorouracil, a form of topical chemotherapy. Other treatments include photodynamic therapy (PDT), laser, topical imiquimod, an immune modulator, and ingenol.

---

The full list of references appears in the digital product found on http://connect.springerpub.com/content/book/978-0-8261-6226-7/part/part03/chapter/ch34

## Functional Prognosis and Outcomes

If recognized and properly monitored and/or treated, the prognosis is often extremely good. It is not uncommon, however, for individuals to continue developing AKs over time, requiring regular intervention.

## DERMATOPHYTE INFECTION

### Core Definitions

Dermatophyte infections affect the skin, hair, and nails and are very common. They are caused by fungus, most often Trichophyton and Microsporum genera, and pose the greatest concern to immunocompromised individuals, where infections can become severe. They are often recalcitrant or recurrent and can cause minor to severe annoyance. Colloquially, the names of dermatophyte infections arise from their appearance or site of manifestation, even for infections caused by different organisms at the same anatomical site. The most common examples include the following: tinea corporis ("ringworm"), tinea pedis ("athlete's foot"), tinea cruris ("jock itch"), tinea capitis ("scalp ringworm"), tinea unguium ("nail fungus"), and tinea incognito.[3]

### Etiology and Pathophysiology

Fungi constitute a component of the human commensal microbiota and the lived environment. Nearly all fungi are nonpathogenic to humans; however, both commensal and environmental pathogenic fungi can lead to infection due to internal or external factors, such as occlusion or moisture retention. Dermatophyte infections seldom involve the epidermis, mostly residing on and within the stratum corneum.

### Diagnostic Approach

Dermatophyte infection presentation is varied. Tinea corporis is an annular lesion, which may be circular, oval, or polycyclic, involving the trunk or extremities and sparing keratinized areas. The border is usually raised and scaly. Tinea pedis is a fungal infection of the foot with scaling or flaking on the soles and between the toes. Symptoms are often mild, and prevalence increases with age. A moccasin distribution may exist with involvement on the medial and lateral aspects of the foot. Interdigital manifestations may be malodorous and weepy. Tinea cruris is another scaly presentation in the groin extending to the medial thighs or buttocks. Diagnosis is based on pronounced pruritus, erythema, and demarcation, sometimes with central clearing. Tinea capitis is a fungal infection of the scalp, more common in children, presenting with scaling and hair loss to the localized area/s. *Trichophyton tonsurans* is the most common, causing black dots on the scalp constituting broken hair shaft fragments (*T. tonsurans* in an endotrix); interestingly, familial adults may serve as asymptomatic carriers, complicating treatment efforts. Tinea unguium or onychomycosis is a dermatophyte infection of the nail, which may become thickened or yellowish in hue. While tolerable if left unresolved for extended durations, pain and secondary infection may result if left unresolved. Lastly, tinea incognito or Majocchi's granuloma is less common and may present as an ill-defined patch or plaque often due to the use of topical steroids.

Diagnosis is usually made clinically based on the previously mentioned symptoms and anatomical sites but often confirmed by dissolving skin scrapings, hair, or nail in potassium hydroxide (KOH) and examining with a microscope looking for hyphae. Of note, however, depending on the severity of symptoms, scrapings may yield a paucity of fungal isolates. For hair, looking for fungal spores within the hair shaft (endothrix) or on the surface of the hair shaft (ectothrix) under magnification with a microscope is a superior diagnostic approach. If index of suspicion is high and KOH is negative, a fungal culture can be obtained.

## Treatment

Skin can usually be treated with topical antifungals, of which there are both over-the-counter (OTC) and prescription options. Oral antifungals include terbinafine, fluconazole, itraconazole, and occasionally griseofulvin in children.

## Functional Prognosis and Outcomes

In otherwise healthy individuals, dermatophyte infections often resolve with appropriate treatment, though some may become more challenging to resolve, depending on patient age, compliance, fungal type, living conditions (e.g., group living), and immunocompetence.

## CONTACT DERMATITIS

### Core Definitions

Contact dermatitis is a direct contact reaction to a chemical or substance in the environment. Skin eruptions are often pruritic and occur in individuals of all ages. Reactions are classified as irritant contact dermatitis (ICD) when the substance is an irritant and allergic contact dermatitis (ACD) when the substance is an allergen.[4]

### Etiology and Pathophysiology

Whereas ICD reactions are characterized by innate immune activation as a result of direct tissue injury and skin barrier disruption, ACD reactions are Type IV reactions, also known as delayed hypersensitivity reactions; both involve immune activation and even education. Accordingly, quantity, duration, and other intrinsic immune conditions or factors can influence the likelihood of contact dermatitis reactions, including genetic predispositions.

### Diagnostic Approach

Diagnosis is often made clinically based on both the site of reaction and patient's recent behavioral history with potential irritants. The rash often presents in a pattern that reflects the area of contact with the causative agent. Classically, ACD presents with erythematous edematous papules and vesicles, often coalescing in a band or linear pattern (streaks). The most well-known ACD is poison ivy, oak, or sumac, all caused by the oily plant resin, urushiol (plants in the genus *Toxicodendron*). For patients experiencing prolonged hospital stays, laundering products and adhesives may also provoke reactions. At times, a skin biopsy is necessary to help confirm the diagnosis when the eruption is atypical in appearance, and patch testing may be useful when the causative agent is unknown. Typical chemical irritants include cosmetics, detergents (soaps), solvents, preservatives (formaldehyde), disinfectants, antiseptics, dusts, pollens, and dander. Long-term repeated friction cause by scratchy clothing, such as wool, may also elicit a reaction as can fine irritants such as sawdust and fiberglass. Of note, the list of potential irritants is extensive. Symptoms include pruritus, pain, and burning.

### Treatment

The mainstay treatment is topical corticosteroids (TCSs) or a tapering course of oral steroids, most commonly prednisone, over a 2- to 3-week duration, depending on the severity of the rash. Antihistamines may also provide relief from pruritus, though side effects from oral treatments may interfere with functional and cognitive ability, temporarily.

### Functional Prognosis and Outcomes

If the causative agent is identified and properly treated, prognosis is good. However, in individuals with underlying atopy, absolute resolution of symptoms may be challenging.

## ATOPIC DERMATITIS

### Core Definitions

Atopic dermatitis (AD or eczema) is a chronic inflammatory skin condition that is very common, involving pruritic, ill-defined, erythematous scaly patches or plaques. Flares may be recurrent and seasonal, worsening in dry weather and decreased natural sunlight. AD can present in individuals of all ages, though peak incidence occurs in early childhood. Allergic rhinitis (asthma) and seasonal allergies are commonly found in individuals with AD, too. Symptoms can be mild to severe, interrupting sleep and qualities of living (QOL).[5]

### Etiology and Pathophysiology

Numerous hereditary, environmental, and biologic factors have been implicated in AD's etiology. These include skin microbiota dysbiosis, maternal allergic history, and skin structural protein (filaggrin) mutations or deficiencies, among others. Collectively, these pathologies result in a disruption of the epidermal barrier function and chronic immune cell infiltration.

### Diagnostic Approach

Diagnosis is often made clinically based on family history, symptoms, and exclusion of more serious skin conditions. Lesions are erythematous, xerotic, scaly, and pruritic, and excoriation may provoke oozing, crusting, and even bleeding. In individuals with darker skin (Fitzpatrick Types V and VI), hyperpigmentation with or without lichenification and striation may also be apparent. While AD shows no anatomical preference and can appear broadly, commonly affected areas include hands, elbows, antecubital fossae, popliteal fossae, and other flexor surfaces.

## Treatment

Nonaqueous moisturizers (emollients), such as petroleum jelly, routinely applied after bathing are the preferred and most effective treatments to improve skin barrier function. In fact, bathing alone with or without bleach has been shown to help. Additionally, TCSs, such as clobetasol are highly effective at controlling flares, when used in short-term higher doses, and others, such as triamcinolone, are highly effective in preventing the recurrence of flares, when used in longer-term maintenance doses, though still with regular holidays to avoid tachyphylaxis and side effects of skin thinning, striae, and telangiectasias, among others. TSCs work by reducing the body's inflammatory response. Rarely, phototherapy is appropriate.

## Functional Prognosis and Outcomes

Long-term prognosis is usually good, however, the high burden on patient compliance to control AD often results in poorer long-term outcomes. Similarly, before appropriate treatment regimens are identified, symptoms can be physically and emotionally burdensome, even disrupting sleep cycles and creating positive feedback loops of stress leading to flares. Uncontrolled AD is especially problematic in children and adolescents, even leading to increases in school absences.

## HIDRADENITIS SUPPURATIVA

### Core Definitions

Hidradenitis suppurativa (HS) is a chronic inflammatory disease of the hair follicle showing female preference (3:1) with hereditary predispositions causing painful lesions, sinus tracts, abscesses, nodules, and cysts in the axillary, inguinal, and anogenital regions. Episodes are recurrent, and onset occurs around puberty, sometimes abating later in life.[6]

### Etiology and Pathophysiology

While further research is needed to fully define the pathophysiology of HS, histological findings demonstrate lymphocyte and neutrophil infiltration and hair follicle and apocrine gland destruction. Aberrant healing results in scarring and abnormal skin tissue restructuring.

### Diagnostic Approach

Diagnosis is made clinically based on symptoms, including draining and nondraining sinus tracts, lesions, abscesses, and double-headed comedones in axillary, inguinal, and anogenital areas. Scarring is also commonly found at these sites, with or without hyperpigmentation, especially in darker individuals (Fitzpatrick Skin Types V and VI). Rarely, secondary bacterial infections may occur, though these may be serious. Misdiagnoses include common boils, folliculitis, cystic acne, and even sexually transmitted diseases, when in the anogenital region.

### Treatment

Treatment is dependent on Hurley's staging of disease (I–III). Stage I disease is defined by single or multiple abscesses, barring sinus tracts or scarring, while stage II involves multiple abscesses with sinus tracts and scarring with normal skin between lesions. For stage I and

II diseases, topical treatments are most appropriate. These include local antimicrobial wash (e.g., Hibiclens), pyrithione zinc shampoo, topical antibiotics (clindamycin), and/or oral antibiotics (including doxycycline, trimethoprim-sulfamethoxazole DS, and rifampin with clindamycin and moxifloxacin). The tumor necrosis factor (TNF) inhibitor adalimumab (Humira) is also FDA approved for stage II or even III disease. Infliximab (Remicade), another TNF inhibitor, has been shown to be of benefit, as well. For stage III disease, which involves more diffuse, chronically recurrent, and debilitating HS, intralesional steroids and surgical intervention are appropriate, including both limited incision and drainage (I&D) and excision of sinus tracts. In severe instances of HS involving the perianal/perineal area, surgical excision and colostomy may be advised. The most effective surgical remedy, in this regard, is to remove the skin covering the entire affected region.

### Functional Prognosis and Outcomes

Functional prognosis is good to poor, depending on a range of factors including patient risk mitigation, patient compliance, and natural disease history. Given anatomical sites affected, mood, sexual function, and other QOLs may be negatively affected.

## SEBORRHEIC DERMATITIS

### Core Definitions

Seborrheic dermatitis (SD/"seb derm") is a common skin condition involving sebum-producing skin via sebaceous glands on the scalp, face, axillae, inframammary trunk, and intercrural folds. Incidence is more prevalent in men and may occur seasonally, with dry winter weather exacerbating symptoms. Presentation occurs as cradle cap in newborns, resolving by 6 to 12 months; in adolescents and adults, SD usually manifests as dandruff on the scalp and central face and can have negative effects on QOLs.[7]

### Etiology and Pathophysiology

Numerous theories have been presented regarding the causes of SD. These involve yeast species (*Malassezia*), chronic inflammation, and keratinocyte proliferation. Some individuals may be genetically predisposed. Given the sex-based bias for men to develop SD, particularly around puberty, androgens have been suspected as causal agents. This aligns with heightened sebaceous gland activity around puberty. Similarly, immunocompetence seems to be a protective factor.

### Diagnostic Approach

The presentation usually occurs symmetrically. In newborns, erythematous, greasy, scaly patches are apparent involving the scalp; this is known as cradle cap. The more widespread disease may present with erythematous, ill-defined scaly patches on the trunk and extremities. In older children and adults, SD presents as diffuse scaling in the scalp with thick plaques in more severe cases. There may be similar scaling in the external ear canals, behind the ears, and in the nasolabial folds. There may also be ill-defined, erythematous scaly patches on the central cheeks as well as the axillae, intercrural folds, and inframammary chest. It may be confused with *Candida albicans* infections but does not have satellite pustules. A KOH stain may help if *C. albicans* or a dermatophyte infection is also suspected as a cause of the skin eruptions. Biopsies are not diagnostic. Relevant to rehabilitation specialists, SD may present bilaterally even in individuals with hemi-paralysis or unilateral Parkinsonism. Additionally, patients using c-collars for spinal cord injuries may develop SD around the neck or beard.

## Treatment

In most instances, treatment consists of topical antifungals, such as ketoconazole shampoo or cream, to prevent flares, along with a topical steroid to control flares; these should be lower potency if on the face or intertriginous areas. When SD is near the eyes or involves concomitant rosacea, a more appropriate treatment may be a topical calcineurin inhibitor, such as Elidel or Protopic.

## Functional Prognosis and Outcomes

Prognosis is good, and treatments are usually effective. Patient compliance poses the greatest clinical hurdle, due to daily regimen for long-term disease management.

## HERPES SIMPLE VIRUS

### Core Definitions

Herpes simple virus (HSV) is a common, contagious pathogen causing an incurable infection in humans that manifests as painful vesicle or vesicles on the skin and mucous membranes, namely the mouth, lips, gums, eyes, genitals, and digits. Increased prevalence is associated with lower socioeconomic statuses and decreased primary care access. Nearly three quarters of retiree-aged adults are seropositive for HSV antibodies. While some individuals are asymptomatic, they can still infect others. HSV itself is caused by HSV1 and HSV2, and it may be latent in individuals after primary infection, though outbreaks within an individual may be recurrent, exacerbated by stress. HSV is of the greatest concern in immunocompromised individuals.[8]

### Etiology and Pathophysiology

Herpesviruses include more than 80 different viruses, many of which cause some of the most common infectious diseases in humans. Herpesviruses have evolved to coexist with humans throughout evolution to remain latent, which increases infection and transmissibility risks. HSV1 and HSV2, in particular, infect individuals through mucous membranes, specifically epithelial cells, that come into direct contact with active lesions or mucosal secretions of infected individuals (either primary or recurrent). Respiratory droplets have also been implicated in viral transmission. Once an individual is infected, the virus migrates to the central nervous system, where it evades the immune system and replicates for life. As such, symptoms may be recurrent due to viral reactivation within the same individual; of note, symptoms are not required during viral reactivation for viral shedding, and transmission may occur from an individual with or without symptoms, though the former is more common. While recurrence may seem random, it is often the result of other underlying factors, such as stress, sleep, sickness, sunlight, or even local trauma, including the nerves.

## Diagnostic Approach

HSV presents as painful, umbilicated, grouped vesicles on an erythematous base, often near the lips. Symptoms often arise only a few days after exposure to an infected individual. Primary infection is also known as "cold sores "or "fever blisters." Recurrent outbreaks may be common, often triggered by stress, viral infection and/or fever, and even UV exposure (sunlight or tanning). Primary HSV can occur on other skin sites, including fingers, in healthcare workers, due to interactions with infected patients, or in children, due to thumb-sucking; this is known as herpes whitlow. HSV may also appear on the genitals (labia, penis) and anogenital regions in both men and women. Transmission may occur through contact of genitals to genitals or through mouth to genitals. Rarely, transmission may occur through other activities associated with skin abrasion and close contact, such as wrestling. After forming, vesicles often rupture, crust over, and heal usually without complication or scarring. Pain and tenderness are often reported. Initially, it was thought that oral HSV was due to HSV1, and genital herpes was due to HSV2; however, now both strains can be found at either site. Diagnosis is most often made clinically but can be confirmed by polymer chain reaction (PCR) or even a culture (swab and transfer to cell culture). PCR is the better test if available.

## Treatment

The most common treatment is valcyclovir (Valtrex) with different dosages depending on whether primary disease, recurrent disease, or suppressive therapy. Other therapeutic options include acyclovir (Zovirax) or Famvir (famciclovir). Topical treatments, although available, are mostly ineffective.

## Functional Prognosis and Outcomes

Prognosis is good in individuals with primary infection, and symptoms should resolve within 1 to 2 weeks. However, even after resolution of symptoms, individuals may still remain contagious. There are many factors that influence the likelihood and severity of recurrence, but this may pose a significant physical and psychological burden on infected individuals, due to the stigma associated with HSV and other sexually transmitted diseases. In cases of ocular herpes, corneal blindness is of great concern.

## HERPES ZOSTER VIRUS

### Core Definitions

Herpes zoster virus (HZV) causes shingles (Herpes zoster [HZV]) after viral reactivation in individuals previously infected with the varicella zoster virus (VZV). Primary VZV infection usually causes varicella (chickenpox). VZV is reactivated in the spinal ganglia due to local immunosuppression and travels down a cutaneous nerve, causing pain that often precedes the onset of the rash. Some reports indicate that in excess of 90% of adults in the United States are infected with VZV. Symptoms resolve by 1-month postinitiation; however, in some individuals, nerve damage and associated pain may be long lasting.[9]

## Etiology and Pathophysiology

Varicella is a respiratory virus and is spread by air droplets. Individuals who have never had varicella or the varicella vaccine are at risk of infection, particularly\immunocompromised individuals. In these individuals, once infected, varicella and not herpes zoster first develops. HZV is also spread by direct contact with the lesions of individuals with varicella. Viral reactivation and resultant herpes zoster are much more common in older individuals, whose immune systems have weakened with age.

## Diagnostic Approach

The rash presents as a linear band of grouped, umbilicated fluid-filled vesicles along a single dermatome—less commonly two or more—of an associated nerve; therefore, the rash is restricted to on one side of the body, though rarely it crosses the midline. HZV in immunocompromised patients may occur in a dermatomal pattern. Pain and/or itching may occur before the presentation of the rash by up to a week. Beyond clinical diagnosis, PCR can confirm findings; viral culture is less sensitive. Though distinct in presentation, confusion between herpes zoster and ACD (such as from poison ivy) may occur. When herpes zoster occurs on the face, the eye, nose, and ear may become affected. Facial weakness may also result. In these cases, it is important to consult with otolaryngologists to avoid long-term symptoms, like hearing loss. Nerve pain that outlasts the symptoms by many months without resolution is referred to postherpetic neuralgia; this increases with age. In young individuals, because herpes zoster often results from a compromised immune system, HIV testing may be appropriate though not necessary.

## Treatment

Antiviral drugs, such as Valtrex 1,000 mg 3 times a day for 7 to 10 days, are most effective at improving herpes zoster and reducing inflammation and pain.

## Functional Prognosis and Outcomes

Depending on the age and severity of symptoms, the prognosis is excellent to okay. In younger individuals without underlying immune conditions, symptoms often resolve without any long-term complications, though postherpetic neuralgia may persist for about a year in some cases. With age, the likelihood of longer-term complications increases. Prognosis can be worst in immunocompromised individuals or when the facial, auditory, or ocular nerves are involved.

## KELOID

### Core Definitions

A keloid is a spontaneous scar developing after trauma to the skin. Onset after trauma is often variable. A hypertrophic scar is similar in appearance but usually limited to the site of damaged skin (often surgical) whereas a keloid extends beyond the margins of trauma.[10]

## Etiology and Pathophysiology

Transforming growth factor-beta (TGF-beta) has been implicated in keloids, along with other fibrotic diseases, and keloid fibroblasts exhibit abnormal TGF-beta signaling. In general, factors affecting keloid scar formation seem to be genetically driven, though inflammation is also involved and spontaneous keloids are also possible. For example, those with African descent have the highest prevalence of keloid formation, and keloid scars exhibit familial inheritance patterns. Some family members even form keloids in the same anatomical location. On the other hand, individuals with spontaneous keloids and no family history often do not form additional keloids.

## Diagnostic Approach

Keloids clinically present as firm, skin-colored, sometimes erythematous or hyperpigmented nodules. Diagnosis is made clinically. Rarely is a skin biopsy needed. Although keloids are commonly seen on the upper trunk, they can occur anywhere. They occur more commonly in patients of color (Fitzpatrick skin types V and VI) and less commonly in whites. Keloids may be pruritic or painful depending on the degree of inflammation or anatomical site of involvement. They may pose psychological distress based on location and severity and be aesthetically displeasing to the individual. Additionally, keloids that occupy flexor regions and joints may interfere with movement.

## Treatment

Treatment options are varied. Potent topical steroids are often used but least effective. Most commonly keloids are treated with repeated intralesional Kenalog (ILK). Other therapies include the following: a combination of Kenalog with 5 fluorouracil (a local chemotherapy), surgical excision followed by ILK after suture removal, and occasionally laser treatment.

## Functional Prognosis and Outcomes

Functional prognosis is varied and depends on the individual, extent of keloid, and family history.

# BASAL CELL CARCINOMA

## Core Definitions

Basal cell carcinomas (BCCs) are the most common cause of skin cancer occurring in approximately 1 out of 3 white Americans and 1 out of 5 in all Americans. It occurs mostly in sun-exposed areas with increased risk in men and with age. Tanning bed use has also increased this frequency, more common in females of age 15 to 25.[11]

## Etiology and Pathophysiology

Skin cancers result from nuclear DNA damage and hyperproliferation of abnormal cells. BCC has been associated with early-life sun exposure of intermittent, high intensity. Individuals with lighter skin colors (Fitzpatrick types I and II) are at greater risk. Because individuals with compromised immune systems have BCCs more commonly, immune system evasion seems to be an underlying mechanism of BCC development. Aberrant hedgehog (HH) signaling has also been implicated in BCCs.

## Diagnostic Approach

BCCs present most commonly as a nonhealing "sore" or enlarging, opalescent, or translucent nodule. When large enough, telangiectasia can be seen on its surface. They are slow growing and may take months to be identified easily. They are often asymptomatic and noticed by the patient or a family member. The larger lesions may bleed intermittently, which is another red flag for malignancy. Clinical appearance alone is usually enough to warrant a skin biopsy. Dermoscopy is a relatively new tool useful for diagnostic confirmation. With polarized light and magnification, patterns and colors help identify subtle features of the lesions, such a crystalline structures, arborizing vessels, spoke wheels, ovoid globules, and leaf-like structures. The histology will categorize the subset of BCC, which will direct the appropriate therapy—these include superficial, pigmented, nodular, morpheaform, and recurrent.

## Treatment

Curettage and electrodessication, excision, Mohs surgery, imiquimod, and 5 fluorouracil have all been approved as appropriate treatments based on anatomical site and BCC subtype. Radiation therapy and brachytherapy (a specific type of radiation) are used less commonly. Advanced disease is treated with vismodegib or sonidegib, which are both HH signaling pathway inhibitors.

## Functional Prognosis and Outcomes

Most BCCs are cured and rarely metastasize but can spread locally.

## SQUAMOUS CELL CARCINOMA

### Core Definitions

SCCs are the second most common cause of skin cancer, though their incidence is increasing rapidly. Like BCCs, SCCs usually occur in sun-exposed areas, though they can also occur in chronic scars and wounds. Although usually curable, SCCs can be aggressive and locally invasive with nerve involvement and metastasizing. SCCs occur more commonly in immunosuppressed patients, especially patients who have undergone bone marrow, stem cell, and organ transplant.[12]

### Etiology and Pathophysiology

SCCs are cancerous skin lesions that contain a high degree of mutation, specifically to tumor mutation genes. Interestingly, therapies for melanomas and BCCs trigger SCC development.

### Diagnostic Approach

SCCs present as erythematous or skin colored, sometimes crusted, nonhealing ulcers; they are often scaly or firm/keratotic nodules. Some lesions rapidly grow in 4 to 6 weeks. Diagnosis is made clinically with pathologic confirmation via skin biopsy. As with BCCs, dermoscopy may be helpful in identifying distinct structures, such as rosettes, crystalline patterns, and hairpin vessels at the periphery. Importantly, while lighter skin (Fitzpatrick types I and II) is a risk factor for SCCs, they are the most common skin cancer in individuals with darker skin (Fitzpatrick types V and VI). SCCs can develop in areas associated with poorer prognoses, such as chronic scars and wounds.

### Treatment

Excision or Mohs surgery is the gold standard. Less commonly, curettage and electrodesiccation are performed.

## MELANOMA

### Core Definitions

Melanoma is the most serious of the more common skin cancers and with other skin cancers increases in frequency with age and history of sun exposure or indoor tanning. Its risk of metastasis is based on its depth in the skin at the time of biopsy, with survival decreasing with tumor thickness and invasion. There are also several genetic mutations associated with a higher risk. Only 18% to 20% develop from prior moles.[13]

### Etiology and Pathophysiology

Melanomas are cancerous skin lesions involving abnormal melanocytes activity and melanin deposition. They have a propensity to spread and even metastasize into surrounding lymph nodes.

### Diagnostic Approach

Melanoma presents as an irregularly pigmented melanocytic nevus (mole) or rapidly enlarging pigmented lesion. A mnemonic for recognizing melanoma is based on its physical features and growth dynamics and is known as the ABCDE's of melanoma: asymmetry, border irregularity, color differences, diameter greater than 6 mm, and evolving (changing). A majority of melanomas are identified by the patient or family member as an "ugly duckling" or mole that does not look like its neighbors. Clinical diagnosis is confirmed by a skin biopsy and hematoxylin–eosin (H&E) staining. As previously discussed, one of the most clinically useful tools is dermoscopy. With this instrument, the clinician can visualize pigment patterns and structures that can confirm a benign mole from melanoma with the goal of fewer unnecessary biopsies. The important histologic criterion is the depth of invasion or Breslow Depth. Sentinel lymph node biopsies are often performed to determine the extent of the spread.

### Treatment

Surgical excision remains the gold standard for melanoma with a 1-cm margin for melanomas less than 1 mm in depth of invasion, 1- to 2-cm margin for melanomas greater than 1 mm in depth but less than 2 mm in depth, and 2 cm margin for melanomas greater than 2 mm in depth. For melanomas 1 mm or greater (and occasionally thinner lesions), a sentinel lymph node biopsy is often recommended at the time of excision. Wider margins are appropriate in certain cases. For metastatic disease, referral to a melanoma center with oncologists familiar with the use of the newer check block inhibitors is recommended.

## WARTS

### Core Definition

Warts are infectious cutaneous lesions that can present on mostly skin but also mucous membranes; they are caused by the human papillomavirus (HPV).[14]

### Etiology and Pathophysiology

HPV is a virus including hundreds of strains, a subset of which are oncogenic. The oncogenic strains are associated with genital cancers (vulva, cervix, anus, penis, and pharynx). HPV viruses can be spread through skin contact or through sexual activity.

### Diagnostic Approach

Common warts (verruca vulgaris) present as skin-colored keratotic papules on any skin site. Pinpoint capillaries may be noted centrally. Plantar warts present on the sole and may coalesce to larger plaques that may become painful when walking or running. Genital warts (condylomata accuminata) may occur on the shaft and glans of the penis, suprapubic area, vulva, intercrural and intergluteal folds, and even extend into the anorectal area. In these areas, warts may be softer/moist due to anatomical site. In individuals with amputations, warts may also be confused with verrucous hyperplasia, particularly on the distal end of the residual limb. Unlike warts, verrucous hyperplasia is not caused by a viral infection but chronic lymphedema resultant from friction, suction, or reduced blood flow.

### Treatment

Common warts may resolve spontaneously so treatment is not always necessary, especially when asymptomatic. The common treatment for warts includes topical salicylic acid, cryosurgery (liquid nitrogen), curettage and electrodesiccation, and laser. Genital warts are usually treated with liquid nitrogen, podophyllin, and imiquimod.

## PSORIASIS

### Core Definitions

Psoriasis is a hereditary, autoimmune skin condition that presents with red, scaly patches and plaques on the scalp, face, trunk, and extremities, including nails. Up to a third of patients will develop psoriatic arthritis, which entails inflammation that may be symptomatic in the joints and often the hands.[15]

### Etiology and Pathophysiology

Psoriasis is an autoimmune disease of unknown etiology and may be triggered by stress, infection, and trauma. Inflammation is associated with a cytokine cascade, including TNF, IL12, IL17, and IL23.

## Diagnostic Approach

Psoriasis presents as erythematous, scaly patches, and plaques causing associated metabolic syndrome (diabetes mellitus, depression, and cardiac disease). Psoriatic lesions, which are chronically inflamed, result in the rapid proliferation of keratinocytes. Pustules may occur on the hands and feet as well as a more serious presentation with generalized pustules.

## Treatment

Prior to 2004, the mainstay of therapy was topical steroids and phototherapy, which continue to be used regularly. We are now able to clear/almost clear many patients since the advent of "biologics" for rheumatoid arthritis in the late 1990s. The therapeutic armamentarium has expanded to include TNF, IL12, IL17, IL23, and PDE4 inhibitors.

## REFERENCES

The full reference list appears in the digital product found on http://connect.springerpub.com/content/book/978-0-8261-6226-7/part/part03/chapter/ch34

# DYSPHAGIA

ALBA AZOLA AND MARLÍS GONZÁLEZ-FERNÁNDEZ

## CORE DEFINITIONS

Dysphagia, or difficulty swallowing, is defined as an impairment in the transport of a bolus of food from the oral cavity into the stomach while protecting the airway. Dysphagia is a common diagnosis encountered by the physical medicine and rehabilitation physician, and it can result in dehydration, malnutrition, pneumonia, airway obstruction, and decreased quality of life. Epidemiologic studies estimate that the prevalence of dysphagia in the general population could be anywhere between 3% and 18%.[1,2] Less than a third of the affected patients report concerns to a physician,[3] highlighting the need to screen for dysphagia during encounters, particularly patients with a diagnosis that puts them at risk for developing dysphagia. In the stroke population, the prevalence of dysphagia is greater than 50%, and they are over three times more likely to develop pneumonia.[4] The presence of clinically relevant anxiety and depression symptoms has been found in 47% of patients with dysphagia.[5] Basic understanding of the risk factors leading to dysphagia is essential to properly assess patients and diagnose them in a timely manner.

## ETIOLOGY AND PATHOPHYSIOLOGY

### Physiology

To diagnose and effectively treat dysphagia, we must understand normal swallow physiology and the mechanisms by which the underlying disorder may disrupt function. A food bolus is transported from the oral cavity into the stomach, through a shared aerodigestive tract by a complex sensorimotor sequence of events that requires the integrity of musculoskeletal structures and the peripheral and central nervous systems.[6] It is important to note that liquid and solid boluses are managed differently. During the oral preparatory stage, liquids stay in the oral cavity as the posterior tongue and soft palate approximating to prevent spillage. The oral propulsive stage starts as liquids are transferred posteriorly through the oropharynx as the tongue approximates the hard palate from anterior to posterior the bolus enters the pharynx. Solids boluses are processed through mastication and mixed with saliva during stage 1 transport until proper consistency is achieved. During stage 2 transport, the tongue

The full list of references appears in the digital product found on http://connect.springerpub.com/content/book/978-0-8261-6226-7/part/part03/chapter/ch35

tip touches the hard palate, transfers processed solids to the oropharynx, and commonly fills the vallecula as the rest of the bolus is being processed.[7]

The pharyngeal phase begins as the soft palate retracts and simultaneous contraction of the superior posterior pharyngeal wall seals the nasal cavity allowing the generation of the pressure gradient needed for bolus propulsion. Simultaneously, airway protection is achieved by the anterosuperior movement of the hyolaryngeal structures, approximation of the true and false vocal folds, and epiglottis inversion closing the laryngeal vestibule. The tongue base and posterior pharyngeal wall contract moving the bolus through the pharynx in a peristaltic-like muscular wave. The upper esophageal sphincter (UES) relaxes allowing passage of the bolus into the esophagus. Finally, during the esophageal phase, the bolus is transported by peristalsis and gravity through the lower esophageal sphincter (LES) into the stomach.

## Pathophysiology

Difficulty swallowing may arise from impairment in the oral, pharyngeal, or esophageal stage of the swallow or more often a combination of these. Difficulties with swallowing can be broadly categorized as affecting airway safety or efficiency of bolus clearance. See Table 35.1 for a summary of the swallowing stages and the potential impairments disrupting functional swallow.

### TABLE 35.1 SWALLOWING PATHOPHYSIOLOGY BY STAGE

| STAGES OF SWALLOWING | EVENTS DURING THE STAGE | COMMON PATHOPHYSIOLOGIC FINDINGS |
|---|---|---|
| Oral preparatory and propulsive (liquids) Oral stage I and stage II transport (solids) | • Bolus held in the oral cavity <br> • Tongue propels bolus into pharynx | • Facial weakness (oral incompetence) <br> • Tongue weakness or impaired movement <br> • Decreased range of motion of the jaw |
| Pharyngeal | • Soft palate elevated to seal nasopharynx <br> • Base of tongue and pharyngeal constrictors sequentially push bolus through pharynx <br> • Airway protected via: <br>   • Elevation of hyolaryngeal complex <br>   • Glottic closure <br>   • Laryngeal vestibule closure <br> • UES opens | • Weakness or structural deficiency at soft palate <br> • Tongue or pharyngeal constrictors weakness <br> • Submental muscle weakness <br> • Peripheral or CNS impairment impacting coordination of events <br> • UES dysfunction or stricture <br> • Pharyngeal diverticula |
| Esophageal | • LES relaxes <br> • Peristaltic wave propels bolus into stomach | • Lower esophageal muscle dysfunction or stricture <br> • Esophageal dysmotility <br> • Obstruction by esophageal or adjacent mass |

CNS, central nervous system; LES, lower esophageal sphincter; UES, upper esophageal sphincter.

## DIAGNOSTIC APPROACH

When assessing a patient with dysphagia, we should understand the particular diagnosis impairing their ability to swallow. A wide variety of diseases and disorders can negatively impact swallowing, including neurologic disorders, structural lesions, connective tissue disorders, and iatrogenic causes (Table 35.2). Another key piece of information to assess is pulmonary status including chronic obstructive pulmonary disease (COPD) or other disorders affecting pulmonary reserve.

### History and Physical Examination

A comprehensive history of the patient with suspected dysphagia should be specific and expand beyond "are you having trouble swallowing?". Important questions include time to finish a meal, bite size, foods or consistencies that they abstain from, self-implemented diet modifications, and avoidance of eating in public places. Several validated questionnaires can be used including the EAT-10[8] and SWAL-QOL.[9] Bedside screening tools may include water swallowing trials such as the 3-oz water swallowing test[10] and the volume viscosity swallow test.[11]

The physical examination can provide clues as to the severity and underlying impairments resulting in swallowing dysfunction. Visual inspection may reveal facial, tongue, or soft palate asymmetry, drooling, or dry mucous membranes. Neurologic examination including cranial nerve, motor, sensory, and coordination testing should be completed. In patients with stroke, the degree of aphasia is associated with severity of dysphagia.[12]

If a diagnosis of dysphagia is suspected (see Figure 35.1), instrumental swallowing evaluation and referral to a speech-language pathologist are indicated. An instrumental swallowing evaluation is imperative to understand the underlying pathophysiology and to design

**TABLE 35.2 DISORDERS ASSOCIATED WITH DYSPHAGIA**

| Neuromuscular | • Stroke<br>• Parkinson's<br>• Multiple sclerosis<br>• Motor neuron disease<br>• Neuromuscular junction disorders<br>• Dementia |
|---|---|
| Structural | • Cervical osteophytes<br>• Zenker's diverticulum<br>• Neoplasm (oropharyngeal)<br>• Cleft palate |
| Connective tissue | • Myositis (Inclusion body myositis)<br>• SLE, Scleroderma, mixed connective tissue disease<br>• Presbyphagia (changes associated with aging) |
| Iatrogenic | • Head and neck radiation<br>• Chemotherapy<br>• Intubation<br>• Resection of head and neck structures |

SLE, systemic lupus erythematosus.

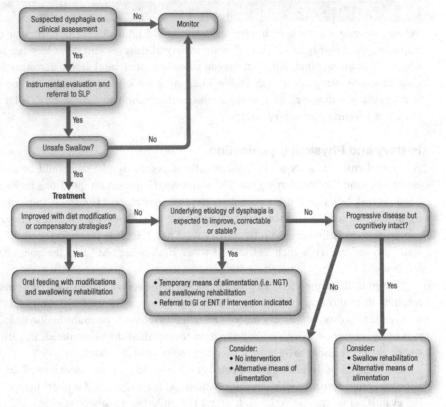

**FIGURE 35.1** Proposed algorithm for dysphagia evaluation and management.

an effective treatment plan. The most widely used instrumental swallowing evaluations are the modified barium swallow (gold standard) and the fiberoptic endoscopic evaluation of swallowing (FEES), usually performed by a speech-language pathologist in conjunction with a radiologist or physiatrist. Other less widely available instrumental evaluations include pharyngeal high-resolution manometry[13] and dynamic CT[14] scan. Based on the history, physical examination, and additional study findings, the patient may require referral to other specialists for further management of identified issues. For example, when esophageal dysmotility or obstruction is suspected, UES stricture, Zenker's diverticula, or oropharyngeal mass or growth is identified, referral to gastroenterology or otolaryngology is indicated.

## TREATMENT

The treatment plan for the patient with dysphagia is tailored to the individual needs based on medical history, goals, impairments, and prognosis. The goal of dysphagia therapy is to return to oral intake while minimizing diet modifications and non-oral feeding. Return to oral feeding is important not only for improved nutrition and hydration but also to improve quality of life, socialization and pleasure during mealtimes, and to prevent disuse atrophy.

In general, the treatment of dysphagia is nonpharmacological and based on diet modifications, exercises, and sensorimotor stimulation.

Compensatory strategies modify the environment and conditions of the swallow, promoting safety and efficiency. Postural changes, such as the chin tuck or head turn, optimize the direction of bolus flow, while changing bolus properties (i.e., consistency) alter sensory input to the swallowing network to modulate how a bolus is swallowed or reduce bolus flow to allow for a safe swallow. This is similar to an assistive device for ambulation, once compensatory strategies are removed, swallowing returns to baseline. Restorative treatment strategies aim to produce lasting improvement in function by addressing mechanisms underlying dysphagia. For example, exercises may be introduced to strengthen weak swallowing musculature or recruit cortical input to improve the timing of swallowing events and to promote coordination of swallowing physiology.

Exercise-based swallowing therapy can be performed at the hospital bedside, outpatient setting, or at home. When indicated, exercises should start as early as possible. Prophylactic swallowing exercises are recommended for head and neck cancer patients prior to chemoradiation or tumor resection.[15] For patients with degenerative disorders, although restoration of function may be limited, treatment of swallowing disorders may allow patients to maintain the current level of function or slow down progression.

Expiratory muscle strength training (EMST) has been shown to improve swallowing outcomes for several patient populations including stroke, amyotrophic lateral sclerosis (ALS), and Parkinson's disease.[16] Electrical stimulation may promote motor function when used in conjunction with swallowing exercises.

Pharmacological and surgical management are utilized when particular causal mechanisms amenable to treatment are identified. A particular challenge in swallowing rehabilitation skill training is the patient's inability to see the laryngeal structures and thus ensure that they are properly performing the exercise. Biofeedback, utilizing surface submental electromyography, has been proposed as a method to surmount this limitation; however, the activation of these muscles is not task specific.[17]

## FUNCTIONAL PROGNOSIS AND OUTCOMES

Predicting functional outcomes in dysphagia is dependent on the severity, underlying etiology, response to treatment, and expected recovery. Intact cognitive function is an important predictor of positive response to swallowing rehabilitation and should be considered in the decision-making process. In the case of the stroke population, a tool has been developed to prognosticate dysphagia outcomes based on age, stroke severity on admission, stroke location, initial risk of aspiration, and initial impairment of oral intake.[18]

## REFERENCES

The full reference list appears in the digital product found on http://connect.springerpub.com/content/book/978-0-8261-6226-7/part/part03/chapter/ch35

# ELECTROLYTE DISTURBANCE

AMY K. UNWIN, ASHLEY M. EAVES, AND AUBREE M. FAIRFULL

## SODIUM DISTURBANCES

### Core Definitions

Derangements in sodium concentration reflect disorders of water/extracellular fluid balance, and renal excretion of water is tightly regulated to maintain body water balance. Normally, when water intake is low or water losses are high, the kidneys conserve water by producing a small volume of urine that is hyperosmotic with respect to plasma; the converse is true when water intake is high.[1]

Antidiuretic hormone (ADH) acts on the kidneys to regulate the volume and osmolality of the urine by stimulating water reabsorption in the renal collecting ducts. ADH is synthesized in hypothalamic neuroendocrine cells and is released by the posterior pituitary when hypothalamic osmoreceptors detect low plasma osmolality or when vascular baroreceptors signal low blood pressure. ADH secretion is suppressed when osmoreceptors detect high plasma osmolality. Normal plasma osmolality is 280 to 295 mOsm/L, and effective osmoles include urea, glucose, and sodium. In a healthy person, urine osmolality can range from approximately 50 to 1,200 mOsm/kg $H_2O$, depending on fluid intake.[1,2]

### Etiology, Pathophysiology, and Treatment
### Hyponatremia

Hyponatremia, or low extracellular sodium concentration (Na < 135), develops if more water is ingested than can be excreted by the kidneys or if the ability to excrete a large volume of dilute urine is compromised because of kidney disease, diuretics, low protein intake (which results in low plasma osmolality), or the presence of ADH.[2]

The overall approach to hyponatremia treatment depends on acuity, severity, and cause. Acute hyponatremia (developing over <48 hours) can lead to cerebral edema and risk of herniation. Etiologies include psychogenic polydipsia, ecstasy use, colonoscopy preparation, and postoperative states. These patients require urgent normalization of their sodium levels, with treatment including hospital/ICU admission or transfer for hypertonic saline infusion if they are symptomatic (e.g., confusion, headache, vomiting, and seizures) or have Na < 125 mEq/L.[2,3]

The full list of resources and references appears in the digital product found on http://connect .springerpub.com/content/book/978-0-8261-6226-7/part/part03/chapter/ch36

As acute hyponatremia is generally managed in the ICU, it is largely beyond the scope of this chapter. However, it should be noted that people who partake in prolonged endurance exercise like marathons are at risk, particularly those who gain weight during the race, have a race time of more than 4 hours, or are at body mass index extremes. Sideline providers should have a high index of suspicion for athletes not feeling well during or after a race. For those with minimal symptoms, close observation and fluid restriction are indicated, with possible hospital observation if the sodium does not improve. If progressive symptoms of encephalopathy develop, treatment entails high-flow oxygen, an initial hypertonic saline bolus of 100 to 150 mL, and quick transport to an emergency facility.[4]

The majority of patients encountered by rehabilitation physicians have subacute/"chronic" hyponatremia. Of note, volume-overload states such as heart failure, cirrhosis with ascites, chronic kidney disease, and nephrotic syndrome all result in chronic hyponatremia because of low blood pressure/cardiac output and impaired renal capacity to eliminate solute-free water.[1] On the other hand, extrarenal losses from vomiting, diarrhea, and sweating also result in hyponatremia, because of decreased effective circulating volume and resultant ADH release. Even mild, chronic cases can have adverse outcomes such as cognitive impairment, osteoporosis, increased risk for falls, and fractures, so hyponatremia should be considered in the differential diagnosis of these conditions. The recommended rate of sodium correction in patients with chronic hyponatremia is 4 to 6 mEq/L per day to prevent osmotic demyelination syndrome.[2]

Several professional organizations have developed algorithms on the comprehensive workup of hyponatremia[2,3,5]; however, the rest of this section focuses on the types of hyponatremia most encountered in inpatient rehab settings (Table 36.1).

### TABLE 36.1 SUMMARY OF TYPICAL LABORATORY FINDINGS AND TREATMENT FOR COMMON SODIUM ABNORMALITIES

|  | SIADH | HYPOVOLEMIA, CSW | PSYCHOGENIC POLYDIPSIA | CENTRAL DIABETES INSIPIDUS |
|---|---|---|---|---|
| VOLUME STATUS | Euvolemic | Hypovolemic | Euvolemic or hypovolemic | Euvolemic |
| SERUM SODIUM | ↓ | ↓ | ↓ | ↑ |
| URINE OSMOLALITY AND SODIUM | ↑ | ↓ (May be normal in CSW) | ↓ | ↑ |
| ADH (NOT TYPICALLY TESTED) | ↑ | ↑ | Normal | ↓ |
| TREATMENT | Fluid restriction <1 L ± salt tabs | Normal saline | Fluid restriction, behavioral modification | Desmopressin |

CSW, cerebral salt wasting.

## Initial Hyponatremia Workup Order Set

Blood: Plasma osmolality, glucose, urea, creatinine, potassium (to assess for pseudohyponatremia [e.g. from hyperglycemia], AKI [suggestive of hypovolemia])[2]

Urine: Osmolality, sodium, ± chloride if the patient is vomiting

See algorithms in references[2,3,5] for further evaluation, depending on the previous results.

### Syndrome of Inappropriate ADH

The syndrome of inappropriate ADH (SIADH) is ADH excess in the setting of plasma hypo-osmolality and euvolemia. Common causes of SIADH are outlined in Box 36.1. Because of inappropriate ADH secretion, these patients typically produce concentrated urine with osmolality >300 mmol/kg.[6] Treatment of SIADH includes discontinuing diuretics and any drug known to cause SIADH, fluid restriction to <1 L per day,[3] and consideration of salt tablets, oral urea supplementation, furosemide with salt tablets, or demeclocycline if water restriction is not effective.[2]

### Hypovolemic Hyponatremia

Many inpatient rehabilitation patients are at risk of hypovolemic hyponatremia due to decreased oral intake, insensible losses in the setting of their illness and hospitalization, and diuretic use. These patients generally produce dilute urine with urine osmolality <150 and urine Na <30, but these numbers are not completely sensitive in detecting hypovolemic hyponatremia. Patients with extrarenal losses due to vomiting are one exception, where urine sodium may be high but urine chloride low. Treatment of hypovolemic hyponatremia consists of administration of normal saline.

Cerebral salt wasting is one subtype of hypovolemic hyponatremia encountered in rehabilitation patients. It is most common after extreme central nervous pathology (e.g., subarachnoid hemorrhage, stroke, TBI) and neurosurgery and usually presents within the first 10 days following the event. It results from renal losses of sodium (and thereby water), possibly from increased brain natriuretic peptide and atrial natriuretic peptide and suppression of the renin–angiotensin system. In response, there is an appropriate rise in ADH. Management involves treatment of the underlying neurologic problem, volume replacement with normal

---

### Box 36.1

#### COMMON CAUSES OF SIADH[2,6]

**1.** *CNS Diseases:* stroke (ischemic or hemorrhagic), infection (encephalitis, meningitis, abscess), neoplasm, demyelinating disorders, TBI, SCI (especially in the first two weeks of traumatic cervical SCI)

**2.** *Malignancy:* especially pulmonary/mediastinal

**3.** *Medications/Drugs:* examples include carbamazepine, ecstasy, desmopressin, narcotics, nicotine, phenothiazines (e.g. prochlorperazine), TCAs, SSRIs/SNRIs, vincristine

**4.** *Pulmonary processes:* infections, COPD, ARDS, asthma, positive pressure ventilation

**5.** *Other:* Colonoscopy preparation, nausea, pain, postoperative state, prolonged strenuous exercise, stress

saline, and possible use of salt tabs and fludrocortisone to encourage volume expansion and sodium retention.[7]

When the underlying cause of hyponatremia is inconclusive between SIADH and hypovolemia (e.g., when volume status is difficult to assess and/or labs are borderline), the urine sodium alone has been found to effectively guide initial fluid management; urine sodium levels up to 50 mEq/L generally have clinically meaningful responses to isotonic saline infusion.[8]

### Psychogenic Polydipsia

Psychogenic polydipsia, resulting in hyponatremia from increased water intake beyond what the kidney can excrete, should be considered in patients presenting with hyponatremia and a history of psychiatric illness or treatment. These patients are clinically euvolemic because of renal excretion of the excess water and generally have otherwise normal laboratory results except for a dilute urine (usually <100 mOsm/kg).[7] Treatment consists of behavioral modification, fluid restriction, and possibly clozapine.[6]

### Hypernatremia

Hypernatremia, or increased serum sodium concentration (>145 mmol/L), is a decrease in total body water relative to electrolyte content, typically from a deficiency of ADH. This is called central diabetes insipidus (DI) and may result from severe head trauma, often with skull fractures at or near the sella turcica, as ADH is secreted from the posterior pituitary. Symptoms include polyuria and polydipsia, and treatment is desmopressin, an ADH analog.[6]

## CALCIUM DISTURBANCES

### Core Definitions

Calcium in the body exists bound to albumin (40%), complexed to anions (15%), and free/ionized (45%). Calcium balance is mediated primarily by parathyroid hormone (PTH) and calcitriol (1,25-dihydroxyvitamin D), which affect intestinal absorption, bone formation and resorption, and urinary excretion.[9] Several patient populations seen by rehabilitation physicians are susceptible to derangements in calcium, namely, hypercalcemia (serum calcium >10.5 mg/dL).[10] Because of the bound and free forms of calcium, hypercalcemia should be confirmed by measuring ionized calcium or correcting for albumin.[10]

### Etiology, Pathophysiology, and Treatment

Many patients with cancer develop hypercalcemia. This is most commonly from osteolytic bone metastases associated with multiple myeloma and breast, lung, and renal cell carcinomas. Cancer-mediated hypercalcemia may also result from paraneoplastic syndromes involving PTH-related peptide (PTHrP) released from tumors such as ovarian, lung, head and neck, esophageal, cervical, pheochromocytoma, and hepatomas.[12]

Other risk factors for hypercalcemia include spinal cord injury (particularly motor complete injury), tetraplegia, dehydration, and prolonged immobilization. These conditions result in increased bone resorption, suppression of the parathyroid-1,25-dihydroxyvitamin D axis, and resorptive hypercalciuria, which predisposes one to kidney stones. Chronic bone resorption may result in osteoporosis.[12]

Signs and symptoms of hypercalcemia are classically thought of as "stones, bones, abdominal groans, and psychiatric overtones." Symptoms can be vague and include anorexia, nausea and vomiting, vague abdominal or flank pain, constipation, lethargy, depression, weakness, muscle and joint aches, polyuria and nocturia, headache, pruritis, and altered mental status. Because young males have an already elevated rate of bone turnover, they are particularly at risk when they sustain a spinal cord injury.[12]

## Evaluation

1. Measurement of calcium, as well as albumin (if not checked recently) or ionized calcium to confirm true hypercalcemia
2. Review of medications, calcium and vitamin D supplementation, and medical conditions to see if it is attributable to one of the entities above
3. Measurement of PTH to distinguish primary hyperparathyroidism (high PTH) from other entities
4. Evaluation for other causes, following an algorithm[10] and/or with nephrology consultation

Patients with acute hypercalcemia are often volume depleted, and treatment entails hydration with normal saline, beginning with a 1- to 2-L bolus of 0.9% saline solution followed by normal saline at 200 to 250 mL/h, with frequent monitoring of calcium levels and monitoring for volume overload (in which case loop diuretics may be used).[10]

High-potency bisphosphonates (pamidronate or zolendronate) are considered first-line therapy for malignancy-associated hypercalcemia and should be initiated as soon as hypercalcemia is identified, as response typically requires 2 to 4 days. Infusion-related fever is a common side effect.[10] Nephrology or oncology consultation may be useful when considering bisphosphonates for malignancy-associated hypercalcemia or for hypercalcemia not resolving with fluids.

## OTHER ELECTROLYTE DISTURBANCES

### Hypokalemia

Patients who are on diuretics (besides potassium-sparing diuretics such as spironolactone or eplerenone) or who have severe or chronic diarrhea are at risk of developing hypokalemia and hypomagnesemia. Transition off the offending diuretic should be considered, but some patients in whom it is needed may require long-term potassium replacement. Of note, if a patient is hypokalemic, magnesium should also be checked and replenished as needed, as hypokalemia will persist if the patient is also hypomagnesemic.

### Hypophosphatemia

Patients with burn injuries are susceptible to hypophosphatemia, for reasons that are multifactorial. Phosphate levels tend to reach a nadir around days 2 to 5 post injury, typically before these patients are seen by physiatrists. Frequent serum phosphate measurement and prompt phosphorus replacement minimize cardiac, neuromuscular, and hematologic effects. Because of the large fluid losses and hypermetabolic state after burn injury, these patients are also subject to derangements in sodium, potassium, magnesium, and calcium. Electrolytes should be monitored closely even as they transition to inpatient rehabilitation.[13]

## Tumor Lysis Syndrome

Patients with cancer, particularly those undergoing chemotherapy for leukemias and lymphomas, are at risk for tumor lysis syndrome, which may result in hyperkalemia, hyperphosphatemia, hypocalcemia, hyperuricemia, and azotemia. Hydration and careful electrolyte monitoring are essential for these patients and should be guided by hematology/oncology teams.[11]

## Acute Kidney Injury

### Core Definitions

Acute kidney injury (AKI) is defined as a change in serum creatinine clearance within 2 to 7 days and oliguria for 6 or more hours. While some patients present with edema, hypertension, or decreased urine output, others have no symptoms. Incidence in hospitalized patients is approximately 20%, and AKI may result in major complications including volume overload, electrolyte disorders (e.g., hyperkalemia), uremic complications (as severe as seizure, coma, cardiac arrest, and death), and drug toxicity.[14]

### Etiology, Pathophysiology, and Treatment

AKI can be classified as prerenal, intrarenal (acute tubular necrosis [ATN] and other parenchymal diseases), and postrenal. The stage of AKI depends on the peak rise in creatinine relative to normal values. Typically, the etiology of AKI can be best determined by patient history and presentation, though the fractional excretion of sodium (FENa) may be helpful in distinguishing prerenal from intrarenal causes; FENa <1% typically suggests prerenal etiology. For patients on diuretics, the fractional excretion of urea (FEUrea) is more reliable. If the cause is not readily determinable, imaging, typically renal ultrasound, is indicated to assess for obstruction/postrenal cause of AKI.[14,15] Common etiologies and clinical presentations of AKI are shown in Table 36.2.

### Diagnostic Approach to Acute Kidney Injury

- Careful review of patient's history, hospital course and medications[13]
- Assessment of volume status and IV fluid replacement if hypovolemic
- Assessment for indications of urgent kidney replacement therapy (volume overload, uremic complications, electrolyte disorders, drug toxicity)
- Urine studies (UA, urine electrolytes)
- Additional lab studies or imaging if etiology unclear

AKI prevention methods include correcting volume, through oral salt and fluid intake or IV normal saline, as well as avoiding diuretics, angiotensin-converting enzyme (ACE) inhibitors, and angiotensin receptor blockers (ARBs) during acute illness. Contrast media, as well as other nephrotoxic medications (Box 36.2), should be avoided as much as possible, and regular vital sign checks should be done on inpatients.[14]

TABLE 36.2 COMMON ETIOLOGIES AND CLINICAL PRESENTATIONS OF ACUTE KIDNEY INJURY[14]

|  | PRERENAL | INTRARENAL: ATN | INTRARENAL: OTHER | POSTRENAL |
|---|---|---|---|---|
| CAUSES | Volume depletion; heart, lung, or liver disease; sepsis; renal artery stenosis | Toxins Ischemia | Glomerulonephritis, interstitial nephritis, pyelonephritis, infarction | Obstructive nephropathy |
| CLINICAL FINDINGS | Volume depletion or overload, SIRS, severe hypertension | Circulatory shock, sepsis, drug exposure, transient hypotension, hemolysis, rhabdomyolysis, tumor lysis | Systemic disease Microangiopathic hemolysis | Urinary tract symptoms, history of urolithiasis, GU tract neoplasia, retroperitoneal disease |
| LAB AND IMAGING FINDINGS | Concentrated urine, no RTE cells or casts | Nonconcentrated urine; RTE cells, granular casts | Hematuria with RBC casts, pyuria with WBC casts, RTE cells | Hydronephrosis, ± stones, hematuria |

GU, genitourinary; RBC, red blood cell; RTE, renal tubular epithelial; SIRS, systemic inflammatory response syndrome; WBC, white blood cell.

## Box 36.2

### COMMON DRUGS CONTRIBUTING TO AKI (MECHANISM)
ACE, ARBs (prerenal)
Acyclovir (crystal nephropathy)
Aminoglycosides (ATN)
Iodinated contrast (ATN)
Methotrexate (crystal nephropathy)
Non-steroidal anti-inflammatory drugs (NSAIDs) (prerenal + tubular toxicity)
Proton pump inhibitors (AIN)
Sulfonamides (AIN)
Tenofovir (tubular toxicity)
Vancomycin (ATN)

ACE, angiotensin-converting enzyme; ARB, angiotensin receptor blocker; ATN, acute tubular necrosis.

Nephrology should be consulted when the cause of AKI is uncertain, for treatment of renal parenchymal disease, or when renal replacement therapy/dialysis may be required (e.g., for volume overload, worsening hyperkalemia, or uremic complications).[14]

## RESOURCES AND REFERENCES

The full list of resources and references appears in the digital product found on http://connect .springerpub.com/content/book/978-0-8261-6226-7/part/part03/chapter/ch36

# FALLS

KATHERINE C. RITCHEY, AMANDA L. OLNEY, AND SCOTT J. CAMPEA

## CORE DEFINITIONS

A fall is defined as "an event which results in a person coming to rest inadvertently on the ground or floor or other lower level not due to an acute event (e.g., syncope)."[1]

A slip is when the leg supporting an individual unintentionally slides a short distance.

A trip is when a person's swinging leg unintentionally encounters an external object or body part.

Both slips and trips typically result in losing one's balance and can result in a fall. Of note, though "slip," "trip," and "fall" are distinct terms, it is important to recognize that patients may use them interchangeably, and each may have identifiable risk factors (i.e., balance or lower extremity impairments). Failure to address a slip, trip, or fall could result in an injury or functional decline, which can be devastating for older adults.

Multifactorial interventions refer to those that are individually tailored to a person's unique risk factors for falling. Multicomponent interventions are those interventions, which provide general fall reduction education, exercises, and prevention strategies, regardless of the individuals' unique risk factors. An example of this would be a group fall prevention class such as Stepping On.

## ETIOLOGY

Falls result from the accumulation and interaction of multiple risk factors, rather than stemming from a single cause. Because they occur frequently in older adults, they are classified as a geriatric syndrome.[2] The more risk factors present in an individual, the greater the risk for falling.[3] A common misconception is that falls are unavoidable and cannot be prevented. But as will be demonstrated later, falls are the result of both nonmodifiable and modifiable factors, which can be intervened upon.

Risk factors can be grouped into intrinsic and extrinsic causes. Intrinsic factors include age-related changes, chronic medical conditions, and behaviors that limit a person's inherent ability to prevent a fall (Table 37.1).[3] Extrinsic factors include environmental hazards, medications, and/or inappropriate footwear (Table 37.1).[4] Falls result from the simultaneous interaction of several intrinsic and extrinsic factors. Risk factors can also be classified as

---

The full list of references appears in the digital product found on http://connect.springerpub.com/content/book/978-0-8261-6226-7/part/part03/chapter/ch37

**TABLE 37.1 INTRINSIC AND EXTRINSIC RISK FACTORS FOR FALLS**

| INTRINSIC RISK FACTORS | EXTRINSIC RISK FACTORS |
| --- | --- |
| Ocular: decreased visual acuity, macular degeneration, glaucoma, cataracts, reduced accommodation, reduced depth perception, vision loss, retinopathy | Medications: anticholinergics, antidepressants, antipsychotics, sedative hypnotics, benzodiazepines, opiates, antihypertensives, alpha- and beta-blockers, antiarrhythmics, use of more than four medications |
| Cardiovascular: bradycardia, tachyarrhythmia, orthostatic hypotension, decompensated heart failure | Footwear: backless shoes and slippers; high heels; shoes lacking dorsum, arch, or heel supports; shoes with heavy soles or a narrow toe box |
| Neurologic: cognitive impairment or dementia, Parkinson's disease, cerebrovascular accident, movement disorder, peripheral neuropathy, gait deficits and imbalance, myelopathy, radiculopathy | Environment: wet or slippery surfaces, lack of grab bars, uneven flooring, floor rugs, poor lighting, lack of handrails for steps, cords, or other walkway hazards |
| Urologic: incontinence (any type), nocturia | |
| Psychological: insomnia/sleep deprivation, depression | |
| Musculoskeletal: osteoarthritis or inflammatory arthritis, joint and spine pain, lower-extremity weakness, postural instability or imbalance, reduced flexibility | |

modifiable and nonmodifiable. The job of the clinician is to identify those intrinsic and extrinsic modifiable risk factors and implement corresponding prevention strategies.

Fear of falling is a common response after a fall. This can create a cycle of deconditioning and social isolation that increases the risk of future falls.[5]

## DIAGNOSTIC APPROACH

The American and British Geriatrics Societies recommend that all community-dwelling persons 65 years and older should be asked annually about whether they have fallen, the number of falls, whether the fall resulted in injury, and whether they have difficulty with walking or balance.[6] If a patient answers affirmatively to any of these questions, further assessment of risk factors is indicated.

The Centers for Disease Control and Prevention (CDC) developed another screening method called the Stopping Elderly Accidents, Deaths, and Injury (STEADI) tool kit.[7] It suggests asking patients the following key questions:

- "Have you fallen in the past 12 months?"
- "Do you feel unsteady when standing or walking?"
- "Do you worry about falling?"

A "yes" to any of the key questions suggests the person is at risk of falling and would benefit from preventative interventions.

Functional assessments are helpful for persons who do not have a history of falling but there is high clinical suspicion that there are gait, lower extremity strength, and/or balance impairments.[8,9] Standardized tests that can be performed include the Timed Up-and-Go (TUG), 30-Second Sit-to-Stand, and Four-Stage Balance Tests, which are all relatively easy to administer in the clinical setting.

■ The TUG has a person rise from a chair, walk 10 feet, turn around, and sit back down in the chair. Persons who complete this in greater than 12 seconds are considered at risk of falling.

■ The 30-Second Sit-to-Stand has a person stand from a seated position as many times a possible in 30 seconds without using their arms. Performing below the number of repetitions expected for age and gender suggests an increased risk of falling and poor leg strength.

■ The Four-Stage Balance Test measures static balance by having a person move through four stances that are each held for 10 seconds. It starts with a parallel stance then transitions to semi-tandem, full tandem, and ending with single-leg stance. Holding less than 10 seconds at any stage indicates impaired balance.

A focused history to identify contributing modifiable risk factors for falls can be performed by following the pneumonic SPLATT.

■ SymPtoms: Dizziness, lightheadedness, palpitations
■ Location: Bedroom, bathroom, other
■ Activity: Details of the fall including the time factors surrounding the event, positional change
■ Timing: Before or after medications, postprandial, outside of the home, nighttime
■ Trauma: Did injury occur?

It is also important to review the patient's past medical history for conditions and medications, which affect balance, gait, strength, or cognition. Examples of classes of medication that increase the risk of falling are listed in Table 37.1 but generally refer to those that are centrally acting neurological agents.[10]

A physical examination should focus on the following regions:

■ Head and eyes: Visual acuity and peripheral vision
■ Cardiovascular: Orthostatic vitals, rate, rhythm
■ Neurological: Cognitive screen, sensory and motor function, proprioception and balance, reflexes and cerebellar function and gait
■ Musculoskeletal: Lower extremity strength, lower extremity joint deformities and swelling, lower extremity alignment, footwear
■ Psychological: Depression

Lastly, fear of falling that is associated with postural changes, reduced balance confidence, activity avoidance, and reduced exercise possibly related to anxiety about falling should be evaluated.[5] Functional impairment associated with a fear of falling can be qualified and quantified using either the long (16-item) or short (7-item) Falls Efficacy Scale International (FES-I) form.[11] This assessment elicits concerns about falling while performing activities of daily living (ADLs), such as getting dressed, preparing meals, or taking a shower. The questionnaire categorizes people into three groups (mild, moderate, or high concern of falling) where higher scores correlate with more concerns and greater risk. It is particularly useful in the outpatient setting for addressing fall-related ADL impairment and identifying older adults who would benefit from durable medical equipment or a home safety assessment.

## TREATMENT

The goal of treatment plans is to prevent future falls. Thus, prevention and treatment for falls are synonymous and utilize the same modalities. These treatment plans can be directed by a geriatrician or specialist in a falls clinic.

Single interventions, especially exercise, offer the same degree of risk reduction as multifactorial interventions. Exercise has also been shown to reduce falls and fall-related injuries including fractures.[12] The exercise program with the greatest evidence as a single intervention is one that includes balance and lower extremity strengthening exercises. These are performed two to three times weekly over six months duration and progresses during that time with higher degrees of exercise challenge. This program, known as OTAGO, has been proven effective either in a group setting or at home and can be initiated by a physical therapist familiar with the exercises.[13]

Alternatively, various forms of Tai Chi have also shown effective in reducing falling risk and rate of falling and may not require a therapist to implement.[14] Other single interventions that have reduced the risk of falling are home hazard removal and reduction of medications.[15] Referral to occupational therapy is recommended to perform a home safety evaluation and hazard removal. Elimination or dose reduction of centrally acting medication is effective and typically is receptive among older adults once they are informed of the correlation between medications and falling.

Lastly, multifactorial (individualized) and multicomponent (standardized, nonindividualized) interventions address more than one risk factor. These should include the aforementioned interventions (exercise; home safety; medication reduction) but may also include some of the following:

- Education on footwear, such as proper shoe fit or heel height, and referral to a podiatrist or medical provider for other foot problems
- Referral to optometrist or ophthalmology or blind therapist for those with severe visual impairment or procurement of special glare-reducing glasses, if appropriate
- Dose reduction or elimination of medications that can contribute to orthostatic hypotension (if found); educate on the importance of exercise such as foot pumps; encourage adequate hydration and consider compression stockings
- Pacemaker or valve replacement surgery for those with symptomatic arrhythmias or stenosis
- Cataract surgery for those with moderate to severe cataracts

## FUNCTIONAL PROGNOSIS AND OUTCOMES

Exercise programs (such as the Otago program) may reduce fall and fall-related injuries by 35%.[12] Improvements may be seen as soon as 8 weeks and are most effective in reducing fall-related injury in those aged 80 years or older.

While Tai Chi reduces the risk of fall, its impact may be less robust than longer, more intense exercise programs especially for high-risk individuals.[14] Home safety modifications are similarly effective, particularly for those at the highest risk.[15]

## BASIC ORDER SETS

### Sample Outpatient Physical Therapy Prescription

Diagnosis: Unsteadiness of gait
Frequency: Two times a week
Duration: 2 to 3 months[16]
Precautions: Falls
Exercise: Strengthening of lower extremities focusing on hip adductors and abductors
Gait, balance, and proprioception training—consider Otago balance program
Evaluation for appropriate assistive device
Set up with a home exercise program

### Sample Home Safety Recommendations

Entrances: Railings and step in good condition, adequate lighting
Kitchen: Common items in reachable places, rubber-backed mats
Bathroom: Nonslip bathmat, grab bars for toilet and bath/shower, raised toilet seat, adequate lighting.
Stairs: Clutter removed, railings in good repair, color contrast strips on steps
Hallways: Clutter removed, night lights

## REFERENCES

The full list of references appears in the digital product found on http://connect.springerpub.com/content/book/978-0-8261-6226-7/part/part03/chapter/ch37

# FATIGUE

GLORIA VON GELDERN AND KEVIN ALSCHULER

## CORE DEFINITIONS

Fatigue is a common symptom seen in neurologic diseases. In this chapter, we will focus on central fatigue. Unlike peripheral fatigue that primarily consists of muscle fatigability, central fatigue is characterized by limited endurance of sustained physical and mental activities including difficulty with concentration and cognition. Central fatigue can be seen in diseases that affect the central, peripheral, and autonomic nervous systems. It is best described in multiple sclerosis (MS) and following stroke but also common in post-polio syndrome and other chronic neurologic diseases. Some studies show that more than 50% of patients with Parkinson's disease report fatigue as one of their three worst symptoms.[1] In MS, a disease primarily diagnosed in young people, fatigue is frequently reported and has been identified as a key risk factor associated with loss of employment.[2] While depression can lead to lack of energy, having fatigue can also worsen mood and impact cognitive abilities and quality of life.

## ETIOLOGY AND PATHOPHYSIOLOGY

Central fatigue can be associated with a disruption in arousal and attention pathways in the limbic system or basal ganglia. However, the exact pathophysiological mechanisms of fatigue in specific neurologic diseases are generally poorly understood. Task-specific fatigue has been described in both MS and stroke. Examples of this are fatigue triggered by speaking in a patient with aphasia or by sustained visual tasks in a patient with impaired vision. Interestingly, it seems that the severity of the fatigue is not necessarily correlated with the severity of the underlying disease. Preexisting low cortisol levels might be a predisposing factor for persistent fatigue following stress.[3]

## DIAGNOSTIC APPROACH

When assessing a patient for fatigue, it is important to rule out other (potentially treatable) conditions that can lead to sleepiness or low energy. As a first step, the quantity and quality of sleep should be assessed. Patients with neurologic conditions may have interrupted sleep due to neurogenic bladder, pain, muscle spasms, or other symptoms. If sleep interruption is

The full list of resources and references appears in the digital product found on http://connect
.springerpub.com/content/book/978-0-8261-6226-7/part/part03/chapter/ch38

present, treating the underlying problems causing insomnia should be the first step when addressing fatigue.

A medication side effect is another common reason for fatigue, and many patients with neurologic conditions are using multiple medications that can cause sleepiness. Common offending agents include benzodiazepines, nonbenzodiazepine sedatives, antihistamines, opioid analgesics, muscle relaxers, anticonvulsants, sedating antidepressants, antianxiety medications, and antipsychotics. Minimizing these medications or changing the timing of when these medications are taken to evening rather than morning time can be helpful in mitigating fatigue.

Additionally, a thorough history and physical examination to screen for medical conditions that can contribute to fatigue is needed, with particular attention to the following conditions:

- Cardiopulmonary conditions: Congestive heart failure, chronic obstructive pulmonary disease
- Sleep disorders: sleep apnea, restless leg syndrome
- Endocrinologic/metabolic conditions: Hypothyroidism, hyperthyroidism, chronic renal disease, chronic hepatic disease, adrenal insufficiency, electrolyte abnormalities, vitamin B12 deficiency
- Hematologic/neoplastic conditions: Anemia, malignancy
- Infectious diseases: Mononucleosis, viral hepatitis, HIV infection
- Rheumatologic conditions: Polymyalgia rheumatica, systemic lupus erythematosus, rheumatoid arthritis, Sjögren's syndrome
- Psychological conditions: Depression, anxiety

The following questionnaires are helpful screening tools when assessing for diseases or conditions that can contribute to fatigue:

- Depression: Patient Health Questionnaire (PHQ)-2 or PHQ-9[4]
- Anxiety: Generalized Anxiety Disorder-7 (GAD-7)[5]
- Sleep apnea: STOP BANG questionnaire[6]

Depending on the history and physical examination as well as the results of screening questionnaires, laboratory and other testing should be considered:

- Thyroid-stimulating hormone (TSH) in blood to assess for thyroid dysfunction
- Complete blood count (CBC) to assess for anemia
- Comprehensive metabolic panel to screen for liver and kidney abnormalities
- Vitamin B12 level and methylmalonic acid to assess for deficiency (goal vitamin B12 level should be >400, even if some labs do not mark levels as abnormal up to 200)
- Age-appropriate cancer screening
- Sleep study to assess for sleep apnea

Finally, there is the assessment of fatigue itself. It is important to evaluate both the individual's self-report of the severity of their fatigue and the impact or interference of their fatigue on their functioning. Importantly, research suggests that fatigue severity and fatigue interference are only moderately correlated, and fatigue interference is often a stronger predictor of quality of life relative to fatigue severity. The following measures capture aspects of fatigue severity and fatigue impact[7,8]:

- Brief Fatigue Inventory (BFI)

- Fatigue Symptom Inventory (FSI)
- Fatigue Severity Scale (FSS)
- Modified Fatigue Impact Scale
- Multidimensional Fatigue Inventory (MFI-20)

## TREATMENT

At the outset of fatigue management, it is essential to identify and prioritize the treatment target. As stated earlier, considering both fatigue severity and fatigue interference is important. Patients may need education on the fact that improving fatigue severity does not automatically cause an increased level of activity or function. In addition to improving fatigue severity, they may also need to make associated behavioral changes to improve their functioning. Additionally, changing behavior patterns will decrease the interference of fatigue and may consequently lessen the self-reported severity of their fatigue.

Interventions should naturally begin by treating causal factors, such as sleep disorders, other fatigue-inducing conditions, and optimizing medications to reduce sedation. An important consideration in the management of fatigue is also to counsel patients regarding the dangers of drowsy driving. The clinician can then engage the patient in any of a number of treatment approaches that may positively impact fatigue severity and/or interference.

While minimizing medications is often an important part of improving fatigue and evidence for the benefits of pharmacologic interventions for fatigue is very limited, several medications have been used to help fatigue in neurologic conditions. An empiric trial of antidepressants, especially selective serotonin reuptake inhibitor or serotonin–norepinephrine reuptake inhibitors, can be helpful for patients with depressive symptoms even if they do not meet the criteria for major depressive disorder. Additionally, there is some limited data to show that treatment of the underlying neurologic disease with immune-modulatory medication in MS (especially with natalizumab) or with dopaminergic medications in Parkinson's disease can have a positive impact on fatigue.[9]

Stimulants have also been used as pharmacologic treatments of fatigue. For MS-related fatigue small randomized controlled trials with some conflicting results provide overall weak evidence to support the use of amantadine[10] or modafinil.[11] Amantadine was originally developed as an antiviral agent against influenza (no longer used due to resistance) and is also a dopamine agonist used to treat Parkinson's disease. For fatigue, typical dosing is 100 mg BID (AM and midday). Amantadine is typically tolerated relatively well but needs to be used with caution in patients with renal insufficiency.

Modafinil has also been studied in small trials with some benefit in post-stroke fatigue and in amyotrophic lateral sclerosis (ALS). Dosing is typically 100 to 400 mg daily, typically given as a single dose in the AM though for some patients split dosing up to 200 mg in the morning and 200 mg midday is beneficial. Armodafinil, the levorotatory enantiomer of modafinil, can be given as 50 to 250 mg a day (once daily in the morning or as divided doses). Both modafinil and armodafinil are controlled substances (schedule IV) and have been approved to treat narcolepsy, shift work sleep disorder, and obstructive sleep apnea. Interaction with hormonal contraceptives is an important consideration in young women and anxiety or headaches are side effects to be aware of.

Other stimulants that are sometimes used off-label to treat excessive daytime sleepiness are methylphenidate and amphetamines. Methylphenidate is usually started at 5 to 10 mg daily in the morning with a maximum daily dose of 60 mg per day in two to three divided doses. Amphetamines used in fatigue are dextroamphetamine-amphetamine (5–40 mg once daily in the morning; maximum daily dose 60 mg given in one to three divided doses) or lis-dexamfetamine (30 mg once daily in the morning, increasing in increments of 10 to 20 mg at weekly intervals, maximum daily dose 70 mg). Both methylphenidate and amphetamines are approved for use in attention deficit hyperactivity disorder (ADHD) and narcolepsy. These stimulants are schedule II controlled substances and carry a risk of abuse and development of tolerance (which may be mitigated by medication vacations). They can have cardiovascular or psychiatric side effects and the benefits need to be balanced with the risks in individual patients.

There is a growing body of evidence that nonpharmacologic symptom self-management interventions effectively improve symptom severity and impact, including in fatigue. Self-management interventions are those that teach individuals cognitive and behavioral skills that can be used to optimize their functioning in the face of interfering symptoms.[12] There are a number of treatment approaches that fit within the self-management intervention context. For example, recent research has demonstrated that self-management interventions that utilize a cognitive behavioral therapy (CBT) approach can have a positive impact on a number of symptoms, including fatigue.[13] This type of intervention focuses on enhancing adaptive or helpful thoughts and decreasing maladaptive or unhelpful thoughts, while similarly growing behaviors that are helpful to improving a person's quality of life and decreasing unhelpful behaviors.

In addition to CBT, a substantial amount of research has focused on the role of optimizing physical activity in improving fatigue management. This includes interventions focused on energy conservation or pacing that seek to modify activity patterns to balance the individual's activity against their need for rest with the goal of promoting consistent engagement with the world around them.[12] This also includes interventions focused on exercise, which have shown that individuals report decreased fatigue despite the paradox of having increased energy expenditure due to exercising.[14]

## FUNCTIONAL PROGNOSIS AND OUTCOMES

As described earlier, management of fatigue requires a broad approach in both diagnosis and treatment and can therefore be challenging. However, addressing this important but often hidden symptom is crucial in preventing loss of employment and negative impacts on the ability to participate in therapies and activities of daily living and on quality of life. In MS, for example, fatigue has been found to be an independent predictor of quality of life.[15]

## RESOURCES AND REFERENCES

The full list of resources and references appears in the digital product found on http://connect .springerpub.com/content/book/978-0-8261-6226-7/part/part03/chapter/ch38

# GAIT DEVIATIONS

KAYLA WILLIAMS AND THIRU ANNASWAMY

## CORE DEFINITION

Gait is a manner of moving on foot using a bipedal system to provide support and propel the body forward. It involves the coordination of motion through the pelvis, hips, knees, and ankles via forces generated by both muscles and momentum to produce a forward translation. This complex process requires a combination of neural and muscular control in addition to multisensory input.

## GAIT CYCLE

Gait is a rhythmic, repetitive pattern involving steps and strides. A cycle of gait is a measure of one step, as a single limb acts as a source of support, and one stride, as the other limb advances forward and becomes a new source of support (see Figure 39.1). This progression is divided into two phases: (a) stance phase during which the foot is in contact with the ground and (b) swing phase where the foot travels through the air as the limb advances. The stance phase begins with weight acceptance during initial contact and loading response. Initial contact most commonly occurs with heel strike while the hip is flexed, knee extended, and ankle dorsiflexed. This facilitates shock absorption, limb stability, and capability for progression. During loading response, the heel is used as a rocker to transfer body weight onto the leading limb. Mid stance begins when the swinging foot is lifted and ends when body weight is aligned over the forefoot with the ankle dorsiflexed and hip and knee extended. Terminal stance begins as the supporting limb heel rises and body weight advances over the forefoot. With pre-swing, the stance limb ankle assumes a plantarflexed position while a simultaneous increase in knee flexion and loss of hip extension occurs to permit a transfer of body weight. During the initial swing, the stance limb ankle partially dorsiflexes and the foot lifts from the floor and is advanced via hip flexion and increased knee flexion. Throughout mid-swing, the hip is further flexed, and the limb is advanced anterior to the body weight line. Terminal swing is marked by the advancement of the swinging limb with the knee flexed, hip flexed, and ankle dorsiflexed until the foot strikes the floor and the tibia becomes vertical to assume the position as the supporting limb once again. In normal circumstances, this cycle is spatially and temporally symmetric.[1]

---

The full list of references appears in the digital product found on http://connect.springerpub.com/content/book/978-0-8261-6226-7/part/part03/chapter/ch39

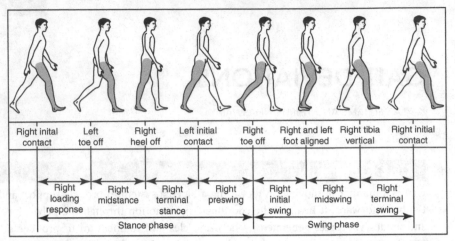

FIGURE 39.1 The gait cycle.

## THE MAKING OF A SMOOTH GAIT—THE DETERMINANTS OF GAIT

The primary goal of human gait is the smooth translation of the body from one point to another, safely and effectively with the least amount of energy expenditure. Energy is conserved by adopting a sinusoidal pathway that reduces the vertical and horizontal displacement of the center of mass. In order to understand how this is achieved, the major determinants of gait must be considered (Table 39.1). The *first* determinant describes the alternating *pelvic rotation* during the stance phase as the hip joint passes from relative internal rotation to relative external rotation. The *second* is *pelvic tilt*, where the pelvis lists downward toward the swinging limb, lowering this hip relative to the contralateral side. As body weight passes over the supporting limb, the *knee flexes* to on average 15 degrees consistent with the *third* determinant. This mechanism allows for shock absorption and maintenance of momentum. The *fourth* and *fifth* determinants describe the intimate relationship between angular *displacements of the ankle, foot, and knee* as the body weight passes over the supporting limb. The *sixth* determinant describes *lateral displacement of the pelvis* creating relative adduction at the hip and occurs twice during the gait cycle. These together are responsible for the smoothness of gait.[2]

## CLINICAL ASSESSMENT OF GAIT

Diagnosis of gait abnormality is based on history and physical findings. Additional elements of history to consider are current medications, history of falls, maximum walking distance, and the use of assistive devices or orthoses. The clinical examination provides a quick, comprehensive assessment of neurologic and musculoskeletal integration. Observation should include an assessment from all sides with examination distance spanning several meters without obstacles, with and without an assistive device and preferably without shoes.

**TABLE 39.1 THE SIX DETERMINANTS OF GAIT**

| REDUCE VERTICAL DISPLACEMENT | 1. PELVIC ROTATION |
|---|---|
| | Allows relative lengthening of the swinging leg in preparation for weight acceptance |
| | 2. PELVIC TILT |
| | Lowers the center of gravity at midstance |
| | 3. KNEE FLEXION IN STANCE |
| | ~15° flexion at footstrike for shock absorption |
| | 4. ANKLE/FOOT MECHANISMS |
| | Ankle plantar flexes to reduce fall of the pelvis |
| | 5. KNEE MECHANISMS |
| | Knee extends to restore length and reduce fall of the pelvis |
| REDUCE HORIZONTAL DISPLACEMENT | 6. LATERAL PELVIC DISPLACEMENT |
| | Displacement toward the stance limb to maintain the center of gravity above the stance foot |

Special attention should be given to posture, stance, initiation, step length, arm swing, turning, and speed.[3] Commonly seen gait abnormalities and their presentations are further described later.

Quantitative gait analysis may be used, but primarily for kinetic and kinematic evaluation in the research setting. In a gait laboratory, in addition to quantitative kinetic and kinematic data, electromyographic activity can be collected to evaluate muscle activation and coordination but may be limited by technical factors such as movement during gait and lactic acid accumulation.[4]

## Common Gait Abnormalities
### Antalgic

Antalgic gait is an adaptive pattern to decrease weight bearing through a painful limb. This is achieved by maintaining a fixed ankle position while lifting and planting the foot. Pain is commonly caused by musculoskeletal conditions including osteoarthritis, fractures, or sprains.[3]

### Genu Recurvatum

Genu recurvatum occurs in the stance phase with characteristic knee hyperextension as the foot strikes the ground causing the ground force reaction to pass well in front of the knee. This is classically caused by knee extensor weakness, knee extensor spasticity, or ankle plantar flexor spasticity. Knee extensor weakness incites a compensatory knee hyperextension to prevent a collapse of the knee. With knee extensor spasticity, the normal knee flexion seen at the initiation of the stance phase is replaced by knee extension, forcing the knee into further hyperextension with heel strike. Ankle plantar flexor spasticity or contracture can also contribute to knee hyperextension by limiting the forward translation of the tibia during the loading response. Genu recurvatum can also less commonly be caused by weakness of the pelvic stabilizers, knee flexors, or ankle dorsiflexors; pain in the ball of the foot; or proprioceptive disorders. It can increase the energy cost of gait and cause stress to ligaments and tendons in the back of the knee, further compromising knee stability.[5]

## Steppage (Neuropathic)

Steppage gait is a common compensation for foot drop. It utilizes excessive hip and knee flexion during the swing phase to functionally shorten the limb and allow for toe clearance. It does not decrease gait speed though is metabolically inefficient. Foot drop is predominantly caused by peripheral neuropathies though can also be seen in gastrocnemius–soleus spasticity secondary to central nervous system disorders or distal predominant myopathies.[6]

## Trendelenburg

Trendelenburg gait is identified during the stance phase when the pelvis tilts down opposite the stance leg as a result of weak ipsilateral hip abductors, primarily gluteus medius. This causes an exaggerated compensatory sway of the trunk toward the stance leg and a contralateral steppage gait to facilitate toe clearance. There also can be a compensatory trunk lean over the affected limb to decrease the hip adductor moment inherent to shifting body weight into single-leg stance. It becomes less evident with increased speed of walking due to decreased time spent in the stance phase.[4]

## Hemiplegic

Hemiplegic gait is often seen in neurologic disorders and is most notable for asymmetry and limb movement patterns, or synergies, on the paretic side. Common leg synergy patterns include hip extension, adduction and internal rotation, knee extension, and foot/ankle plantarflexion/inversion. Associated compensatory changes involving the hip and nonparetic side along with absent or diminished arm motion can also be seen. These changes may include prolonged paretic limb swing time and decreased paretic limb stance time, relative increase in paretic step length, and increase in double support periods. There is a decrease in hip extension that most often is caused by overactivation of the plantar flexor muscles that limits ankle dorsiflexion in the stance phase. Hip flexion at initial contact is similarly decreased, which may be attributed to overactive hip extensor or limited activity of hip flexors. In hemiplegic gait, the knee can either have increased knee flexion, reduced knee flexion followed by knee hyperextension, or excessive knee hyperextension during the stance phase. To compensate for decreased knee flexion, elevation of the hip and pelvis, or hip hiking, may be employed. Typically, there is an overall decreased cadence related to the degree of motor strength and balance.[7,8]

## Myopathic

Myopathic gait occurs with diffuse muscle weakness and is often associated with contracture formation. There is a characteristic wide base of support and decreased cadence with knee hyperextension used to compensate for knee instability. Toe walking patterns may be adopted to engage distal muscles for added muscle strength. As weakness progresses, lordosis increases, and lateral trunk deviations become more exaggerated due to weak pelvic girdle muscles.[9]

## Spastic Diplegic

Spastic diplegic gait is often seen in cerebral palsy and has an unsteady, decreased cadence with a characteristic crouch gait pattern. There is sustained knee flexion and toe walking, termed crouched gait, due to contractures of the hamstring and gastrocnemius–soleus complex. Hip internal rotation and flexion are also common as a result of spasticity and contracture. Gait is often symmetric, but very metabolically inefficient.[9]

## Ataxic

Ataxic gait is described as disorderly, uncoordinated movement and can be due to cerebellar or sensory deficits. Cerebellar ataxia displays as a broad-based gait with variable step lengths and leg movements. It is often paired with a slight stoop and bends at the hip to steady the stance limb. There is great difficulty with higher-level gait tasks such as tandem walking or walking on uneven surfaces. In sensory ataxia, there is loss of proprioception most commonly caused by sensory polyneuropathy or dorsal column lesion. This can similarly lead to a broad-based stance with shortened step length and slow, cautious progression. It may also feature a stomping quality as the feet are lifted high and strike the ground forcefully due to decreased proprioceptive input. The two can be distinguished clinically as with sensory ataxia, visual input can be used to compensate and thus symptoms worsen with the eyes closed whereas, in cerebellar ataxia, symptoms are static with eyes open or closed.[3]

## Parkinsonian

Parkinsonian gait is a rigid akinetic gait most classically seen in Parkinson's disease with slowed walking speed even in the early stages of the disease process. There is decreased lifting of the feet commonly termed shuffling gait, and increased variability in step-to-step patterns. Characteristic festinating gait is apparent with a leaned forward posture with decreasing stride length as step frequency increases. Freezing, or difficulty with initiation of gait, turning or approaching perceived obstacles can also be seen. In the early stages, freezing is typically responsive to antiparkinson's medication, though as the disease progresses, freezing may become resistant to levodopa replacement. It is important to note that antiparkinson's medication may exacerbate orthostatic hypotension leading to a more cautious, insecure gait as well.[3]

## Psychogenic

Psychogenic, or functional gait, is a commonly diagnosed abnormality of gait. Its etiology is poorly understood and is a diagnosis of exclusion. Gait is characterized as slow and hesitant with a wide base and bizarre irregular strides. Astasia-abasia is a commonly used term to describe the inability to stand or walk with characteristic bouncing or buckling of the knees without falls. Functional lower limb dystonia can also be seen along with huffing and puffing. It is largely distractible and associated with exaggerated effort out of proportion to movement. Psychogenic gait can interfere significantly with normal gait and normal function. Early diagnosis and appropriate treatment have been shown to improve gait and prevent wheelchair dependence.[10]

### Senile

Gait impairments are common in the aging population due to decreased muscle power, impaired proprioceptive function, poor vision, frontal disorders, and musculoskeletal disorders. There is a change in gait pattern in the older adults notable for decreased step length and gait speed (though cadence remains stable), a wider step width, reduced arm swing, and stooped posture. Irrespective of underlying comorbid conditions, there is increased relative fear and actual risk of falls. Gait pattern often improves significantly with a small amount of assistance, even as little as handheld support. In the aging population, self-selected walking speed is a sensitive marker of overall health status and life expectancy.[3]

## TREATMENT

Functional ambulation is an ability that is desired despite the diagnosis, prognosis, or degree of deficit. Pathologic gait deviations are a subconscious compensation to promote upright stability at the expense of metabolic efficiency. The goal of treating gait abnormalities is to regain stable, confident ambulation that allows for the highest level of functional independence within varied environments. This is best achieved by a multidimensional, multidisciplinary approach.[9]

Gait training provides a transition to ease the process of acquiring new walking skills in preparation for ongoing progression and maintenance through a home exercise program. Initial gait training should include practice with varied environmental barriers such as curbs, steps, inclines, or uneven terrain to prepare for obstacles that may be encountered in the future.[9] Training may utilize technology such as body weight-supported treadmill training or other electromechanical assisted gait training systems that have been shown to facilitate neuromotor recovery.[4]

Orthoses perform several functions including support and alignment, prevention of deformity, correction of deformity, substitution for function, or reduction of discomfort. When used correctly, they influence functional capability and musculoskeletal alignment for more optimal ambulation.[9] Consideration must be taken after prescribing a new orthosis, progressing slowly into full-time use, and planning for annual to biannual follow-up to monitor wear, ensure adequate fit, and re-evaluate necessity.

Assistive devices can aid in stability, assist in propulsion, and transmit sensory cues, making safe upright ambulation feasible. A cane is the simplest device and primarily enhances balance and provides sensory feedback from the environment. Walkers have a framed base providing bilateral support and can provide varying stability depending on the combination of tips and wheels for base construction. Various types of crutches may be used to provide stability and decrease weight bearing, though do not necessarily address gait asymmetry.[11] Functional electrical stimulation of the peroneal nerve has been used for foot drop and is effective in persons with stroke.[12]

Medical treatment of underlying condition must be considered. Treatment of spasticity with botulinum toxin and other chemodenervation options has been shown to improve walking speed and step length and has largely replaced tendon transfer or surgical release procedures.[4]

## FUNCTIONAL PROGNOSIS AND OUTCOMES

Due to varying etiologies of gait abnormalities, prognosis and outcomes vary, depending on the underlying condition. Gait abnormalities should be addressed early to potentially prevent establishing inefficient compensations and significant asymmetry. Typically, the goal is to limit energy inefficiency and pain due to abnormal gait; however, in the chronic stage, interfering with the adapted asymmetric gait can cause a decrease in functional ambulation at the optimal level.[8]

## REFERENCES

The full reference list appears in the digital product found on http://connect.springerpub.com/content/book/978-0-8261-6226-7/part/part03/chapter/ch39

# HETEROTOPIC OSSIFICATION

KENDL M. SANKARY AND KATE E. DELANEY

## CORE DEFINITIONS

Heterotopic ossification (HO) is the formation of extraskeletal lamellar bone in muscle and soft tissue, thought to be caused by an aberrant tissue repair process. This can occur in certain neurologic diagnoses including stroke, traumatic brain injury (TBI), spinal cord injury (SCI), and brain tumor. HO is also associated with nonneurologic diagnoses including amputation, fracture, arthroplasty (most commonly total hip arthroplasty [THA] and total knee arthroplasty [TKA]), muscular trauma, burns, and some genetic disorders. This condition can greatly impact patients' functional recovery from injury, leading to joint contractures, chronic pain, and nearby nerve and vessel injury.

Numerous grading scales have been proposed to classify the severity of HO using x-ray findings at specific joints, including the Brooker classification system for the hip (see Box 40.1), the Hastings and Graham system at the elbow, and the De Valle classification, which is a modified Brooker classification. These scales have been developed for clinical research and surgical planning and are not typically used for diagnosis or prognostication for patients with HO.

### BOX 40.1

**BROOKER CLASSIFICATION SYSTEM FOR HETEROTOPIC OSSIFICATION AT THE HIP[1]**

| Class | Definition |
|-------|------------|
| I | Islands of bone within soft tissues of the hip |
| II | Bone spurs in the pelvis or femur but with ≥1 cm between bone surfaces |
| III | Bone spurs within the pelvis or femur but with <1 cm between bone surfaces |
| IV | Ankylosis of the hip |

The full list of resources and references appears in the digital product found on http://connect.springerpub.com/content/book/978-0-8261-6226-7/part/part03/chapter/ch40

## ETIOLOGY AND PATHOPHYSIOLOGY

The exact mechanism for HO development is not fully understood. It is thought that increased activity of osteoblasts and increased mesenchymal stem cell differentiation into osteoblasts can lead to HO development. The trigger for this process can be neurologic, traumatic, or genetic, as previously described. Research suggests that an exaggerated inflammatory response increases tissue expression of bone morphogenic proteins (BMPs) recruiting mesenchymal stem cells to the affected area and facilitating their transformation into osteoblasts, which form the bone matrix. Osteoblasts produce alkaline phosphatase, which inactivates pyrophosphate, promoting calcium deposition and mineralization of the bone matrix. As with normal bone formation, heterotopic bone goes through predictable stages as it matures. In the early stage, immature bone is composed of a collagen matrix with sparse calcification. At this stage, x-rays are unable to detect HO; only bone scan, MRI, or ultrasound can detect early HO. In the intermediate stage, there is increased inflammation, vascularity, and continued calcification and typically HO can be seen on x-ray at this time. The final stage is mature lamellar bone, at which point, histological examination closely resembles normal bone.[2-4] The disease progression of HO allows for multiple possible treatment targets (see Figure 40.1).

In the case of TBI, SCI, and burns, the risk of developing HO increases with the severity of injury. Between 8% and 20% of patients with TBI develop clinically significant HO. With TBI, the risk of HO increases with any associated polytrauma. In SCI, clinically significant HO develops in about 20% of patients. Patients with cervical or thoracic level of injury, more complete injury, severe spasticity, impaired cognition, tracheostomy, pneumonia, and UTI are at higher risk.[3] Burns involving >20% of the body substantially increase the likelihood of HO formation.[6]

In the orthopedic population, HO is most often due to fracture or surgical intervention. The overall rate of HO development in patients undergoing THA is 53%, with a significantly higher risk in bilateral THA, prior history of HO, ankylosing spondylitis, diffuse idiopathic

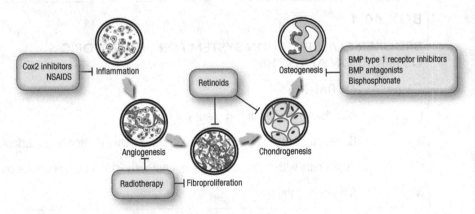

**FIGURE 40.1** Progression of heterotopic ossification and treatment targets.[5]

*Source*: Reprinted by permission from Shimono K, Uchibe K, Kuboki T, Iwamoto M. The pathophysiology of heterotopic ossification: current treatment considerations in dentistry. *Jpn Dental Sci Rev.* 2014;50(1):1–8. doi:10.1016/j.jdsr.2013.07.003

skeletal hyperostosis (DISH), and Paget's disease.[7] In traumatic fractures, HO at the hip and elbow have been studied most, with an incidence of about 40% at each joint. Risk factors include concomitant neurologic injury, delayed internal fixation, and the use of bone graft. In patients with acetabular fractures, the risk is increased in patients who need long-term mechanical ventilation. Injury severity, sex, and fracture type do not affect the risk of developing HO in patients with acetabular fractures. In elbow fractures, HO most commonly develops posteromedially. There does appear to be a relationship between specific surgical interventions for fracture fixation and development of HO.[6]

HO has been shown to form in 23% of the residual limbs of lower extremity amputees, regardless of the cause for amputation. When studied in the civilian population, there is no difference in the prevalence of HO in patients with traumatic versus nontraumatic amputations. Risk factors for the development of HO in amputation are blast injury and concomitant neurologic injury.[8]

## DIAGNOSTIC APPROACH

HO most frequently presents as decreasing range of motion (ROM), pain, or stiffness at the affected joint and can be accompanied by localized swelling, erythema, warmth, and low-grade fever.[9] There should be a heightened suspicion of HO in patients with an associated neurologic injury, burn injury, recent THA, or orthopedic trauma. Differential diagnosis often includes deep venous thrombosis (DVT), hematoma, tumor, cellulitis, hardware infection, osteomyelitis, thrombophlebitis, and fracture. The highest risk of HO is 3 to 4 months out from injury, though it can develop as early as 3 weeks up to about 6 months after the injury. The location of HO formation follows specific patterns depending on the underlying diagnosis. In SCI and TBI, the hip joints are most commonly affected, and in burns, it is the elbow (see Exhibit 40.1). In SCI, the site of HO formation is always caudal to the level of injury, whereas in TBI HO can occur anywhere in the body.

Initial laboratory workup should include serum alkaline phosphatase, erythrocyte sedimentation rate (ESR), C-reactive protein (CRP), creatine phosphokinase (CK), and white blood cell count (WBC). Alkaline phosphatase may take 2 weeks to elevate and reaches a maximum value at 10 weeks after HO begins to develop. Alkaline phosphatase >250 IU/L is associated with HO in THA patients. Of note, the level of serum alkaline phosphatase does not correlate with the maturity of HO. ESR and CRP are inflammatory markers that can be elevated in early HO but are not specific for HO. Elevated CK is associated with a more aggressive course of HO and may correlate with resistance to etidronate therapy.

In addition to the previous laboratory evaluation, imaging modalities including x-ray, Techneitium-99 bone scan, ultrasound, CT scan, and MRI can be helpful for diagnosis and evaluating the severity of HO. X-rays begin to show HO starting 3 to 4 weeks after bone begins to form. Classically, Technetium-99 bone scans have been thought of as the most sensitive method of evaluating for HO as they reveal changes as early as 2.5 weeks. However, recent studies have revealed that MRI can show changes consistent with HO within 1 to 2 days of the start of symptoms. Obtaining a CT scan may be recommended for surgical planning but is not used for initial evaluation.[3,6]

**EXHIBIT 40.1** Common locations of heterotopic ossification per injury type.[6]

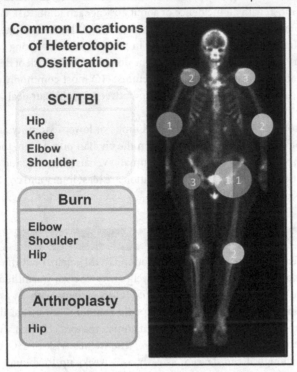

**Common Locations of Heterotopic Ossification**

**SCI/TBI**

Hip
Knee
Elbow
Shoulder

**Burn**

Elbow
Shoulder
Hip

**Arthroplasty**

Hip

*Source*: Reprinted by permission from Ranganathan K, Loder S, Agarwal S, et al. Heterotopic ossification: basic-science principles and clinical correlates. *J Bone Joint Surg Am*. 2015;97:1101–1111.

## TREATMENT

Once HO is already present, several studies have looked at the effect of bisphosphonates or disphosphonates in preventing expansion. These medications are thought to prevent mineralization of the osteoid matrix.[10] In SCI, Stover's protocol has classically been used for the treatment of HO that consists of etidronate 20 mg/kg for 2 weeks followed by 10 mg/kg for 10 weeks. In a study using this protocol, there was a pretreatment HO rate of 22% to 25% seen on x-ray; whereas, at follow-up, the incidence of HO seen on x-ray in the treatment group was 30% while it was 41% in the placebo group.[11] Finerman et al. treated patients with SCI or THA with clinical signs but no x-ray evidence of HO with the same protocol. After the treatment course, 6% had HO on x-ray in the treatment group (2% was clinically significant) versus 27% in the placebo group (13% clinically significant). After etidronate treatment stopped, the incidence did increase in the treatment group but the lesions were less extensive.[12] Garland et al. found that using 20 mg/kg for 6 months is also effective.[13]

For burn patients, although a number of case studies have reported that etidronate could be used to treat or prevent HO, a study evaluating etidronate in fact showed a higher incidence of HO in the treatment group (46.4%) as compared to the control group (13.8%).

However, in this study, the total body surface area was higher in the treatment group, and treatment was given for 39 days on average, which is shorter than the typical duration of treatment that has been found to be effective in other diagnoses.[14]

In one study of HO in severe TBI, etidronate 20 mg/kg per day for 3 months followed by 10 mg/kg per day for an additional 3 months was used in 10 patients and HO was found in 20% of those who had been treated compared to 70% of injury-matched controls.[15]

Radiation can be used as a primary treatment of HO in SCI. In a study by Sautter-Bihl et al., in 33 joints with HO, 50% showed absence of radiographic abnormalities after radiation and <10% showed progression of HO.[16]

Surgical indications for resection include loss of function, difficulty with seating or positioning, and pressure injury/ulceration related to the HO.[17] Approximately 5% of SCI patients with HO will require surgical resection.[18]

It has historically been thought that surgical resection of HO should be done after maturation of HO in order to prevent recurrence as well as to allow for maximal neurologic recovery. For this reason, some have recommended visualization of mature bone on bone scan or x-ray and normal serum alkaline phosphatase prior to operating.[6,13,18] Therefore, preferred timing for surgical resection may occur at 6 to 9 months in traumatic HO, 12 months in SCI, and 18 months in TBI, though the average time to surgery is often longer.[7,13]

Postoperatively, rehabilitation goals are to regain and maintain ROM, with passive ROM up to several times a day starting at least 48 hours postop for the hip and until soft tissue swelling improves in the elbow.[10,18]

## FUNCTIONAL PROGNOSIS AND OUTCOMES

For all diagnoses and joints, on average, there are reported improvements in ROM after surgical intervention. In TBI, postoperative recurrence may be associated with spasticity and there may be a higher risk of recurrence in patients with more severe neurologic deficits, longer duration of coma, and more severe HO. Recurrence rates have been reported to be around 20% in a meta-analysis. The rate of recurrence was not significantly different when surgery was performed at 13, 21, or 30 months postdiagnosis of HO.[19] For burn patients treated with surgery, recurrence has been reported at 6.7%.[20] Postoperative medical or radiation treatment may be helpful to prevent recurrence.[17,21]

Medically, NSAIDs have been found to reduce the incidence and severity of HO in spinal cord injury (SCI) and total hip arthroplasty (THA).[22,23] It is thought that NSAIDs suppress mesenchymal cell proliferation into osteoblasts.[24] In THA, indomethacin 75 mg total daily for 2 to 6 weeks was found to reduce incidence and severity of HO.[23] In SCI, indomethacin 75 mg daily for a 3-week course found a higher incidence of HO in the placebo group (65%) versus the treatment group (25%).[22] In TBI, indomethacin 75 mg daily or etidronate 20 mg/kg daily for 3 months at a minimum and up to 6 months if there is evidence of recurrence can help prevent expansion.[25] Additionally, warfarin may prevent HO formation via inhibiting vitamin K-dependent synthesis of osteocalcin.[26]

Postoperatively, radiation treatment is used to prevent recurrence of HO. Thus far, there is no evidence that there is an increased risk of cancer from radiation treatment in this population.[23,24]

## BASIC ORDER SETS

### Initial Evaluation of HO
### Laboratory Studies

Serum alkaline phosphatase

Erythrocyte sedimentation rate (ESR)

C-reactive protein (CRP)

Creatine phosphokinase (CK)

White blood cell count (WBC)

### Imaging Studies

Plain x-ray *(if negative, consider Technetium-99 bone scan, ultrasound, or MRI)*

## RESOURCES AND REFERENCES

The full list of resources and references appears in the digital product found on http://connect
.springerpub.com/content/book/978-0-8261-6226-7/part/part03/chapter/ch40

# HYDROCEPHALUS

CLAUSYL (CJ) PLUMMER II

## CORE DEFINITIONS

"Hydrocephalus" originates from the Greek words "hydro," meaning water, and "cephalus," meaning head.[1,2] It is defined as the accumulation of cerebrospinal fluid (CSF) in the various cavities within the intracranial space.[1] The potential spaces in which this accumulation can occur to include the third ventricle, fourth ventricle, and the lateral ventricles. According to the American Association of Neurological Surgeons, hydrocephalus is defined as "a condition in which excess CSF builds up within the ventricles of the brain and may increase pressure within the head."[3]

## ETIOLOGY AND PATHOPHYSIOLOGY

Noncommunicating or obstructive hydrocephalus occurs when an intraventricular obstruction impedes CSF flow.[4] It is typically caused by blood (i.e., interventricular hemorrhage), external compression (e.g., tumors), or a congenital condition (i.e., stenosis). The obstruction can occur in several locations to include the Foramen of Monro (between the lateral ventricles and the third ventricle), aqueduct of Sylvius (between the third and fourth ventricle), or the various foramina distal to the fourth ventricle.[4,5] Intraventricular hemorrhages, infections (such as meningitis), and traumatic brain injury result in scarring of the meningeal lining or damage to the arachnoid villi, which then inhibit reabsorption of CSF, thus leading to enlarged ventricles.[2,5]

Normal-pressure hydrocephalus (NPH) involves accumulation of CSF in the ventricles without an increase in intracranial pressure. Ventriculomegaly may be present. The classic triad associated with NPH, Hakim's triad, is gait abnormality, dementia-like impairment, and urinary incontinence. This triad is thought to be pathognomonic for NPH, though patients do not always have all three findings. The abnormal gait pattern typically seen in NPH is a broad-based shuffling gait. NPH can be further divided into idiopathic NPH and secondary NPH, with the latter being the result of traumatic brain injury, subarachnoid hemorrhage, and/or meningitis.[4,6]

The etiology of NPH is less straightforward. There are several theories about its etiology, including impaired CSF flow, vascular anomalies, and, to a lesser degree, neurodegeneration, inflammation, and hereditary factors.[4] The impairment in CSF flow is thought to be related

The full list of resources and references appears in the digital product found on http://connect .springerpub.com/content/book/978-0-8261-6226-7/part/part03/chapter/ch41

to alterations in CSF pulsations that occur after chronic systolic–diastolic changes that affect cerebral perfusion. The vascular anomalies thought to be related to NPH involve arterial hypertension and/or venous pressure abnormalities (choroidal venous pressures) leading to enlarged ventricles.[4]

Congenital hydrocephalus is thought to be present at birth and involves blockage at the Sylvian aqueduct located between the third and fourth ventricle.[2,7] According to the Hydrocephalus Association, the most common cause of congenital hydrocephalus is aqueductal stenosis.[2] Neural tube defects are another common cause of congenital hydrocephalus.[2] Other possible causes include arachnoid cysts, Chiari malformation, and Dandy–Walker syndrome (characterized by deformity of the fourth ventricle, large posterior fossa, and hypoplasia of the cerebellar vermis).[2,8]

The term "hydrocephalus ex vacuo" is used to describe ventricular enlargement in the setting of brain tissue loss after traumatic brain injury or stroke.[3]

## DIAGNOSTIC APPROACH

### History

The signs and symptoms associated with hydrocephalus vary depending on type and patient's age. The most common signs and symptoms in infants and young children include bulging fontanels, enlarged head circumference, irritability, vomiting, and headache. For young and middle-aged adults, the more common symptoms include long-standing headaches, gait abnormalities, cognitive impairment, and urinary urgency or incontinence.[2]

Older adults, who are typically affected by NPH, exhibit gait disturbances, cognitive impairment, and urinary incontinence (i.e., Hakim's triad).[2,6,9] The gait disturbances classically seen are symmetrical, hypokinetic, wide-based movement with shuffling, impaired foot clearance, multistep turns with instability, and poor gait initiation.[4,6] Gait may also be described as magnetic, where the feet appear to be "magnetically" attached to the floor with poor ground clearance during the swing phase. There is typically also evidence of motor apraxia and difficulties with changes in position (e.g., sit to stand).[4] The cognitive impairments typically involve learning difficulties, recall disturbances, executive function deficits, and reduced processing speed with psychomotor issues.[4] It is important to evaluate cognitive performance during the physical examination (Mini-Mental Status Examination or Montreal Cognitive Assessment [MoCA]) with subsequent neuropsychological testing to differentiate the types of cognitive deficits present. The urinary complaints typically start with urinary urgency in early stages and progress to urge incontinence.[3,4,6]

Other common signs and symptoms include pain, headaches, changes in mood, nausea, drowsiness, and balance issues.[1,4,6,9] If a patient has already been diagnosed or has a shunt for hydrocephalus, it is important to gain an understanding of what combination of symptoms they typically present with in times of worsening hydrocephalus. This information can also be obtained by inquiring about the type of signs/symptoms present during past shunt failures/malfunction. The clinical challenge of hydrocephalus is that these findings are nonspecific and further complicated by comorbidities that may confound the clinical presentation.

## Physical Examination

The clinical examination should work to not only identify classic findings observed in hydrocephalus but also gain an understanding of confounding aspects of the clinical picture. For this reason, it is recommended that individuals undergo a full neurologic examination coupled with manual muscle testing of the upper and lower extremities. The fundoscopic examination is also important, as papilledema should be ruled out. As mentioned previously, the gait assessment is very important, as is the cognitive assessment with the Mini-Mental Status Examination or the MoCA.[6] In the case of the pediatric population, an inspection of the head (circumference with growth charting, presence of fontanels) is important to track.[8]

## Diagnostic Testing

Congenital hydrocephalus is typically assessed by antenatal ultrasonography (US) to evaluate ventricular size. In pediatric obstructive hydrocephalus, US is the modality of choice to prevent ionizing radiation exposure and the need for sedation/anesthesia.[2,7,8] If abnormalities are found on US, MRI is warranted for categorization. For older children, brain MRI is preferred, as it is a comprehensive evaluation that can evaluate CSF flow and flow dynamics.[8] Brain MRI is also preferred for adults who have a suspected obstructive pattern. Head CT may be performed, but visualization is better with MRI, and it requires radiation exposure.[2,6,9]

The modified Evans ratio is a screening evaluation for enlarged ventricles. It is determined by calculating the ratio between the maximum width of the frontal horns (lateral ventricles) and the widest diameter of the brain on the same axial CT or MRI images.[6] Generally, ventriculomegaly is considered present when the ratio is greater or equal to 0.3, but more accurate age cutoffs have been proposed, particularly for those over the age of 65.[6,9,10]

A lumbar puncture (LP) is not required for the diagnosis of hydrocephalus but is helpful in the evaluation for potential shunt placement.[4,6,9] Neuroimaging to rule out herniation should be obtained prior to LP. The assessment involves LP for drainage of up to 50 mL of CSF and monitoring gait and subjective symptom improvement over the next 30 to 60 minutes or several days.[6] Objective gait function evaluations such as the *Tinetti score* or the Timed Up and Go Test should be used to monitor improvement instead of relying on subjective symptom reports.[6] The latter test has a strong positive predictive value for a response after shunt placement, although other studies that have demonstrated improvement in gait after shunt placement when LP screening results were equivocal or negative.[6]

An external lumbar drain catheter may be placed and left in place to drain CSF at a set rate (typically at 10 mL per hour).[2,4,6] This method requires hospitalization for approximately 72 hours for monitoring. Gait assessments and cognitive testing are performed before, during, and after the drain is removed.[2,6]

## TREATMENT

The definitive treatment of hydrocephalus is surgical placement of a shunt to divert CSF flow. Shunt placement is indicated in congenital hydrocephalus, obstructive hydrocephalus, and NPH.[2,4] The most common catheter used is a ventriculoperitoneal (VP) shunt, but ventriculoatrial (VA) shunts and lumboperitoneal shunts may also be used.[2,11] VP shunts divert CSF fluid from the ventricles (most commonly, R lateral ventricle) to the abdomen. The three major types of shunt valves include slit valves, diaphragm valves, and spring-loaded ball in cone valves.[2] Programmable shunts allow for adjusting the amount of CSF to be drained and have become more common, as there is no need for surgical intervention to make adjustments.[2]

An endoscopic third ventriculostomy is a surgical procedure that creates an opening on the floor of the third ventricle to allow for CSF drainage into the lower cavities of the brain, thus effectively bypassing the aqueduct of Sylvius (which connects the third and fourth ventricle).[2,3,12] This surgery is an alternative to traditional shunting and is indicated in patients who have obstructive hydrocephalus.[2,12]

## FUNCTIONAL PROGNOSIS AND OUTCOMES

The prognosis for individuals with hydrocephalus is favorable, assuming definitive treatment is appropriately established.[13,14] There have been studies that have demonstrated functional recovery in gait, ambulation, and cognition after shunt placement. The challenge of predicting the degree of functional improvement after shunting remains.[2,4,6]

## RESOURCES AND REFERENCES

The full list of resources and references appears in the digital product found on http://connect .springerpub.com/content/book/978-0-8261-6226-7/part/part03/chapter/ch41

# INFECTIONS

AUBREE M. FAIRFULL AND AARON E. BUNNELL

Rehabilitation populations are at high risk of morbidity and mortality from infectious disease. This is due to high rates of neurogenic bladder and bowel, impaired pulmonary function, aspiration, skin breakdown, colonization with multidrug resistant organisms and surgical procedures. Physiatrists have a key role in the prevention, diagnosis and treatment of infections. This chapter will plan to cover the most common infections in the rehabilitation population including urinary tract infections, pneumonia, sepsis, and meningitis.

For all infections, the use of institution-specific antibiograms and antibiotic stewardship is recommended to minimize patient harm, decrease exposure to unnecessary antibiotics, and reduce the development of antibiotic resistance.

## URINARY TRACT INFECTIONS

### Core Definitions

*Asymptomatic bacteriuria*—urine culture growing more than 100,000 CFU/mL of bacteria in a patient without urinary tract symptoms or signs; however, for those with indwelling catheters, any detectable concentration of bacteria is considered bacteriuria.[1,2]

*Urinary tract infection*—significant bacteriuria (urine culture growing more than 100,000 CFU/mL) with symptoms or signs attributable to the urinary tract without alternate source of infection.

*Cystitis*—infection of the bladder or lower urinary tract.

*Acute uncomplicated cystitis*—cystitis in a patient without associated catherization, immunocompromised status, urologic abnormalities, or pregnancy.[3]

*Pyelonephritis*—infection of the kidney and upper urinary tract.

*Urosepsis*—clinically evident severe infection of the urinary tract and/or the male genital tract including the prostate, with features consistent with systemic inflammatory response syndrome.[4]

*Catheter-associated urinary tract infection (CAUTI)*—Involves the following parameters[5]:

1. Signs/symptoms consistent with UTI
2. No other identified source of infection
3. ≥100,000 CFU/mL of ≥1 bacterial species in a urine specimen from a patient in whom an indwelling urinary catheter was in place for more than two consecutive days AND an indwelling urinary catheter was in place on the date of event or the day before.

---

The full list of resources and references appears in the digital product found on http://connect .springerpub.com/content/book/978-0-8261-6226-7/part/part03/chapter/ch42

## Etiology and Pathophysiology

The most common pathogens seen in UTI and various clinical populations are described in Table 42.1 below.

Many rehabilitation patients have injuries resulting in neurogenic bladder, which places them at significantly increased risk for recurrent urinary tract infections compared to the general population. Factors that contribute to this include chronic indwelling catheter use, bladder stasis and overdistention, vesicoureteral reflux, and nephrolithiasis.[6] The primary risk factor for catheter-associated bacteriuria is duration of catheter use, with an increased incidence of 3–8% per day.[7]

## Diagnostic Approach
### History

In women, the new onset of frequency and dysuria, with the absence of vaginal discharge or irritation, has a positive predictive value of 90 percent for UTI.[3] CAUTI most commonly presents with symptoms such as fever, rigors, altered mental status, malaise, flank pain, costovertebral angle tenderness, acute hematuria, and/or pelvic discomfort.[5] When the catheter has been removed, the patient may experience dysuria, urgency or frequency of urination, or suprapubic tenderness.

In the rehabilitation population, it is important to consider that limited reporting of UTI symptoms can occur in patients with neurogenic bladder due to abnormal or absent sensation. An indication of a UTI may be worsening of the patient's underlying functional impairments such as weakness or cognitive status. Patients with a spinal cord injury (SCI) may develop signs and symptoms such as increased spasticity, autonomic dysreflexia, bladder spasms, or sense of unease.[5]

### Testing

Urine cultures are recommended in patients with suspected pyelonephritis, UTI symptoms that do not resolve or that recur within two to four weeks after completing treatment, and for those who present with atypical symptoms like flank pain or delirium.[3]

Urine analysis and urine culture should be obtained for suspected UTI in a patient with an indwelling urinary catheter if:

### TABLE 42.1 COMMON UTI PATHOGENS[2,5]

| CONDITION | PRIMARY CAUSE | OTHER CAUSES |
|---|---|---|
| Uncomplicated cystitis | Escherichia coli | Proteus mirabilis, Klebsiella pneumoniae, and Staphylococcus saprophyticus |
| UTI with long-term catheterization | Polymicrobial | Serratia, Citrobacter, P. aeruginosa, and coagulase-negative staphylococci. |
| UTI in spinal cord injury | Gram-negative bacilli, Enterococci | |

UTI, urinary tract infection.

## TABLE 42.2 CRITERIA FOR SIGNIFICANT BACTERIURIA IN SCI

| BLADDER MANAGEMENT METHOD | COLONY FORMING UNITS |
|---|---|
| Intermittent catheterization | $10^2$ + |
| Clean-void specimens from patients who use external condom collecting devices | $10^4$ + |
| Indwelling catheters | Any detection |

SCI, spinal cord injury.

1. The catheter was in place for more than two consecutive days the catheter was in place during onset of symptoms or removed the day before onset

   For presumed CAUTI, a urine specimen for culture should be obtained prior to initiating antimicrobial therapy and after replacing the catheter.[5]

   The diagnosis of UTI in patients with SCI is based the following criteria[2]:

1. Significant bacteriuria as defined in Table 42.2
2. Pyuria
3. Signs and symptoms such as fever, malaise, dysuria, urinary incontinence, spasticity, autonomic dysreflexia or lethargy

## Imaging

Genitourinary ultrasound may be considered for patients who do not respond to treatment to evaluate for pyelonephritis, abscesses, stones, and urine flow blockage. MRI or CT may be performed to evaluate for stones or obstruction. An intravenous pyelogram or voiding cystourethrogram may be used to examine the urinary tract for structural abnormalities, urethral narrowing, or incomplete emptying. Cystoscopy can be used to detect structural abnormalities and interstitial cystitis in individuals with recurrent UTI, particularly those with SCI.[2]

## Treatment

*Asymptomatic bacteriuria:* No treatment is required for asymptomatic patients including those with long-term indwelling catheters or SCI.[6] In patients with neurogenic bladder, asymptomatic bacteriuria is not typically treated unless stone-forming bacteria such as Proteus, Klebsiella, or Serratia are present.[3] For elderly patients with cognitive impairment or delirium, who have bacteriuria but lack genitourinary symptoms or systemic signs of infection, best practice suggests assessment for other causes and careful observation, rather than immediate antimicrobial treatment.[6] However, it is important to consider whether accurate symptoms can be reported based on the patient's cognitive condition.

*Uncomplicated UTI:* Recommended antibiotic treatment for patients with an uncomplicated UTI can be seen in Table 42.3.

*CAUTI:* Empiric therapy depends on the severity of illness and on the extent of the infection. Narrower spectrum agents such as Bactrim or ceftriaxone is appropriate empiric treat-

**TABLE 42.3 UNCOMPLICATED UTI ANTIBIOTIC TREATMENT[6]**

| ANTIBIOTIC AGENT | DOSAGE | DURATION |
|---|---|---|
| Trimethoprim-sulfamethoxazole | 160/800 mg twice-daily | 3 days |
| Nitrofurantoin monohydrate/ macrocrystals | 100 mg twice daily | 5 days |
| *Alternates: amoxicillin-clavulanate, cefdinir, cefaclor, and cefpodoxime-proxetil | | 3–7 days |

*Alternate choices when recommended agents cannot be used.
UTI, urinary tract infection.

ment for lower tract infections. Broad spectrum antibiotic with anti-pseudomonal should be started for septic patients or if pyelonephritis is suspected.

The urine culture results should be used to ensure empirical regimen provides appropriate coverage and to allow tailoring of the regimen on the basis of antimicrobial susceptibility data. Initial antimicrobial treatment duration is typically 7 days if prompt resolution of symptoms is observed; treatment extension to 10–14 days is recommended for those with a delayed response (febrile >72 hrs on appropriate treatment), regardless of continued catheterization. If an indwelling catheter has been in place for >2 weeks at the onset of CAUTI, the catheter should be removed or replaced to hasten resolution of symptoms and to reduce the risk of subsequent infection.[5]

*Urosepsis*: If suspected, empiric broad-spectrum intravenous antimicrobial therapy should be initiated.[4] As with CAUTI, urine culture results should be followed to guide treatment.

### Functional Prognosis and Outcomes

Patients with neurogenic bladder and frequent recurrent UTI should be investigated with urodynamic studies, ultrasound, or cystoscopy to identify modifiable causes of UTI such as calculi, bladder debris, poor bladder compliance, or detrusor sphincter dyssynergia.

## PNEUMONIA

### Core Definitions

*Aspiration pneumonia*—pneumonia due to aspiration of bacteria into the lungs. Associated with compromise of airway defenses often due to due to dysphagia, altered consciousness, or use of sedatives.

*Aspiration pneumonitis*—aspiration of gastric contents or chemicals without pulmonary infection.

*Hospital acquired pneumonia (HAP)*—pneumonia not present at the time of hospital admission and occurring 48 hours or more after admission.

*Ventilator acquired pneumonia (VAP)*—a subset of hospital-acquired pneumonia occurring >48 hours after endotracheal intubation with mechanical ventilation.

## Risk Factors

Baseline respiratory dysfunction may result in atelectasis and subsequent pneumonia. Dysphagia, altered mental status, and decreased respiratory drive is frequently seen in the rehabilitation population which places this population at high risk for aspiration. Medications that are deliriogenic or impair respiratory drive can also increase a patient's risk of respiratory dysfunction.

Specific risk factors for aspiration in the SCI population include supine position, gastric reflux, decreased ability to expectorate or swallow saliva, medications that decrease gastrointestinal (GI) motility or cause nausea/vomiting. The presence of a trachcostomy is the strongest predictor of dysphagia in this population.[8]

Major risk factors for VAP include the supine positioning, extensive burns, cardiothoracic surgery, acute respiratory distress syndrome (ARDS), head trauma, presence of tracheostomy, anterior approach to spinal stabilization, and ongoing mechanical ventilation.[9]

## Etiology

Bacterial aspiration pneumonia in the hospital is mostly due to gram-negative organisms, including P. aeruginosa. S. pneumoniae, S. aureus, H. influenzae, and Enterobacteriaceae. HAP and VAP may be caused by a variety of aerobic and anaerobic gram-positive cocci and gram-negative bacilli. The most common pathogens in HAP and VAP are similar including Acinetobacter baumannii, Pseudomonas aeruginosa, and Klebsiella pneumoniae.[10]

## Diagnostic Approach
### History, Physical Examination, Labs, and Imaging

Signs and symptoms of aspiration pneumonia can include cough, dyspnea, pleuritic pain, fever or chills, acute functional or cognitive decline, and tachycardia. It is important to note that clinical manifestations of pneumonia may be delayed 24–48 hours after a suspected or witnessed aspiration event. Intensive oral care and pulmonary toilet are crucial in the first 24 hours after a suspected event. Signs of pulmonary compromise should be closely monitored including increased respiratory rate, hypercapnia, fatigue, tachycardia, vital capacity < 15 cc/kg, or negative inspiratory force < 20 cm $H_2O$. Chest radiograph should be performed if any of these changes are present.[8] The diagnosis of aspiration pneumonia must be inferred when an at-risk patient has radiographic evidence of a bronchopulmonary infiltrate.

There is no gold standard for the diagnosis of HAP or VAP. VAP is suspected when the individual develops a new or progressive infiltrate on chest radiograph, leukocytosis, and purulent tracheobronchial secretions.[11]

Due to the growing frequency of MDROs and the risks of initial ineffective therapy, cultures of respiratory secretions should be obtained from all patients with suspected VAP.[12] Endotracheal aspiration with semiquantitative cultures is preferred to diagnose VAP, rather than invasive methods such as bronchoalveolar lavage or blind bronchial sampling. Additionally, blood cultures should be collected for all patients with suspected VAP.

## Treatment

*Aspiration pneumonia*—Antibiotic agents of choice include those with activity against gram-negative organisms such as third generation cephalosporins, fluoroquinolones, and piperacillin.[13] Current guidelines suggest not routinely adding anaerobic coverage for suspected aspiration pneumonia unless there is suspected lung abscess or empyema. The duration of antibiotic therapy should be guided by signs of clinical stability, such as resolution of vital sign abnormalities.

*HAP*—Antibiotics with activity against S. aureus, such as piperacillin-tazobactam, cefepime, levofloxacin, imipenem, or meropenem are recommended.[13] Vancomycin or linezolid should be added for patients who have risk factors for MRSA infection. The addition of two antibiotics from different classes with activity against P. aeruginosa is recommended for patients at high risk for Pseudomonas or other gram-negative infection (for example, prior intravenous antibiotic use within 90 days) or high risk for mortality.[13] Best practice is a 7-day course of antimicrobial therapy.[9]

*VAP*—In patients with suspected VAP, coverage for *S. aureus, Pseudomonas aeruginosa,* and other gram-negative bacilli for initial treatment is recommended.[13] Vancomycin or linezolid should be added for patients at risk for antimicrobial resistance or if admitted in units where >10%–20% of S. aureus isolates are methicillin-resistant.[13] Best practice is a 7-day course.

## Functional Outcomes

Serious complications such as pleural effusions, respiratory failure, renal failure, and septic shock can occur in patients with HAP. Risk factors for mortality include need for ventilatory support due to HAP and septic shock.[12]

All-cause mortality associated with VAP has been reported to range from 20% to 50%.[12] Higher mortality rates are seen in VAP caused by *Pseudomonas aeruginosa, Acinetobacter* spp., and *Stenotrophomonas maltophilia.*

## SEPSIS/CRBSI/CLABSI

### Core Definitions

Sepsis is a life-threatening condition caused by a dysregulated response to infection, resulting in organ injury.

*Catheter-related bloodstream infection (CRBSI)* is defined as the presence of bacteremia originating from an intravenous catheter.

*Central line-associated bloodstream infection (CLABSI)* is defined as a laboratory-confirmed bloodstream infection not related to an infection at another site that develops within 48 hours of central line placement.

### Risk Factors

Risk factors for sepsis include immune system compromise/neutropenia, severe burns, malnutrition, and prolonged hospital stay prior to catheter placement. Related to CRBSI and CLABSI, situational risk factors include emergency insertion, number of device lumens, incomplete adherence to safe insertion practice, and diligence of catheter hub care.

## Etiology

Any type of infection can lead to sepsis, though pulmonary, GI, and genitourinary infections are some of the most common causes. CRBSI is often due to catheter contamination. According to the Infectious Diseases Society of America, there are four recognized routes of catheter contamination[14]:

1. Migration of skin organisms from the insertion site into the cutaneous catheter tract with colonization of the catheter tip
2. Direct contamination of the catheter or hub by contact with hands or contaminated fluids/devices
3. Hematogenous seeding from another focus of infection
4. Contamination of the infusing fluid

## Diagnosis

Sepsis can be diagnosed in the setting of a suspected or confirmed infection with 2 or more of the following criteria:

- Temperature < 36 °C or > 38 °C
- Heart rate > 90/minute
- Respiratory rate > 20/minute, or arterial partial pressure of $CO_2$ less than 32 mmHg
- White blood cell count < 4 × 109/L or > 12 × 109/L, or > 10% bands.

The clinical definition of CLABSI is met by the following criteria[15]:

1. Presence of clinical signs of infection: fever, rigors, altered mental status, hypotension
2. No alternate source of bloodstream infection
3. Positive blood culture from a peripheral vein with any one of the following:

- Catheter tip/segment culture matches organism grown from the blood
- At least threefold higher number of organisms grown from the catheter versus the peripheral blood culture on simultaneously drawn cultures
- Growth from the catheter-drawn blood culture occurs at least two hours before growth of the same organism from a percutaneous blood culture

CRBSI will present with similar clinical signs of infection (fever, rigors, altered mental status, and hypotension). Blood cultures should be obtained peripherally and from the indwelling catheter. For diagnosis both of these cultures are required to be positive with clear evidence that the catheter is the source of infection.

## Treatment

It is first important to identify the source of infection by a thorough examination with appropriate lab and imaging studies. Vancomycin is recommended for empirical therapy. Empirical coverage for gram-negative bacilli should be based on local antimicrobial susceptibility data and the severity of disease. Neutropenic patients, severely ill patients with sepsis, or patients known to be colonized with MDRO should receive antibiotic coverage for multidrug-resistant gram-negative bacilli, such as Pseudomonas aeruginosa when CRBSI is suspected.[16] Blood cultures should be followed to guide treatment. It is best practice for any catheter or central line that are suspected as the source of infection to be removed and exchanged.

## MENINGITIS

### Diagnosis

Meningitis is an infection involving the cerebrospinal fluid (CSF) of the leptomeninges which surrounds the brain and spinal cord.

### Etiology and Pathophysiology

Viral meningitis is more common than bacterial meningitis, though often has less severe symptoms. The three most common pathogens of meningitis in adults are *Neisseria meningitides, Streptococcus pneumoniae* and *Listeria monocytogenes*.[17] Meningitis can be transmitted via the respiratory or throat secretions as well as some invasive procedure. Those with neurosurgery or head trauma are at increased risk of developing meningitis due to the risk direct contamination of the central nervous system associated with these surgeries. Factors associated with an increased risk of postoperative cranial meningitis are intraventricular or subarachnoid hemorrhage, cranial fracture with CSF leak, catheter irrigation, craniotomy, and duration of catheterization (greater than 5 days).[12]

### Diagnostic Approach

Clinical features of meningitis include new headache, fever, nausea, lethargy, seizures, or worsening mental status. Lumber puncture and CSF analysis is the best diagnostic tool to confirm the diagnosis of meningitis.[17] CSF findings depend on whether the cause of meningitis is bacterial or viral. CSF cultures are critical to confirm the diagnosis of bacterial meningitis. Blood cultures should also be obtained. More advanced cranial imaging can be considered which may demonstrate meningeal inflammation or evaluate for postoperative cranial complications.

### Treatment

Vancomycin plus an anti-pseudomonal beta-lactam (cefepime, ceftazidime, or meropenem) is recommended as empiric therapy. For patients who have experienced anaphylaxis to beta-lactam antimicrobial agents and in whom meropenem is contraindicated, aztreonam or ciprofloxacin is recommended for gram-negative coverage.[18] CSF and blood cultures should be followed to guide and ensure adequate antibiotic treatment. In cases of postoperative cranial meningitis neurosurgery should be consulted and any hardware removed as indicated.

### Functional Prognosis and Outcomes

Even when treatment with appropriate antibiotics is given, about half of patients with acute bacterial meningitis suffer severe complications, most often during the first week. These complications can include brain edema, hydrocephalus, stroke, cerebral hemorrhage, septic thrombosis, epileptic seizures, cerebritis and brain abscesses. In the perspective of the rehabilitation population, the most serious sequelae after acute bacterial meningitis are neurological including motor impairment, epilepsy, vision loss, speech disorder and hearing loss.

## RESOURCES AND REFERENCES

The full list of resources and references appears in the digital product found on http://connect.springerpub.com/content/book/978-0-8261-6226-7/part/part03/chapter/ch42

# PAIN MANAGEMENT PRINCIPLES

DANIEL EZIDIEGWU AND SOO YEON KIM

## CORE DEFINITIONS

The International Association for the Study of Pain (IASP) defines pain as "An unpleasant sensory and emotional experience associated with actual or potential tissue damage or described in terms of such damage."[1] Acute pain is a normal physiologic response to a noxious stimulus from a tissue injury. However, in its chronic stage, "it no longer serves a useful purpose and then becomes, through its mental and physical effects, a destructive force," as stated by Dr. Bonica in 1953.[2] While the acknowledgment of chronic pain as a disease in its own right can be debatable, there is no doubt that chronic pain has become a significant healthcare burden worldwide. Understanding of pain mechanisms is essential in the development of an evidence-based treatment approach and to optimize choice and selection of pharmacological therapy.

## ETIOLOGY AND PATHOPHYSIOLOGY

### Nociceptive Pathway

Acute pain is initiated by the transduction of energy from noxious stimuli (mechanical, thermal, or chemical) to electrical action potentials via nociceptors within the skin, muscle, tendons, and joints. Action potentials are transmitted through primary afferent fibers to the dorsal horn of the spinal cord, where they synapse to second-order neurons. They are further transmitted to the thalamus via second-order neurons which form a spinothalamic tract and then are projected to the multiple areas in the brain by third-order neurons. Perception happens when the electrical signals reach the brain and are converted to subjective sensory and emotional responses to be recognized as pain. Although the detailed mechanism is not well understood, the sensory-discriminative component, which gives information about the location, quality, and intensity of pain, is known to be processed in the somatosensory cortex while the limbic system mediates the affective-emotional response. Modulation occurs at multiple different levels, but it is often described as descending pathways that originate from the brain stem to the dorsal horn which controls nociceptive ascending pathways via endogenous opioid, serotonin, or norepinephrine. This pathway is often targeted in chronic pain management.

The full list of resources and references appears in the digital product found on http://connect .springerpub.com/content/book/978-0-8261-6226-7/part/part03/chapter/ch43

## Neuropathic Pain

Unlike nociceptive pain that arises from damage to nonneural tissue and processed by the normal nociceptive pathway described earlier, neuropathic pain is caused by a disease of the somatosensory nervous system (Table 43.1). Postherpetic neuralgia and entrapment neuropathies are examples of conditions that may cause neuropathic pain. Neuropathic pain is commonly burning, or pins-and-needles like in nature, and often occurs spontaneously without any triggering noxious stimulus. Neuropathic pain tends to become chronic as a result of the peripheral and central sensitization.

## Chronic Pain

Chronic pain was once defined by a duration of pain over 3 months. However, with a better understanding of the chronification of acute pain, chronic pain is more than just the difference in duration. Acute pain is a physiologic protective mechanism in response to tissue trauma expected to return to normal with resolution of the underlying cause. Chronic pain not only extends beyond the period of normal healing[3] but is also disproportionate to the original pathology (Table 43.2). This hyperactivity occurs at both peripheral and central levels. Peripherally, nociceptors are upregulated due to increased inflammatory cytokines (prostaglandins, substance P) released by the injured tissue that become sensitive to normally non-noxious stimuli. Central sensitization involves chronic activation of spinal and

## TABLE 43.1 PAIN CHARACTERISTICS BY UNDERLYING DISEASE PROCESS

| PRIMARY NOCICEPTIVE | NOCICEPTIVE AND NEUROPATHIC | PRIMARY NEUROPATHIC | |
|---|---|---|---|
| | | Peripheral | Central |
| Osteoarthritis | Chronic back pain (Nerve lesion and nociceptive input from soft tissue) | Back pain | Post stroke |
| Visceral pain | Cancer pain (with nerve infiltration) | PHN | Multiple strokes |
| Headache | CRPS I (without nerve injury) | Trigeminal neuralgia | Spinal cord injury |
| Ischemic pain | | HIV | |
| Cancer pain (without nerve injury) | | CRPS II | |
| Back pain (without nerve injury) | | Phantom pain | |
| **Injured/irritated somatic or visceral structure** | **Nociceptive and neuropathic components** | **Injury of neural structure** | |

CRPS, complex regional pain syndrome; PHN, postherpetic neuralgia.

## TABLE 43.2 CHARACTERISTICS OF ACUTE VERSUS CHRONIC PAIN

| ACUTE PAIN | CHRONIC PAIN |
|---|---|
| Sudden, short duration<br>Resolves when tissue heals | Insidious<br>Pain persists despite tissue healing |
| Protective response to actual or potential tissue damage | Poor |
| Severity correlates with the degree of injury | Severity not correlated with the degree of injury |
| Pain pathway intact | Altered pain pathway in both CNS and PNS |

CNS, central nervous system; PNS, peripheral nervous system.

supraspinal neurons. Increased neurotransmitters from primary afferent neurons increase the responsiveness of postsynaptic receptors, especially *N*-methyl-D-aspartate (NMDA) receptors. At this stage, the nociceptive pathway may become spontaneously activated without stimuli due to reduced activation threshold. A hyperexcitable state is further maintained by decreased activity of inhibitory nonadrenergic and opioid modulatory pathways.

## DIAGNOSTIC APPROACH

The first step is to identify the type of pain the patient is experiencing as each type of pain should be managed differently. The pain history should include "the 4 A's"[4]:

**Analgesia:** Here, we assess the underlying conditions causing pain (e.g., osteoarthritis, neuropathy), type (nociceptive, neuropathic), intensity, and duration of pain. An initial pain assessment form can be used to measure intensity, function, and mood.

**Activities of daily living (ADLs):** This will help clarify the current functional status and realistic goals.

**Adverse event:** It is vital to understand side effects to assess barriers to treatment, that is, cognitive impairment, missing doses, expectations of faster analgesia onset, causing early termination before adequate time.

**Aberrant behavior:** Assess for dependence/addiction with questionable behaviors such as early refills, demands for additional medication, or use with other substances. Patients should also be assessed for a mood disorder.

## TREATMENT

### Pain Management Planning

Proper pain management may be achieved by understanding patient goals and expectations, available resources to meet those expectations, and time tables of treatment. Establishing a clear and realistic goal is important as they can differ between patients based on chronicity and etiology (neuropathic vs. nociceptive). Once goals are set, expectations of treatment can be assessed, and discussion of the various methods of treatment and proper the time required for effective treatment ensue.

## Acute Pain

Treatment should aim to control acute pain effectively to prevent progression to chronic pain. This strategy should include investigating and treating the underlying process while controlling the pain. Analgesic medications are essential but should be accompanied by other modalities.

## Chronic Pain

This is more difficult to treat and requires the understanding that pain may not be completely eliminated. The goal should be a reduction in pain enough to improve function and quality of life. The mechanisms underlying chronic pain are often multifactorial and involve both nociceptive and neuropathic elements. Thus, multiple analgesic medications to treat various pain pathways are necessary. In most cases, multimodal approaches, including medications, injections, physical therapy, behavioral therapy, and vocational interventions, are required.

## Pharmacologic Interventions

Many factors must be taken into account with regard to analgesia such as the type of pain, the response to prior medications, comorbidities (gastrointestinal [GI] bleed, heart disease, chronic kidney disease [CKD]/end-stage renal disease [ESRD]), and current medications. Proper administration routes (oral, transmucosal, transdermal, intravenous), dosing, and interval should be considered.

## Treatments for Nociceptive Pain

Non-opioid analgesics (Table 43.3): Non-steroidal anti-inflammatory drugs (NSAIDs) inhibit cyclooxygenase, which results in inhibition of prostaglandin synthesis. NSAIDs only act on nociceptive pain and are not effective in neuropathic pain. NSAIDs must be used with caution in patients with renal and cardiovascular risks. Acetaminophen is another widely used non-opioid analgesic, but the mechanism of action is unclear. It is thought to work on the descending inhibitory pathways and does not have anti-inflammatory action.

Opioids (Table 43.4): Opioids are natural ligands for the opioid receptors found throughout the nociceptive pathway centrally and peripherally. Opioids act mainly via μ receptors, reducing the pain signal transmission by inhibiting the presynaptic release of excitatory neurotransmitters and causing postsynaptic hyperpolarization. Opioids work on both nociceptive and neuropathic pain. Due to abuse potential, opioids should not be considered as first-line therapy. When opioids are being used for acute pain, immediate-release preparations are first choice. When a long-acting opioid is considered, the total daily dose (TDD) of short-acting opioids is calculated. Then 60% of the TDD can be converted to a long-acting preparation and 40% remains short-acting divided into appropriate dosing intervals. To prevent withdrawal, patients typically need about one fourth of the previous daily dose given in four divided parts.[5]

Antispasmodics (Table 43.5): Useful in patients with acute musculoskeletal pain syndromes and not recommended for chronic pain. While there is much diversity to this groups' mechanism of action, in animal models, they have been shown to inhibit interneuronal activity at the descending reticular formation blocking polysynaptic neurons in the spinal cord.

## TABLE 43.3 COMMONLY USED NON-OPIOID ANALGESICS FOR ADULTS

| MEDICATION | HALF-LIFE | DAILY MAXIMUM (PO) | DOSAGE (PO) | DETAILS |
|---|---|---|---|---|
| Acetaminophen | 2 hours | 3,250 mg Extra strength: 3,000 mg | 650 mg q4–6h prn Extra strength: 1 g q6h prn | Peak concentration in 2 hours. CYP-450 inducers (EtOH) increase metabolites and hepatotoxicity. Less nephrotoxic than NSAIDs. |
| Aspirin | 2–3 hours | 3,900 mg | 325–650 mg q4h prn | Irreversible COX inhibitor. 10–14-day platelet inhibition. Reyes syndrome if given to children with viral illness. |
| Ibuprofen | 3.5 hours | 3,200 mg | 400–600–800 mg TID–QID prn | Peaks in 1–2 hours, hepatic excretion. Renal side effects >1,600 mg/day in older adults, low-volume patients. Antagonizes ASA platelet inhibition and may limit cardioprotective effects. Aseptic meningitis risk. |
| Naproxen | 14 hours | 1,500 mg | 250, 375, 500 mg q6–8h prn | Superior efficacy and less GI effect compared to Aspirin. Safe cardiovascular profile. Aseptic meningitis risk. Renal excretion. |
| Diclofenac | 1–2 hours | 200 mg | 50 mg TID prn 75 mg BID prn | Good synovial fluid buildup. Higher hepatotoxicity than other NSAIDs. Renal excretion; metabolites accumulate in renal disease. |
| Ketorolac | 4–6 hours | 40 mg/day | 10 mg q4–6h prn for 5 days only | Onset 30 minutes; peak 1–2 hours. 60 mg associated with acute tubular necrosis. |
| Meloxicam | 15–20 hours | 15 mg | 7.5 mg BID prn 15 mg QD prn | No reported effect on renal function. Interacts with cholestyramine, lithium, CYP 450,2C9 & 34A inhibitors. Excreted by urine and feces. |

*(continued)*

**TABLE 43.3 COMMONLY USED NON-OPIOID ANALGESICS FOR ADULTS (continued)**

| MEDICATION | HALF-LIFE | DAILY MAXIMUM (PO) | DOSAGE (PO) | DETAILS |
|---|---|---|---|---|
| Nabumetone | 24 hours | 2000 mg | 1,000 mg daily or BID prn | |
| Indomethacin | 2–4.5 hours | 200 mg | 25–50 mg. TID prn | Used in OA and gout. Risk of gastritis and renal dysfunction. Metabolized in liver, excrete in liver and urine. |
| Celecoxib (COX-2 only) | 6–12 hours | 400 mg | 100–200 mg BID prn 400 mg for acute pain | Used for OA, RA, acute pain. Peaks at 3 hours. No platelet effect. Less GI irritation than diclofenac or naproxen. Contraindicated in sulfonamide allergy or ASA/NSAID allergy. Eliminated by liver. |

ASA, acetylsalicylic acid; COX, cyclooxygenase; CYP, cytochromes P; GI, gastrointestinal; NSAIDs, non-steroidal anti-inflammatory drugs; OA, osteoarthritis.

## Treatments for Neuropathic Pain

The use of two or more agents with different mechanism of action increases the likelihood that pain signals will be interrupted.

### Anticonvulsants

Gabapentin and pregabalin are most commonly used and recommended as first-line agents in the treatment of neuropathic pain. They selectively bind to the alpha-2-delta subunit of calcium channels and reduce presynaptic excitatory neurotransmitter release by stabilizing presynaptic membranes. An effective dose of gabapentin can range from 900 to 3,600 mg/day, but it may take weeks to reach an effective dose. Pregabalin has a higher bioavailability and can reach an effective dose within a day. There are no known drug interactions, but side effects include dizziness, somnolence, dry mouth, and edema.[6-8]

### Antidepressants

Antidepressants inhibit pain signals by enhancing descending inhibitory pathways: noradrenergic and serotonergic. Both tricyclic antidepressants (TCAs) and serotonin norepinephrine reuptake inhibitors (SNRIs) inhibit the reuptake of serotonin and norepinephrine. Their analgesic effect is mainly due to noradrenergic reuptake inhibition; therefore, more effective than selective serotonin reuptake inhibitors (SSRIs). TCAs (amitriptyline, nortriptyline) are typically cheaper, and side effects like sedation may assist sleep. They are effective at much lower doses in pain than in depression. For example, amitriptyline is effective in neuropathic pain at 25 to 75 mg/day, while the recommended dose for depression is 150 to 300 mg/day. TCAs have anticholinergic and antihistamine effects

## TABLE 43.4 OPIOID ANALGESICS

The maximum dose of an opioid PRN should not be greater than four times the minimum dose.

| MEDICATION | IV | PO (IV EQUIVALENT DOSE) | RELATIVE STRENGTH | HALF-LIFE | STARTING DOSE | |
|---|---|---|---|---|---|---|
| Morphine | 10 mg | 30 mg | 1 | 2–3.5 hours | 30–60 mg | Morphine sulfate:4–6 hours analgesia; metabolite (morphine-6-glucuronide) will accumulate in renal insufficiency. MS Contin: 8–12 hours analgesia. True allergy rare, usually related to opium-related plant protein. Renal elimination |
| Codeine | 100 mg | 200 mg | 0.15 | 3 hours | 15–60 mg | Prodrug; metabolized to morphine in liver. Limited analgesic effect. More CNS effects and nausea than morphine. Abuse common. Renal elimination |
| Methadone | 10 mg | 37.5–75 mg | 3 | 13–50 hours | 5–10 mg | 4–8 hour analgesia but long half-life increases risk of drug accumulation. Watch for central sleep apnea, prolonged QTc and torsades. Renal and fecal elimination |
| Oxycodone | 10 mg | 20 mg | 1.5 | 2–4 hours | 5–20 mg | May induce constriction of ampulla of Vater worsening gallbladder and pancreatic disease. |
| Oxymorphone | 1 mg | 10 mg | 3 | 7.5–9.5 hours | 5 –10 mg | 18:10 morphine:oxymorphone ratio 12:10 oxycodone:oxymorphone ratio Contraindicated in liver disease. Food improves absorption, take 1 hour prior to or 2 hours after a meal. Alcohol increases plasma levels. |
| Hydromorphone | 1.5 mg | 7.5 mg | 3.75 | 2–3 hours | 4–8 mg | Semisynthetic, smaller volumes than morphine Renal elimination |

*(continued)*

**TABLE 43.4 OPIOID ANALGESICS** (*continued*)

| MEDICATION | IV | PO (IV EQUIVALENT DOSE) | RELATIVE STRENGTH | HALF-LIFE | STARTING DOSE | |
|---|---|---|---|---|---|---|
| Hydrocodone | NA | 30 mg | 1.5 | – | 2.5–10 mg | Mu agonist like morphine. Schedule 2 if alone. Schedule 3 with combined with Acetaminophen. |
| Fentanyl | 0.1 mg | NA | 150 | 3–7 hours | | Lag time benefit of 12 hours and max concentration at 36 hours. Takes 24 hours for 50% reduction after patch removal. For Opioid tolerant patients only Metabolized to despropionyl fentanyl which may cause neurotoxic side effects like normeperidine. Reduced systemic circulation in cachectic or hypoalbuminemic patients. Renal and hepatic elimination. |
| Tramadol | NA | 120 mg | 0.22 | 9 hours | 25–50 mg | >100 mg QID offers no advantage and causes higher toxicity. Lowers seizure threshold. More neuropathic effect than nociceptive. Slow titration recommended. |

PRN, pro re nata.

## TABLE 43.5 ANTISPASMODICS

| MEDICATION (PO) | ONSET | DURATION | DOSING | SIDE EFFECT | DETAILS |
|---|---|---|---|---|---|
| Carisoprodol | 30 minutes | 4–6 hours | 250 mg, 350 mg TID | Ataxia, dizziness, drowsiness, nausea, vomiting, withdrawal potential | CNS depressant. Addictive potential Max duration, 2–3 weeks |
| Metaxalone | 1 hour | 4–6 hours | 400–800 mg TID-QID | Dizziness, drowsiness, headache, nausea, vomiting, rash | CNS depressant. Contraindicated in severe renal or hepatic impairment. |
| Methocarbamol | 30 minutes | N/A | 750 mg–1 g TID | Blurred vision, drowsiness | CNS depressant |
| Cyclobenzaprine (TCA-like) | 1 hour | 12–24 hours | 5–10 mg PO TID | Drowsiness, dizziness, dry mouth | Contraindicated in arrhythmias, CHF, hyperthyroidism or during acute MI. Caution with SSRI as risk serotonin syndrome. Risk of seizure with tramadol. Do not use with MAOi or within 14 days of stopping. Older adults may have hallucinations and confusion. Should be tapered to avoid withdrawal symptoms. |
| Diazepam (Gaba agonist) | 30 minutes | Variable | 2–10 mg PO TID | Sedation, fatigue, hypotension, ataxia, respiratory depression | Potentiation of effects with opioids, barbiturates, MAOis. Requires slow taper. Caution in older adults and renal impairment |
| Baclofen (Gaba B agonist) | 3–4 days | Variable | 5 mg PO TID titrated up to 40–80 mg/day | Drowsiness, slurred speech, hypotension, constipation, urinary retention | Antidepressants (short-term memory loss) Additive effects with imipramine |
| Tizanidine (Alpha 2 agonist) | 2 weeks | Variable | 2–8 mg PO TID-QID | Drowsiness, dry mouth, dizziness, hypotension, increased spasm/tone | CNS depressant. Additive effects with alcohol. Caution in renal impairment, 50% reduction in clearance if GFR <25 m/min. Reduced clearance with oral contraceptives |

CHF, congestive heart failure; CNS, central nervous system; GFR, glomerular filtration rate; MAOI, monoamine oxidase inhibitors; MI, myocardial infarction; SSRI, selective serotonin reuptake inhibitor.

and may cause dry mouth, urinary retention, and orthostatic hypotension. Cardiotoxicity attributed to anticholinergic effects prohibits this use in patients with ischemic heart. EKG in patients >40 years old is recommended. SNRIs (duloxetine, venlafaxine) are not associated with anticholinergic and antihistamine side effects, thus better tolerated than TCAs. Side effects include nausea, somnolence, dizziness, and constipation, which may resolve over time.[6,9]

### Topical Lidocaine

Lidocaine blocks overexcitable Na+ channels on damaged nociceptors and stabilizes membrane potentials of primary afferent neurons, resulting in a reduction of ectopic activities. Reduced peripheral input may counteract central sensitization.

## FUNCTIONAL PROGNOSIS AND OUTCOMES

Nociceptive pain will improve once the pain stimulus is eliminated.

Musculoskeletal injuries should improve with a period of rest/immobilization if indicated, physical therapy, stretching, oral medications, or potentially surgical intervention. The prognosis and outcome will be specific to each etiology (muscle strain, muscle tears, ligament sprain or tears, tendonitis, tendon rupture, bone bruises, bone fractures, and disc herniation).

Muscle spasms may improve with postural changes, proper alignment, physical therapy and their modalities, oral medications, dry needling, and trigger point. Ultimately, the outcome will depend on the ability to remove the cause of muscle spasm.

In neuropathic pain, pain may continue or worsen over time, even after the initial stimulus subsides. Chronic neuropathic pain should be treated as its own disease entity, focusing on pain management rather than the original etiology, with emphasis on functional restoration and improvement in quality of life, using multimodal approaches. In some acute neuropathies, such as idiopathic brachial plexopathy, symptoms may appear suddenly, especially for neuropraxic lesions, but resolve as damaged nerves recover. It is important to maintain the mobility of the joint involved during the recovery period to prevent any permanent contracture.

## RESOURCES AND REFERENCES

The full list of resources and references appears in the digital product found on http://connect .springerpub.com/content/book/978-0-8261-6226-7/part/part03/chapter/ch43

# PAROXYSMAL SYMPATHETIC HYPERACTIVITY

LESLEY ABRAHAM, KAYLI GIMARC, AND CHERRY JUNN

## CORE DEFINITIONS

Paroxysmal sympathetic hyperactivity (PSH) is a syndrome of simultaneous, paroxysmal, and transient increases in sympathetic overreaction after an acquired brain injury.[1] It is characterized by repeated episodes of rapid-onset simultaneous tachycardia, fever, hypertension, tachypnea, and diaphoresis, and rigidity with dystonic posturing.[2] PSH has been referred to by at least 31 separate terms in literature, including "autonomic seizures," "autonomic storming," "paroxysmal hyperthermic autonomic dysregulation," and "dysautonomia." The term PSH is preferred, as it is specific and accurately portrays the conceptual definition.[1]

## ETIOLOGY AND PATHOPHYSIOLOGY

PSH can occur after any brain lesions, including trauma, infection, hemorrhage, infarction, brain tumor, global anoxia-ischemia, autoimmune encephalitis, or degeneration. Generally, the clinical presentation does not differ depending on the underlying etiology.[3]

The precise pathophysiology of PSH is still not completely understood. It is thought that injury to the neuraxis at various levels may lead to PSH. In PSH, an excess activation of the sympathetic system, without parasympathetic activation, is noted. Generally, it is thought that an injury can lead to (a) increased activation of excitatory pathways, (b) inhibition of descending inhibitory pathways leading to releasing excitatory reflexes, or (c) a combination of both of these mechanisms.

It is hypothesized that structural damage sustained after acquired brain injury results in disruption of autonomic regulatory centers, including the hypothalamus, the rostral ventrolateral medulla, midbrain, and cortical centers.[4,5]

A second hypothesis includes the excitatory:inhibitory (EIR) model. A lesion in the inhibitory centers in the brainstems and diencephalon reduces tonic descending inhibition to afferent sensory information from spinal cord circuits. This disruption of inhibitory centers results in the amplification of normally nonnociceptive afferent sensory information from the periphery and leads to overexcitation of the sympathetic nervous system response.[4,6] A combination of these two hypotheses may explain PSH.

The full list of references appears in the digital product found on http://connect.springerpub.com/content/book/978-0-8261-6226-7/part/part03/chapter/ch44

## DIAGNOSTIC APPROACH

PSH is a diagnosis of exclusion. PSH should be considered after excluding conditions that present similarly, such as systemic inflammatory response syndrome, infection, noxious stimuli causing discomfort (fracture, heterotopic ossification, pressure wounds, constipation), seizures, intracranial hypertension, hydrocephalus, medication or substance withdrawal, serotonin syndrome, or neuroleptic malignant syndrome.[4]

History should assess repeated episodes of rapid-onset tachycardia, hypertension, tachypnea, fever, diaphoresis, and rigidity with dystonic posturing. Not all features have to be present, but several must be observed simultaneously. Possible triggers should also be assessed during history gathering. Triggers can be painful or nonpainful, such as touching, passive movements, turning, significant gastroesophageal reflux, and endotracheal tube suctioning.[1] The paroxysmal features can occur spontaneously without external stimulation. PSH can develop within the first week after trauma or illness but can also start later. These episodes typically resolve spontaneously but can last up to 20 to 30 minutes. Patients with PSH may have more deep structural lesions.[7]

Physical examination during the episodes may reveal worsened level of consciousness and dilated pupils.[1,3,6] Assessment for skin breakdown and heterotopic ossification should be done to identify possible triggers.

PSH cannot be diagnosed based on laboratory studies, but these can be helpful in assessing for infection. Imaging studies can be used to help identify causes of pain. As PSH leads to increased energy expenditure, nutritional deficiencies may occur and should be assessed.

In 2014, the paroxysmal sympathetic hyperactivity assessment measure was developed by an international expert group to help determine PSH diagnostic likelihood.[1] The first section of this assessment measure, the diagnostic likelihood tool, assesses the presence of PSH features. The second section, the Clinical Feature Scale, measures the severity of PSH features. One study found that this tool helps to reduce misdiagnosis of PSH, which may lead to favorable impacts on length of hospital stay and hospitalization costs.[8]

## TREATMENT

PSH treatment should start with minimizing avoidable stimulation and reducing noxious stimulation. Pharmacological treatment should be used to abort paroxysms and also to prevent further episodes (Table 44.1). All treatment trials are empirical but are supported by clinical experience.

One study found that antipsychotics/dopamine antagonists such as haloperidol are not useful and may even worsen PSH.[10] For severe dystonia or rigidity, treatment with intrathecal baclofen and botulinum toxin injection may be beneficial.

In the subacute and chronic stage, continue passive range of motion and position changes to prevent decubitus ulcer, deep vein thrombosis, joint contractures, and heterotopic ossifications. As vital signs stabilize, mobility should be increased. Aggressive treatment for dystonia should be considered.

## TABLE 44.1 MEDICATIONS FOR PAROXYSMAL SYMPATHETIC HYPERACTIVITY[2,9]

| MEDICATION | MECHANISM | DOSE | CLINICAL EFFECT | SIDE EFFECTS |
|---|---|---|---|---|
| Propranolol | Noncardioselective beta-blocker | Start: 10 mg TID by enteral route Max: 320 mg/day | Preventive; effective for tachycardia, hypertension, and diaphoresis Less effective for fever | Bradycardia, hypotension, sleep disturbance Contraindicated: asthma, heart block |
| Labetalol | Noncardioselective beta-blocker; selective alpha(1)-adrenergic receptor antagonist | Start: 50 mg BID by enteral route (IV option available) | Preventive; effective for tachycardia and hypertension | Bradycardia, hypotension Contraindicated: asthma, heart block |
| Gabapentin | Interacts with α2delta subunit of voltage-gated calcium channels in brain and spinal cord | Start: 100–300 mg TID by enteral route Max: up to 3600–4800 mg/day | Preventive; improves most features | Sedation |
| Clonidine | Central $\alpha_2$-adrenergic receptor agonist | Start: 0.1–0.3 mg BID by enteral route Max: 2.4 mg/day | Abortive and preventive; mostly improves tachycardia and hypertension | Bradycardia, hypotension, sedation |
| Bromocriptine | Dopamine D2 receptor agonist | Start: 1.25–2.5 mg q12h by enteral route Max: 20–40 mg/day | Preventive; effect tends to be modest and delayed | Confusion, agitation, dyskinesia, nausea/emesis, orthostatic hypotension, could reduce seizure threshold |
| Dantrolene | Inhibits calcium release from sarcoplasmic reticulum | Start: 0.5–2 mg/kg/IV q6–12h or 25 mg daily by enteral route Max: 10 mg/kg/IV or 400 mg QID by enteral route | Abortive; improves hypertonicity and dystonia | Hepatotoxicity (can be severe), respiratory depression, muscle weakness |

(continued)

**TABLE 44.1 MEDICATIONS FOR PAROXYSMAL SYMPATHETIC HYPERACTIVITY[2,9]** (*continued*)

| MEDICATION | MECHANISM | DOSE | CLINICAL EFFECT | SIDE EFFECTS |
|---|---|---|---|---|
| Baclofen | $GABA_B$ agonist | Start: 5 mg q8h by enteral route Max: 80 mg/day | Preventive; improves hypertonicity and dystonia | Sedation, muscle weakness |
| Morphine | Opioid agonist | 2–8 mg IV bolus | Abortive; improves most features | Respiratory depression, sedation, hypotension, ileus, emesis, histamine release, developing of tolerance |

GABA, gamma-aminobutyric acid; IV, intravenous.

## REFERENCES

The full list of references appears in the digital product found on http://connect.springerpub.com/content/book/978-0-8261-6226-7/part/part03/chapter/ch44

# PELVIC PAIN

MELISSA OSBORN AND SARAH HWANG

## CORE DEFINITIONS

The pelvic floor is a group of muscles, fascia, and ligaments that support the internal pelvic organs and help to provide bowel and bladder control. When the pelvic floor muscles are functioning normally, the muscles voluntarily and involuntarily contract with normal strength and relax completely.[1] Pelvic floor dysfunction (PFD) is the inability of the pelvic floor muscles to properly contract and relax.

Overactive or high-tone pelvic floor muscles do not relax and may paradoxically contract when relaxation is needed.[1] Underactive or noncontracting pelvic floor muscles cannot voluntarily contract when desired.[1] Noncontracting, nonrelaxing pelvic floor occurs when the pelvic floor muscles are both weak and hypertonic.[1]

Pelvic floor myofascial pain is defined as a regional condition of myofascial pain and tightness caused by chronic muscle contraction. It is characterized by tender points, taut bands, and trigger points within the pelvic floor muscles.[2]

## ETIOLOGY AND PATHOPHYSIOLOGY

The differential diagnosis of pelvic pain is vast and includes gynecologic, gastrointestinal, urologic, musculoskeletal, and neurologic causes. Women with pelvic pain often seek care from multiple providers and may have multifactorial etiologies for their pain. If a patient is presenting to a physiatry office first, referrals to gynecology, urogynecology, gastroenterology, and urology should be considered to rule out other causes of pain. Common comorbid conditions that occur in patients with PFD include vulvodynia, irritable bowel syndrome, endometriosis, interstitial cystitis, pudendal neuralgia, chronic prostatitis (in men), anxiety, depression, central sensitization, and a history of trauma/sexual abuse.

Primary musculoskeletal causes of pelvic pain are common, especially with high-tone PFD. Painful pelvic floor muscles can occur as a result of musculoskeletal injury within the pelvic floor (muscles, fascia, and ligaments) or as an adaptation to other problems within the pelvis/spine/hip complex.[3] Studies have shown that women with endometriosis often develop spasm of the pelvic floor muscles that is likely an adaptive response.

Underactive pelvic floor muscles can lead to urinary stress incontinence, pelvic organ prolapse, and fecal incontinence. The prevalence of these disorders is estimated to affect about 25% of women and become more prevalent with age.[4]

---

The full list of resources and references appears in the digital product found on http://connect.springerpub.com/content/book/978-0-8261-6226-7/part/part03/chapter/ch45

## DIAGNOSTIC APPROACH

### History

- *Setting*: Private examination room with the patient fully clothed[5]
- *HPI*: Obtain a standard pain history, including the onset of pain, location of pain, description of pain, duration and frequency of pain, pain intensity (e.g., numerical pain score currently, at best, and at worst over the past 2–4 weeks), and associated symptoms. Pertinent questions to ask for pelvic pain include variability in intensity with menses/ovulation, dyspareunia (pain with intercourse), and bowel/bladder symptoms (see Table 45.1).
- *Review of systems (ROS):* Should be thorough in order to bring to light other system-based causes of the pain.
- *PMH*: Be aware of common comorbid conditions (listed earlier). Also, take detailed obstetric and gynecologic histories including number of past pregnancies and deliveries (vaginal or cesarean), use of forceps during labor, and complications during labor or delivery.
- *Past surgical history (PSH)*: Inquire specifically about prior abdominal or pelvic surgeries, which could be associated with pelvic complications including adhesions or nerve damage.
- *Family Hx*: Include history of endometriosis, chronic pain conditions, or gynecologic cancer.
- *Social Hx*: Inquire about sexual history and history of trauma or abuse given the high prevalence of this among patients with chronic pelvic pain.
- *Goals*: Understand how the pain is interfering with the patient's life and everyday function, as well as the patient's individual goals, in order to guide the treatment plan.
- *Transition to physical examination: Describe the physical examination and ask for permission to proceed. This aspect of the encounter is considered especially important by the authors to establish an environment of security and support for this patient population, in which there is a high prevalence of history or trauma and abuse.*

### Physical Examination

Once the patient has given permission for the physical examination, the physician steps out of the room and allows the patient to remove underwear (may keep bra on) and change into a gown open to the back. A general screening examination including basic musculoskeletal and neurologic examinations focused on the lumbar spine, pelvis, and lower extremities (primarily hips) is performed as detailed later. Based on clinical suspicion, more extensive and nuanced examination maneuvers may be added for determining the diagnosis.[3,5] Throughout the examination, the physician should stay attuned to the patient's nonverbal communication, including guarding, grimacing, and hesitancy.

- *Standing*: Include lumbar spine inspection and ROM. Important areas to palpate for tenderness include the L-S spinous processes, lumbosacral paraspinal muscles, posterior superior iliac spine (PSIS), long dorsal ligaments, gluteal muscles.
- *Sitting*: Basic neurologic examination including lower extremity manual muscle testing, sensation to light touch, reflexes, and seated slump (if suspicious for a radiculopathy).

## TABLE 45.1 QUESTIONS TO ASK DURING HISTORY EXAMINATION

| SYSTEM | QUESTIONS | FEATURES CONSISTENT WITH PELVIC FLOOR DYSFUNCTION |
|---|---|---|
| BLADDER | • Do you have any urinary frequency or urgency?<br>• How often do you go to the bathroom in 1 day?<br>• Do you ever notice leakage of urine? How much? Do you wear pads or panty liners for this reason? How many pads do you use on a typical day?<br>• Do you have a history of frequent UTIs with negative cultures? | *High tone:*<br>Urinary frequency and urgency ± urinary leakage<br>*Low tone:*<br>Loss of urine with coughing, sneezing, laughing (may soak pad) ± urinary urgency |
| BOWEL | • Do you feel constipated often?<br>• Do you strain to have a bowel movement?<br>• Do you have difficulty passing all of your stool?<br>• Do you notice loss of stool that you cannot control?<br>• Do you have pelvic or abdominal pain that is worse during or after a bowel movement? | *High tone:*<br>Constipation, straining, incomplete evacuation of stool, pain worse after bowel movement<br>*Low tone:*<br>Fecal incontinence, need to splint (e.g., place finger in vagina) to pass stool |
| SEXUAL FUNCTION | • Do you have pain with sexual intercourse? Does the pain occur with superficial penetration, deep penetration, or both?<br>• Have you ever had nonpainful intercourse?<br>• Does the pain continue after intercourse? How long?<br>• Do you have pain with inserting a tampon or speculum examinations? | *High tone:*<br>Dyspareunia, pain with penetration (should evaluate for other diagnoses as well, including vaginismus, vulvodynia, endometriosis)<br>*Low tone:*<br>NA |
| PSYCHOLOGY | • Do you feel down or depressed often?<br>• Do you feel anxious or on edge often?<br>• Do you have a history of trauma or abuse? | *High tone:*<br>Anxiety, depression, history of trauma<br>*Low tone:*<br>NA |

NA, not applicable; PFD, pelvic floor dysfunction; UTI, urinary tract infection.

■ *Laying supine:* Abdominal examination including inspection (note any scars or hernia), tenderness to light and deep palpation, and evaluation of rectus diastasis with abdominal crunch (if the patient has a history of pregnancy). Hip examination includes ROM, palpation (make note if the patient reports focal pain overlying a muscle, tendon, or greater trochanter), and special tests including log roll, Scour, FABER, FADIR, AP glide, Stinchfield's, and sacroiliac (SI) joint maneuvers.[5]

■ *Laying supine with knees flexed and hips abducted/externally rotated (no stirrups):* Let the patient know that the vaginal portion of the examination is about to begin and give clear verbal cues throughout the vaginal examination. Perform external examination including inspection (note rash, hyper- or hypopigmentation, hair loss, high-grade pelvic organ prolapse). If the patient is reporting symptoms consistent with vulvodynia (hypersensitivity, burning, superficial pain at the level of the skin), perform a more extensive neurologic examination including the Q tip test to assess for allodynia. Next, palpate the superficial muscles, including ischiocavernosus, bulbospongiosus, and superficial transverse perineal, externally and note muscle tension as well as reported pain. Then, place lubrication on the gloved index finger and insert it into the vagina while spreading the labia with the other hand. Palpate the superficial pelvic floor muscles again internally and then advance deeper to the levator ani. Imagining the pelvic floor as a clockface with the urethra at noon and the rectum at 6 o'clock, palpate the levator ani from 3 to 5 o'clock and 7 to 9 o'clock. Note whether there are trigger points or diffusely increased tone. Also, note whether palpation of these muscles is painful to the patient or if it provokes the patient's presenting symptoms. Next, palpate the obturator internus bilaterally (may be found by asking the patient to perform resisted hip external rotation with the ipsilateral thigh). Assess for pelvic floor muscle strength and coordination by asking the patient to squeeze as though trying to hold in urine. Assess ability to actively relax the pelvic floor by having the patient Valsalva (asking the patient to bear down as though having a bowel movement). Coordination can be assessed by asking the patient to quickly squeeze (quick flicks). A rectal examination may be performed for examination of the pelvic floor in men and for further evaluation of the pelvic floor in women.[5]

■ The diagnosis of PFD is confirmed with the following examination findings:
  ❏ High-tone PFD: Muscle spasm and/or muscle shortening, trigger points, taut bands, pain with palpation, lack of relaxation after muscle contraction
  ❏ Low-tone PFD: Weakness of the pelvic floor muscle contraction, deficiencies in coordinating a muscle contraction

## DIAGNOSTIC APPROACH

PFD is a clinical diagnosis based on the combination of findings on history and physical examination. Other diagnoses considered in the differential for pelvic pain, such as endometriosis and interstitial cystitis, may require imaging such as pelvic ultrasound and/or MRI, cystoscopy, or urinalysis and culture.

*Scales:* Strength of the pelvic floor musculature may be assessed using the Oxford, Modified Oxford, and/or International Continence Society criteria.[5]

## TREATMENT

Multidisciplinary treatment of pelvic pain and PFD is crucial, and this approach should incorporate pelvic floor physical therapy with a trained physical therapist. As always, physical therapy should be tailored to each individual patient. When the pelvic floor muscles are high tone, therapy focuses on relaxation, down-training, and myofascial release. When the pelvic floor muscles are weak or noncontracting, physical therapy focuses on pelvic floor muscle strengthening. Often, patients with PFD will also have weak core and weak hip girdle muscles, so strengthening of these areas should be included. Bowel and bladder retraining should be incorporated into pelvic floor physical therapy if the patient presents with these problems. This may include training on proper techniques for defecation and/or techniques for suppression of urinary frequency/urgency. Pelvic floor physical therapy should always be explained to patients prior to referral, as these therapists do internal vaginal muscle examination, and part of the treatment may include myofascial release that is done from a vaginal approach. Of note, for patients that have a history of abuse, this type of physical therapy may be retraumatizing, thus it may be beneficial to start with external therapy only and progress to internal pelvic floor physical therapy after the patient develops a relationship with the therapist.

Medications can be helpful in the management of myofascial pelvic pain and high-tone PFD. These may include intravaginal compounded muscle relaxant suppositories (such as baclofen) or oral medications aimed at chronic pain or central sensitization (such as antidepressants or neuromodulators).

Injections can also be utilized as an adjunctive therapy option when treating myofascial pelvic pain and high-tone PFD. Clinically, these injections are most beneficial when combined with physical therapy. Trigger point injections can be utilized when there are palpable trigger points in the pelvic floor muscles. Botulinum toxin injections can be utilized for recalcitrant diffuse muscle spasms.

Psychotherapy can be an important part of treatment for patients, especially in those with a history of trauma or abuse. Sex therapy can also be helpful for patients that have dyspareunia or vaginismus or have trouble tolerating physical examination or physical therapy due to prior sexual trauma or abuse. Cognitive-behavioral therapy can be utilized for the treatment of chronic pain and central sensitization.

## FUNCTIONAL PROGNOSIS AND OUTCOMES

Given the complex nature of chronic pelvic pain and PFD, a multifactorial approach is generally considered to be the most efficacious for treatment, especially, in chronic cases.[3]

There is moderate-to-strong evidence supporting the use of pelvic floor physical therapy for the treatment of both high- and low-tone PFD, including cases involving pelvic floor myofascial pain, vaginismus, vulvodynia, stress urinary incontinence, interstitial cystitis, and pelvic organ prolapse.[6] See the following points for more details:

- *Pelvic floor myofascial pain and vaginismus*: Single studies have demonstrated improvement in pelvic pain in 59% to 80% of patients with pelvic floor myofascial pain[7] and 45% of patients with dyspareunia and vaginismus after a course of pelvic floor physical therapy.[8]

- *Stress and mixed urinary incontinence*: Patients with stress urinary incontinence were 6 to 8 times more likely to report resolution after completing pelvic floor physical therapy rather than placebo or no treatment groups.[9] Short-term improvement in patients with stress urinary incontinence and mixed urinary incontinence has been estimated to vary between 56% and 70% based on self-report and 44% and 80% based on leakage less than 2 g on two pad tests. This benefit was shown to be sustained at 1 year or longer for 41% to 85% of patients.[10]

- **Interstitial cystitis**: A prospective randomized control trial of patients with interstitial cystitis/painful bladder syndrome and pelvic floor tenderness showed a trend toward improvement with myofascial physical therapy.[11]
- **Pelvic organ prolapse**: Patients with pelvic organ prolapse stages I to III have been shown to have a reduction in symptom scores at 1 year after pelvic floor physical therapy.[12,13]

## BASIC ORDER SET(S)

Sample PT orders

- *Case 1:* A 35-year-old G2P2 female presents for evaluation of urinary incontinence worse with coughing and sneezing. Physical examination shows grade II cystocele, pelvic floor weakness, and impaired coordination.
  - ❏ PT order: Start pelvic floor physical therapy to focus on core and pelvic floor strengthening and pelvic floor neuromuscular training. May incorporate biofeedback/electrical stimulation, bladder diary, and dietary habits. 1 session per week for 8 weeks.
- *Case 2:* A 22-year-old nulliparous female presents for the evaluation of chronic pelvic pain that started as cyclic pelvic pain with her menstrual cycles 8 years ago and now occurs daily. Physical examination reveals pelvic pain that is provoked by the entire internal pelvic examination including palpation of superficial and deep pelvic floor muscles. The patient has a palpable trigger point in the right obturator internus as well as tight bands throughout the levator ani bilaterally. The patient appears very hesitant regarding internal pelvic floor therapy.
  - ❏ PT order: Start pelvic floor physical therapy to focus on pelvic floor down-training including reverse kegels, myofascial release, stretching, desensitization, and general relaxation techniques including deep breathing. May incorporate biofeedback. Begin with external PT and start to incorporate internal PT when the patient is comfortable. 1 session per week for 8 to 12 weeks.

## RESOURCES AND REFERENCES

The full list of resources and references appears in the digital product found on http://connect.springerpub.com/content/book/978-0-8261-6226-7/part/part03/chapter/ch45

# POSTTRAUMATIC STRESS DISORDER

LAKEYA S. MCGILL AND RACHEL V. AARON

## CORE DEFINITIONS

In the context of posttraumatic stress disorder (PTSD) and acute stress disorder (ASD), a traumatic event is defined as exposure to actual or threatened death, serious injury, or sexual violence.[1] An individual may directly experience a traumatic event themselves or learn that such an event occurred to a friend or relative. A formal diagnosis of PTSD or ASD requires the presence of four categories of distressing or functionally impairing symptoms. The specific symptoms within each category are diverse, and symptom profiles vary across individuals; thus, the presentation of PTSD and ASD is heterogeneous. ASD refers to these symptoms when they occur within the first month following a traumatic event, and PTSD involves symptoms that persist for more than one month. In the current review, we focus on PTSD and ASD symptom profiles for adults and children over six; specific symptoms profiles for children 6 years old and younger differ slightly and can be found in the *Diagnostic and Statistical Manual of Mental Disorders, Fifth Edition* (*DSM-5*).

The first symptom category, intrusions, entails re-experiencing aspects of the traumatic event.[1] Specific symptoms within this category include unwanted trauma-related memories, nightmares, flashbacks, and intense psychological or physiological responses at reminders of the traumatic event. The second category, avoidance, entails avoiding internal or external reminders of the traumatic event. For example, an individual may actively avoid distressing memories of the trauma or avoid places or objects that remind them of the event. The third category, negative alterations in cognitions and mood, entails changes that occur or worsen following the traumatic event. Specific symptoms include excessive blame of self or others about the cause or consequences of the traumatic event, and exaggerated or distorted negative beliefs about oneself, others, or the world. Finally, hyperarousal and reactivity entail arousal symptoms that begin or worsen after the trauma. Specific symptoms include sleep disturbance, hypervigilance, difficulty concentrating, reckless behavior, and irritable or aggressive behavior.

## ETIOLOGY AND PATHOPHYSIOLOGY

The primary etiological factor of PTSD and ASD is exposure to a traumatic event. Epidemiological studies have demonstrated that exposure to a traumatic event is common;

---

The full list of resources and references appears in the digital product found on http://connect.springerpub.com/content/book/978-0-8261-6226-7/part/part03/chapter/ch46

approximately 90% of adults in the United States have experienced at least one traumatic event in their lifetime.[2] The presence of symptoms across all four categories and that cause significant distress or functional impairment—meeting the criteria for a formal PTSD diagnosis—is less common, with a 12-month prevalence of 5% in the United States. The presence of some PTSD and ASD symptoms in the days and weeks following a traumatic event is normal and expected, and early assessment can help determine whether these symptoms are distressing or impairing, requiring formal intervention.

Other factors are associated with increased risk of PTSD and ASD following exposure to a traumatic event. Individuals with ASD versus those without are more likely to eventually meet diagnostic criteria for PTSD.[1] Across the lifespan, females have a higher prevalence of PTSD and ASD compared to males. Rates of PTSD and ASD vary across cultural groups. Compared to non-Latinx Whites, African Americans, American Indians, and Latinxs have higher rates of PTSD, and Asian Americans have a lower rate of PTSD. Within a rehabilitation population, other factors increase the risk of developing PTSD, including sustaining a mild traumatic brain injury or being admitted to an intensive care unit.[3] Individuals who experience major life stressors such as unemployment and financial strain in the aftermath of a traumatic event are also at greater risk of developing PTSD.[1]

In addition to risk factors, several protective factors that reduce the likelihood of developing PTSD and ASD have been identified. Individuals with greater levels of hope, optimism, and self-efficacy tend to have lower levels of PTSD.[4] Those who rely on more adaptive coping strategies to manage stress, such as adopting an active and solution-focused approach to managing stressors, are also less likely to develop PTSD and ASD.[1] The presence of adequate social support both before and following a traumatic event is associated with lower rates of PTSD and ASD. In summary, the etiology of PTSD and ASD is complex, involving interacting biopsychosocial factors; ongoing research is needed to understand more fully who is at lower or higher risk for developing PTSD or ASD and why.

## DIAGNOSTIC APPROACH

A formal diagnosis of PTSD requires an in-depth clinical interview and assessment by a mental health professional to understand the nature of an individual's trauma exposure and to fully characterize their symptom profile and the impact of these symptoms on their life. During rehabilitation, healthcare providers can facilitate the process by identifying patients who may be experiencing PTSD or ASD symptoms. Routine screening for PTSD and ASD symptoms is the best way to identify those at risk and is the best practice in settings where patients have a high likelihood of trauma exposure (e.g., veterans affairs, trauma hospitals). In the absence of a routine screening practice, healthcare providers should ensure that any patient with known trauma exposure (recent or remote) or any patient demonstrating symptoms consistent with PTSD or ASD is screened for PTSD or ASD using a standardized instrument.

In some—but not all—cases, recent or remote trauma exposure will be readily identifiable, for example, if a patient's rehabilitation is directly related to a traumatic injury such as an assault, motor vehicle crash, or lifesaving medical intervention. However, it is important to note that even remote exposure to traumatic events that are not directly related to medical care could result in PTSD symptoms that interfere with rehabilitation. Moreover, the experience of an event as traumatic is highly subjective and nuanced and may not be readily obvious in the absence of in-depth clinical interview, such as that conducted by a mental health professional. PTSD and ASD symptoms manifest in myriad ways throughout rehabilitation; for example, a patient may become distressed when describing the event that contributed to their current rehabilitation or altogether avoids providing specific details, complains of impaired sleep or nightmares that began after the onset of the traumatic event, describes negative changes in mood, or voices strong feelings of self-blame for the occurrence of the negative event.

Standardized screening tools exist to assess PTSD and ASD in medical settings. The primary care PTSD screen for *DSM-5* (PC-PTSD-5)[5] is a widely used 5-item measure that was developed to identify individuals with probable PTSD in medical settings. Respondents who endorse recent or remote exposure to a traumatic event indicate whether they are experiencing symptoms in the four primary symptom categories previously delineated. A positive screen on this measure indicates the need for comprehensive assessment with a mental health provider. For a list of more PTSD and ASD screening and assessment tools, please refer to the websites of the National Child Traumatic Stress Network, the American Psychiatric Association, the American Psychological Association, or the US Department of Veteran Affairs National Center for PTSD.

## TREATMENT

The first-line treatment for PTSD and ASD is evidence-based psychological intervention.[6] These interventions are delivered by a mental health professional and target PTSD-related symptoms, usually in a one-on-one format. The course of treatment is typically 8 to 12 sessions that are approximately 50 minutes in length. Mental health professionals who provide psychological intervention for PTSD and ASD include psychologists, psychiatrists, counselors, and clinical social workers. Ideally, medical providers would refer patients to a mental health professional with expertise in providing treatment for PTSD among rehabilitation populations. In many cases, however, this may not be a viable option; for example, in rural areas, it can be more difficult to find specialty providers. In the absence of PTSD or rehabilitation specialists, referral to a general mental health provider is appropriate.

Several psychological interventions have demonstrated efficacy in reducing PTSD symptomatology. Key approaches to PTSD intervention include exposure and cognitive restructuring.[7,8] Exposure-based interventions target avoidance of internal and external reminders of a traumatic event, which maintain and exacerbate fear.[7] For example, a patient who recently sustained orthopedic injuries in a motor vehicle accident may become distressed at the prospect of riding in a car and thus avoid doing so. Avoiding riding in a car could interfere with attending medical appointments and engagement in other valued activities. In a safe and structured environment, mental health professionals facilitate exposure to feared stimuli, such as riding in a car. Exposure results in the reduction of fear and anxiety and, ultimately, a decrease in PTSD symptomatology. Specific examples of empirically supported exposure-based PTSD treatments include prolonged exposure and eye movement desensitization and reprocessing.[9]

Cognitive behavioral therapy (CBT)-based approaches target alterations in mood and cognition related to ASD or PTSD. With the support of a mental health provider, patients learn to identify maladaptive trauma-related thoughts and beliefs and reframe them to be more helpful and realistic.[8] For example, a victim of domestic violence may experience pervading thoughts of guilt and self-blame for the endured abuse. They may ruminate on thoughts of how they might have prevented the abuse and seek evidence that they are blame-worthy. Over time, these cognitions contribute to harmful beliefs that maintain PTSD, such as beliefs that one is unlovable, unworthy, or inherently flawed. Using a systematic CBT-based approach, mental health professionals provide tools to help patients identify, examine, and restructure these negative distorted beliefs to be more realistic; for example, a restructured thought would be "I cannot control the actions of other people. Although I've received messages that I'm unlovable from some people, I know that's untrue. I am a good friend and parent, and the people who matter most to me love me for who I am." Restructuring negative thoughts in this way can help reduce PTSD and ASD symptoms. Specific examples of evidence-based CBT approaches for treating PTSD include cognitive processing therapy for adults and trauma-focused CBT for children.[9,10]

Some forms of pharmacotherapy have demonstrated efficacy in reducing PTSD symptoms in adults and are most effective when paired with psychotherapy.[6] Antidepressants have the most robust evidence base for the treatment of PTSD symptoms, particularly paroxetine and sertraline; trazodone has also been shown to reduce nightmares and improve sleep onset and maintenance. Some initial evidence suggests that prazosin has evidence for reducing PTSD-related nightmares and insomnia.[11] PTSD often co-occurs with psychological and medical comorbidities, such as substance-related disorder and traumatic brain injury, which require distinct pharmacological management. More complex cases may necessitate a referral to psychiatry or neuropsychiatry.

Emerging evidence highlights the preliminary efficacy of novel PTSD prevention efforts; however, additional research is needed to develop and test effective prevention programs. Some research suggests that a single session of eye movement desensitization and reprocessing (EMDR) or online psychoeducation provided within the first three months of a traumatic event may lower the likelihood of developing PTSD and ASD symptoms.[6] Mobile health interventions for PTSD and ASD have demonstrated promising but limited efficacy for symptom management.[12] Online and mobile applications are available, including PTSD Coach and CRAFT-PTSD.

## FUNCTIONAL PROGNOSIS AND OUTCOMES

Prognosis and outcomes following a traumatic event vary across individuals. Following a traumatic event, most individuals will experience few or no PTSD symptoms. Some will experience subclinical symptoms that resolve on their own within months following the trauma.[13] A smaller group of individuals will develop PTSD: within this group, some will develop symptoms immediately following exposure to the traumatic event, and others will develop symptoms in the months that follow.[3] In the absence of intervention, persistent or worsening symptoms of PTSD are likely to endure. PTSD commonly co-occurs with other mental health disorders.[1] The most common comorbid disorders include major depressive disorder, anxiety disorders, and substance use disorders. There is some evidence that PTSD is associated with physical health comorbidities, including poorer physical health-related quality of life, chronic pain, and cardiorespiratory, gastrointestinal, and general health complaints.[14]

PTSD and ASD are distressing and impairing conditions that can occur in rehabilitation populations. Whether these symptoms are related to recent or remote traumatic events, they can interfere with full engagement in rehabilitation and contribute to poor long-term health outcomes. The best treatment for PTSD and ASD is psychological intervention; fortunately, a number of evidence-based approaches, delivered by mental health care professionals, are effective in reducing PTSD and ASD symptoms. Across the continuum of rehabilitation care, medical providers can identify patients in need of psychological intervention by routinely screening for PTSD and ASD. Several empirically supported and brief assessment tools are available for this purpose. Ultimately, the timely identification of patients experiencing PTSD and ASD symptoms and subsequent referral to a mental health professional for targeted and evidence-based treatment can maximize engagement in rehabilitation and enhance an individuals' well-being and overall quality of life.

## RESOURCES AND REFERENCES

The full list of resources and references appears in the digital product found on http://connect .springerpub.com/content/book/978-0-8261-6226-7/part/part03/chapter/ch46

# RHEUMATOLOGICAL DISEASES

IRVIN J. HUANG, JENNA L. THOMASON, AND ALISON M. BAYS

## AXIAL SPONDYLOARTHRITIS (ANKYLOSING SPONDYLITIS)

### Core Definitions

Spondyloarthritis comprises a group of conditions characterized by inflammation of the sacroiliac joints, spine, or peripheral joints. Spondyloarthritis includes axial spondyloarthritis (also known as ankylosing spondylitis [AS]), psoriatic arthritis, inflammatory bowel disease-associated arthritis, and reactive arthritis. Patients can either have an axial or peripheral predominance. Axial spondyloarthritis can be further differentiated into AS and nonradiographic spondyloarthritis based on the presence or absence of radiographic evidence of damage in the sacroiliac joints on x-ray. AS is more prevalent in men and is often diagnosed at a younger age (<45 years).[1]

### Etiology and Pathophysiology

The tendon enthesis (connective tissue between tendon and bone) is the target of inflammation. The inflammation is related to the interactions of immune cells, microbiome, and mechanical stress at the enthesis in individuals with genetic predisposition.[1] Given that this disease is not an autoimmune condition with an autoantigen, autoantibody testing is not available.

### Diagnostic Approach

The hallmark feature of AS is inflammatory back pain that improves with physical activity and worsens with rest. Patients report prolonged low back stiffness in the morning, typically lasting greater than an hour. Patients can also have features shared with other spondyloarthritides including peripheral arthritis, dactylitis, enthesitis, psoriasis, inflammatory bowel disease, and inflammatory eye disease. Special examination techniques can be utilized to assess mobility including the lateral lumbar flexion, anterior lumbar flexion (modified Schober test), occiput-to-wall test, and chest wall expansion measurements. Laboratory studies are limited but include inflammatory markers (C-reactive protein [CRP] and erythrocyte sedimentation rate [ESR]) and the HLA-B27 test. Inflammatory markers are elevated in about half of patients with AS. While HLA-B27 can be diagnostically helpful, a negative test does not rule out the disease particularly in patients who are not White. Imaging studies should be considered

The full list of references appears in the digital product found on http://connect.springerpub.com/content/book/978-0-8261-6226-7/part/part03/chapter/ch47

as part of the workup. Conventional radiography (anterior–posterior view of the pelvis or dedicated sacroiliac joint film) to evaluate the sacroiliac joints is a good starting point given much lower radiation, cost, and simplicity of the test in comparison to advanced imaging. X-ray of the spine may also show syndesmophytes. If the study is negative or inconclusive despite convincing history and/or physical examination, advanced imaging can be considered. MRI of the pelvis with T1-weighted and short tau inversion recovery (STIR) sequences and semicoronal views is the current gold standard imaging modality, which can assess for both acute and chronic evidence of sacroiliac inflammation and the extent of structural damage.[2] If the patient is unable to tolerate an MRI or has contraindications, CT can be considered to evaluate for sclerosis and erosions, although it is unable to demonstrate active inflammatory changes.

## Treatment

Early initiation of exercise and physical therapy is key to preserving mobility and function. Non-steroidal anti-inflammatory drugs (NSAIDs) remain the first-line of therapy. Unlike most rheumatologic diseases, systemic steroids provide little benefit and are not recommended. Patients with peripheral arthritis who are symptomatic despite adequate NSAIDs use or have contraindications can be treated with sulfasalazine. Tumor necrosis factor (TNF) and IL-17 inhibitors can be used to treat those with refractory disease.[3]

## Functional Prognosis and Outcomes

Functional prognosis and outcomes can be highly variable depending on the individual's genetic predisposition, disease progression, and time of diagnosis. AS can result in significant disability. Morbidity includes significant ankylosis of the spine resulting in severe limitation in range of motion and increased risk of fractures.

## Basic Order Sets

X-ray of sacroiliac joints and other symptomatic regions, CRP, and ESR. Consider the HLA-B27 test.

## PSORIATIC ARTHRITIS

### Core Definitions

Psoriatic arthritis is a chronic inflammatory joint disease associated with psoriasis. Recent studies found psoriatic arthritis occurs in up to 30% of the patients with psoriasis.[4] Manifestations of psoriatic arthritis include peripheral arthritis, enthesitis, dactylitis, spondylitis, and nail pitting and onycholysis.

### Etiology and Pathophysiology

Psoriatic arthritis is believed to be a highly heritable polygenic disease associated with class I major histocompatibility complex (MHC) alleles where T cells play an important role in the pathogenesis. Risk factors include obesity, severe psoriasis, and psoriasis involving the scalp, genital, and intertriginous regions.[4] The tendon enthesis is the target of inflammation and the initial site of musculoskeletal disease.

## Diagnostic Approach

There are five clinical subtypes of psoriatic arthritis: oligoarticular (≤4 joints), polyarticular (≥5 joints), distal (affects the distal interphalangeal joints), arthritis mutilans (deforming and destructive), and axial (involves the spine and sacroiliac joints).[4] Clinical features of psoriatic arthritis include inflammatory arthritis, enthesitis, dactylitis, and nail dystrophy. Enthesitis most commonly involves the plantar fascia and Achilles' tendon, although tendons around the knees, elbows, shoulders, and pelvis can also be affected. Dactylitis can be acute (swelling, erythema, and pain) or chronic (swelling without erythema or pain). The third and fourth toes are most commonly affected.[4] Nail dystrophy includes onycholysis, pitting, or hyperkeratosis. The polyarticular subtype can sometimes be confused for rheumatoid arthritis (RA), but the rheumatoid factor should be negative. The arthritis mutilans subtype is the most deforming, causing destruction of the bone and cartilage. Peripheral joint radiographs often show bone loss with eccentric erosions and joint-space loss. New bone formation with periostitis, ankylosis, and enthesophytes can be observed. The "pencil-in-cup" deformity is a classic finding in arthritis mutilans subtype. Those with axial subtype can have unilateral sacroiliitis and spinal paramarginal and vertical syndesmophytes.[4] Diagnosis of psoriatic arthritis is based on clinical and imaging features as discussed earlier. MRI may show synovitis and bone marrow edema. Musculoskeletal ultrasound can be employed to evaluate for synovitis, enthesitis, enthesophytes, and erosions. There are no specific serology or antibody tests for psoriatic arthritis.

## Treatment

NSAIDs are the first-line therapy for both peripheral and axial symptoms. Nonpharmacologic therapies, such as physical therapy and weight loss, should be initiated early especially for those with axial involvement. Local glucocorticoid injections can be used for monoarticular arthritis. While systemic glucocorticoids can be effective for joint symptoms, discontinuation can exacerbate psoriasis, so it should be used with caution. Conventional disease-modifying antirheumatic drugs (DMARDs), anti-TNF agents, anti-IL-17 agents, and anti-IL-12/23 agents can be considered for more severe disease.[5]

## Functional Prognosis and Outcomes

Functional prognosis and outcomes can be highly variable depending on the subtype of psoriatic arthritis. Arthritis mutilans can result in a significant reduction of hand function, and axial involvement can lead to mobility restriction and increased risk of fractures.

## Basic Order Sets

X-ray imaging of hands, feet, sacroiliac joints, and other symptomatic regions. CRP and ESR can sometimes be elevated. Musculoskeletal ultrasound examination for enthesitis evaluation can be considered in more diagnostically challenging cases.

# SYSTEMIC LUPUS ERYTHEMATOSUS

## Core Definitions

Systemic lupus erythematosus (SLE) is a chronic, multisystemic autoimmune disorder that can affect virtually any organ in the body. The prevalence in women is much higher with the vast majority being women of childbearing age.[6] The prevalence among non-White race/ethnicity (African American, Asian, or Hispanic) is three to four times higher than in the White population.[7]

### Etiology/Pathophysiology

While the etiology is unclear, it is believed to be multifactorial including immunologic, genetic, hormonal, and environmental components.[6] Many of the clinical manifestations are mediated by antibody formation resulting in immune complexes. These immune complexes can deposit in various organs, such as the kidneys, leading to complement activation and subsequent tissue damage.

### Diagnostic Approach

Diagnosis of this complex and variable disease necessitates a complete history and physical examination. Major clinical features include constitutional symptoms, arthritis, oral or nasal ulcerations, rash, cardiac manifestations, Raynaud phenomenon, renal involvement, hematologic abnormalities, and neuropsychiatric manifestations.[7] Antinuclear antibody (ANA) by immunofluorescence is considered the hallmark laboratory test and can be considered if clinical suspicion for SLE is high. While a titer of $\geq 1:80$ suggests clinical significance, a positive test alone is not diagnostic of SLE. Patients can have SLE-specific antibodies including anti-dsDNA and anti-Smith antibodies. During active disease, patients can have hypocomplementemia with low C3 and/or C4. SLE is sometimes accompanied by antiphospholipid antibodies (anticardiolipin antibodies, anti-$\beta$2GP1 antibodies, or lupus anticoagulants). Given the multisystemic nature of the disease, in addition to the above antibody tests, patients should also have a complete blood count (CBC) with differential (cytopenias), comprehensive metabolic panel (CMP; renal insufficiency or elevated liver enzyme), and urinalysis with protein to creatinine ratio (proteinuria or hematuria).[7]

### Treatment

Hydroxychloroquine is the mainstay therapy for all SLE patients given recognized mortality benefits. Life or organ-threatening presentation of SLE is treated with high-dose steroids (1 mg/kg body weight), along with steroid-sparing therapies including cyclophosphamide, mycophenolate, azathioprine, or calcineurin inhibitors depending on organ involvement.[6] Belimumab, the only biologic medication currently approved for SLE, can be helpful for musculoskeletal and mucocutaneous manifestations.

### Functional Prognosis and Outcomes

Functional prognosis is excellent when disease remission is achieved.

### Basic Order Sets

ANA with reflex panel, CBC with differential, CMP, urinalysis (with protein/creatinine ratio), C3, C4, ESR, and CRP.

# SYSTEMIC SCLEROSIS (SCLERODERMA)

## Core Definitions

Systemic sclerosis (SSc) is a chronic multisystemic disease characterized by progressive fibrosis of the skin, vasculature, and internal organs.[8] The term scleroderma describes the thickened and hardened skin that is a hallmark of the disease. SSc can be divided into limited cutaneous SSc (formerly known as CREST [calcinosis, Raynaud's phenomenon, esophageal dysmotility, sclerodactyly, telangiectasia]) and diffuse cutaneous SSc.

## Etiology and Pathophysiology

While the etiology is unknown, the pathogenesis is believed to be centralized in early immunological events and vascular changes leading to the production of activated fibrogenic fibroblasts.[8] This results in the development of fibrosis in the skin and organs with vasculopathy.

## Diagnostic Approach

Raynaud phenomenon and skin thickening are the hallmark manifestations of this disease. Skin thickening can affect the hands, arms, feet, and face. Examination of the nailfold capillaries with capillaroscopy reveals abnormal features such as dilated capillary loops, capillary dropout, and hemorrhages. Laboratory tests include ANA reflexive panel, CBC with differential, urinalysis, and creatine kinase. Anti-Scl-70 (anti-topoisomerase I) antibodies are generally associated with diffuse cutaneous SSc, which has a higher risk for interstitial lung disease.[8] Anticentromere antibodies are typically associated with limited cutaneous SSc. Anti-RNA polymerase III antibodies are typically found in patients with diffuse cutaneous SSc and is associated with rapid skin thickening and the development of scleroderma renal crisis. Scleroderma renal crisis is heralded by the new onset of hypertension and renal insufficiency that can rapidly lead to renal failure if treatment is delayed. Antegrade colonic enema (ACE) inhibitors are effective treatments and can reduce mortality.[9]

## Treatment

There is no standard treatment. Treatment is primarily focused on symptomatic control of Raynaud's phenomenon and reflux. In certain cases, patients may receive immunosuppression, as with interstitial lung disease and rapidly progressive skin involvement.[9] Patients with the Raynaud phenomenon should be encouraged to stay warm by maintaining a good core body and digit temperature.

## Functional Prognosis and Outcomes

Individuals with extensive skin involvement as well as those with visceral involvements (cardiac, pulmonary, and/or renal) have a higher risk of mortality. Extensive skin involvement can lead to contractures resulting in significant mobility impairment.

## Basic Order Sets

ANA with reflex panel, CBC with differential, and CMP.

## RHEUMATOID ARTHRITIS

### Core Definitions

RA is an inflammatory arthritis characterized by inflammation of the synovial lining of joints resulting in erosions and destruction if left untreated. It commonly affects the metacarpophalangeal (MCP) joints, proximal interphalangeal (PIP) joints, wrists, knees, and metatarsophalangeal (MTP) joints, though it may affect other joints as well. Patients often complain of prolonged morning stiffness (usually greater than 1 hour) and swelling, and improvement in symptoms with activity and NSAID use. This is in contrast to mechanical causes of joint pain, which are worse at the end of the day and after prolonged use, typically without significant swelling and morning stiffness.

### Etiology and Pathophysiology

The synovium is the target of inflammation, which is driven by CD4+ T cells and macrophages.[10] The synovium expands when proinflammatory cytokines are present. With untreated disease, there is damage to cartilage and bone due to synovial invasion.

RA typically onsets between ages 45 and 65, though patients of any age can be affected. RA is more common in women by 2 to 3:1. There is a higher prevalence in the Native American population (5%–6%).[10] Although there is a strong genetic component, twin studies only show concordance of 12% to 15%.[10] There is a shared epitope located in the HLA-DR region, significantly associated with the development of RA.

### Diagnostic Approach

The hallmark feature is symmetrically swollen peripheral joints, often MCPs, PIPs, wrists, and MTP joints but larger joints can also be affected. Patients complain of inflammatory joint symptoms as described previously, slightly improved by NSAIDs. Workup includes rheumatoid factor and anticyclic citrullinated peptide (anti-CCP) antibody testing. Inflammatory markers (ESR and CRP) are often elevated. X-rays of bilateral hands and feet should be obtained to look for marginal joint erosions, which may not be present in early disease. Periarticular osteopenia is the earliest radiographic finding in RA. Ultrasound may be used to assess for subclinical synovitis.

### Treatment

Early initiation of DMARDs is critical.[11] Triple therapy includes methotrexate, sulfasalazine, and hydroxychloroquine. If the patient has an inadequate response to DMARDs, therapy is quickly escalated to biologic medications, often starting with anti-TNF therapy. Patients are responsive to 10 to 15 mg of prednisone daily, which can be used as a bridge until DMARDs take effect.

### Functional Prognosis and Outcomes

Functional prognosis and outcomes can be excellent if the disease is recognized early and there is good adherence to medication. With later diagnosis or lack of access to medications, significant disability can result.

## Basic Order Sets

X-ray imaging of bilateral hands and feet to look for marginal erosions, RF, anti-CCP, ESR, and CRP.

## DERMATOMYOSITIS AND POLYMYOSITIS

### Core Definitions

Dermatomyositis (DM) and polymyositis (PM) are idiopathic inflammatory myopathies resulting in muscle inflammation and proximal muscle weakness. DM is also associated with a number of skin manifestations. While the clinical presentations between DM and PM are similar, the histology on muscle biopsy is distinct.

### Etiology and Pathophysiology

DM and PM are both autoimmune inflammatory conditions, although the exact pathogenic mechanisms are unknown. Women are affected more often than men with onset at any age.[12] Juvenile DM and PM are both rare, with the former being far more common than the latter.

### Diagnostic Approach

Patients present with subacute proximal symmetric weakness affecting deltoids, hip flexors, and neck flexors. Dysphagia, arthralgia/arthritis, Raynaud's phenomenon, and interstitial lung disease may also be present. Myalgia, if present at all, is usually mild.

In DM, cutaneous manifestations often precede or accompany weakness. A subset of patients have amyopathic disease (ADM).[13] Cutaneous manifestations include Gottron's papules, Heliotrope rash, Shawl sign, V sign, Holster sign, raggedy cuticles, dilated nailfold capillaries, facial erythema, and calcinosis cutis.[13] DM rashes have a violaceous appearance, and the hands are almost always involved.

The creatine kinase level is often elevated, which can be as high as 50 times the upper limit of normal (except in ADM).[13] Elevated levels of serum and urine myoglobin, aspartate aminotransferase (AST), alanine aminotransferase (ALT), aldolase, and lactate dehydrogenase (LDH) are also typically observed due to muscle inflammation. A positive ANA is often present, and myositis-specific antibodies are sometimes seen as well.

EMG and MRI may show similar findings for these two conditions, but the histopathologic findings on biopsy are distinct. EMG shows a myopathic pattern with insertional activity, spontaneous fibrillation, myopathic low amplitude and short duration action potentials, and complex repetitive discharges.[14] MRI of affected muscles may show edema, fibrosis, calcification, and/or muscle atrophy; these findings are nonspecific but MRI is helpful for surveying a large territory. In both conditions, muscle biopsy reveals muscle fiber necrosis, degeneration, regeneration, and an inflammatory cell infiltrate.[14] In PM, the inflammation is perivascular, observed in multiple foci within the endomysium, and consists mostly of CD8+ cytotoxic T lymphocytes invading healthy fibers expressing MHC class I antigen. In DM, muscle biopsy reveals injury in both capillaries and myofibers, particularly perifascicular myofibers; the inflammatory infiltrate consists primarily of CD4+ cells.[14] Also in DM, skin biopsy reveals interface dermatitis.

## Treatment

Patients are treated with high-dose steroids (1 mg/kg of body weight) with a slow taper. A steroid-sparing agent, such as azathioprine or methotrexate, is started concurrently to facilitate steroid taper. Mycophenolate can also be used, though the data are more limited. For refractory disease, rituximab or IVIG may be added.

## Functional Prognosis and Outcomes

Patients are typically responsive to immunosuppression, with the exception of anti-melanoma differentiation-associated protein 5 (MDA-5) positive DM patients, who have a high mortality rate due to rapidly progressive interstitial lung disease (ILD). Notably, both DM and PM have been associated with malignancy, with the risk being greater in DM (particularly in patients with transcription intermediary factor 1-gamma [TIF1-gamma] or nuclear matrix protein-2 [NXP-2] antibodies).[14]

## Basic Order Sets

ANA with reflex panel, myositis antibody panel, CK level, serum and urine myoglobin, aldolase, AST, ALT, and LDH. Consider MRI, electromyography and nerve conduction study (EMG/NCS), or muscle biopsy to aid with diagnosis.

## REFERENCES

The full list of references appears in the digital product found on http://connect.springerpub.com/content/book/978-0-8261-6226-7/part/part03/chapter/ch47

# SEIZURES

LESLEY C. KAYE AND SHAHIN HAKIMIAN

## CORE DEFINITIONS

A seizure is defined as "a transient occurrence of signs and/or symptoms due to abnormal excessive or synchronous neuronal activity in the brain," or more simply, a clinical manifestation of storms of excessive neuronal activity in the brain. The lifetime cumulative risk of a seizure is nearly 10%.[1] Seizures can be provoked or can occur spontaneously in patients with epilepsy. Provoked seizures can happen in many circumstances, and these are discussed later.

Epilepsy is defined as two unprovoked seizures more than 24 hours apart, or a single seizure with a high probability of a second seizure based on MRI, EEG, or epilepsy syndrome.[2] Epilepsy affects about 1% of the population. In a patient without risk factors for epilepsy, a first unprovoked seizure has a 30% to 40% chance of recurrence, with the highest risk in the first 6 months.[1] Patients with structural brain lesions (e.g., prior stroke, tumor, or trauma) or an abnormal EEG have a higher risk of second seizure and thus may have a diagnosis of epilepsy after a single clinical event.[2,3] In the rehab setting, patients with recent brain injuries, strokes, or brain surgery have an elevated risk of having a seizure.

Status epilepticus is a convulsive seizure lasting more than 5 minutes (or nonconvulsive seizures lasting more than 10 minutes). This is a neurologic emergency.

## ETIOLOGY AND PATHOPHYSIOLOGY

### Seizure Classification and Presentation

Seizures have different manifestations depending on which parts of the brain are involved and the pattern of abnormal brain activity. Seizures can start focally (classified as "focal onset seizures") or start more diffusely across the brain (classified as "generalized onset seizures"). The description of the seizure, the neurologic examination, prior imaging, and EEG findings can all help with seizure classification.

Symptoms of a focal seizure depend very much on where in the brain it starts, which may correspond to an area of structural abnormality. Focal seizures may or may not have "focal motor signs" (i.e., focal twitching) or other more complex movements (called "automatisms"). Non-motor signs and symptoms can include behavioral arrest, emotional change, cognitive changes, unusual internal feelings (e.g., déjà vu, weird smell, nausea, etc.), or autonomic manifestations

---

The full list of resources and references appears in the digital product found on http://connect
.springerpub.com/content/book/978-0-8261-6226-7/part/part03/chapter/ch48

(e.g., drooling). Focal seizures commonly spread to parts of the brain that result in impaired awareness. As impaired awareness has implications for patient safety, these focal seizures have a unique designation called "focal onset with impaired awareness" (previously called "complex partial" seizures). Focal seizures can subsequently spread from the area of onset and generalize to bilateral hemispheres, leading to bilateral generalized tonic-clonic seizures, also called secondarily generalized seizures. Some seizures may generalize quickly, making it difficult to determine how they started. Patients with epilepsy may have one or multiple different seizure types.

Generalized onset seizures occur commonly as well. Some occur in specific epilepsy syndromes, though they can also be provoked (e.g., drug intoxication or withdrawal). Typical generalized onset seizure types include primary generalized tonic-clonic seizures, clonic, tonic, myoclonic, atonic, and absence seizures.[4]

## Epilepsy Syndromes

Patients with recurrent focal onset seizures are classified as having "focal onset epilepsy." There are acquired conditions (e.g., trauma), genetic syndromes (e.g., tuberous sclerosis or focal cortical dysplasia), or unknown presumed structural (formerly called cryptogenic) etiologies for focal epilepsy syndromes. Idiopathic generalized epilepsy syndromes are common and occur in people who are otherwise neurologically intact. These syndromes include childhood absence epilepsy, juvenile myoclonic epilepsy, juvenile absence epilepsy, and epilepsy with generalized tonic-clonic seizures alone. A third major category of epilepsy syndromes is "epileptic encephalopathies" or "symptomatic generalized onset epilepsies." These often manifest in infancy or early childhood and are accompanied by developmental delay and refractory epilepsy. This category includes Lennox-Gastaut syndrome, though there are many other examples of these syndromes.

## DIAGNOSTIC APPROACH

### Ongoing Seizures

Most important is to ensure patient safety. Remove sharp objects and lower the patient to bed or ground if possible. A pillow/soft object under the patient's head is advisable but any item in their mouth is not. If convulsing, evaluate for airway and breathing. Roll the patient on their side to improve breathing mechanics and to avoid aspiration. Administer oxygen and suction the oral cavity if possible. Restraints are not advisable. The duration and behaviors observed during the seizure should be recorded. If a convulsion is lasting more than 5 minutes or another seizure type is lasting more than 10 minutes, then initiate status epilepticus treatment.

Immediately after a seizure evaluation of the airway, breathing, pulse, and oxygenation is recommended. A brief period of postictal apnea or hypopnea after a convulsion is common, though prolonged hypopnea can cause SUDEP (sudden unexpected death in epilepsy patient). Physically stimulate the patient to encourage breathing. Oxygen may be administered if needed. Arrhythmias may occur thus clinicians should be vigilant.

### Postictal State

Patients may be agitated, confused, or even aggressive. If a patient continues to be confused for several minutes, they may be experiencing ongoing subtle focal seizures. Postictal transient focal motor weakness, referred to as "Todd's paralysis," or exacerbation of prior neurologic deficits may occur. Postictal deficits should improve over a few minutes to hours and suggest brain area of seizure onset contralateral to the weakness. Persistent new deficits warrant an evaluation.

Musculoskeletal injuries including spinous process fractures, subdural hematomas, neck injuries, and shoulder dislocations may happen after seizures. New posterior shoulder dislocation is nearly pathognomonic for a seizure. Tongue lacerations, chipped teeth, or facial and corneal abrasion may all occur and deserve attention. Recurrent seizures, even in the acute setting, deserve abortive therapy and acute medical evaluation.

## Seizure History

Often seizures are not witnessed and have varied manifestations. Understanding what happened and determining whether an event was a seizure can be difficult. Important questions to ask include the duration and sequence of events. The signs and symptoms of a seizure at its onset and progression, including any sensation that the patient may recall, provide important clues to the diagnosis. Important characteristics include whether the patient was responsive or aware at some point during the event and the description of any movements including the timing and occurrence of tonic-clonic movements. Features such as unilateral shaking at onset, forced head-turning, or eye deviation provide clues from which hemisphere the seizure started. Automatisms, or automatic movements, such as picking, fidgeting, or lip-smacking are frequently seen in temporal lobe seizures. Incontinence and tongue biting are often clues to convulsive seizures. Stereotyped events are more likely to be seizures, so one should ask if recurrent events are like each other. Medical history of prior central nervous system (CNS) infection, prior seizures, brain injury, stroke, developmental delay, or family history of epilepsy are risk factors that provide clues to the diagnosis.

## Evaluation

A thorough neurologic examination can provide clues as to the diagnosis and localization of seizure. Bedside EEG is helpful to determine an underlying seizure focus, to detect any ongoing subclinical seizures, and gauge the risk of subsequent seizures. Longer EEG studies are needed if the diagnosis is uncertain for recurrent events or there is suspicion for ongoing seizures.

For patients without a prior neurologic injury or deficit, a brain MRI with and without contrast (or at least a contrasted head CT) is necessary to rule out a new lesion as the cause of the first-time seizure.

Many first-time seizures are provoked. An important step involves a review of any recent medication changes or concurrent health problems that may increase seizure (see Table 48.1). Laboratory evaluation including complete blood count (CBC), comprehensive metabolic panel (CMP), urine drug screen, and urine analysis may be indicated for identifying a provoking factor. Prolonged convulsions can lead to elevated creatine phosphokinase (CK) and rhabdomyolysis, thus attention should be paid to renal function.[5] If there is any concern for CNS infection, a lumbar puncture and rapid initiation of treatment for the infection is indicated.

**TABLE 48.1 MOST COMMON CAUSES OF ACUTE SYMPTOMATIC SEIZURES[6]**

| | |
|---|---|
| ELECTROLYTE ABNORMALITIES | Hypoglycemia, severe hyperglycemia, hypocalcemia, hyponatremia, hypernatremia, hypomagnesemia, hypophosphatemia |
| MEDICATIONS (IATROGENIC) | Bupropion, clozapine, cephalosporins, quinolone antibiotics (esp. ciprofloxacin), Baclofen, tramadol, theophylline, withdrawal from antiseizure drugs, and rarely other antipsychotics or antidepressants |
| RECREATIONAL DRUGS | Withdrawal: benzodiazepines, alcohol, or barbiturates Overdose: cocaine, ethamphetamine, other stimulants and hallucinogens |
| DIFFUSE/SYSTEMIC BRAIN | Sepsis/infection, eclampsia, anoxic brain injury, PRES |
| BRAIN LESIONS | Trauma, tumors, stroke, hemorrhage, abscess, vascular malformations, congenital malformation, venous thrombosis |
| INFLAMMATORY | Encephalitis, meningitis, autoimmune encephalitis |

PRES, posterior reversible encephalopathy syndrome.

## Differential Diagnosis

Any convulsive like event, transient alteration of mental status, paroxysmal behavioral spell, or episodic abnormal movement can be misidentified as a seizure. There are often strong clues in history and tests that can distinguish them. Epileptic seizures are typically stereotyped (if recurrent), may show rhythmic involuntary twitching-type movements, and often progress and end between 30 seconds to 2 minutes. They are often followed by a postictal recovery phase that can last several minutes.

By contrast, syncope or near syncope often occurs immediately after standing, may have palpitations, sensation of lightheadedness, or appearance of skin pallor at the onset. There is a more clear early loss of muscle tone. After the loss of tone, patients may briefly stiffen and have transient irregular whole-body jerking movements (sometimes called 'convulsive syncope'), which can be especially misleading. Recovery from syncope is often very quick. Evaluation with EKG and orthostatic vital signs may be helpful, but the distinction is best based on history.

Psychogenic nonepileptic spells (PNES), colloquially known as "pseudoseizures," commonly mimic epileptic seizures. Clues to PNES include hip thrusting movements, eye closure (particularly during a convulsive phase of an event), prolonged episodes with fluctuating or nonrhythmic movements, ictal or postictal sobbing, and quick return to baseline.

Transient ischemic attacks (TIAs) may be differentiated from seizures in that they cause transient loss rather than the gain of neurologic function (e.g., flaccid loss of unilateral muscle tone). TIAs generally last many minutes (more than 5 minutes) and often have a more gradual onset. Tremor or other movement disorders are typically more continuous or provoked with action, and often bilateral.

Multifocal myoclonus can be caused by metabolic derangements or by postanoxic brain injury. Jerks can occur in any limb, are not stereotyped or rhythmic, and are often provoked by the stimulus. Importantly, a patient's mental status often does not change during these movements, although patients may be confused for other reasons.

Delirium may be difficult to differentiate from nonconvulsive seizure but timing and progression are different. Parasomnias causing abnormal movements such as periodic limb movement disorder, REM behavior disorders, or even hypnic jerks may be misinterpreted by patients or families as a seizure. A key difference is that in epilepsy, the specific movements are often stereotyped, while parasomnias have more variability in motor signs but tend to be tied to specific stages of sleep.

## TREATMENT OF ACUTE SEIZURES

Acute abortive treatment for self-limited seizures lasting less than 5 minutes is generally not necessary. Prolonged seizures or status epilepticus require timely acute treatment typically using a well-established protocol. A timeline of the treatment protocol for status epilepticus is in Figure 48.1.

For new provoked seizures, an important step is eliminating provoking factors (such as a new medication or electrolyte abnormalities) if possible. In patients with a reversible provoking cause, long-term treatment is not indicated. Long-term treatment with an antiepileptic drug is necessary for patients who are at high risk of having additional seizures, such as those with an underlying CNS cause or epilepsy. For a patient with a first-time seizure with no clear underlying risk, normal EEG, and normal MRI, treatment is generally deferred until a second seizure, though a discussion of risk and benefit should be hard with the patient.[8]

### Breakthrough Seizures in Epilepsy Patients

Patients with epilepsy are at risk of having breakthrough seizures.[9] Common provoking factors include sleep deprivation, systemic infection or acute illness, drugs/alcohol, new medications such as antibiotics, and changes to antiepileptic drug levels due to drug interactions or missed medication doses. In the setting of known epilepsy, EEG and head imaging are not necessarily required. Medications may or may not need to be adjusted based on baseline seizure frequency, presence of clear provoking factor, and levels of medications. Even with optimal treatment, 30% of patients with epilepsy are refractory to medical treatment and liable to sporadic unprovoked breakthrough seizures.[10]

For patients with epilepsy, an acute treatment plan should be in place. A seizure action plan should include instructions for care providers for acute management of seizures, instructions on the use of rescue drugs, and directions on when to call for emergency help (9-1-1). Rectal diazepam gel for prolonged convulsions, oral lorazepam for clusters of seizures, and nasal midazolam are good options (Table 48.2).

### Antiepileptic Drugs

Patients with epilepsy should be on an antiepileptic drug to reduce the risk of seizure recurrence. With an increasing number of antiepileptic drugs (AEDs) on the market, the choice of which agent to start can be intimidating. Initial drug choice is usually based more on tolerability (which varies by comorbid conditions), drug interaction considerations, and availability of a drug for a patient (related to affordability), than on effectiveness. In contrast, for patients with chronic epilepsy, medication changes are not trivial. A simple inappropriate substitution can lead to dangerous seizures and injury. Common AEDs are listed in Table 48.3.

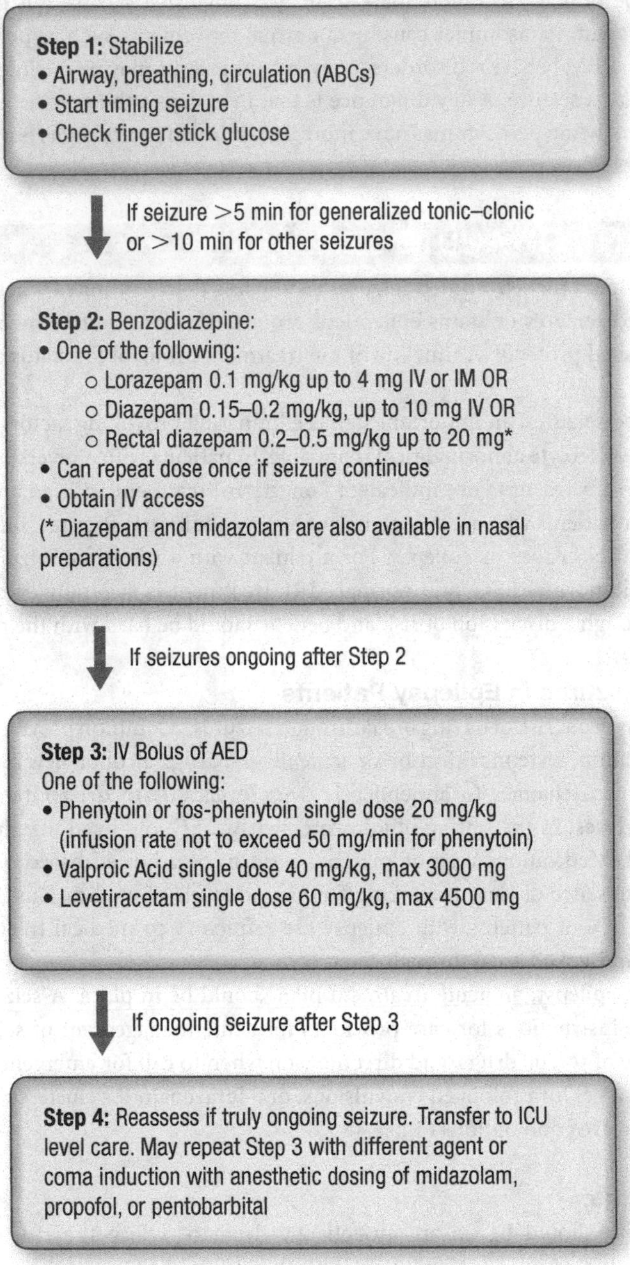

**Step 1:** Stabilize
- Airway, breathing, circulation (ABCs)
- Start timing seizure
- Check finger stick glucose

If seizure >5 min for generalized tonic–clonic
or >10 min for other seizures

**Step 2:** Benzodiazepine:
- One of the following:
  - Lorazepam 0.1 mg/kg up to 4 mg IV or IM OR
  - Diazepam 0.15–0.2 mg/kg, up to 10 mg IV OR
  - Rectal diazepam 0.2–0.5 mg/kg up to 20 mg*
- Can repeat dose once if seizure continues
- Obtain IV access

(* Diazepam and midazolam are also available in nasal preparations)

If seizures ongoing after Step 2

**Step 3:** IV Bolus of AED
One of the following:
- Phenytoin or fos-phenytoin single dose 20 mg/kg
  (infusion rate not to exceed 50 mg/min for phenytoin)
- Valproic Acid single dose 40 mg/kg, max 3000 mg
- Levetiracetam single dose 60 mg/kg, max 4500 mg

If ongoing seizure after Step 3

**Step 4:** Reassess if truly ongoing seizure. Transfer to ICU level care. May repeat Step 3 with different agent or coma induction with anesthetic dosing of midazolam, propofol, or pentobarbital

**FIGURE 48.1** Status epilepticus flow sheet.[7]

## TABLE 48.2 ACUTE PROLONGED SEIZURE OR SEIZURE CLUSTER RESCUE DRUGS

| MEDICATION (BRAND NAME(S)) | INDICATION | DOSING |
|---|---|---|
| Lorazepam—po or iv (Ativan) | PO—seizure clusters IV—status epilepticus/ prolonged seizures | 2 mg tablet PO/IV/IM or per G-tube with flush, may repeat × 2 in a day |
| Rectal diazepam (Diastat or Acudial) | Seizure clusters (or prolonged seizure) | Up to 10 mg rectal gel. May repeat × 1 |
| Intranasal midazolam (Nayzilam) | Seizure clusters (or prolonged seizure) | 5 mg intranasally. May repeat × 1 |
| Intranasal diazepam (Valtoco) | Seizure clusters (or prolonged seizure) | 10 to 20 mg nasally (0.2 mg/kg). May repeat × 1 after 4 hours. Limit to 1 episode per 5 days or 5 episodes/month |

Rescue medications are intended for acute treatment of seizure clusters, or prolonged convulsive seizures lasting more than 5 minutes, or other seizure types lasting more than 10 minutes.

## TABLE 48.3 MOST COMMONLY USED ANTIEPILEPTIC DRUGS[11]

| DRUG (MAJOR BRANDS)— FORMULATIONS | RX INTERACTIONS | CAUTIONS/ADVERSE EFFECTS |
|---|---|---|
| Carbamazepine (Tegretol, Carbatrol, Epitol) as tablet, ER tablet, capsules chewable tablet, suspension | **High interaction risk.** CYP3A4 inducer and substrate with many interactions including warfarin, other oral anticoagulants, and macrolides | **Caution:** risk of Steven Johnson/TEN when initiating (must check for HLA-B*1502 haplotype in Asians). Some risk of aplastic anemia/agranulocytosis. **Avoid:** generalized onset epilepsy (may worsen seizures in primary generalized epilepsy). **Possible adverse effects:** ataxia, diplopia, sedation, hyponatremia (SIADH). **Monitor:** check CMP and CBC after initiating |
| Clonazepam (Klonopin) as tablet, ODT | Levels lowered by other hepatic enzyme-inducing drugs | **Caution:** sedative and high risk of habituation/ tolerance and withdrawal. Can depress respiration particularly if combined with opioids. **Avoid** in narrow angle glaucoma or liver disease. **Possible adverse effects:** sedation, impaired cognition or motor skills **Note:** mainly used for myoclonic seizures |
| Lacosamide (Vimpat) as IV, tablet, oral solution | Use caution if combined with other drugs that prolong PR interval | **Caution:** prolongs PR interval, risk of atrial arrhythmias. Also, use caution in primary generalized epilepsies. **Possible adverse effects:** ataxia, diplopia, sedation. Usually well tolerated. **Note:** $$ only available as brand Vimpat (as of 2020). |

(continued)

**TABLE 48.3 MOST COMMONLY USED ANTIEPILEPTIC DRUGS[11] (*continued*)**

| DRUG (MAJOR BRANDS)— FORMULATIONS | RX INTERACTIONS | CAUTIONS/ADVERSE EFFECTS |
|---|---|---|
| Lamotrigine (Lamictal) as tablet, ODT, dispersible or chewable tablet | Metabolism is inhibited by valproic acid. Levels lowered with hepatic enzyme-inducing drugs including contraceptive pills (or pregnancy). | **Caution:** risk of SJS/TEN. Rare risk of HLH and aseptic meningitis. May affect cardiac conduction (prolonged QRS or heart block) **Possible adverse effects:** insomnia (or sedation), ataxia/dizziness (usually at high doses). May exacerbate myoclonus. **Note:** *must* titrate slowly due to the risk of SJS. Risk higher if on divalproex. |
| Levetiracetam (Keppra) as IV, tablet, oral suspension, chewable or ODT tablet | None | **Caution:** depression **Possible adverse effects:** risk of agitation, depression, and rarely psychotic symptoms. May cause sedation. **Note:** low systemic toxicity and broad spectrum. |
| Oxcarbazepine (Trileptal) as tablet, ER, oral suspension | Induces: weakly CYP3A4, UGT Inhibits: CYP2C19 | Similar to carbamazepine (see earlier description). Most adverse effects are milder than carbamazepine except higher risk for hyponatremia. **Avoid** in generalized epilepsy. **Monitor:** serum sodium |
| Phenobarbital as IV, tablet, elixir | **High interaction risk.** Strong inducer of several hepatic enzymes with a high risk of drug interactions. | **Caution:** risk of SJS/TEN, DRESS, respiratory depression (worsened with concurrent EtOH or sedatives). Osteoporosis. **Avoid** in hepatic dysfunction. **Possible adverse effects:** sedation, mood, impaired cognition, tolerance/dependence, nausea, headache **Note:** high risk of withdrawal (including seizures). Requires very slow taper. |
| Phenytoin (Dilantin) as IV, tablet, chewable, capsules, and suspension Fos-phenytoin as IV | **High interaction risk.** Enzyme inducer; can decrease levels of other drugs. Has nonlinear pharmacokinetics | **Caution**: IV infusion has a risk of hypotension and bradyarrhythmias and thrombophlebitis. **Possible adverse effects:** nystagmus, ataxia, gingival hyperplasia, osteoporosis, sedation **Avoid:** generalized onset epilepsy |
| Pregabalin (Lyrica) as capsules and | No significant interactions. | **Possible adverse effects:** weight gain, peripheral edema, sedation, dizziness. **Avoid**: generalized onset epilepsy **Note:** related drug, gabapentin, has limited efficacy for epilepsy but a similar profile. |

(continued)

## TABLE 48.3 MOST COMMONLY USED ANTIEPILEPTIC DRUGS[11] (continued)

| DRUG (MAJOR BRANDS)— FORMULATIONS | RX INTERACTIONS | CAUTIONS/ADVERSE EFFECTS |
|---|---|---|
| Topiramate (Topamax, Trokendi XR) as tablet, extended release, sprinkle | Enzyme inducer at high doses (may decrease the efficacy of hormonal contraception) | **Caution:** risk of kidney stones, glaucoma, elevated ammonia<br>**Possible adverse effects:** depressed mood, paresthesias, decreased appetite, cognitive/ language impairment |
| Valproic acid/ divalproex (Depakote) as IV, tablet, EC tablet, extended release, capsule, sprinkles | Can block some hepatically metabolized drugs (esp. UGT/CYP2C2) | **Caution:** Risk of hepatotoxicity, hyperammonemia, pancreatitis (can be fatal), high teratogenicity risk<br>**Possible adverse effects:** alopecia, weight gain, tremor.<br>**Avoid** in woman of childbearing potential and liver disease.<br>**Monitor** CBC (particularly platelets) and hepatic function panel. May need monitoring of ammonia (slight elevation is expected). |
| Zonisamide (Zonergan) as capsule | Enzyme-inducing AEDs will decrease its half-life. | **Caution**: kidney stones, rare sulfa allergies, rare elevated ammonia.<br>**Possible adverse effects:** decreased sweat, weight loss, agitation/irritability, elevated ammonia.<br>**Avoid** combining with other carbonic anhydrase inhibitors |

AED, antiepileptic drug; CBC, complete blood count; CMP, comprehensive metabolic panel; EC, enteric coated; ER, extended release; EtOH, ethyl alcohol; HLH, hemophagocytic lymphohistiocytosis; IV, intravenous; ODT, orally disintegrating tablet.

## Instructions for Patients

Patients and care providers should be educated about seizures, seizure symptoms, safety precautions, medication use, and acute treatment plan. Patients with epilepsy should have follow-ups with a neurologist. Special populations (such as women with epilepsy and the older adults) may require complex management including considerations for family planning and teratogenicity for antiseizure drugs. Families and patients should be instructed on basic seizure first aid.

**Driving:** Drivers licensing regulations and physician-mandated reporting vary per state. Due to the high initial risk of recurrence, patients should not drive a car for some time after a seizure. Depending on the state, 3 to 12 months of seizure freedom is typically required by law before a patient is allowed to return to driving.[12]

**Other seizure precautions:** Patients should be cautioned not to bathe in a bathtub, swim, operate heavy machinery, cook over open flames, climb ladders, or do other activities in which the safety of themselves or others would be affected if they had a seizure.

## RESOURCES AND REFERENCES

The full list of resources and references appears in the digital product found on http://connect
.springerpub.com/content/book/978-0-8261-6226-7/part/part03/chapter/ch48

# SLEEP

CRAIG DITOMMASO, NATHAN DARJI, TONY NGUYEN, AND ABANA AZARIAH

## CORE DEFINITIONS

**Sleep disorders**: Medically recognized problems with sleep affecting the quality, timing, and/or amount of sleep, which cause problems with functioning and distress during the daytime.

## ETIOLOGY AND PATHOPHYSIOLOGY

### Traumatic Brain Injury

Sleep issues are commonly reported within many rehabilitation populations. Arguably, the most complex issues may occur after traumatic brain injury (TBI). The complexity of the sleep issues in this population likely represents both intrinsic changes in sleep due to the TBI and an increased number of sleep disorders after TBI. Please see Table 49.1 for more information about the collected epidemiology of sleep disorders after TBI. Objectively, individuals with TBI have demonstrated the following:

- More apneic periods[1]
- Longer sleep latencies[1]
- More and longer-lasting nocturnal awakenings[1]
- Abnormal NREM and REM sleep[1]
- Global endocrine changes that may be related to sleep[2]

The pathophysiology of sleep disorders in the TBI population is likely multifactorial, involving neurochemical, structural, and metabolic changes. This may account for the high prevalence of sleep disorders that occur after TBI. Common sleep disorders that have been diagnosed after TBI include the following:

- Obstructive sleep apnea (OSA)[3,4]
- Central sleep apnea[3]
- Posttraumatic hypersomnia[3,4]
- Periodic limb movement disorder[3,4]
- Narcolepsy[3,4]
- Circadian rhythm sleep disorders (CRSD)[3]

### Spinal Cord Injury

The primary sleep disorder in the spinal cord injury (SCI) population is typically sleep-disordered breathing (SDB). Epidemiology indicates that 9% to 68% of the SCI population

---

The full list of resources and references appears in the digital product found on http://connect.springerpub.com/content/book/978-0-8261-6226-7/part/part03/chapter/ch49

**TABLE 49.1 COLLECTED EPIDEMIOLOGY OF SLEEP DISORDERS IN REHABILITATION POPULATIONS**

| DIAGNOSIS | PREVALENCE | NOTES |
|---|---|---|
| TBI | 25%–50% (Mathias) | Prevalence not related to the severity of injury per GCS |
| SCI | 83% for cervical injuries (Berlowitz) | Level of injury is important |
| STROKE | 73% develop OSA, and 7% develop central sleep apnea (Johnson) | May improve over the first 3 months |

GCS, Glasgow Coma Scale; OSA, obstructive sleep apnea; SCI, spinal cord injury; TBI, traumatic brain injury.

has SDB after injury, and that number may be as high as 83% in the cervical SCI population.[5,6] This is notably higher than the general population. The pathophysiology of SDB in the SCI population is multifactorial and likely involves intrinsic changes to the intercostal and abdominal musculature in addition to possible neurologic changes. Of note, the risk of SDB is correlated with changes in abdominal girth but not neck circumference.[6]

## Stroke

SDB such as OSA is common not only with SCI but also after stroke. The estimated prevalence of OSA after stroke or transient ischemic attack (TIA) is >70%.[7] The epidemiology data indicates stroke survivors are at an increased risk for OSA with an incidence of 50% to 70% within the first 3 months following stroke. One reason for the high prevalence of SDB is that the same risk factors that apply to OSA, such as obesity and cardiovascular disease, are also risk factors for stroke. Other explanations for the high prevalence are post-stroke changes in positioning, stroke-related changes to the muscles of the upper airway, and possibly untreated OSA preceding the stroke.[7]

## Other Populations

It is impossible to cover every possible sleep disorder and patient population within this chapter. There are a few disorders that will present to most rehabilitation physicians that have associated with sleep disorders. Parkinson's disease is prevalent in rehabilitation centers and rapid eye movement behavior disorder (RBD) is common for these patients.[8] This may be due to pathological changes within the dorsal mesopontine tegmentum or changes in dopamine within the striatum.[9] Sleep dysfunction can occur in patients with seizure disorders, especially if associated with frequent nocturnal seizures. Patients with Alzheimer's disease often have CRSD, and the sleep disorder typically worsens as the disease progresses.[8]

## DIAGNOSTIC APPROACH

### History

The first step in diagnosing sleep disorders is to obtain a thorough history including the following:

- Pre-injury and current sleep–wake patterns
- Frequency of sleep issues

- Duration of sleep issues
- Severity of sleep dysfunction
- Fluctuations of sleep difficulties at night
- Reported daytime sleepiness[10]

Other considerations include the following:

- Assessing potential contributing factors (e.g., pain, spasticity)
- Correlating core symptoms of sleep disorders such as snoring, breathing interruptions, nightmare, and limb movements
- Discussing substances that may interfere with sleep such as caffeine, alcohol, or recreational drugs
- Examining environmental factors
- Exploring psychiatric conditions (i.e., anxiety and depression)
- Reviewing prescription and over the counter drugs[10]

It is also important to note whether the patient is using light-emitting devices prior to bedtime. Studies have shown the use of these devices prolong sleep onset, decrease REM sleep, disrupt the circadian clock, and decrease the production of melatonin.[11]

## Objective Evaluation

The findings of the history should then guide a focused examination. Please see Sampathkumar et al.[10] and Figure 49.1 for more information.

Several questionnaires for evaluating sleep disorders are available. These include questionnaires:

- Subjective sleep problems focused
  - ❏ Pittsburgh Sleep Quality Index (PSQI)
  - ❏ Morningness–Eveningness Questionnaire (MEQ).
- Condition-specific measures
  - ❏ Insomnia Severity Index (ISI)
  - ❏ Swiss Narcolepsy Scale (SNS).
- Symptom-related measures
  - ❏ Epworth Sleepiness Scale (ESS)
  - ❏ Fatigue Severity Scale (FSS).

## Specific Testing

*Polysomnography (PSG)* is the gold standard test for sleep disorders. It includes an overnight assessment of EEG, electromyography (EMG), electrooculography (EOG), EKG, respiratory effort, respiratory flow, oxygen saturation, video monitoring, and additional variables like end-tidal capnography during sleep. PSG is indicated for diagnoses such as sleep-related breathing disorders, parasomnias, restless leg syndrome, periodic limb movement disorder, circadian rhythm disorder, and nocturnal seizures. It is typically performed in an outpatient sleep laboratory, but home PSG is sometimes available.

*Multiple Sleep Latency Testing (MSLT)* is an extended form of PSG that continues during the daytime and is used to quantify daytime sleepiness. The polysomnogram is done first to rule out nocturnal sleep disruption causing excessive daytime sleepiness. The MSLT can also be used to differentiate between excessive daytime fatigue from excessive daytime

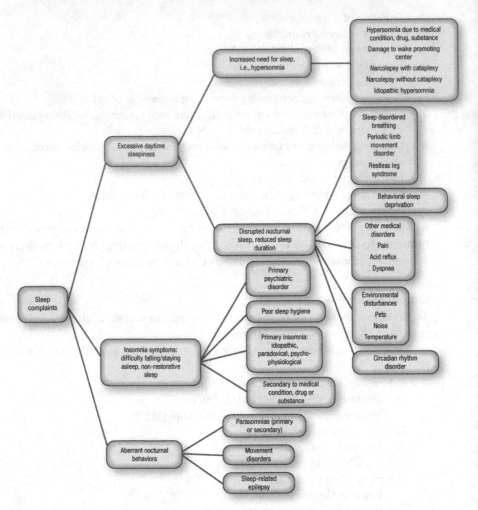

**FIGURE 49.1** A Conceptual framework to approach sleep–wake disturbances.

*Source:* Reproduced with permission from Sampathkumar H, DiTommaso C, Holcomb E, Tallavajhula S. Assessment of sleep after traumatic brain injury. *NeuroRehabilitation.* 2018;4(3):267–276.

sleepiness. Although some clinical centers offer this evaluation, it is typically reserved for research studies.

*Actigraphy* is accelerometer-based testing that estimates sleep time based on movement patterns. It is a particularly useful test to monitor a patient over a prolonged period of time because it is portable and can be used for diagnosis and treatment monitoring. This technology is becoming more available with smartphones and watches, but it lacks the ability to detect certain sleep disorders such as obstructive and central sleep apnea.

*Brain imaging* can be useful since there are radiological correlations associated with sleep disorders after TBI. Midbrain, pons, lateral medulla, and cerebellum damage can be related to central sleep apnea. However, it is not routinely used as a diagnostic tool.

## TREATMENT

Numerous treatment options exist for patients suffering from sleep disturbances. The proper treatment may include nonpharmacologic as well as pharmacologic measures. Good sleep hygiene, assessment for sleep disorders, such as OSA, environmental changes, and ruling out other causes of sleep disturbances is recommended before pharmacologic interventions.

### Nonpharmacological Interventions

*Sleep hygiene:* Implementing sleep hygiene measures is appropriate whenever possible. Patients should be counseled on sleep hygiene with the goal of improving poor sleep–wake schedules. This includes the following:

- Keeping the bedroom dark
- Limiting noise
- Setting a sleep schedule
- Limiting the use of television and other electronics in the evening
- Appropriate exercise

*Continuous positive airway pressure (CPAP):* The standard treatment option for OSA in the general population is CPAP. There are very few studies exploring the treatment of OSA in the rehab populations—especially SCI. Also, studies have shown poor compliance with CPAP therapy in the SCI population. Alternative treatment includes oral appliances and weight loss. Uvulopalatopharyngoplasty is effective but is associated with complications, such as velopharyngeal insufficiency. In addition, sedative medications, such as benzodiazepines and opioids, should be minimized when possible to prevent further apneic episodes.[5]

In central sleep apnea, CPAP and bilevel positive airway pressure are the treatment of choice but were found to be effective in only 50% of patients with the cross-sectional area (CSA) in one study.[12] Another option is transvenous phrenic nerve stimulation. Theophylline anhydrous and acetazolamide have been used with inconsistent results. Again, avoidance of sedating medication is important within this diagnosis.

*Cognitive behavioral therapy (CBT):* CBT is commonly advocated as a standard of care for patients suffering from insomnia. It involves techniques that utilize relaxation, sleep restriction, and stimulus control with the goal of recognizing and diminishing negative associations surrounding sleep.

### Pharmacological Interventions

If pharmacological intervention is needed, treatment should be appropriate for the specific sleep disorder, selected for fewer side effects, tailored to specific sleep complaints, and consider treatment of comorbid conditions.

*Melatonin:* For example, post-TBI patients who have irregular sleep–wake patterns may have a circadian sleep disturbance. If this is the case, melatonin and/or bright light therapy, rather than hypnotic drugs, are appropriate treatment options.[13] A randomized placebo-controlled trial reported that TBI patients given melatonin had improved sleep quality, efficiency, and decreased anxiety without a difference in sleep latency compared to placebo.[14]

*Trazodone:* A heterocyclic atypical antidepressant, trazodone may be used for patients with difficulty initiating sleep with concurrent depression. Although it is widely used in patients with insomnia after TBI, clinical trials studying trazodone's use in the TBI population are scarce. However, patients with insomnia and depression have been found to exhibit improved sleep duration with trazodone,[15] and depression is a common comorbidity in rehabilitation patients. Trazodone must be used with caution given the risk of increased falls and QT prolongation.[16]

*Benzodiazepines*: Benzodiazepines are effective for short-term sleep initiation but should be limited due to adverse effects such as the following:

- Dependency
- Daytime sedation
- Cognitive impairment
- Increased risk of falls (especially in older adult patients)

In addition, as mentioned earlier, these medications can worsen sleep disorders such as central and OSA.

*Z-drugs*: Drugs such as zolpidem tartrate are better alternatives to benzodiazepines. Due to their more specific action on type 1 GABA receptors, these drugs have a more favorable side effect profile, although they are not completely without adverse effects (sedation and sensory impairment). While their side effect profiles are favorable compared to benzodiazepines, patients with a history of drug abuse or psychiatric disorders should be treated cautiously due to their risk of dependency.

*Modafinil:* For patients with daytime hypersomnia, a stimulant such as modafinil may be beneficial, although mixed outcomes of efficacy in patients with TBI have been shown.[17] Other stimulants such as amantadine and methylphenidate can also be used to improve daytime wakefulness and alertness.

## FUNCTIONAL PROGNOSIS AND OUTCOMES

Long-term outcome likely depends more on the severity of the underlying condition and socioeconomic factors than specific sleep issues.

### Traumatic Brain Injury

Several studies suggest that issues with sleep after a TBI are likely to persist for years after the injury, regardless of the patient population.[18]

In acute rehabilitation, however, individuals with TBI and sleep disorders have the following:

- Slower reaction times[3]
- Poorer vigilance on psychological testing[3]
- Increased behavioral disorders[19]
- Decreased memory

when compared to other TBI subjects not diagnosed with a sleep disorder. While little evidence exists that improving sleep will result in better performance, it is reasonable to hope that better sleep will result in better performance.

### Spinal Cord Injury

The primary predictor of sleep disorder and severity in this population is abdominal circumference. Also, in general, the chronological age of the patient has a greater correlation with sleep dysfunction than the length of time after injury. The correlation seems to change after 65 years of age, however, as there are fewer sleep problems in the geriatric population.

## Stroke

SDB is a harbinger for recurrent ischemic stroke but not mortality.[20] Luckily, SDB seems to improve during the first 3 months after stroke with a strong reduction in central sleep apnea.[21] Long-term prognosis is multifactorial depending on the location of the stroke and change in weight.

## BASIC ORDER SET

- Sleep hygiene
  - ❏ Lights on and window shades open QAM
  - ❏ Lights off and television off QPM
  - ❏ No caffeine after 2 PM
- Nurses to keep a sleep log at night
  - ❏ Identify hours awake and asleep
  - ❏ Note any complaints or issues at night
  - ❏ Mark snoring, apneic spells, or movements during sleep
- Notify physician if patient unable to initiate sleep by 10 pm

## RESOURCES AND REFERENCES

The full list of resources and references appears in the digital product found on http://connect .springerpub.com/content/book/978-0-8261-6226-7/part/part03/chapter/ch49

# SPASTICITY AND CONTRACTURE

MADELINE A. DICKS AND MONICA VERDUZCO-GUTIERREZ

## CORE DEFINITIONS

Spasticity is a common disorder that affects individuals with neurologic conditions such as stroke, cerebral palsy, multiple sclerosis, traumatic brain, and spinal cord injuries. Often described as muscle overactivity, spasticity, has been defined as a velocity-dependent increase in muscle tone with exaggerated tendon jerks due to the hyperexcitability of stretch reflexes.[1] This suggests that the faster the passive movement of the limb through its range of motion, the greater the increase in muscle tone. Spasticity is recognized as a component of the upper motor neuron syndrome, which is characterized as disordered sensorimotor changes that occur after injury to an upper motor neuron controlling voluntary skeletal muscle movement.[2]

### Clinical Features of Spasticity

The changes seen in spasticity often manifest as increased tone, spasms, clonus, spastic dystonia, and/or joint immobility. It characteristically affects the antigravity muscle groups in the upper and lower limbs.[3] In the upper limbs, the excessive tone is commonly seen in the shoulder adductors, elbow, wrist and finger flexors, forearm pronators, and thumb adductors. In the lower extremities, increased muscle tone is prominent in the hip adductors, knee and plantar flexors, and ankle invertors.

The influence of spasticity varies widely from it being a subtle neurologic symptom to a condition that generates severe pain, contractures, and poor quality of life. The debilitating nature of spasticity can directly impact a person's independence and their ability to perform activities of daily living (ADL), including self-care tasks such as bathing, toileting, and grooming. As a result, the caregiver burden and the utilization of healthcare resources rise. Therefore, effective management of spasticity is essential to improve patient satisfaction in life and opportunities to participate within the community.

## ETIOLOGY AND PATHOPHYSIOLOGY

Spasticity is commonly associated with a lesion (or lesions) causing disruption of the inhibitory descending pathways including the corticoreticular pathways at the level of the cortex or internal capsule and the reticulospinal and vestibulospinal tracts at the level of the spinal cord.[2] In order to properly appreciate the physiology of abnormal muscle tone

The full list of resources and references appears in the digital product found on http://connect.springerpub.com/content/book/978-0-8261-6226-7/part/part03/chapter/ch50

and spasticity, it is imperative to understand the mechanics of the normal stretch reflex. The stretch reflex is a monosynaptic reflex that automatically regulates skeletal muscle length.[4] When a muscle is passively lengthened, the muscle spindles are excited triggering Ia fibers to discharge and send inputs to the alpha-motoneurons which in turn send an efferent impulse to the muscle, causing it to contract. Meanwhile, Ia afferent fibers also synapse with Ia inhibitory interneurons, producing relaxation of the antagonist muscles.[5] This is known as reciprocal inhibition.

Thilmann et al. demonstrated that spasticity is due to an exaggerated stretch reflex.[6] Surface electromyography (EMG) recordings in normal subjects at rest showed that passive muscle stretch at velocities performed in clinical practice does not produce any reflex contraction of the stretched muscle. In contrast, patients with spasticity showed a positive correlation between passive stretch and stretch velocity. When the muscle is stretched slowly, the stretch reflex is small, and the examiner perceives minimal to normal tone. When the passive stretch is quick, the stretch reflex increases and the perceived tone is large.

The exaggerated stretch reflex in patients with spasticity is likely due to abnormal intraspinal sensory input processing.[4] Several mechanisms have been proposed including (a) increased sensitivity of muscle spindles that increase afferent inputs to spinal motor neurons, (b) abnormal sensory input processing of muscle spindles resulting in enhanced motor neuronal reflex activation, and (c) intrinsic changes to soft tissue and motor neurons. These reflex pathway deviations and intrinsic anatomical changes can cause decreased reflex threshold, thus leading to spasticity.

## DIAGNOSTIC APPROACH

A comprehensive history and physical examination are essential when evaluating for spasticity. Spasticity is a clinical diagnosis, without any specific laboratory confirmation. Evaluation should include a strict analysis of the etiology of the spasticity, including any reversible causes (i.e., urinary tract infection, stool impaction, or skin pressure injury) and how it is influencing mobility, self-care and ability to perform ADL. When monitoring chronic spasticity, the examiner should compare findings with previous evaluations. If there be evidence of symptom worsening, the practitioner must further evaluate for a deterioration of the original cause or determine if there is a new injury.

Clinical measurement scales may be useful to quantify the severity of spasticity and monitor treatment efficacy. The most commonly used scales in clinical practice are the Modified Ashworth Scale,[7] which measures the resistance of the muscle to passive stretch, and the Penn Spasm Frequency Scale, which characterizes the frequency of muscle spasms[8] (Table 50.1). The Tardieu scale is another clinical method that is often used in research to specifically measure spasticity, which is based on comparing the threshold angles of muscle reaction to passive stretch at predefined velocities[9] (Table 50.2).

## TREATMENT

Any approach to the treatment of spasticity or contractures should be multidisciplinary involving physical and occupational therapy, pharmacotherapy, and consideration of possible surgical intervention. Management should be tailored to the individual patient with realistic goals kept in mind. The treatment of spasticity solely on its presence is not recommended as often increased muscle tone may serve as a partial substitute for voluntary muscle contraction and used to the patients' advantage (i.e., ambulation in the setting of hip and knee extensor spasticity seen after stroke). Therefore, the risk of complications of both treating and not treating spasticity should be considered.

Treatment should be initiated when spasticity starts to interfere with self-care and functional goals or if it causes skin breakdown and pain. Establishing common goals between the patients, families, and providers is a cornerstone to treatment that can assist in both planning management strategies and therapeutic interventions.[10] The following are common interventions that aid in the treatment of spasticity.

## Therapeutic Interventions

The foundation of a successful spasticity management program is a regime of strength and active/passive range of motion exercise and stretching initiated by trained physical and occupational therapists that can be transitioned to a home-based environment where the patient and/or caregiver can continue the independent practice.[10] Stretching and range of motion aid in the prevention of contracture formation and may temporarily reduce increased muscle tone. It is also a useful adjunct for other treatment options such as chemodenervation with botulinum toxins and oral antispasmodic medications. Standing has shown to be beneficial, with changes in passive range of motion, spasticity, and psychological well-being.[11] Aquatic therapy has proven beneficial in the treatment of spasticity as well and may decrease the amount of oral antispasmodic required when compared to passive range of motion exercise alone.[12]

## Physical Modalities

It has been shown that the efficacy of passive stretching in the conservative treatment of spasticity can be augmented when cold or heat is applied.[13] It has been shown that several physical modalities, including ultrasonography (US), functional electrical stimulation (FES), and biofeedback, are used to help facilitate stretching. The energy from ultrasound is absorbed by tissue and converted to heat, thus allowing the muscles to relax. One trial, however, demonstrated that US in combination with passive stretching of the ankle plantar muscles had no effect on the stretching treatment in diminishing spasticity.[13] FES has proven beneficial in reducing spasticity, improving range of motion, facilitating stretching in persons with neurologic conditions as well.[14] In addition, when FES is used to stimulate the common peroneal nerve, dorsiflexion and eversion of the foot occur, and when timed appropriately in the gait cycle, walking performance can be improved. The application of biofeedback techniques by providing an appropriate visual or auditory signal can reduce spasticity.[15]

## Positioning/Orthotics

Serial casting with and without chemodenervation has been utilized to restore proper biomechanics to the joint. Several studies have reported a significant benefit of serial casting post toxin injection in children and in persons with traumatic brain injury.[10] Practitioners should be conscious of the possible complications serial casting carries including pressure injuries and circulation impairment. Taping, orthotics, and bivalve casts are additional strategies to support the joint.

## Pharmacotherapy

There are several oral antispasmodic medications available for the treatment of generalized spasticity including centrally acting drugs, alpha-2 agonists, anticonvulsants, and peripherally acting drugs (Table 50.3).[16]

### Centrally Acting Medications

1. Baclofen: A common first-line treatment that works pre- and postsynaptically as a gamma aminobutylic acid (GABA) B agonist at the spinal level. Side effects include systemic muscle relaxation, sedation, and lethargy. Liver function tests should be monitored due to the risk of hepatotoxicity.
2. Tizanidine: An imidazoline alpha-2 agonist that increases the presynaptic inhibition of motor neurons thereby decreasing the release of excitatory amino acids and reducing tone.[17] This medication is a common second-line agent that is often used in addition to other oral medications for additive effects. The most common adverse events are somnolence, xerostomia, and hypotension. Liver function tests should be monitored due to the risk of hepatotoxicity.

### Anticonvulsants

1. Benzodiazepines: Anticonvulsants that work postsynaptically as a GABA-A agonist. The most commonly used benzodiazepines are diazepam and clonazepam. Side effects include respiratory depression and significant sedation; therefore, it is recommended to use only at night.
2. Gabapentin: An anticonvulsant that inhibits the alpha 2-delta subunit of voltage-gated calcium channels, thus inhibiting calcium currents. This medication is rarely used as monotherapy in the treatment of spasticity. Side effects include somnolence, tremor, and nystagmus.

### Peripherally Acting Medications

1. Dantrolene: A peripherally acting medication that inhibits calcium release at the sarcoplasmic reticulum in the muscle. Side effects include general muscle weakness. Liver function tests should be monitored due to the risk of hepatotoxicity and liver failure.

These medications have had mixed results in the treatment of spasticity with differing etiology including spinal cord injury, traumatic brain injury, and stroke. The centrally acting medications cause significant sedation, which limits the dosage that can be tolerated.[16] This sedative side effect can hinder rehabilitation goals and further impair cognition in persons with preexisting cognitive impairment (i.e., stroke, traumatic brain injury). Moreover, the maximally tolerated dosage may not be sufficient to control the spasticity. In addition, diazepam is better suited for spasticity due to spinal cord injury compared to cerebral spasticity as it has a greater effect on flexor reflexes, which is commonly seen in spinal cord injury.

## Injectable Medications

Treatment with injectable medication such as botulinum toxins and phenol are effective methods for reducing focal spasticity while minimizing the systemic side effects of oral antispasmodics. As discussed earlier, with all injection procedures, physical and occupational therapy should be utilized as adjunctive treatment to enhance the delivery of the medication and improve patient outcomes.

Botulinum toxin is the treatment of choice for focal spasticity and acts by blocking neuromuscular transmission by inhibiting acetylcholine release.[18] There are seven serologically distinct toxins, but the most used on the market today are type A (onabotulinumtoxin A, incobotulinumtoxin A, and abobotulinumtoxin A) and B (rimabotulinumtoxin B). The effect of botulinum toxin injection reaches its peak at 2 to 3 weeks with local relief of spasticity lasting 3 to 4 months. Botulinum toxin is typically well tolerated in therapeutic doses; however, it does carry an Food and Drug Administration (FDA)-mandated black box warning of the rare, but potentially life-threatening complication of systemic weakness, vision changes, dysarthria, dysphonia, dysphagia, and respiratory compromise should the toxin spread beyond the site of injection. Therefore, it is recommended the practitioner have a comprehensive understanding of muscle anatomy and use appropriate guidance via EMG, electrical stimulation, or ultrasound to localize the targeted muscle prior to injection.

Chemical neurolysis with phenol in concentrations ranging from 3% to 7% and alcohol in concentrations of 50% to 100% is utilized to destroy the nerve that is causing spasticity.[16] The result can last days to years due to the partial nerve regeneration and sprouting that may ensue after treatment. Adverse events include painful dysesthesias and muscle fibrosis.

## Surgical Interventions

Intrathecal baclofen (ITB) is a common intervention that has the same mechanism of action as oral baclofen, but instead it is delivered via an intrathecal catheter directly into the cerebrospinal fluid.[8,19] This delivery method allows for higher concentrations of the drug directly at the spinal level while avoiding the systemic complications that may be caused by oral baclofen. Individuals being considered for this intervention must first undergo an ITB trial prior to permanent pump implantation to confirm the efficacy of the medication at the spinal level and evaluate the safety profile of the medication. The main disadvantage, though relatively uncommon, is device failure leading to overdose, which causes respiratory depression and coma, or withdrawal, resulting in hyperthermia, rhabdomyolysis, and disseminated intravascular coagulation.[16]

Other neurosurgical techniques that can be considered if treatment alternatives do not provide adequate control of spasticity include selective dorsal rhizotomies and myelotomies. These procedures interrupt nerve signal transduction by removing the peripheral nerve thereby reducing spasms and pain.[16] In addition, and especially in cases with contracture, neuro-orthopedic procedures such as tendon release or lengthening, tenotomy, and joint fusion can be performed to correct limb deformities, improve function outcome, and reduce pain and spasticity.[20]

## FUNCTIONAL PROGNOSIS AND OUTCOMES

Spasticity and resultant contractures can cause profound functional limitations. Poor posture due to spasticity can make transfers, wheelchair positioning, and changes in a position difficult, all of which contribute to the development of pressure injuries. Spasticity can interfere with daily hygiene such as washing the hands, axillae, and genital areas. It can also make bladder and bowel programs particularly difficult to accomplish and interfere with sexual relationships.

Poorly controlled spasticity or insufficient stretching may lead to permanent loss of range of motion or contracture that are associated with devastating consequences. To name a few, these include skin issues (i.e., excessive moisture accumulation, skin irritation and breakdown, bacterial overgrowth, infection) and joint abnormalities (i.e., adhesive capsulitis, joint subluxation). Treatment should be aimed at the prevention of these complications.

Spasticity, however, can be valuable for some patients. For example, it can aid in sitting stability, transfers, standing, and walking. Therefore, it is critical for treatment to be individualized to each patient as spasticity may be used as a strategy to compensate for weakness. With this in mind, the practitioner should be able to develop an appropriate treatment protocol that maximizes functional goals and outcomes.

## BASIC ORDER SET

### Sample Therapy Orders

Evaluate and treat with focus on (chose all that apply): neuromuscular reeducation, stretching, splinting, modalities, serial casting, positioning, standing program, FES/therapy, strengthening, constraint-induced movement therapy, body weight-supported ambulation, gait training, aquatic therapy, and ADL training.

Goals: Restore functional alignment, improve selective motor control, improve strength, improve functional performance, and facilitate activity and community participation.

### TABLE 50.1 MODIFIED ASHWORTH SCALE[2]

| 0 | No increase in muscle tone |
|---|---|
| 1 | Slight increase in muscle tone, manifested by a catch and release or by minimal resistance at the end range of motion when the part is moved in flexion or extension/abduction or adduction |
| 1+ | Slight increase in muscle tone, manifested by a catch, followed by minimal resistance throughout the remainder (less than half) of the range of motion |
| 2 | More marked increase in muscle tone through most of the range of motion, but the affected part is easily moved |
| 3 | Considerable increase in muscle tone, passive movement is difficult |
| 4 | Affected part is rigid in flexion or extension (abduction or adduction) |

## TABLE 50.2 TARDIEU SCALE

| 0 | No resistance throughout the course of the passive movement |
|---|---|
| 1 | Slight resistance throughout the course of the passive movement |
| 2 | Clear catch at precise angle, interrupting the passive movement, followed by release |
| 3 | Unsustained clonus (less than 10 seconds when maintaining pressure) occurring at a precise angle, followed by release |
| 4 | Sustained clonus (more than 10 seconds when maintaining pressure) occurring at a precise angle |

The angle of muscle action is measured relative to the position of a minimal stretch of the muscle (corresponding to angle zero) for all joints except the hip where it is relative to the resting anatomical position.

## TABLE 50.3 ORAL ANTISPASMODIC MEDICATIONS

| MEDICATION | MECHANISM OF ACTION | STARTING DOSE | COMMON SIDE EFFECTS | RELATIVE CONTRAINDICATIONS |
|---|---|---|---|---|
| Baclofen | GABA-B agonist | 5–10 mg TID Max dose 80 mg/day | Sedation, lethargy, rare hepatotoxicity, withdrawal symptoms | Cognitive impairment, seizures |
| Tizanidine | Alpha-2 agonist | 2 mg TID Max dose 32 mg/day | Sedation, hypotension, hepatotoxicity | Cognitive impairment |
| Benzodiazepines | GABA-A agonist | 2 mg TID | Sedation, respiratory | History of benzodiazepine or other substance abuse |
| Gabapentin | Inhibits alpha 2-delta subunit of voltage-gated calcium channels | 300 mg daily Max dose 2400 mg/day | Somnolence, tremor, nystagmus | Renal impairment |
| Dantrolene | Inhibits calcium release at the sarcoplasmic reticulum in the muscle | 25 mg daily | Weakness, hepatotoxicity, occasional sedation | Liver disease |

GABA, gamma-aminobutyric acid.

## RESOURCES AND REFERENCES

The full list of resources and references appears in the digital product found on http://connect
.springerpub.com/content/book/978-0-8261-6226-7/part/part03/chapter/ch50

# SPEECH AND LANGUAGE DISORDERS

AMANDA K. GALLAGHER, SHAUNA K. BERUBE, AND MARTIN B. BRODSKY

## COMMUNICATION DISORDERS

Communication disorders are common side effects following neurologic injury or impairment. A speech-language pathologist (SLP) is trained in the assessment and rehabilitation of disorders impacting communication. Communication disorders are generally divided into three domains: language, speech, and voice. Each of these systems is distinct and requires specific evaluation and treatment.

Language skills include word finding, grammar, and understanding information that is seen (reading comprehension) or heard (auditory comprehension). Speech skills include clear pronunciation of sounds and words, coordinating breath support for speaking, fluency, and maintaining an appropriate speaking volume. Vocal skills include the quality, pitch, and tone of our voice in conveying information and emotion.

Regardless of the communication system impacted, the resulting deficits can be devastating. Communication is integral to an individual's safety and quality of life as communication disorders impact our ability to clearly communicate wants and needs, build and maintain relationships with family and friends, and maintain employment.

## MOTOR SPEECH DISORDERS

Motor speech disorders (MSDs), specifically dysarthria and apraxia, are a group of neurogenic speech disorders resulting from sensorimotor damage to the brain. They are caused by impairments of strength, range of motion, coordination, and/or planning of the muscles used to produce speech. These muscles include the lips, tongue, soft palate, muscles of the larynx, and respiratory muscles. MSDs commonly occur in stroke, TBI, multiple sclerosis, Parkinson's disease, ALS, and various other neurologic disorders including brain tumors and degenerative disease. SLPs specialize in the diagnosis and treatment of MSDs.

### Dysarthria
### Core Definitions

Dysarthria refers to a group of speech impairments caused by damage to the central or peripheral nervous system that impacts the sensorimotor function of the lips, tongue, velum,

---

The full list of references appears in the digital product found on http://connect.springerpub.com/content/book/978-0-8261-6226-7/part/part03/chapter/ch51

larynx, or respiratory system. Dysarthria results from changes in the speed, strength, range of motion, and/or coordination of the speech system affecting at least one of the five speech systems: respiration (i.e., support for voice), phonation (voice), resonance (e.g., nasality), articulation, and prosody (i.e., the rhythm of speech output). Damage to these systems impacts the clarity of speech, or intelligibility. The most commonly reported dysarthria symptom is "slurred speech."

There are seven major types of dysarthria (Table 51.1). The type of dysarthria is dependent upon the location and extent of the injury.

## Diagnostic Approach

Assessment of dysarthria should include a cranial nerve examination, objective strength testing,[1] diadochokinetic speech tasks including alternating motion rates (/pa-pa-pa/, /ta-ta-ta/, /ka-ka-ka/) and sequential motor rates (pa-ta-ka), instrumental and clinical

### TABLE 51.1 DYSARTHRIA CLASSIFICATIONS

| TYPE | LOCATION OF INJURY | NEUROMOTOR BASIS | COMMON CHARACTERISTICS |
|---|---|---|---|
| FLACCID | Lower motor neuron damage | Weakness including forehead, face, and jaw | Facial droop, fasciculations, atrophy, synkinesis (e.g., smiling causes an eye twitch), breathy voice |
| SPASTIC | Bilateral upper motor neuron damage | Spasticity | Slow speech rate, strained vocal quality, labile facial expression (smile/grimace), pathological oral reflexes (e.g., sucking, snout, jaw jerk reflexes) |
| ATAXIC | Cerebellar control circuit | Incoordination | Irregular sound errors, difficulty regulating/controlling speaking volume |
| HYPOKINETIC | Basal ganglia | Reduced range of motion, rigidity | Resting tremor, decreased speaking volume, poor verbal initiation, rapid speech rate, tremors, masked facial expression |
| HYPERKINETIC | Basal ganglia control circuit | Involuntary movements | Inconsistent breathiness, excessive loudness, sudden forced inhalation/exhalation, multiple motor tics, facial grimace while talking |
| UNILATERAL UPPER MOTOR NEURON | Unilateral upper motor neuron damage | Weakness | Unilateral weakness involving the lower face, jaw and/or tongue, slow rate or speech, decreased volume |
| MIXED DYSARTHRIA | Multifocal damage | Variable | Mixed dysarthria includes features of two or more dysarthria types |

Adapted from Duffy[1]; https://www.asha.org/Practice-Portal/Clinical-Topics/Dysarthria-in-Adults/

measurement of respiratory capacity/coordination, and subjective measurements of intelligibility via oral reading and spontaneous speech samples. While the standardized measures most commonly used are the Frenchay Dysarthria Assessment and Assessment of Intelligibility in Dysarthric Speakers (AIDS), assessment is often informal.[2] Whether standardized or informal, assessment should also include a variety of tools that include patient-reported measures of impairment.

## Treatment

Treatment of dysarthria may include isotonic and isokinetic exercises of the facial, oral, and laryngeal musculature, oral reading of sounds and words, and training of compensatory strategies such as decreased rate, increased volume, increased pitch, or breaking words into single syllables for improved accuracy of individual sounds.[3] Treatment may include modalities such as neuromuscular electrical stimulation for the facial muscles, thermal tactile stimulation to the face, tongue, soft palate and throat, manual massage, and myofascial release.

The Lee Silverman LOUD™ program, designed to treat hypokinetic dysarthria in Parkinson's disease,[4] has also been found effective for individuals who have difficulty coordinating breathing for speech following TBI and stroke.[5] Although quality literature for specific treatment approaches for dysarthria is limited, the available evidence suggests that best practice includes rehabilitation with an SLP to implement exercises and compensatory strategies for improved intelligibility.[6,7]

## Apraxia
### Core Definitions

Apraxia occurs with damage to the left premotor and motor cortices,[8] resulting in difficulty with motor planning/programming of the muscles of the mouth, face, and throat. The two subtypes of apraxia include oral apraxia (difficulty with volitional planning/programming of the facial muscles, tongue, soft palate, or laryngeal muscles) and verbal apraxia (difficulty with planning/programming the production of sounds and words for communication). Verbal apraxia, also called apraxia of speech (AOS), is characterized by a slow speech rate, segmentation of syllables, sound distortions, distorted substitutions, trial-and-error articulatory movements (i.e., groping), and increased difficulty with increased length and complexity of utterances.[9] AOS is not a language disorder although it commonly occurs in conjunction with aphasia.

### Diagnostic Approach

If a patient is suspected to have AOS, an SLP should be consulted for evaluation. Assessment should include a cranial nerve examination, alternating and sequential motion rates, and repetition and oral reading of sounds, words, and sentences. There are standardized measures such as the Apraxia Battery for Adults-2 (ABA-2) and embedded measures within standardized language assessments (e.g., Western Aphasia Battery). Differential diagnosis of AOS versus dysarthria includes intact strength of the oral musculature, inconsistent error patterns across sounds produced, difficulty maintaining prosody (rate/rhythm/intonation), and groping produced by the articulatory muscles.

The symptoms of apraxia can range in severity. Mild symptoms may include inconsistent errors with sounds or occasional word substitution in conversation. A patient with severe apraxia may present as aphonic (without voice). It is common for individuals with apraxia to become frustrated while communicating because they are often aware of the errors that they make. Increased focus and effort on a specific sound may make speaking more difficult, which makes correction of errors challenging. Oftentimes, automatic speech tasks like counting, singing, or spontaneous small talk, such as "hello", remain intact. This occurs because automatic speech does not require a high level of cognitive or motor planning to execute. In the absence of a coexisting aphasia, written communication is an excellent option for patients with AOS.

## Treatment

Treatment of apraxia targets motor planning and control at the various levels of speech complexity. This may include repetition of gross oral movements, training of individual sounds and words,[10,11] and training of compensatory strategies such as pacing.[11] Biofeedback may also aid in the treatment of AOS.[12]

## Prognosis

Recent literature continues to support a positive prognosis for improvement via therapeutic rehabilitation for adults with acquired AOS.[13]

## Aphasia

### Core Definitions

Aphasia is an acquired condition that affects a person's ability to express and/or understand language. Aphasia occurs as a result of neurologic damage to the language centers of the brain, such as from a stroke, TBI, brain tumor, or neurodegenerative conditions such as primary progressive aphasia (PPA). Aphasia may impact any of the four modalities of language: (1) verbal expression, (2) written expression, (3) auditory comprehension, or (4) reading comprehension. Anomia, difficulty accessing words, is both a hallmark characteristic of aphasia and a type of aphasia (i.e., anomic aphasia).

A number of characterizations that may accompany verbal expression may be further characterized by paraphasias, neologisms, or circumlocution. Paraphasias are phonemic (i.e., sound) substitutions (e.g., "bog" for "dog") or semantic (i.e., meaning) substitutions (e.g., "spoon" for "knife"), neologisms are nonsense words, and circumlocution is being vague or talking around a word. Aphasia types are characterized based on fluency, naming, repetition, and comprehension (Table 51.2).

### Diagnostic Approach

Patients suspected to have aphasia should be referred to an SLP for further evaluation and treatment. The SLP will complete a comprehensive, standardized language assessment, most commonly the Western Aphasia Battery Revised (WAB) and the Boston Diagnostic Aphasia Examination (BDAE). Each of these test assessments probes all four modalities of language.

## TABLE 51.2 APHASIA CLASSIFICATIONS[14,15]

| APHASIA TYPE | AREA OF THE BRAIN LESION | CHARACTERISTICS OF EXPRESSIVE LANGUAGE | CHARACTERISTICS OF RECEPTIVE LANGUAGE |
|---|---|---|---|
| ANOMIC | No specific lesion | Naming impaired more for nouns compared to verbs. Spelling mostly intact | Generally intact auditory and reading comprehension |
| BROCA'S | Broca's area: posterior, inferior frontal gyrus | Nonfluent spontaneous speech, impaired repetition. More difficulty naming verbs compared to nouns. Often agrammatic. impaired spelling | Difficulty comprehending complex grammar (i.e., metaphorical language, lengthy phrases, and clauses). Impaired reading |
| WERNICKE'S | Wernicke's area: posterior, superior temporal gyrus | Fluent spontaneous speech that lacks meaning and may consist of neologisms or jargon. Poor repetition. Impaired spelling | Poor auditory and reading comprehension across words, sentences, and conversation. Generally unaware of errors |
| TRANSCORTICAL SENSORY | Damage to areas surrounding Wernicke's area in the posterior cerebral artery area | Fluent spontaneous speech lacking meaning. Intact repetition. Impaired spelling | Impaired auditory and reading comprehension |
| TRANSCORTICAL MOTOR | Damage to area anterior or superior to Broca's area often from occlusion of anterior cerebral artery | Nonfluent spontaneous speech. fluent and grammatical repetition. May have intact spelling | Auditory comprehension is generally intact, though impaired for complex grammar structures. May have intact reading comprehension |
| MIXED TRANSCORTICAL | Damage to areas around Broca's and Wernicke's | Echolalia, empty speech. Intact sentence repetition. Poor spelling | Severely impaired reading and auditory comprehension |
| CONDUCTION | Damage to the supramarginal gyrus | Generally fluent and meaningful spontaneous speech that may consist of phonemic paraphasias. Impaired repetition. Spelling may be intact | Intact auditory comprehension for words and simple sentences. May have intact reading comprehension |
| GLOBAL | Damage to both Broca's and Wernicke's areas | Severely impaired verbal and written expression. Often perseverative on single words | Severely impaired comprehension |

The SLP may supplement these test batteries with specialized assessments, such as the Boston Naming Test (BNT) used to assess naming, and/or informal tasks to gather additional information regarding verbal expression, written expression, reading comprehension, and auditory comprehension.

## Treatment

*Rehabilitation:* Aphasia is treated behaviorally by an SLP. An SLP uses a number of evidence-based behavioral interventions to strengthen language skills through principles of neuroplasticity, specifically by retraining unaffected parts of the brain to compensate for impairments. The majority of aphasia research has been done in post-stroke aphasia (PSA), although treatment techniques are used to treat aphasia across patient populations despite the etiology of deficits. Treatment may be impairment-based or compensatory. Evidence supports that frequent and intensive therapy in both subacute and chronic aphasia results in positive outcomes.[16] Noninvasive brain stimulation techniques, including transcranial direct current stimulation and transcranial magnetic stimulation paired with speech-language treatment, may enhance treatment outcomes through an increase in cortical excitability in PSA and PPA, and has the potential to be beneficial in the TBI population.[16-19]

*Medical:* Some research suggests that medications can be used as an adjunct to behavioral therapy in PSA, although clinical trials have had poor designs and limited participants.[16,20] One of the more recent studies suggests that *memantine* may have positive effects on language performance when paired with speech-language therapy, though further research is needed.[21]

## Prognosis

Prognosis is dependent on the etiology of aphasia and underlying disease. In stroke, the severity of aphasia correlates to the lesion location and volume,[22] whereas the presence and severity of aphasia in patients with brain tumors are associated with age and grade of the tumor.[23] Given the heterogeneous nature of TBI, the prognosis is dependent on the location and severity of the injury. Individuals with severe TBI often require long-term rehabilitation, whereas patients with mild TBI may only require only short-term rehabilitation or no rehabilitation.[24] For neurodegenerative conditions, the prognosis is poor though SLP intervention may be beneficial.[17]

## SPECIAL CONSIDERATIONS

The previously mentioned rehabilitation techniques for individuals with MSDs and aphasia are effective for improving a person's ability to communicate effectively. For those who continue to be limited in their ability to independently communicate, there are a variety of low-tech and high-tech augmentative and alternative communication options available. A referral to an SLP is appropriate to determine and implement the most effective form of communication.

## REFERENCES

The full list of references appears in the digital product found on http://connect.springerpub.com/content/book/978-0-8261-6226-7/part/part03/chapter/ch51

# SUBSTANCE USE

KATHERINE STREETER WRIGHT AND MICHELLE ACCARDI-RAVID

## CORE DEFINITIONS

The *Diagnostic and Statistical Manual of Mental Disorders, 5th Edition* (*DSM-5*) describes the essential feature of a substance use disorder (SUD) as "a cluster of cognitive, behavioral, and physiologic symptoms indicating that the individual continues using the substance despite significant substance-related problems" (p. 483).[1]

When the *DSM* was updated in 2013 to the fifth edition, the categories of "abuse" and "dependence" were eliminated, and instead, diagnoses now specify substance type and severity along a continuum based on the number of symptoms present. For *mild* substance use, two to three symptoms are present; for *moderate*, four to five symptoms; and for *severe*, six or more symptoms. Course specifiers can also be added to the diagnosis now and include the following: "in early remission," "in sustained remission," "on maintenance therapy," and "in a controlled environment."

The substances in question comprise 10 separate classes of drugs: (a) alcohol, (b) caffeine, (c) cannabis, (d) phencyclidine (or similarly acting arylcyclohexylamines), (e) other hallucinogens, (f) inhalants, (g) opioids, (h) sedatives, hypnotics, or anxiolytics, (i) stimulants (amphetamine-type substances, cocaine, and other stimulants) (j) tobacco, and other (or unknown) substances.

SUDs and substance-induced disorders (e.g., "intoxication, withdrawal, and other substance-/medication-induced mental disorders)" are different entities (p. 481).[1]

## ETIOLOGY AND PATHOPHYSIOLOGY

The development of SUDs is multifactorial, often involving some interaction or combination of genetic predisposition (e.g., family history, lower levels of self-control/higher impulsivity), activation of the brain's reward system, trait differences, cognitive factors, social and environmental cues and reinforcement, and brain changes that occur as a result of ongoing substance use.[1] Given that the factors that contribute to the initiation and maintenance of addiction are multifaceted, the majority of treatments with the best evidence are similarly complex and guided by biopsychosocial models,[2] such as the Transtheoretical Model (TTM) of intentional behavior change.[3]

The National Survey on Drug Use and Health (NSDUH) estimated that 58.8 million people (23.8% of the total population) were current (i.e., past month) tobacco users and that 19.3

The full list of resources and references appears in the digital product found on http://connect
.springerpub.com/content/book/978-0-8261-6226-7/part/part03/chapter/ch52

million people aged 18 and older (7.8% of the population) had problems with SUD of which 38.3% or 7.4 million struggled with illicit drugs, 74.5% or 14.4 million struggled with alcohol, and 12.9% or 2.5 million struggled with both illicit drugs and alcohol. Additionally, 10.3 million people or 3.7% of the total population struggled with opioid misuse.[4]

Tobacco, alcohol, and drug use contribute the largest percentage of preventable causes of death in the United States,[5] and thus integration of evidence-based practices for identification and treatment for SUD is critical for all healthcare settings, including rehabilitation. SUD may be present at the onset of a medical condition or injury, may complicate the course of treatment and rehabilitation, and/or may continue or start after medical rehabilitation.

In rehabilitation patient populations, the rate of substance use has been found to be higher than in the general public. For instance, estimates of preinjury alcohol use disorders (AUD) in patients with traumatic brain injuries (TBI) range from 16% to 66%[6] and estimates of preinjury AUD in patients with spinal cord injuries (SCI) range from 35% to 49%.[7]

Substance use may contribute to eventual medical conditions seen in rehabilitation settings or may play a role at the time of injury. The rate of alcohol intoxication for patients who sustained a TBI has been found to range between 36% and 51%.[6] In another sample of patients with TBI, 23.7% of patients were positive for marijuana, 13.2% for cocaine, and 8.8% for amphetamine.[8] Rate of alcohol intoxication at the time of a new SCI was found to be approximately 37%.[9]

SUD severity and outcomes are affected by the type and number of substances used and duration and frequency of use. Co-occurring mental health conditions can contribute to the initiation and/or maintenance of SUD and complicate recovery efforts bidirectionally. Pain management may also be more complicated when SUD is co-occurring, lowering pain thresholds and changing tolerance for medications. When patients are contending with physical or cognitive deficits or disabilities, co-occurring SUD can have significant effects on one's medical and rehabilitation outcomes, and vice versa. This underscores the importance of a biopsychosocial approach to assessment and treatment.[10]

## DIAGNOSTIC APPROACH

### Screening

Screening for substance use has several significant goals: (a) to detect current at-risk use at an early stage before substance use results in more serious disease or other health problems; (b) to connect substance use to current health problems and future health risks; (c) to identify how a patient's substance use could interfere with other treatments; and (d) to identify a patient's willingness to consider substance use behavior change and treatment options.

The clinical interview should start with asking about specific substances the patient uses and their substances of choice. Open-ended questions and clarifying questions should be used. For the substances patients identify, providers should delve into the assessment of routes of administration, age of first use, if/when use became regular, amount and frequency of use, any periods of abstinence and for how long, evidence of dependence (e.g., symptoms of withdrawal, hospitalizations), and ways in which SUD has affected a patient's life, such as interference with work, hobbies, and relationships. In rehabilitation settings, assessing the impact of SUD may also mean discussing the ways in which substance use has affected medical

## TABLE 52.1 IMPORTANT PRIMARY AND SECONDARY SCREENING TOOLS

| SUBSTANCE | PRIMARY SCREENING | SECONDARY SCREENING | ADDITIONAL COMMENTS |
|---|---|---|---|
| Tobacco | "Have you ever smoked cigarettes or used other tobacco products?" "Have you smoked even a puff of a cigarette or used other tobacco products in the past 30 days?"[12] | If yes: "On average, how many cigarettes did/do you smoke per day?" If yes: "How long have you been smoking at that rate (in years)?"[12] | Any positive answer about tobacco or other nicotine use warrants secondary screening and/or intervention Assessment is also part of the "5 A's" approach (ask, advise, assess, assist, arrange), a step-by-step assessment and brief intervention that is augmented by use of MI[13] |
| Alcohol | NIAAA single question screen: "On any single occasion during the past 3 months, have you had more than 5 drinks containing alcohol?"[14] | AUDIT[15] The CAGE Questionnaire[16] | It is important to know what constitutes a "standard drink," which pocket cards often illustrate to help providers and patients quantify the amount The AUDIT is 10 items and takes 2–5 minutes. A shorter version is the AUDIT-C, which is three items and takes 1 minute, but does not measure consequences. |
| Illicit substances | NIDA Quick Screen: "How many times in the past year have you used an illegal drug or used a prescription medication for nonmedical reasons?"[17] | World Health Organization ASSIST[18] DAST-10[19] | The ASSIST is an 8-item screening tool that covers tobacco, alcohol, use of prescription drugs for non-medical reasons, and illicit substances. The DAST-10 is a 10-item screening tool for substances other than alcohol in the 12 months. |

ASSIST, Alcohol, Smoking, and Substance Involvement Screening Test; AUDIT, Alcohol Use Disorders Identification Test; DAST-10, Drug Abuse Screening Test; MI, motivational interviewing; NIAAA, National Institute on Alcohol Abuse and Alcoholism; NIDA, National Institute on Drug Abuse.

conditions, access or adherence to treatment, and self-care. Primary screening helps identify whether or not a substance is used at all and at a potentially risky level. Positive answers to these questions warrant additional or secondary follow-up screening (Table 52.1).

Secondary screening involves the use of formal measures to identify the level of risk of a person's behavior. Secondary screening is important as clinicians have been found to be very poor at detecting SUD without the use of such measures.[11]

## Assessment

A critical part of the assessment is "staging" such that the clinician determines a patient's readiness for change in order to match the appropriate intervention (Table 52.2). The theory of matching a patient's stage of change is part of the TTM of intentional behavior change.[3] Stage of change is assessed by asking how ready a patient is to change the behavior in question.

## TREATMENT

### Brief Interventions

Screening, brief intervention, and referral to treatment (SBIRT) was developed as an evidence-based protocol for clinicians in medical settings to identify those with tobacco, alcohol, or other SUDs, or are misusing prescription medication, acts as a guide for initial treatment, and assists with medical decision making with regard to escalating treatment needs and resources. SBIRT pocket cards can be a helpful tool for clinicians to carry with them as a reference for the validated screening questions and identifying varying levels of risk so that the appropriate steps for intervention can be taken (see Online Resources).

### Behavioral Treatments

Although not a formal treatment, motivational interviewing (MI) is a style of communication that aims to enhance a patient's intrinsic motivation for behavior change and resolving ambivalence, often paired with the stages of change model (Table 52.2). MI techniques can be used to augment other behavioral treatments.

Harm reduction is a set of principles and interventions to promote safety and reduce the harm of ongoing substance use (such as overdose, transmitted diseases). Examples include needle and syringe exchange or access programs, naloxone distribution, Good Samaritan Laws, supervised injection facilities, or drug/pill checking.

Cognitive Behavioral Therapy (CBT) or cognitive behavioral coping skills training helps patients learn to change thinking and behavior related to substance use. Strategies include monitoring antecedents and consequences of thinking or behavior, cognitive restructuring, strengthening coping skills, and social support.

Relapse prevention (RP) teaches patients a number of cognitive and behavioral strategies to prevent or handle high-risk situations, recognize warning signs, emphasize positive lifestyle changes, interrupt lapses, and use lapses/relapse as an opportunity for self-knowledge.

### TABLE 52.2 STAGES OF THE TRANSTHEORETICAL MODEL OF INTENTIONAL BEHAVIOR CHANGE

| STAGE OF CHANGE | DESCRIPTION | ASSOCIATED TASKS |
|---|---|---|
| Precontemplation | Not ready to consider changing in the next month | To build interest and concern for behavior change |
| Contemplation | Aware and considering behavior change | Risk-reward analysis and decision making |
| Preparation | Intending to take action in the next month | Commitment and creating an effective and acceptable plan |
| Action | Already begun behavior change | Implementation of the plan and revising as needed |
| Maintenance | Actively engaged in behavior change for at least 3–6 months | Consolidating change into a lifestyle |

**TABLE 52.3 PHARMACOLOGICAL TREATMENTS FOR TOBACCO, ALCOHOL, AND OPIOID USE DISORDERS**

| DISORDER | STRONG EVIDENCE | WEAK EVIDENCE | INSUFFICIENT EVIDENCE |
|---|---|---|---|
| Tobacco use disorder | NRT (patch, gum, inhaler, spray, tablets, lozenges), combined NRT, Bupropion, Varenicline | Cytisine, Nortriptyline, Clonidine | Mecamylamine with NRT |
| Alcohol use disorder | Acamprosate, Disulfiram, Naltrexone (oral or extended release), Topiramate | Gabapentin | Baclofen, Valproic Acid, Buspirone, Citalopram, Fluoxetine, Quetiapine |
| Opioid use disorder | Buprenorphine/naloxone, Methadone (in an OTP), extended-release injectable Naltrexone ("for whom opioid agonist treatment is contraindicated, unacceptable, unavailable, or discontinued and who have established abstinence for a sufficient period of time.") | Buprenorphine (without Naloxone in pregnant women) | Naltrexone, Dihydrocodeine |

NRT, nicotine replacement therapy; OTP, opioid treatment program

See Online Resources for more information.

Self-help or 12-step facilitation (TSF) aims to engage patients in the 12-step model for self-help, and focuses on acceptance, surrender, and active involvement. Well-known 12-step groups include alcoholics anonymous (AA), narcotics anonymous (NA), cocaine anonymous, marijuana anonymous, self-management and recovery training (SMART), and women for sobriety.

## Pharmacological Treatments

The treatments listed earlier are the most common, evidence-based behavioral treatments for SUD. Pharmacological treatments for substance use disorders can be used as stand-alone treatments or can be used in conjunction with behavioral treatments, with the latter having more evidence of success (Table 52.3). There are a number of other treatments that use some of the previously mentioned principles and are tailored for couples or families, or involve treatment communities.

## FUNCTIONAL PROGNOSIS AND OUTCOMES

SUD, whether preinjury, intoxication at the time of injury, or postinjury, has been found to negatively impact the course of recovery and functioning in both the short and long term. Effects are often dose dependent, both in substance quantity and duration (e.g., years) of misuse (see Table 52.4). However, more research is needed in this area, particularly on the effects of other substances than alcohol.

Cognitive deficits will affect patients' ability to plan and be self-directed in SUD recovery, so treating SUD may be more challenging for patients with stroke, TBI/ABI, or other long-standing vascular problems that may contribute to cognitive changes over time.

## TABLE 52.4 OUTCOMES IN DIFFERENT MEDICAL REHABILITATION POPULATIONS

| OUTCOME | TBI | SCI | AMPUTATION |
|---------|-----|-----|------------|
| Physical health effects | *Preinjury alcohol use:*<br>• Increased risk of mortality<br>• More severe brain lesions<br>• Higher risk of recurrent TBI<br>*Alcohol intoxication during the initial injury*<br>• Longer length of coma<br>• Longer period of agitation<br>• Less cerebral blood flow<br>• Greater cerebral atrophy[11] | *Preinjury alcohol use:*<br>• Increased risk of pressure sores in the first 3 years<br>*Alcohol intoxication during the initial injury*<br>• More severe SCI<br>• Higher rates of cervical SCI<br>*Alcohol use postinjury*<br>• Greater likelihood of being hospitalized with a pressure ulcer<br>• Increased risk of sustaining injuries necessitating medical treatment[11] | *Pre- and postamputation alcohol misuse:*<br>• Associated with medical disorders that can contribute to limb loss or complicate recovery (e.g., diabetes, obesity, hypertension, cardiovascular disease)<br>• Risk factor for foot ulceration<br>*Cigarette smoking:*<br>• Risk factor for amputation<br>• Poorer healing<br>• Higher risk of revision surgery[20] |
| Mental health effects | *Preinjury alcohol use disorder:*<br>• Greater risk of emotional and behavioral problems[11] | *Preinjury alcohol use disorder:*<br>• Higher rates of depression and suicide[11] | • SUD is associated with less engagement with hobbies or therapies, which in turn is associated with poorer mental health[10] |
| SUD outcomes | • May continue heavy alcohol consumption<br>• Alcohol use disorders were the second most common psychiatric diagnosis 30 years post-TBI[11] | • Alcohol consumption may be higher than in the general population[11] | |
| Pain management | *Considerations for all populations:*<br>• Lower pain thresholds<br>• Differential tolerance of pain meds<br>• Higher chronic pain ratings[10] | | |

(continued)

**TABLE 52.4 OUTCOMES IN DIFFERENT MEDICAL REHABILITATION POPULATIONS (*continued*)**

| OUTCOME | TBI | SCI | AMPUTATION |
|---|---|---|---|
| Social and other functional domains | *Preinjury alcohol use:*<br>• Reduced community integration<br>• Less likely to return to productive activity<br>• Poorer vocational outcomes[11] | *Preinjury alcohol use:*<br>• Spend less time in rehabilitation therapies<br>*Alcohol use postinjury*<br>• May interfere with health maintenance behaviors (e.g., judgment, coordination, memory)[11] | *Pre- and postlimb loss alcohol misuse:*<br>• Risk factor for either not receiving or failing to use a prosthetic<br>• Reduced likelihood of pre-amputation mobility levels<br>*Cigarette smoking:*<br>• Reduced walking distances with a prosthetic[20] |

SCI, spinal cord injury; SUD, substance use disorder; TBI, traumatic brain injury.

## RESOURCES AND REFERENCES

The full list of resources and references appears in the digital product found on http://connect .springerpub.com/content/book/978-0-8261-6226-7/part/part03/chapter/ch52

# SYRINGOMYELIA

AUDREY S. LEUNG AND KATE E. DELANEY

## CORE DEFINITIONS

Syringomyelia, often termed a syrinx, is defined as a fluid-filled cyst lined by gliotic tissue within the spinal cord parenchyma. Hydromyelia refers to a focal dilatation of the central canal lined by ependymal cells.[1] Additional terminology to describe these similar conditions includes hydrosyringomyelia. Typically, these are progressive, chronic conditions that most commonly develop at levels C2 to T9, but can ascend up to the brain stem (termed "syringobulbia") or descend caudally into the conus medullaris.

## ETIOLOGY AND PATHOPHYSIOLOGY

Although there is no consensus on the categorization of syringomyelia, this is often broadly separated into congenital syringomyelia and acquired syringomyelia. Congenital syringomyelia is present at birth and caused either by an abnormality of primary neurulation or by other congenital malformations that cause a disturbance to the normal cerebrospinal fluid (CSF) circulation. The latter is commonly associated with Chiari malformations and tethered cord syndrome. In Chiari malformation syndromes, it is thought that the downward herniation of the cerebellar tonsils results in obstruction of normal CSF flow from the cranial to the spinal compartments, leading to accumulation of fluid in the central canal or spinal cord parenchyma.[2] With tethered cord syndrome, the mechanical effects and/or metabolic and ischemic changes in the distal cord are likely contributing factors to syrinx formation.[3]

Acquired syringomyelia is caused by any lesion or disease resulting in a disturbance to normal CSF dynamics. Etiologies of acquired syringomyelia are diverse and include hydrocephalus, postinfectious (i.e., meningitis leading to arachnoid scarring), postinflammatory (i.e., transverse myelitis, sarcoidosis, multiple sclerosis), posttraumatic, spinal cord tumors (i.e., ependymomas, hemangioblastomas), extramedullary tumors, and spinal canal stenosis.[4]

Posttraumatic syringomyelia, in particular, is an important cause of neurologic deterioration after traumatic spinal cord injury (SCI). It is estimated to be present in a little over half of all patients with traumatic SCI.[5,6] However, the presence of clinically symptomatic posttraumatic syringomyelia is much less frequent, ranging from <1% to 7% of all traumatic SCI.[7] Posttraumatic syringomyelia can present at any time after initial SCI, but are most common 5 to 15 years after SCI.[7] Risk factors for early syrinx formation are complete motor

---

The full list of resources and references appears in the digital product found on http://connect
.springerpub.com/content/book/978-0-8261-6226-7/part/part03/chapter/ch53

and sensory SCI (American Spinal Injury Association Impairment Scale [AIS] A) and older age at the time of SCI (age > 30 years).[7]

In some cases, no underlying cause can be identified, although it is thought that this condition may represent a fetal configuration of the central canal of the spinal cord and is sometimes referred to as a "persistent central canal." To make a diagnosis of the persistent central canal, there should be no other factors predisposing to syringomyelia and it should be located at the junction of the ventral one-third and dorsal two-thirds of the spinal cord, be filiform in shape, and not eccentrically located. A persistent central canal is considered a normal anatomical variant and typically does not warrant treatment.[4] These lesions are typically small and asymptomatic, and two small case studies have so far shown that these lesions do not progress in size.[8,9]

## DIAGNOSTIC APPROACH

### Evaluation

Syringomyelia may be asymptomatic, however, classic symptoms described are cape-like pain and loss of temperature sensation along the back and arms, caused by damage to the fibers of the spinothalamic tracts. Patients also often present with weakness and increased muscle tone in the back and extremities. In acquired syringomyelia, autonomic bladder and bowel dysfunction are uncommon until end-stage spinal cord dysfunction. In contrast, patients with congenital syringomyelia secondary to neural tube defects usually present differently.[4] In these patients, neurologic deficits in the lower extremities along with bowel and bladder dysfunction are common and may be difficult to distinguish from tethered cord syndrome. With children, in particular, progressive scoliosis may be the only presenting sign of syringomyelia. Overall, clinical manifestations of syringomyelia are typically slow and progressive.

In patients with suspected syringomyelia, a thorough history with particular attention to the individual's neurodevelopmental status, medical conditions, neurologic disorders, and details of prior injuries and surgeries should be obtained. Baseline functional history and changes in function should be noted, as well as relevant family and social history. Pertinent symptoms to elicit include new onset or worsening pain (which often presents unilaterally), progressive weakness in the arms or legs, stiffness, headaches, vision changes, cranial nerve palsies, new or worsening autonomic dysreflexia, loss of or abnormal sensation (particularly in the hands), loss of bowel/bladder control, problems with sexual function, muscle wasting, changes in muscle tone, ataxia, and progressive scoliosis. Decline in respiratory function and dysphagia should also be assessed, as syringomyelia extending into the brain stem can impact respiratory control of the diaphragm and would be a cause for urgent neurosurgical evaluation. If available, prior neuroimaging studies and electrodiagnostic studies should be reviewed.

In most respects, the physical examination is similar to that performed in other neurologic conditions and should include testing of the cranial nerves, motor and sensory function, reflexes, balance, and gait. Of note, the International Standards for Neurological Classification of SCI (ISNCSCI) examination can be helpful. This detailed examination is not only useful for serial monitoring for any motor or sensory changes but can be helpful in noting any neurologic changes in the thoracic region where no key muscle groups are otherwise available for testing as well as to assess for improvement if surgical intervention is performed. Musculoskeletal findings may include scoliosis and Charcot arthropathy.

### Differential Diagnosis

Other causes of a patient's neurologic changes must be considered before a definitive diagnosis of syringomyelia is made. Spinal etiologies such as radiculopathy, myelopathy, hardware failure, or tethered cord syndrome can lead to progressive neurologic symptoms and should be considered. Neurodegenerative diseases such as multiple sclerosis and motor neuron diseases, as well as peripheral nerve injuries, should also be on the differential based on the patient's history and presenting symptoms.

### Neuroimaging

MRI of the spine is the gold standard for the evaluation of syringomyelia and is also used to evaluate for other possible causative spinal lesions. MRI of the brain should be obtained to rule out hydrocephalus or shunt malfunction if the patient has a history of shunt placement. If there are contraindications to MR imaging, delayed CT myelography may be considered and can be helpful in identifying cavitations within the spinal cord as well as cord tethering.[10]

## TREATMENT

If a syrinx is noted on imaging but does not have associated symptoms, no intervention is needed. However, the natural course of asymptomatic syringomyelia is not well understood.[11] For those who have mild symptoms or who do not wish to pursue surgical intervention, re-evaluation of functional needs is appropriate, including equipment, medications, physical or occupational therapy, and caregiver support required. Serial physical examinations can be helpful to assess for any progression and new functional needs.

The goal of surgical intervention is to alter the CSF flow. Surgery may be indicated if there is a deterioration of motor function, but not solely for sensory abnormalities or pain.[11] If the altered flow is thought to be from spinal canal stenosis, laminectomy may be warranted.[4] Shunting can redirect CSF to either the subarachnoid space or to the pleural or peritoneal cavities. If the tethered cord has resulted from spinal cord scarring and appears to be contributing to cystic cavity formation, detethering surgery may be needed.[11]

For posttraumatic syringomyelia, a syringosubarachnoid shunt may be pursued if the syrinx is confluent and if there is no cord tethering. If both are present, the cord detethering may be performed first and a shunt can be placed if the cyst does not improve in size with that intervention alone, which may occur in about 60% of cases. In one retrospective study, surgery was performed on average 6.5 years after the initial presenting symptom, which was most commonly pain.[12]

For syringomyelia associated with Chiari I malformation (CIM), the surgical options include posterior fossa bony decompression (PFBD), typically involving a C1 laminectomy, or PFBD with duraplasty (PFBDD). The presence of syringomyelia with CIM increases the risk of reoperation in the PFBD cases and can lead to longer postoperative hospitalization. It may take months to years for the syringomyelia to improve or resolve after either procedure. In one recent study, a fourth ventricle shunt was placed in patients with syringomyelia and CIM who had prior treatment failure from surgical decompression. In total, 93% of patients did have significant improvement or resolution of the syringomyelia over the follow-up period (mean 8 years), with 14% of patients first requiring reshunting after syrinx recurred.[13]

Syringomyelia may also be associated with acquired Chiari malformations (ACM), for example, due to posterior fossa tumor. In these cases, the syringomyelia may resolve with resection of the space-occupying lesion and shunting alone was not effective.[14]

Complications from these surgeries can include neurologic worsening, CSF leak, headache, infection, hematoma, and shunt malfunction.[4]

## FUNCTIONAL PROGNOSIS AND OUTCOMES

For those who do not have symptoms necessitating surgical intervention, the natural course of posttraumatic syringomyelia is a slow progression of symptoms. Based on a small case series, it is possible that up to 50% of patients will not have progression of symptoms over a decade-long period. There have been a few reports of spontaneous resolution.[15]

Surgical intervention for posttraumatic syringomyelia is most likely to result in improvement in motor function as opposed to sensory abnormalities or pain. Overall, the surgical intervention depends on the underlying etiology and no one surgical technique has been found to be superior.[11]

In posttraumatic syringomyelia treated with shunt and/or de-tethering, resolution of the cyst occurred in 93% to 95% of cases for both interventions, although that did not necessarily correlate with improvement in function or pain.[12] Overall, shunting the syrinx alone in posttraumatic syringomyelia has a failure rate of about 50% and high rates of revision.[12] This is also the case for syringomyelia without Chiari malformation.[16]

For syringomyelia associated with CIM, PFBD has fewer complications at the time of the procedure while the PFBDD is overall more successful, although riskier, including higher risk of CSF leak and mortality. The PFBDD has >85% rate of clinical improvement, likely due to increasing the posterior fossa and CSF spaces, versus >80% in the PFBD and recurrence of syrinx in 2% to 4% as opposed to 2% to 12% in the PFBD.[13]

## BASIC ORDER SETS

Imaging modalities: MRI with contrast if concern for syringomyelia without known etiology. If not available, consider CT myelogram. Posttraumatic syringomyelia can be evaluated with MRI without contrast.

## RESOURCES AND REFERENCES

The full list of resources and references appears in the digital product found on http://connect.springerpub.com/content/book/978-0-8261-6226-7/part/part03/chapter/ch53

# VENOUS THROMBOEMBOLISM

DORIANNE FELDMAN AND CHENG-CHUAN CHIANG

## CORE DEFINITIONS

Venous thromboembolism (VTE) is a collective term that includes deep venous thrombosis (DVT) in the upper or lower extremities and pulmonary embolism (PE) in the lungs. After acute coronary syndrome and stroke, VTE is the third most common cardiovascular disease.[1]

## ETIOLOGY AND PATHOPHYSIOLOGY

The pathophysiology of thrombosis can be explained by Virchow's Triad, where clotting occurs as a result of changes in blood circulation, blood vessel architecture, and blood composition. Any one of these factors increases the risk for thrombosis.

Risk factors for VTE include major surgery, cancer, immobility, trauma, pregnancy, hormonal therapies, obesity, advanced age, varicosities, family history, central venous catheters, and transvenous pacemaker placement. Other etiologies such as heparin-induced thrombocytopenia (HIT), nephrotic syndrome, immune thrombocytopenia purpura, hyperthyroidism, homocystinuria, inflammatory bowel disease and chronic kidney disease, rheumatoid arthritis and Lupus, sickle cell disease, and obstructive sleep apnea are also associated with VTE.[2]

## DIAGNOSTIC APPROACH

### History

Diagnosing VTE can be challenging because DVT presents similarly to cellulitis, hematoma, peripheral edema, and superficial thrombophlebitis, whereas PE is difficult to distinguish from other cardiopulmonary disorders.[3] It is important to conduct a comprehensive medical history, review of symptoms, and the risk factors listed earlier.

### Physical Examination

Thoroughly examine the limb for changes in size, color, temperature, and any vein abnormalities. Heart and lung examination is particularly important if PE is suspected.

Signs of DVT include the following:

- Warmth, erythema, tenderness, and palpable cords.
- Limb circumference measured at 10 cm below the tibial tuberosity is greater than 3 cm from the contralateral limb.

---

The full list of references appears in the digital product found on http://connect.springerpub.com/content/book/978-0-8261-6226-7/part/part03/chapter/ch54

■ Homan's sign, which is calf pain elicited by passive dorsiflexion with knee extension and the leg raised to approximately 10°.

## Laboratory Testing

D-dimer has high sensitivity and negative predictive value with low specificity, where a negative test rules out PE, but a positive test cannot confirm the diagnosis.[3,4]

## Imaging

Ultrasonography has a high sensitivity and specificity. It is recommended as the first line for diagnosing DVT.[3]

Magnetic resonance venography with high sensitivity and specificity has not been validated, but it has been employed as a diagnostic option for DVT if ultrasound is not definitive.[3]

Computed tomography pulmonary angiography (CTPA) has high specificity, sensitivity, and negative predictive value. It is the first-line imaging modality to diagnose PE despite the radiation exposure and contrast to visualize the vasculature. CTPA is avoided in significant renal disease due to contrast-associated nephrotoxicity.[3]

Magnetic resonance imaging has been found inconclusive for its ability to diagnose PE.[5]

V/Q scintigraphy is an alternative to CTPA for patients with renal impairment and contrast allergy. It is a nuclear medicine scan of the pulmonary vasculature and ventilation between the upper airway and lung parenchyma.[3,6]

## TREATMENT

### Upper Extremity Deep Venous Thrombosis

Upper extremity DVT is often related to central venous catheter, pacemaker, implanted cardiac defibrillator, or vascular procedure. For catheter-associated thrombus, the catheter should not be removed for 1 week after starting anticoagulation to eliminate PE risks. The duration of anticoagulation is for at least 3 months or for the duration of catheter existence. Immediate removal is preferred if anticoagulation is contraindicated. If the thrombus is associated with a pacemaker or implanted defibrillator, anticoagulation is also administered without removing the device.[7]

### Lower Extremity
### Distal Deep Venous Thrombosis

Defined as a thrombus below the knee, it has a lower risk for PE compared to proximal DVT. The concern is propagation to proximal deep vessels, PE, and postthrombotic syndrome (PTS). Treatment with anticoagulation is recommended for 3 months. If anticoagulation is not feasible, venous duplex ultrasound is repeated in 1 week to evaluate for thrombus propagation. The risk of PE is even higher if there is also an elevated D-dimer, significant thrombosis (based on length, 7 mm diameter, thrombus in more than 1 vein, clotting near the proximal deep veins), known history of DVT, active cancer, or hospitalization.[4]

## Proximal Deep Venous Thrombosis

Defined as a thrombus above the knee, the risk for PE is very high. Similar to distal DVT, anticoagulation is preferred for the same minimal duration. If there is a concern for limb viability or if iliofemoral DVT is present in younger patients without significant bleeding risk, thrombolysis may be considered.[4]

## Pulmonary Embolism

Treatment with anticoagulation is first line unless contraindications exist. The medications and timeline recommendations for anticoagulation agent selection are the same as for treatment of proximal and distal DVT.[4]

### Pharmacologic Interventions

Systemic or catheter-directed thrombolysis with mechanical thrombectomy is considered for significant thrombus burden, hemodynamically instability, or limb-loss risk. Thrombolysis is less effective after thrombi stabilize.[6]

Oral anticoagulation for a minimum of 3 months is the mainstay treatment. The pharmacologic options for anticoagulation include unfractionated heparin (UFH), low molecular weight heparin (LMWH), fondaparinux, vitamin K antagonists (VKA) (i.e., Coumadin), and direct oral anticoagulants (DOACs) (i.e., rivaroxaban, apixaban, dabigatran).

Subcutaneous UFH and LMWH are recommended for hospitalized patients due to their shorter half-lives. UFH has a shorter half-life (1 hr) and complete reversibility, so it is preferred for patients who need procedures, are at high risk for bleeding, have severe kidney disease, and those who have morbid obesity or are underweight. Outside of these patients, LMWH (half-life 3–5 hr) is more commonly used because UFH has eight- to tenfold increased risk for HIT. Subcutaneous fondaparinux is rarely used due to its longer half-life (17–21 hr) compared to UFH and LMWH. However, fondaparinux has extremely low HIT risk, so when patients develop HIT with UFH or LMWH, fondaparinux is an alternative.

When transitioning to oral medications, DOACs are first line over VKA because monitoring is not necessary. However, it is more challenging to reverse DOACs due to their longer half-lives (7–15 hr) and the novelty of the reversal agents. It is also contraindicated for those with moderate-to-severe hepatic disease or creatinine clearance (CrCl) less than 30 mL/min.

In the situation that VKAs are considered, it is started once UFH/LMWH reaches therapeutic levels. UFH/LMWH can be stopped after 5 days of overlap and when VKA reaches therapeutic INR levels of 2 to 3 for 24 hours.

### Contraindications

The relative contraindications to anticoagulation including gastrointestinal bleeding, thrombocytopenia, anemia, dementia, advanced age, intracranial hemorrhage (ICH), and hematologic malignancy. Active and major bleeding is an absolute contraindication.[6]

### Monitoring

PT and INR levels must be monitored with VKAs and checked daily in the inpatient setting. Once the INR is therapeutic, weekly and later monthly monitoring is recommended. When necessary, activated partial thromboplastin time (aPTT) is used to monitor UFH. It is important to know that aPTT is often prolonged by liver disease, coagulation factor deficiencies, and antiphospholipid antibodies. As for LMWH, fondaparinux, or heparin infusion, antifactor Xa can be used to monitor therapeutic levels.[6,8]

### Overdose and Reversal of Anticoagulation

Protamine sulfate can completely reverse UFH, but it only partially reverses LMWH. It has severe side effect profiles of cardiovascular and pulmonary complications.[8]

For vitamin K antagonist reversals, there are IV or oral vitamin K and vitamin K-dependent procoagulant factors including fresh frozen plasma (FFP), recombinant factor VIIa (rFVIIa), and three or four-factor prothrombin complex concentrates (PCC). Four-factor PCC has prothrombin and factors VII, IX, and X, where three-factor PCC does not have factor VII. PCCs are preferred over FFP because FFP requires large volume infusions and can easily cause volume overload. However, PCCs are associated with thrombotic complications and disseminated intravascular coagulation. The normal hemostasis is not restored by rFVIIa so it is not Food and Drug Administration (FDA) approved.[8,9]

There are no specific reversal agents for DOACs. However, PCC is most commonly considered. Promising novel reversal agents such as idarucizumab is FDA approved to reverse Dabigatran, but andexanet alfa is not FDA approved for apixaban or rivaroxaban reversal.

Careful consideration of initiating reversal agents should be given to patients without serious life-threatening bleeds. If there is no major or intracranial bleeding, the preferred management is to discontinue anticoagulation and to provide supportive care as there are serious risks when using reversal agents.[8]

## SPECIAL CONSIDERATIONS

### Superior Vena Cava Filters

Superior vena cava (SVC) filters are not recommended for distal DVT, superficial vein thrombosis, VTE duration greater than 1 month, or upper extremity DVT. If anticoagulation is contraindicated due to bleeding risks and if the thrombus is no older than 4 weeks, filter placement is considered with a plan for removal within 6 months or when anticoagulation is possible. The risks of SVC filter-associated thrombosis, thoracic vasculature injury, or other complications should be considered.[4]

### Surveillance Ultrasound

The practice of surveillance US remains controversial and may be clinically indicated in high-risk populations based on cost and significance of results and in spinal cord injured patients upon admission to rehabilitation.[10,11]

## REHABILITATION CONSIDERATIONS

### Spinal Cord Injury

The majority of VTE in patients with spinal cord injury (SCI) occurs within the first two weeks of injury. LMWH is superior and preferred over UFH in this population. Intermittent pneumatic devices and compression stockings are often concomitantly used to increase lower extremity venous return. It is recommended to combine both pharmacological and mechanical methods of prophylaxis in this population. The minimal duration of VTE prophylaxis is 8 weeks and up to 12 weeks for those with risk factors such as complete injuries, older age, previous VTE, cancer, and obesity. Despite no clinical trials in patients with SCI, transition to DOACs can be considered given its ease of use.[12,13]

## Cancer

VTE is the second most common cause of death among cancer patients. Cancer is an independent factor predicting VTE prophylaxis failure. It also predicts an increased risk of VTE recurrence. The preferred treatment for cancer-associated thrombosis is LMWH due to its ease of use and lower risks for bleeding. DOACs have a higher bleeding profile, but they can be considered in patients not on systemic therapy. Duration of treatment is a minimum of 3 months up to 6 months. Termination or continuation is based on individual benefit-to-risk ratio, tolerability, drug availability, patient preference, and cancer activity. Primary VTE prophylaxis is recommended for 7 to 10 days within 12 to 24 hours after cancer surgery up to 5 weeks, but there are unclear benefits for patients on chemotherapy given the increased bleeding risks associated with cancer.[12,14-16]

### Neurosurgery, Stroke, and Traumatic Brain Injury

Patients with stroke, traumatic brain injury (TBI), and neurosurgical patients require a careful consideration as they are at increased risks for ICH and VTE. Severe brain injuries are considered an independent risk factor for DVT. The more severe the neurologic impairments, the higher the risk for DVT.[12]

Both pharmacologic prophylaxis and mechanical prophylaxis are recommended. There is a debate between LMWH or UFH as the preferred agent. Some studies showed lower risks of ICH with UFH in TBI patients. The earliest time to safely start anticoagulation for TBI is 24 to 72 hours with stable CT head imaging.[5] After intracranial or spine procedures, VTE prophylaxis can be administered 24 hours following surgery with the transition to therapeutic anticoagulation after 72 hours.[6] It is important to note that low dose antiplatelet agents do not have benefits for VTE prophylaxis. There is no specific indication for continuing VTE prophylaxis after inpatient stay.

### Orthopedic

Postop VTE prophylaxis is recommended for major orthopedic surgeries (i.e., Total hip arthroplasty, total knee arthroplasty, hip fracture surgery). DVTs most commonly occur in the operative limb, but they can also occur in the contralateral limb. LMWH is the preferred agent, and it can be started at 12 to 24 hours following surgery for the recommended duration of 35 days. No prophylaxis is suggested for isolated lower-extremity injuries requiring immobilization or knee arthroscopy.[6,17]

### Burn

In those with thermal injuries, there is an elevated VTE risk due to burn-associated hypercoagulable state, prolonged bed rest, multiple surgeries, and the potential for critical infection. Additional risk factors include morbid obesity, extensive or lower extremity burns, femoral venous catheter, prolonged immobility, and lower extremity trauma. Those with a total body surface area of 40% to 59% burn are at the highest VTE risks. Pharmacologic and or mechanical prophylaxis should be initiated when it is safe and is to be continued until mobility is sufficient.[12,18]

## Amputees

Patients with major lower limb amputations (hip disarticulation, transfemoral, knee disarticulation, and transtibial) have higher VTE risks. DVTs can occur in both the residual and contralateral limb. Among those with a more proximal amputation level, above knee amputees are at the greatest risk. Additional factors including advanced age, lower functional independence measure score, prolonged hospitalization, and chronic vascular diseases increase the risks for DVT. There are no current guidelines for continuing VTE prophylaxis after discharging from inpatient rehabilitation.[12,19]

## COMPLICATIONS

PTS is a result of damaged venous valves that causes venous reflux, leading to venous hypertension and edema. Symptoms include cramping, dull pain with standing, pruritus, and skin changes such as hyperpigmentation. Cellulitis and venous ulceration can also occur. This condition can present within 2 years of a DVT diagnosis or earlier in those with proximal and recurrent DVTs. Early ambulation during the acute stage of DVT and wearing graded compression stockings for 2 years post-DVT decreases the risk of developing PTS.[12]

## Recurrence

Approximately 30% of patients have VTE recurrence within 10 years of the initial event.[2] Specific risk factors are advanced age, higher body mass index, male, active cancer, immobility, hypercoagulable disorders, idiopathic VTE, and residual vein thrombosis.[4]

## BASIC ORDER SET

Table 54.1 provides recommendations for VTE prophylaxis based on level of risk.

### TABLE 54.1 VENOUS THROMBOEMBOLISM PROPHYLAXIS[20]

| RISK LEVEL | PROPHYLAXIS REGIMEN |
|---|---|
| Low | SCD, sequential compression device. |
| Moderate | Select one of the medications ± compression devices<br>■ SCDs—optional<br>■ Unfractionated Heparin 5,000 units SQ TID<br>■ Enoxaparin/Lovenox<br>  ❑ 40 mg SQ daily (CrCl >30 mL/min)<br>  ❑ 30 mg SQ daily (CrCl 10–29 mL/min)<br>  ❑ 40 mg SQ BID (BMI >40 kg/m², CrCl >30 mL/min) |
| High | Select one of the medications AND compression devices<br>■ SCDs—required<br>■ Unfractionated Heparin 5,000 units SQ TID<br>■ Enoxaparin/Lovenox (preferred)<br>  ❑ 40 mg SQ daily (Wt <150 kg, CrCl >30 mL/min)<br>  ❑ 30 mg SQ daily (Wt <150 kg, CrCl >30 mL/min)<br>  ❑ 30 mg SQ daily (Wt <150 kg, CrCl >30 mL/min) |

*(continued)*

**TABLE 54.1 VENOUS THROMBOEMBOLISM PROPHYLAXIS[20] (*continued*)**

GENERAL GUIDELINES
ORTHOPEDIC GUIDELINES[17]

| SURGERY | PROPHYLAXIS DOSING |
|---------|-------------------|
| Total knee replacement/ Major trauma | Select one of the medications below<br>■ Aspirin 325 mg PO BID<br>■ Lovenox<br>  ❑ 30 mg SQ BID (CrCl >30 mL/min)<br>  ❑ 30 mg SQ daily (CrCl <30 mL/min) |
| Total knee replacement | Select one of the following medications:<br>■ Aspirin 325 mg PO BID<br>■ Lovenox<br>  ❑ 40 mg SQ daily (CrCl >30 mL/min)<br>  ❑ 30 mg SQ daily (CrCl <30 mL/min) |

CrCl, creatinine clearance.

## REFERENCES

The full list of references appears in the digital product found on http://connect.springerpub.com/content/book/978-0-8261-6226-7/part/part03/chapter/ch54

# VENTILATOR MANAGEMENT

DOMINIQUE VINH

## CORE DEFINITIONS

The most important concept to recognize is that mechanical ventilation—no matter how sophisticated the ventilatory strategy is—remains a supportive intervention, and the underlying primary cause for the respiratory compromise must be addressed.

### Respiratory Failure

Respiratory failure is defined as impaired gas exchange, in which $PaO_2$ is lower than 60 mmHg, often associated with $PaCO_2$ higher than 50 mmHg. Respiratory failure can be thought of as a syndrome, based on the underlying primary or contributing factors (e.g., central nervous system, peripheral nervous system, respiratory muscles, chest wall, airways, and alveoli). Significant mortality has been associated with acute respiratory syndrome (ARDS) and chronic obstructive pulmonary disease (COPD) exacerbation. While acute respiratory failure can develop quickly with serious arterial blood gases and acid–base abnormalities, chronic respiratory failure is more insidious in nature, allowing for physiologic compensations to take place. There are two types of respiratory failure—hypoxemic respiratory failure (Type 1) and hypercapnic respiratory failure (Type 2).

### Type 1 Respiratory Failure: Hypoxia

Hypoxemic respiratory failure (Type 1) represents a failure of oxygen exchange at the level of the aveolo-capillary membrane, where $PaO_2$ is less than 60 mmHg with normal or low $PaCO_2$. Ventilation/perfusion mismatching is the most common pathophysiologic mechanism for hypoxemia, and other etiologies include increased shunt, diffusion impairment, and alveolar hypoventilation.[2] Common causes include cardiogenic or noncardiogenic pulmonary edema and severe pneumonia. In addition to assessing the underlying causes, the treatment approach for hypoxemia is to carefully up-titrate the concentration of oxygen ($FiO_2$) in order to recruit the collapsed alveoli.

### Type 2 Respiratory Failure: Hypercapnia

Hypercapnic respiratory failure (Type 2), on the other hand, represents a ventilatory problem with a failure to remove $CO_2$, where $PaCO_2$ is greater than 50 mmHg, often associated with hypoxemia. Common causes include defects in the central nervous system, impairment of

The full list of references appears in the digital product found on http://connect.springerpub.com/content/book/978-0-8261-6226-7/part/part03/chapter/ch55

neuromuscular transmission, mechanical defect of the ribcage, and fatigue of the respiratory muscles.[2] Once the underlying conditions are addressed, the strategy to correct the hypercapnia is to improve ventilation by increasing the minute ventilation.

## Acute Respiratory Distress Syndrome

ARDS represents a life-threatening physiologic inflammatory response resulting in hypoxic lung injury with increased pulmonary vascular permeability, requiring mechanical ventilation support. The 2011 consensus-based Berlin Definition of ARDS relies on four criteria: timing, chest imaging, origin of edema, and oxygenation. The degree of hypoxemia characterizes ARDS as mild, moderate, or severe. Compared with earlier criteria, the Berlin Definition is better at predicting mortality at different stages of ARDS.[3] The current recommended approach to management includes low-tidal volume mechanical ventilation, prone ventilation, and extracorporeal membrane oxygenation (ECMO) as a bridging intervention for specific situations.[4]

## Noninvasive Ventilation

Noninvasive ventilation (NIV) provides positive pressure ventilatory support for patients with respiratory failure through noninvasive interface (e.g., nasal mask, face mask, or nasal cannula). Noninvasive positive pressure ventilation (NPPV) benefits primarily medically stable patients who are alert, cooperative with minimal airway secretions.

NPPV is provided as continuous positive airway pressure (CPAP), where constant pressure is maintained, or as bilevel positive airway pressure (BiPAP), where the patient initiates the breaths within a predetermined expiratory positive airway pressure (EPAP) and inspiratory positive airway pressure (IPAP). NPPV is contraindicated in patients who are obtunded, hemodynamically unstable, with high aspiration risks, or with impaired gastric emptying.

## Invasive Mechanical Ventilation

Invasive mechanical ventilation (IMV) provides respiratory support for patients who can no longer maintain an airway for adequate oxygenation or ventilation through improving the work of breathing and gas exchange, as well as protecting the lungs from iatrogenic injuries. Mechanical ventilation allows the patient time to recover from the underlying medical condition. It is imperative to aggressively assess and treat the underlying illness or injury.

There are emergent (e.g., cardiac or respiratory arrest, coma, drowning, traumas, head or spinal cord injuries [SCIs]) and urgent situations (e.g., respiratory failures) requiring immediate airway control.[5] The most common indications for IMV include airway protection for patients with decreased level of consciousness, hypercapnic respiratory failure, hypoxemic respiratory failure, and circulatory failure.[6] The general accepted guidelines for mechanical ventilation include respiratory rate greater than 30/minute, inability to maintain arterial oxygen saturation greater than 90%, fractional inspired oxygen ($FIO_2$) greater than 0.60, pH greater than 7.25, and $PaCO_2$ greater than 50 mmHg acutely.[7] To minimize potential complications, as soon as mechanical ventilation is initiated, it is prudent to consider strategies to minimize the duration and to initiate weaning as soon as clinically appropriate.[6]

## PHYSIOLOGY

The two primary categories of ventilation include negative pressure ventilation and positive pressure ventilation. The negative pressure ventilation relies on decreasing extrathoracic pressure, which causes the chest to expand, drawing air into the lungs (e.g., iron lung). Modern mechanical ventilation predominantly uses positive pressure, expanding the lungs during inspiration by positive pressure delivery. Mechanical ventilation effectiveness is affected by lung pressure and lung compliance, which represent intricate interplays between tidal volume, alveolar pressure, the positive pressure administered, and lung volume. In addition, underlying conditions will also affect lung compliance. Diseases that damage lung parenchyma (e.g., emphysema) will increase compliance, while those that generate stiffer lungs (e.g., ARDS, pneumonia, pulmonary edema, pulmonary fibrosis) will decrease lung compliance. Stiff lungs are prone to barotrauma due to a disproportionate increase in pressure with only a small increase in volume. During inspiration, the peak pressure measures airway resistance to the PPV. At the end of a full inspiration, the plateau pressure during the inspiratory hold by the ventilator is a measure of alveolar pressure and lung compliance. Plateau pressure must be monitored, as above 30 cm $H_2O$ it can cause barotrauma.[8]

### Basic Modes of Mechanical Ventilation

Virtually all modern ventilators deliver positive pressure. Ventilator settings are guided by intended therapeutic endpoints. Although there are many different modes, the most commonly selected initial modes of mechanical ventilation include volume-limited assist control (AC) ventilation and pressure-limited AC ventilation. The overall approach to choosing a ventilation mode involves how the patient's spontaneous breaths are managed, which ranged from providing full support to the patient's work of breathing to allowing the patient to determine the size of their breaths. The complexity of evolving ventilatory protocols often obscures the traditional pressure or volume-controlled modes, with the focus on phase variables in mechanical ventilation: triggering, limits, cycling, and positive end-expiratory pressure (PEEP). Patients on mechanical ventilation for respiratory failure need more support than those ventilated for airway protection. Volume- or pressure-limited AC ventilation provides the most support in resting respiratory muscles and eases the work of breathing.

### Volume Control Mode

In volume control mode, there is a predetermined tidal volume at a set ventilator rate to ensure minimum minute ventilation. Once the set tidal volume is delivered, inspiration stops. Although the volume remains constant, pressure can change from breath to breath and from patient to patient, due to airway resistance, lung compliance, and chest wall compliance. This means poor lung compliance will elevate pressure, risking barotrauma. The delivery of breaths can be ventilator initiated or patient initiated.

### Pressure Control Mode

In pressure control mode, the flow of air into the lung is determined by a set pressure limit and a set ventilator rate. Once the set inspiratory time has passed, inspiration ends. In this situation, the pressure remains constant, but the tidal volume can vary due to compliance, airway resistance, or tubing resistance. As a result, specific minute ventilation cannot be assured. This means that in certain conditions such as asthma where compliance varies, fluctuating tidal volumes will affect $CO_2$ clearance. The pressure-limited breaths can also be ventilator initiated or patient initiated.

## Assist Control Ventilation

AC is often the initial mode chosen in order to manage the minute volume and work of breathing. In volume-limited AC ventilation, a predetermined tidal volume is set for each breath, along with $FiO_2$ and PEEP. If the patient attempts to take a spontaneous breath, the ventilator will deliver a full breath. This approach can lead to excess ventilation, especially when the patient is tachypneic from pain or anxiety, with a risk for respiratory alkalosis. In AC mode, the ventilator delivers support for every breath (assist) and controls the set respiratory rate independent of the spontaneous respiratory rate.

## Volume Modes
### Volume-Limited Assist Control Ventilation

Volume-limited AC ventilation (ACV)—also referred to as continuous mandatory ventilation (CMV)—is the preferred mode of ventilation for most situations. Volume control ensures that the patient receives a set volume of air each minute. Settings involve tidal volume, frequency or respiratory rate, oxygen concentration, and positive end-expiratory pressure. Tidal volume (Vt) represents the volume of air set to be delivered with each breath, based on lean body weight. The respiratory rate, or frequency (f), indicates the number of breaths delivered per minute. The breath-to-breath time trigger interval is calculated by dividing the respiratory rate by 60. The oxygen concentration ($FiO_2$) represents the fraction of inspired oxygen. $FiO_2$ setting ranges from 35% ($FiO_2$ 0.35) to 100% ($FiO_2$ 1.0). $FIO_2$ is set to reach an $SpO_2$ of 92% to 96%.

### Synchronized Intermittent-Mandatory Ventilation

In synchronized intermittent-mandatory ventilation (SIMV), the ventilator will deliver a predetermined number of breaths, synchronized to the patient's spontaneous respirations. Not all spontaneous breaths are supported, minimizing risks of hyperinflation or alkalosis. SIMV increases the work of breathing and decreases cardiac output. The addition of pressure support (PS) to spontaneous breaths can improve the work of breathing.

## Pressure Modes
### Pressure-Limited Assist-Controlled Ventilation

Pressure-limited assist-controlled ventilation (PCV) is the preferred mode for patients with neuromuscular disease but normal lungs. PCV does not allow spontaneous breaths. It has less barotrauma risk, with lower peak pressure. The disadvantage is that minute volumes can be variable.[9]

### Pressure Support Ventilation

Pressure support ventilation (PSV) is used only to augment spontaneous breathing, as it depends on patient-triggered breaths. There is no backup rate, and this mode should not be used in patients with decreased consciousness. As tidal volumes are a function of the patient's effort and lung compliance, PSV is often used for ventilator weaning. PSV enhances breathing efforts but has no effects on tidal volume or respiratory rate. As a result, variable tidal volumes may worsen the work of breathing.

## Positive End Expiratory Pressure

PEEP keeps airways and alveoli open to improve ventilation. PEEP is not specifically a ventilatory mode. Physiologic PEEP is 5 cm $H_2O$, and PEEP setting range is between 5 and 20 cm $H_2O$. PS can be used to augment the patient's spontaneous breaths—the larger the PS, the larger spontaneous breaths the patient can take with assistance. The setting for PS ranges from 5 to 20 cm $H_2O$, with typical values 8 to 10 cm $H_2O$, primarily to correct the ET tube resistance.

## TREATMENT

### Weaning

Readiness to wean from mechanical ventilation must be proactively planned on a daily basis.[10] Timely weaning decreases morbidity and mortality while optimizing resource utilization; conversely, prolonged mechanical ventilation (PMV) will worsen mortality.[11] Prior to initiating the weaning process, one must resolve the underlying medical condition, eliminate the need for positive pressure, maintain the cardiovascular reserve, clear obstructions, and protect the airway. Once ready, the amount of ventilator support can be slowly withdrawn or abruptly in short periods of spontaneous breathing without ventilator support.[12]

Current recommendations suggest once daily spontaneous breathing trials (SBTs), where the patient breathes spontaneously through the endotracheal tube through a T-piece or with minimal ventilator support.[13] Prior to performing an SBT, protocolized daily sedation holiday should be adhered until the patient remains alert of all sedatives while continuing to meet the criteria for extubation.

During the SBT, ventilator support is reduced to a minimum via T-piece or PS. For simple weaning, PS appears to be superior with a shorter weaning time. SBT is performed for 30 to 120 minutes, with close monitoring of signs of respiratory distress. Symptoms and signs of unsuccessful weaning include tachypnea (heart rate greater than 140 bpm), respiratory distress (respiratory rate greater than 35 breaths/minute, with the use of accessory muscles), hemodynamic changes (systolic blood pressure greater than 180 mmHg or less than 90 mmHg, marked diaphoresis), oxyhemoglobin desaturation (pulse oxygen saturation less than 90%, $PaO_2$ less than 50 mmHg, pH less than 7.32), and changes in mental status (somnolence, agitation).[13] If these signs are found, the patient should be placed back on the prior ventilator settings.

## SPECIAL CONSIDERATIONS

Early rehabilitation in the ICU can reduce the complications associated with postintensive care syndrome (PICS). Critically ill patients are at risk for chronic neuromuscular weakness, critical illness polyneuropathy, anxiety, depression, and posttraumatic stress disorder (PTSD). Potential benefits of early rehabilitation include improved muscle strength, physical function, and quality of life, reduced healthcare costs, and hospital length of stay. ICU-based rehabilitation interventions require a multidisciplinary team approach, as rehabilitation may take place as soon as medical stability has been achieved, while patients are still on mechanical ventilation.[14]

PMV is defined as mechanical ventilation that is expected to last for at least 21 days, for at least 6 hours per day.[15] In the setting of a chronic ventilation facility, the physiatrist's role is to maximize the individual's function, within the context of a chronic disabling medical condition. The physiatrist provides an expert opinion on the medical and functional management of certain neurologic conditions such as SCI or neuromuscular disease, in addition to addressing primary or secondary musculoskeletal problems such as spasticity or rotator cuff injury. Ongoing efforts at diagnosing, treating, and preventing recurrent injuries that could further hamper the patient's progress are also important.

Respiratory therapists may perform manually assisted coughing, endotracheal suctioning, mechanical insufflator–exsufflator, mechanical percussion and vibration, and postural drainage. Respiratory muscle training will improve deep breathing and coughing, intermittent positive pressure breathing will maximize tidal volumes, and intrapulmonary percussive ventilation will minimize risks of mucus plugging.[16] During these respiratory interventions, one must monitor for potential hypoxemia, reflexive hypotension, vasal nerve irritation, tracheal mucosal injury, pneumothorax, pneumomediastinum, and barotrauma. Trendelenburg positioning can be helpful, particularly in SCI tetraplegia, as gravity displaces abdominal contents toward the diaphragm increasing vital capacity and functional expiratory volume.[1] The same effects may be achieved with an abdominal binder during supine sitting.

Pulmonary rehabilitation is beneficial in maximizing patients' functional capacity when on or off a ventilator, whether partially or completely. In patients on chronic mechanical ventilation, pulmonary rehabilitation promotes independence and autonomy through self-directed care. A successful rehabilitation program for mechanically ventilated patients requires well-coordinated interdisciplinary team interactions between physiatrists, pulmonologists, respiratory therapists, physical therapists, occupational therapists, speech pathologists, registered dieticians, and social workers.[17]

## MECHANICAL VENTILATION RISKS

Hemodynamic compromise may occur with mechanical ventilation. Positive pressure ventilation may result in impaired venous return and secondarily decreased cardiac output, with tachycardia, hypotension, and decreased perfusion. Barotrauma can result on rare instances when the alveoli are ruptured under high pressure, with clinical findings of pneumothorax, pneumomediastinum, and pneumoperitoneum. Cardiac compromise may result if tension pneumothorax ensues. Precautionary steps involve avoiding large tidal volumes, judicious use of PEEP, and alleviating high airway pressure. In a parallel process, ARDS patients may experience volutrauma where large volume ventilation may cause alveolar damage due to high pressure. This can be prevented by using smaller tidal volumes. Finally, the occurrence of ventilator-associated pneumonia (VAP) increases risks for morbidity and mortality. Prevention of aspiration, avoiding trauma to airways, active oral care, minimizing sedatives, and regular assessment for readiness to extubate will help decrease the risks for VAP.

Comprehensive interdisciplinary pulmonary rehabilitation programs result in better survival rates, quality of life, and functional outcomes. The success of these programs depends on strong pulmonary and physiatric leaderships, an interdisciplinary staff specialized in the management of ventilated patients, respiratory therapists, comprehensive rehabilitative team, psychologists, and nutritional support.[18]

## REFERENCES

The full list of references appears in the digital product found on http://connect.springerpub.com/content/book/978-0-8261-6226-7/part/part03/chapter/ch55

# WOUND CARE

HOLLY VANCE

## CORE DEFINITIONS

### Pressure Injuries

Previously called pressure ulcers or decubitus ulcers, a pressure injury occurs when there is prolonged pressure over a localized area of the skin and soft tissue.[1-3] Pressure injuries, usually over an area of bony prominence or under a medical device, can also occur as a combination of shear and/or pressure.[1-3] It is considered a "bottom-up" type of skin damage, with damage beginning at the muscle or bone and progressing out toward the skin.[1,4]

### Moisture-Associated Skin Damage

This type of skin damage is a result of repeated or prolonged exposure of the skin to moisture including water, urine, stool, mucus, saliva, perspiration, bowel effluence, and wound exudate.[5,6] This is considered "top-down" skin damage, as it begins at the surface of the skin.[7,8]

### Traumatic Wounds

Traumatic wounds include burns, skin tears, medical adhesive-related skin injury (MARSI), and surgery-related wounds.

### Lower Extremity Ulcers

Leg ulcers are typically associated with arterial or venous disease and neuropathy.[9-12] Sensory and vascular deficits predispose patients to skin breakdown and infections.[9,12-14]

## ETIOLOGY AND PATHOPHYSIOLOGY

### Pressure Injuries

The development of pressure injuries is influenced by multiple factors, including but not limited to the patient's overall health status, nutrition, condition of the soft tissue, and microclimate.[1,3] There are multiple pressure injury stages, described in Table 56.1.[2]

---

The full list of resources and references appears in the digital product found on http://connect .springerpub.com/content/book/978-0-8261-6226-7/part/part03/chapter/ch56

## TABLE 56.1 PRESSURE INJURY STAGES

| STAGE | DESCRIPTION |
|---|---|
| Stage 1 | *Intact* skin that is erythematous and not blanching.[2] May be difficult to assess in patients with darker skin tones.[2] |
| Stage 2 | Tissue damage that is partial thickness and without measurable depth, with a red or pink wound bed.[2] May also present as a serum-filled blister.[2] |
| Stage 3 | Tissue damage that is full thickness with visible adipose and granulation tissue.[2] May also present with rolled edges.[2] |
| Stage 4 | Tissue damage that is full thickness, with exposed or directly palpable muscle, tendon, fascia, ligament, cartilage, or bone.[2] |
| Unstageable | Full-thickness tissue damage obscured by eschar or slough, unable to confirm the true depth of the tissue loss and damage, though will reveal a stage 3 or 4 pressure injury once the slough and eschar are removed.[2] |
| Deep tissue | Tissue damage that appears to be maroon, purple, or a deep red that is not blanching.[2] It may evolve to reveal the true depth and damage (progress to stages 2, 3, 4, or unstageable), or may resolve without tissue loss.[2] |
| Mucosal membrane | Mucosal membrane pressure injury is on mucous membranes with a history of a medical device pressure at the location of the injury.[2] Due to the anatomy of the tissue these ulcers cannot be staged with the 1,2,3,4, and unstageable stage system.[2] |

## Moisture-Associated Skin Damage

*Incontinence-associated dermatitis (IAD)*: Most common form of moisture-associated skin damage (MASD); it is defined as "an irritant dermatitis that develops from chronic exposure to urine or liquid stool."[15–17] Ammonia is produced when urea in urine breaks down, and prolonged exposure of the skin to urine causes the acidic nature of skin to become more alkaline, thus compromising the acid mantle/protective barrier of the skin.[5,16,17] Skin exposed to liquid stool is at higher risk for IAD because the enzymes present in liquid stool are activated when the excessive moisture causes the skin to become more alkaline, resulting in proteolytic damage and possible tissue loss to the skin.[5,16,17] Skin at risk for IAD includes all areas that can be exposed to liquid stool or urine.[16] Often confused for a pressure injury, IAD presents as more diffuse and pressure injuries are more localized.[4,16–18]

*Intertriginous dermatitis (ITD)*: Also known as intertrigo; ITD is found in skin folds and related to moisture and friction within the skin folds.[5,6,19] ITD is caused by a combination of moisture that is trapped within skin folds causing the skin to become overhydrated, and friction of the skin folds rubbing against each other.[5,6] It is linear in presentation and may coexist with IAD. At-risk areas include skin located within the abdominal folds, under the breasts, and within the axillae, intergluteal cleft, or inguinal region.[5,6]

*Periwound MASD*: Skin damage that is a result of skin exposure to wound exudate.[5,6] Pathophysiology of this is thought due to a combination of maceration, inflammation, and friction.[5,6] Excessive wound exudate drains from a wound or incision, causing the skin to become overhydrated or macerated.[5,6] The skin is then at higher risk for damage from friction as well as pathogen and irritant penetration.[5,6]

## Traumatic Wounds

*Burns*: The mechanisms of burn injury include thermal, chemical, electrical, and radiation (Table 56.2).[20–22] Severity of burns is typically measured either with the hand method, rule of nines, or Lund–Browder chart to determine the total area of the body affected by burns (see Exhibit 56.1).[20,21,23]

*Skin tears*: Separation of skin layers occurs as a result of shear, friction, and/or trauma.[5,6] People most at risk include the elderly or the very young, critically or chronically ill patients, and patients with fragile skin related to medications (e.g., steroids).[5,6]

*MARSI*: Occurs when redness or other skin abnormalities (including, but not limited to, vesicle, bulla, erosion, or tear) persists after 30 or more minutes post removal of the adhesive.[5,6,19] Common mechanisms of injury include the following: irritant contact dermatitis, allergic contact dermatitis, maceration, mechanical trauma, tension blisters, and folliculitis.[5,6,19]

*Surgical incisions*: Surgical incisions may heal through primary closure (with glue, staples, or sutures), delayed primary closure (left open with packing for a period of time to monitor for infection and then sutured closed), or secondary intention (with wound care

## TABLE 56.2 BURN MECHANISMS AND PATHOPHYSIOLOGY

| MECHANISM | PATHOPHYSIOLOGY |
|---|---|
| Thermal | The result of heat transfer either directly or indirectly (e.g., stove, boiling water, or steam), through conversion of kinetic energy to electromagnetic energy and back to kinetic energy (e.g., tanning bed, or through heat carried by air currents (e.g., flash explosions).[20–22] The heated temperature of the tissue and duration of the exposure determine severity.[20,21] |
| Chemical | The result of tissue exposure to a noxious substance.[20–22] The concentration and quantity of the substance, duration of exposure, and the cutaneous toxicity of the substance determine the severity of the burn.[20,21] The substances may be alkaline (e.g., industrial cleaning agents), acidic (e.g., household bathroom cleansers), or vesicant (e.g., nerve gas).[20–22] |
| Electrical | These include high voltage (>1,000 V) (e.g., alternating current) or low voltage (<1,000 V) (e.g., lightning strikes, electric arc injuries—electricity flows adjacent to the body but the body is never in contact with the electric current) burns.[20–22] Severity is determined by the type of the electric current, direction of flow, resistance of the tissue to the electricity, and exposure duration.[20,21] Electrical current flows from the entry wound in the patient to the ground or from the path of least resistance.[20,21] These types of burns are often associated with compartment syndrome, neurologic symptoms, and delayed healing complications.[20–22] |
| Radiation (rare) | The result of excessive ionizing radiation exposure.[20,21] When radiant energy transfers to the body, it stimulates the formation of reactive chemicals and toxins that target rapidly growing cells.[20,21] |

**EXHIBIT 56.1** Lund and Browder Chart for TBSA Calculation

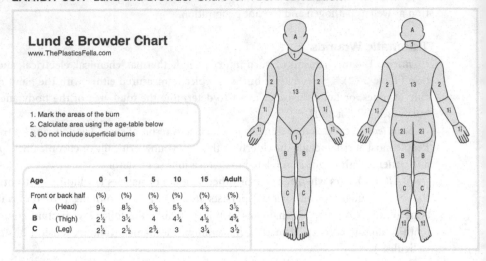

TBSA, total body surface area.
*Source*: Reprinted by permission from https://www.theplasticsfella.com/staging/7660/wp-content/uploads/2020/05/Burns-TBSA-Calculator.png

management).[24] Flaps (using skin and soft tissue from one area of the body to close the defect) or grafts (using tissue or skin from the patient, a donor, or animal) may be used.[24]

## Lower Extremity Ulcers

*Venous*: Ulcers occur as a result of venous hypertension or venous system functional abnormalities (i.e., including edema, skin changes, and ulceration).[11] Valve dysfunction and ambulatory venous hypertension lead to ulcerations and tissue changes.[11] These are the most common types of lower extremity wounds.[11] Venous wound characteristics include moist red wound beds and serpiginous edges.[11] The surrounding skin may be edematous and hemosiderin stained with lipodermatosclerosis, varicose veins, and/or atrophie blanche.[11]

*Arterial*: These ulcers occur in the setting of arterial insufficiency and progressive arterial occlusion.[10] They may occur spontaneously or due to trauma when the damaged arteries and vessels are unable to meet the increased oxygenation demands required for wound healing.[10] They typically have a "punched out" appearance with well-defined edges, and the wound bed may be red, pale pink, or have signs of ischemic damage such as eschar or slough.[10] The leg of a person with arterial disease generally appears pale, with thin and shiny skin, cool or cold to the touch, hairless, and diminished or absent pulses, with dependent rubor/elevational pallor.[10]

*Neuropathic*: Neuropathic foot ulcers develop due to sensory (i.e., decreased sensation and injury awareness), autonomic (resulting in drying of the skin), and mechanical (i.e., structural deformities) factors.[9,14] These types of ulcers are usually seen in patients with diabetes.[9,14] Callus formation (i.e., hyperkeratotic patches) is common in high-pressure areas and may be associated with subcutaneous ulcer formation.[9,14] Skin cracks and fissures are common due to xerosis.[14,25] There are multiple scales used to classify the diabetic foot ulcer, including the Wagner Ulcer Classification System and the University of Texas system.[9] Most classification systems evaluate location, depth, necrotic skin changes, infection, ischemia, and neuropathy in their staging.[9]

## DIAGNOSTIC APPROACH

### Pressure Injuries

The diagnosis of pressure injuries relies on visual inspection of the skin to assess color and blanching, anatomical structures, induration, and pain.[3] Pressure injury risk should be evaluated.[3] Assessment tools, such as the Braden Scale©, Waterloo Score©, or Norton Scale©, may be used to determine a patient's risk for pressure injury and to develop patient-specific prevention interventions.[3]

### Moisture-Associated Skin Damage

The diagnosis is based on the overall presentation of the skin, the history of moisture retained against the skin, and the type of moisture causing the skin damage.[6,19] For instance, diffuse blanching skin breakdown in an area affected by urine or stool in a patient with incontinence leads to a diagnosis of IAD.[6,7] Skin breakdown on the area around a wound (periwound skin) or around an incision with drainage leads to a diagnosis of periwound MASD.[6] ITD is diagnosed when there is linear skin breakdown within a skin fold.[6,19]

### Traumatic Wounds

#### Burns

Burns are diagnosed based on the type of burn sustained.[20,21] They are also classified by the depth of the skin damage, partial versus full thickness, and quantified by the percentage of total body surface area damage (TBSA%; a patient's hand represents approximately 1% of the TBSA—Figure 56.1).[20,21,23,26] They were previously classified in stages, but more recently have started to be classified as superficial, superficial partial thickness, deep partial thickness, and full thickness.[20,21] According to the American Burn Association (ABS), minor burns in adults encompass 15% TBSA, moderate burns encompass 15% to 25% TBSA, and major burns encompass >25% TBSA.[20,21] There are also considerations made for the location and depth of the burns as to whether or not they are considered minor, moderate, or major.[20,21,23]

#### Skin Tears

Skin tears can be classified as partial thickness or full thickness and as type 1, 2, or 3 using the ISTAP classification system.[5,6] Use of this system can help guide the management and treatment of skin tears.[5,6] Type 1 skin tears have no skin loss, and the skin flap or area of loose skin can be placed back over the wound bed.[5,6] Type 2 skin tears have a partial flap loss that is

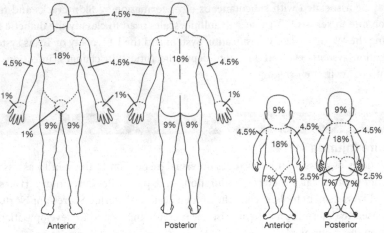

**FIGURE 56.1** Rule of nine's calculator.

*Source:* Reprinted from Veenema TG, ed. *Disaster Nursing and Emergency Preparedness: For Chemical, Biological, and Radiological Terrorism and Other Hazards.* 4th ed. Springer Publishing Company; 2019:432.

not able to be placed back over the wound bed.[5,6] Type 3 skin tears have total loss of the flap, and the entire wound bed is exposed.[5,6]

## Medical Adhesive-Related Skin Injury

Diagnoses are based on a patient's health history, presentation of the skin injury, and the patients' contact with medical adhesive products.[5,6] A definitive diagnosis can only be determined 30 minutes after removal of the medial adhesive, as transient hyperemia is commonly misdiagnosed as MARSI.[5,6]

## Surgical Incisions

Treatment and management is based on whether the incision was able to be closed by primary intension with sutures, staples, or glue or by secondary intention to heal with topical wound management.[24]

## Lower Extremity Ulcers
### Arterial

Noninvasive diagnostics to assess for the presence of arterial disease include ankle-brachial indexes (ABI) or toe-brachial indexes (TBI), used to assess the oxygen perfusion in the lower extremities.[10,13] Toe brachial indexes are recommended in diabetics due to the increased risk for noncompressible vessels secondary to vessel calcification in the ankle region.[10,13] Normal ankle-brachial indexes are >0.90 to 1.3; >1.3 is abnormally high, and therefore a toe-brachial index is recommended. ABI values ≤0.9 are indicative of lower extremity arterial disease; 0.6 to 0.8 indicates borderline perfusion; and ≤0.5 is indicative of severe ischemia.[10,13] Other diagnostic tools include exercise stress testing, waveform studies, segmental limb pressures, TcPO$_2$ measurements, and angiography.[10,13]

### Neuropathic/Diabetic

The Semmes-Weinstein or 10-g monofilament examination is a useful tool to assess loss of protective sensation (LOPS).[9,12] Vibratory sense test with a 128-Hz tuning fork can assess the loss of vibratory sensation, a LOPS precursor.[9,12,14] Impaired proprioception, common in lower extremity neuropathic disease, increases fall risk and can be evaluated with a position sense test using the great toe.[9] Assessment of the patient's footwear can assist with assessing high-pressure points and anatomical areas at risk for ulcerations.[9,14]

### Venous

On physical assessment, hemosiderin staining, edema, lipodermatosclerosis, varicose veins, and ankle flaring may be apparent and indicative of venous insufficiency.[11,12] Noninvasive vascular tests of the lower extremity, such as the Ankle-Brachial Index, are recommended to rule out coexisting peripheral arterial disease, as compression therapy is contraindicated in cases of comorbid peripheral arterial disease.[11,12] A duplex ultrasound may be used to scan for venous reflux or obstruction and has a high degree of sensitivity to assist in the diagnosis of venous insufficiency.[11,12]

## TREATMENT

### General Principles of Wound Care

The four phases of wound healing include hemostasis, inflammation, proliferation, and remodeling.[27] Factors that may affect wound healing include tissue perfusion and oxygenation, nutritional status, presence of infection, diabetes, medications, aging, immunosuppression, and stress.[27]

Factors to consider when choosing a dressing include etiology, location, appearance of the wound bed, amount and type of drainage, appearance of the periwound skin, presence of infection, frequency of dressing changes, patient goals and preferences, caregiver abilities, product availability, cost, and reimbursement.[28,29] If wound healing is unlikely, preventing infection, odor and exudate control, minimizing deterioration of the wound bed, and decreasing frequency of dressing changes are appropriate goals.[28] Wound care goals may differ for patients receiving palliative care and should focus on comfort thus a dressing plan that decreases pain and minimizes wound deterioration is recommended.[28,30,31] Other considerations include nutrition and diabetes management, pressure redistribution, edema control, microclimate control, and pain control.[28]

When developing a wound treatment plan, it is important to consider who will be performing care (i.e., patient, family, staff), how often dressings should be changed, and patient access to the recommended dressings. If inpatient, the patient and/or family members should be taught how to perform dressing changes prior to discharge. Home health nursing may be an option for patients unable to perform wound care independently or without caregivers to assist. Some patients may require dressing changes and wound management to be performed by primary care providers or at specialized wound care clinics. Most home health agencies and clinics are unable to see patients daily, thus a treatment plan that includes multiday dressing products is important when the patient or caregivers cannot assist in wound care.

Dressing changes should include wound cleansing (soap and water, normal saline, or a commercial wound cleanser) and application of a skin barrier for periwound skin protection against moisture and irritation. The most common dressings are summarized in Table 56.3.

### TABLE 56.3 COMMON WOUND CARE DRESSINGS

| DRESSING | CHARACTERISTICS AND COMMON USE |
| --- | --- |
| Gauze | These dressings absorb minimal-to-moderate exudate.[29] They are changed daily or more often. Available in fine mesh and large mesh in multiple sizes.[29] It is also available in rolls and packing strips.[29] May also be impregnated with a variety of antimicrobial agents.[29] |
| Contact layers | Generally placed over exposed muscle, tendon, bone, or other organs to maintain a moist wound bed and to decrease pain with dressing changes. They have minimal absorption and are meant to allow drainage to pass through.[29] They come impregnated with silicone, petrolatum, and multiple other types of ointments meant to help maintain a moist wound bed.[29] Depending on the brand and the type of ointment, these dressings may be changed every 1 to 7 days and should be covered with a secondary dressing such as gauze or a bordered foam.[29] There are a variety of versions of contact layers. Examples include Mepitel by Molnlycke, Restore TRIACT technology by Hollister, Adaptic by Acelity, and Cuticerin by Smith & Nephew. |
| Hydrocolloids | Indicated for partial- and full-thickness wounds with minimal-to-moderate exudate.[29] They can be combined with wound fillers, including alginates and hydrofibers.[29] They are changed at least weekly.[29] Examples include Duoderm by ConvaTec, Exuderm by Medline, and Replicare by Smith & Nephew. |
| Foam dressings | These come in a variety of shapes and sizes, with and without adhesive borders.[29] They may be used for moderate to large amounts of drainage and may also be combined with other dressings such as alginates.[29] Foam dressings are typically indicated for multiple days.[29] There are a variety of foam dressings available. Examples include Mepilex by Molnlycke, Allevyn by Smith & Nephew, Optifoam by Medline, and Aquacel by ConvaTec. |
| Calcium alginate and hydrofiber dressings | Indicated for moderate to largely exudative wounds.[29] These highly absorptive dressings act as a wound bed filler and assist with light packing of undermining or tunneling areas.[29] Some versions are antimicrobial, and some may facilitate autolytic debridement.[29] Require coverage by a secondary dressing and can be changed at least weekly or more frequently when needed.[29] Multiple pieces should not be used in areas of undermining and tunneling due to the risk of being retained in the wound bed. Examples of calcium alginates include Kaltostat by ConvaTec, Medihoney alginate by Derma Sciences, Algisite by Smith & Nephew, and Maxorb alginate by Medline. Examples of hydrofibers include Aquacel Ag by ConvaTec, Aquacel by ConvaTec, and Versiva® XC™ by ConvaTec. |

(continued)

**TABLE 56.3 COMMON WOUND CARE DRESSINGS (continued)**

| | |
|---|---|
| Honey | Products with honey help maintain a moist wound environment and facilitate autolytic debridement.[29] Gels should be reapplied daily, and hydrocolloid and alginate dressings are indicated for multiple day use. The first two or three applications of honey can increase exudate within the wound beds and require more frequent dressing changes. Examples of honey products include Medihoney by Derma Sciences, Manukapli by ManukaMed, or TheraHoney by Medline. |
| Hydrogels | Gels are used to donate moisture to wound beds and maintain a moist environment.[29] Indicated for full- and partial-thickness wounds that have minimal to no exudate.[29] Intended for daily application to achieve a moist wound bed.[29] An example includes DuoDerm Hydroactive sterile gel by ConvaTec, Skintegrity by Medline, and Vigilon by Bard. |
| Transparent films | Nonabsorptive impermeable dressing commonly used for securing IV sites. These occlusive dressings can increase the risk for moisture-related skin damage as excessive moisture can be trapped under the dressing. They are not indicated for skin tears, as they may worsen skin damage upon removal. Examples include 3M Tegaderm and Opsite by Smith & Nephew. |
| Skin barrier products | Liquid barriers that when applied topically dry to form a breathable transparent coating meant to protect intact or damaged skin. Skin barriers should be allowed to dry before applying creams or dressings. Examples include 3M Cavilon No Sting Barrier Film, Smith & Nephew Skin-Prep, Safe n Simple Skin Barrier Sheet, and ConvaTec AllKare protective barrier wipes. |

## SPECIAL CONSIDERATIONS

### Pressure Injuries

Treatment should focus on ways to prevent pressure over the wound to promote healing.[3] For patients with impaired mobility and sensation (e.g., spinal cord injuries), seating restrictions and bowel and bladder management to prevent wound contamination is paramount.[3] In some cases, referral for surgical debridement and possible flap closure is necessary. If the pressure injury is related to a medical device, consider modification or discontinuation of the device.[3] Pressure redistribution interventions, such as a turning schedule, are needed to promote healing.[3]

### Moisture-Associated Skin Damage

Topical products that protect against moisture, for instance a barrier cream with zinc oxide and dimethicone, are important if the patient is experiencing incontinence.[6,7,17] Skin barrier sprays or wipes may be used to protect periwound skin against drainage.[6,17] When choosing a dressing, the amount of drainage should be considered as the appropriate dressing will absorb drainage and prevent excessive periwound moisture.[6,17]

## Burns

Urgent surgical intervention may be required for escharotomy and fasciotomy, and continued surgical intervention may be indicated for debridement, wound care, and skin grafting.[20,21,23,26,32] Ongoing treatment with nutritional support, physical therapy, occupational therapy, speech therapy, rehabilitation medicine, and rehabilitation psychology is needed for ongoing medical and psychosocial needs.[21,23,32]

When significant surface area is affected by burns, patients are at risk for shock due to increased capillary permeability at the injury site and throughout the body as inflammatory mediators are released.[20,21,32] In patients with more than 20% TBSA burns, this is most severe within the first 24 hours.[20,21,32] Intravascular volume deficits and local or systemic edema follow a flood of fluids, electrolytes, and protein into the interstitial space.[20,21,32] This is followed by decreased cardiac output, metabolic rate, oxygen consumption, and blood pressure, as well as continued fluid imbalance and cellular shock for 3 to 7 days.[20,21] Patients with these types of burns face long recovery periods, due to treatment of shock and fluid imbalance in addition to the burns themselves.[20,21]

Criteria for referral to burn specialty centers include the following: partial-thickness burns that have >10% TBSA; burns of the face, hands, genitalia, feet, joints, or perineum; full-thickness burns; electrical or chemical burns; inhalation injury; burns co-occurring with trauma such as fractures in which the burn is the greater risk to the patient; burned patients with comorbidities that may delay burn healing or affect mortality; and children.[20,23]

## Skin Tears

Treatment considerations depend on the type of skin tear present.[5,6] If the skin flap is intact and able to be placed back over the wound bed or partially placed back over the wound bed, a nonadhesive dressing may be placed over it.[5,6] To protect the skin flap, an arrow should be drawn on the dressing to indicate the direction in which the dressing should be removed.[5,6] If possible, the dressing should be secured with tubular netting to prevent using medical adhesive on fragile skin.[5,6] If an adhesive is needed, a skin barrier should be applied prior to placing the dressing.[5,6]

## Medical Adhesive-Related Skin Injuries

Application of a skin barrier prior to applying an adhesive can be beneficial toward preventing further skin injury from adhesive removal.[5,6]

## Surgical Incisions

Dressings are typically at the discretion of the surgeon; however, periwound skin protection (skin barrier use), infection prevention (antimicrobial infused dressings), dehiscence prevention (incisional negative pressure wound therapy), and prevention of medical adhesive-related skin injury (use of adhesive removing products) are important.[5,6]

## Venous Ulcers

The mainstay for the treatment of venous ulcerations is compression therapy; however, this is contraindicated in patients with infection, uncontrolled heart failure, and coexisting peripheral arterial disease.[11,12] It should be used with caution with patients with neuropathy, as the LOPS associated with neuropathy impairs the patient's ability to discern if the compression is too tight.[11,12] If a patient is not amenable or unable to wear compression therapy, the limbs should be elevated.[11,12] Patients should be encouraged to lie down and elevate their legs above the level of the heart for 1 to 2 hours twice a day and when they are sleeping.[11,12] If the patient is unable to lie flat, they should be encouraged to avoid prolonged standing or sitting with their legs in a dependent position.[11,12] Ambulation is encouraged as the calf-muscle pump helps initiate a venous return.[11,12] When choosing a dressing, a high absorption dressing should be considered as venous wounds typically have a high volume of exudate.[11,12]

### Arterial Ulcers

Treatment for patients with severe arterial disease should focus on the prevention of infection and wound progression.[10,13] Dry, stable eschar that is attributed to arterial disease should be kept dry until the patient can be surgically revascularized or until the eschar is no longer dry or stable.[10,13] Povidone-Iodine is often used to maintain a dry wound bed and prevent infection.[10]

### Neuropathic Ulcers

Management of diabetes is important in treating wounds, as elevated glucose can impede wound healing.[9,14] Diabetic wounds have a high risk for infection and wound deterioration, thus the need for topical and systemic antimicrobial agents should be evaluated.[9,14] Offloading the wound with appropriate footwear or orthotic devices minimizes pressure and sheer to the area and can help prevent deterioration of the wound.[14] Offloading and pressure reduction devices include the following: crutches, felt pads, removal cast walker, and total contact casts.[9] As these wounds can have a deep wound bed, consider imaging such as x-ray or MRI to assess for osteomyelitis, especially when the wound bed depth probes to the bone.[9,14] The removal of the hyperkeratotic rim of the wound edges, a common finding, can assist with wound healing.[9]

## BASIC ORDER SETS

Wound care orders should include the following:

1. Cleaning instructions
2. Peri-wound skin protection agents
3. Dressing(s) to be used
4. Frequency of dressing changes

## RESOURCES AND REFERENCES

The full list of resources and references appears in the digital product found on http://connect .springerpub.com/content/book/978-0-8261-6226-7/part/part03/chapter/ch56

# Section 4

# DIAGNOSTICS, MODALITIES, EQUIPMENT, AND TECHNOLOGY

## 57

# ELECTROENCEPHALOGRAPHY

DEREK YU AND JEFFREY TSAI

## CORE DEFINITIONS

EEG measures the summated membrane potentials of large populations of neurons in the neocortex using surface electrodes placed on the scalp. It provides a window to the electrical activity of the brain in real time and with high temporal resolution. EEG has been in use in humans since 1924.[1] Modern digital EEG techniques allow flexible reformatting and analysis of the data. EEG is an important tool that can aid in diagnosis and evaluation in a number of conditions. The sensitivity and specificity of EEG findings vary with respect to the following indications.

## INDICATIONS

**Classify and characterize seizures:** When seizures are suspected, EEG provides information on the risk of seizures and regions of the brain involved. EEG is only moderately sensitive, but highly specific, for diagnosing seizures.

**Evaluate intermittent or persistent encephalopathy:** EEG is a sensitive measure of encephalopathy but not specific to the underlying etiology. Moreover, EEG is particularly useful for ruling out a role of seizures contributing to encephalopathy. EEG can also assess the degree of encephalopathy, as well as regions of the brain affected.

The full list of references appears in the digital product found on http://connect.springerpub.com/content/book/978-0-8261-6226-7/part/part04/chapter/ch57

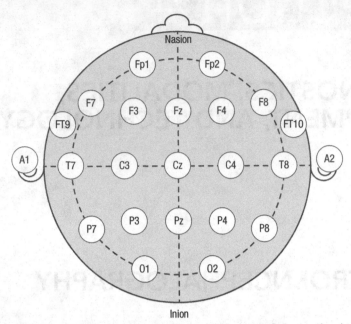

**FIGURE 57.1** The international 10–20 system of electrode placement on the scalp schematized. The letter of the electrode name designates the region of the brain where the electrode is placed (Fp—frontopolar, F—frontal, FT—frontotemporal, C—central, T—temporal, P—parietal, O—occipital). The electrodes with an odd number are placed on the left, and those with an even number are placed on the right. Electrodes with a larger number are further from midline. The letter "z" denotes midline electrodes.

**Diagnose nonepileptic conditions:** Paroxysmal events, including functional disorders and other mimics of epilepsy, may be difficult to ascertain clinically. Capturing an episode on EEG is the gold standard for diagnosis.

## RELATIVE CONTRAINDICATIONS

EEG requires a patient's ability to tolerate electrode placement and to hold still. On the other hand, excessive pharmacologic sedation may limit the information obtained from EEG. Also, certain electrodes may not be CT or MRI compatible, so imaging will need to be obtained either before or after the study is performed. Extensive lesions or extraneous material on the scalp may preclude the placement of electrodes.

## TYPES OF EEG

### Routine Outpatient EEG (Ordered as "Awake/Sleep" Study)

There are several different types of EEGs, each with particular applications. This is usually ordered for initial evaluation of suspected seizures. In addition to scalp electrodes, an EKG lead and video are recorded. The technologist attempts to capture sleep so as to increase the likelihood of detecting seizures or epileptiform abnormalities[2]; thus, it is helpful if the patient is sleep deprived the night prior. Typically, the study lasts from 30 minutes to 1 hour.

## Ambulatory EEG

This is often an outpatient study where a longer period of recording or a patient's habitual environment is conducive to capture events of interest. Other advantages include higher sensitivity to detect epileptiform activity and quantifying the burden of such activity.[3] For this study, the patient will come to the EEG lab and have electrodes applied. The patient will then go home with a recorder and go about their normal routine for a period of time (often 24 hours) before returning to the lab for removal of electrodes and download of data. During the test, the patient is asked to keep a diary of events of interest. Potential limitations of this study are as follows: (a) lack of concurrent video, (b) patient must be reliable enough to keep an accurate diary, (c) artifacts may obscure the study as the recording takes place outside of a controlled lab setting.

## Inpatient Routine EEG (Often Ordered as an "Awake/Drowsy" or "Sleep/Coma" Study Depending on the Patient's Mental Status)

This is similar to the routine outpatient EEG but is performed on hospitalized patients. The technologist will perform the study in the patient's room with a portable EEG machine.

## Extended Video EEG Monitoring

Extended monitoring may also be performed for hospitalized patients. This can occur in a dedicated epilepsy monitoring unit or in other locations in the hospital (which varies by availability in different hospitals). An epilepsy monitoring unit would have staff that are specially trained to monitor for clinical signs of seizures and rapidly respond to seizures. This is the only safe way to withhold antiseizure medications to induce seizures. Extended monitoring in the ICU has also become more widely used as studies have shown that subclinical seizures, which are often unrecognized, affect a significant portion of this patient population.[4]

## Ordering EEG

The most important aspect of the order is to specify the type of EEG that is needed. Also, detailed indications help the technologist and EEG reader look for events of interest, and triage the urgency of the study. In some hospitals, extended EEG monitoring may need a separate discontinue order when the EEG is ready to be removed.

EEG captured in different states (awake, drowsy, sleep) and for longer durations increases the yield (sensitivity) of the study.

## INTERPRETATION OF EEG

Electrodes are applied on the scalp according to a standardized system of electrode placement (see Figure 57.1). Data are visualized as the potential difference between two electrodes, each pair forming a channel. Multichannel data are organized into montages for interpretation.

EEG is interpreted based on several features, such as the frequency, voltage, and morphology of the waveforms, which vary depending on the patient's clinical state. Hemispheric asymmetry or specific regional differences are noted. Age is important in pediatric EEG, though the EEG does not usually change significantly due to age alone as an adult. While the interpretation of EEG may vary depending on the experience of the interpreter, the interrater reliability among experts is fair to substantial in recognizing epileptiform discharges.[5]

## Provocation Techniques

Typically, two activation procedures are performed during the study, if possible:

*Hyperventilation*: Patient is asked to breathe slowly and deeply for several minutes. Hyperventilation may not be performed if the patient cannot cooperate, or has certain medical conditions (e.g., respiratory or cerebrovascular disease).

*Intermittent photic stimulation*: Patient is exposed to a strobe light at various flash frequencies.

These procedures are designed to provoke certain generalized seizures, such as childhood absence epilepsy or juvenile myoclonic epilepsy.[6]

## Normal EEG

The normal EEG will usually demonstrate certain waking or sleep rhythms (see Figure 57.2). When a healthy subject is in a relaxed, waking state with eyes closed, a posterior dominant alpha rhythm will usually be present. The posterior dominant rhythm is characterized by several features: (a) 8.5 to 12 Hz activity in an adult, (b) prominence in the back of the head, (c) symmetry, (d) attenuation with eye opening.

The drowsy state is marked by the emergence of lower frequency activities and decreased muscle artifact and eye blinks. Sleep is characterized by the appearance of patterns such as positive occipital sharp transients of sleep (POSTS), vertex waves, K-complexes, and sleep spindles.

A normal EEG does not rule out a diagnosis of epilepsy, as the sensitivity of a single outpatient routine EEG for diagnosing epilepsy is only about 50%.[7]

## Common Abnormal Findings

Nonepileptiform abnormalities are nonspecific with regards to etiology and do not indicate an increased risk of seizures.

Focal slowing on EEG indicates localized cerebral dysfunction that is etiologically nonspecific and may be due to many potential causes (ischemic stroke, hemorrhage, tumor, traumatic injury, other focal lesions). Focal slowing can be persistent (such as after a stroke) or transient (after a TIA or a seizure). See Figure 57.3.

Generalized slowing is a marker of encephalopathy, but etiologically nonspecific (see Figure 57.4). Common etiologies include, but are not limited to, toxic-metabolic, infectious, neurodegenerative, or sedative medications.

Triphasic waves are traditionally associated with encephalopathy due to hepatic or renal impairment but may also be seen in other causes of generalized cerebral dysfunction.

Burst suppression is a pattern only seen in patients who are in a deep coma. It indicates severe global cerebral dysfunction. Burst suppression may be a result of anoxic-ischemic encephalopathy from cardiopulmonary arrest or from the use of sedative medications.

Epileptiform patterns are seizures (ictal) or correlated with an increased risk of seizures (interictal).

Epileptiform discharges (spikes or sharp waves) are specific findings associated with an increased risk of seizures (see Figure 57.5). These can be either focal or generalized, corresponding to an increased risk of focal or generalized seizures, respectively.

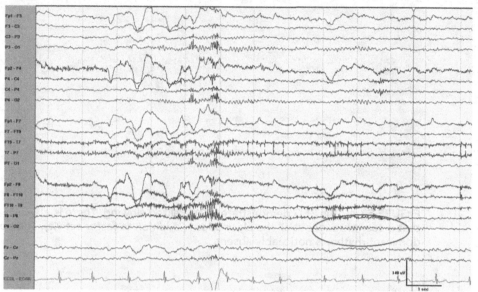

**FIGURE 57.2** This EEG demonstrates a normal waking background. There is the emergence of a 10–11-Hz posterior dominant rhythm (circled) with eye closure that is bilaterally symmetric.

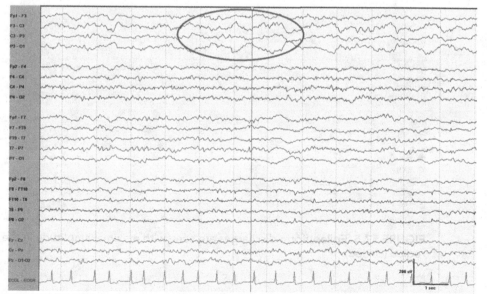

**FIGURE 57.3** This EEG demonstrates focal slowing in the left hemisphere. There is continuous 0.5–2-Hz activity (circled) seen on the left that is mostly absent on the right.

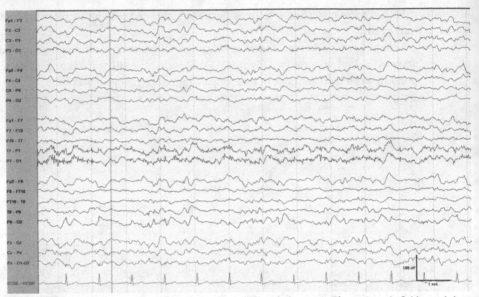

**FIGURE 57.4** This EEG demonstrates generalized slowing. There is a 1–3-Hz activity that is seen throughout all the electrodes in addition to faster activity. The posterior dominant rhythm is noticeably absent.

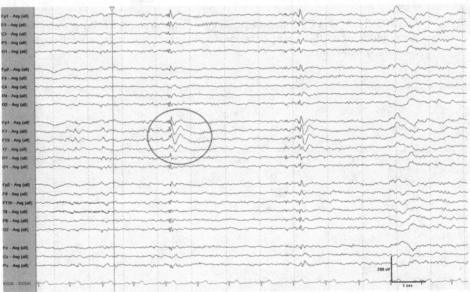

**FIGURE 57.5** Epileptiform discharges are seen with maximal amplitude in the left FT region (circled).

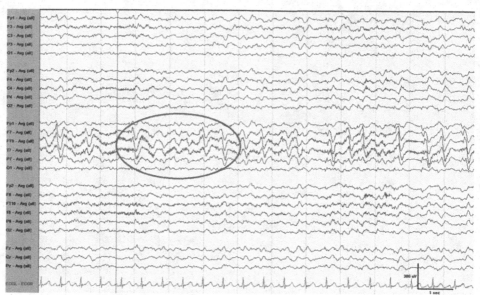

**FIGURE 57.6** Left temporal lobe seizure. There are sharp waves and evolving rhythmic activity in the left temporal electrodes (circled).

Lateralized periodic discharges (or periodic lateralized epileptiform discharges) are associated with a high risk of seizures, often from a focal structural lesion.

Seizures may be focal or generalized and may be clinical or subclinical/electrographic (seen only on the EEG without apparent clinical manifestations). Electrographically, they may take different forms, including spikes, sharp waves, and rhythmic activities. See Figure 57.6.

Focal seizures limited to a small area may not show up on scalp EEG. Previous studies with concurrent intracranial and scalp EEG suggest that an area of the brain up to 10–20 cm² may need to be involved before changes on the scalp are seen.[8]

## REFERENCES

The full list of references appears in the digital product found on http://connect.springerpub.com/content/book/978-0-8261-6226-7/part/part04/chapter/ch57

# ELECTROMYOGRAPHY AND NERVE CONDUCTION STUDIES

ILEANA HOWARD, KEVIN HAKIMI, AND MARLÍS GONZÁLEZ-FERNÁNDEZ

## CORE DEFINITIONS

The American Association of Electrodiagnostic Medicine (AAEM)—now known as the American Association of Electrodiagnostic and Neuromuscular Medicine (AAENM)—published a comprehensive glossary of electrodiagnostic terminology in 2001.[1] The following is an abbreviated list of core terminology.

**Nerve conduction studies (NCS):** Recording and analysis of peripheral nervous system electric waveforms elicited in response to electric stimuli. They include compound sensory nerve action potentials (SNAP), compound muscle action potentials (CMAP), or mixed nerve action potentials.

**Nerve conduction velocity (NCV):** The speed of action potential propagation along a nerve fiber or nerve trunk. Generally assumed to refer to the maximum speed of propagation unless otherwise specified.

**CMAP:** The summation of muscle fiber action potentials recorded from a muscle produced by stimulation of the nerve supplying the muscle. Baseline-to-peak amplitude, duration, and latency of the negative phase are usually described. Usually recorded in millivolts (mV).

**Compound SNAP:** A compound nerve action potential recorded from the afferent fibers of a sensory nerve. Peak-to-peak amplitude, latency, duration, and configuration of the SNAP should be described. Usually recorded in microvolts (μV)

**Amplitude:** The maximum voltage difference between two points ($y$-axis), usually baseline-to-peak or peak-to-peak.

**Latency:** The time between the stimulus and a response. May be measured to the onset or peak of the response.

**Duration:** The time from the beginning of the response (deflection from the baseline) to its final return to baseline.

**Electromyography:** The practice of recording electrical impulses from muscle.

**Gain:** Also referred to as "sensitivity," this is the $y$-axis on the visual EMG display, usually

The full list of references and Table 58.5 appear in the digital product found on http://connect .springerpub.com/content/book/978-0-8261-6226-7/part/part04/chapter/ch58

recorded as microvolts (µV)/division. This scale is important to determining the amplitude of waveforms.

**Sweep:** This refers to the *x*-axis on the electromyography (EMG) display, recorded as millisecond (msec)/division. This scale is critical to understanding the duration and frequency of waveforms.

**Insertional activity:** Electrical activity observed in a muscle with the movement of an electrodiagnostic needle. This may be normal, increased/prolonged, or decreased.

**Motor unit action potential (MUAP):** Waveform created by a single terminal nerve branch and all of the muscle fibers it innervates. Normal MUAPs are semi-regular and have three or less phases.

**Phasicity:** Number of segments of the MUAP above or below the baseline. This can also be calculated as follows:

$$(\text{\# of baseline crossings}) + 1$$

**Frequency:** The number of repetitions of a waveform over a period of time, usually recorded in hertz (Hz) or waveforms per second

$$\text{frequency} = \frac{\text{\# times waveform seen on the computer display} \times [1000 \text{ msec}]}{[(\text{sweep}) \times (\text{\#boxes on the computer display screen})]}$$

**Recruitment:** Quantitative or qualitative reflection on a variety of MUAPs activated during voluntary muscle contraction. Recruitment may be reported as normal, reduced, or increased (early). The recruitment ratio is a quantitative expression of this phenomenon, expressed as follows:

$$\text{recruitment ratio} = \frac{\text{firing frequency of fastest MUAP}}{\text{\# distinct MUAPs on the screen}}$$

**Fibrillation:** Waveform caused by spontaneous contraction of a single muscle fiber

**Positive sharp wave:** A biphasic action potential created from a single muscle fiber, generally an abnormal finding

**Complex repetitive discharge:** A spontaneous train of regular, repeating trains of complex potentials that begin and end abruptly. Typically seen in chronic neuropathic/myopathic conditions, thought to be due to ephaptic transmission

**Myotonic discharge:** Repetitive discharges occurring from muscle fibers that wax and wane in frequency and amplitude

**Myokymic discharge:** Repetitive spontaneous discharges of MUAPs

## NERVE CONDUCTION STUDIES

NCSs seek to evaluate the health and integrity of peripheral nerves. During an NCS, electrical impulses are applied through the skin to stimulate a peripheral nerve. Stimulation can be orthodromic—same direction as physiologic conduction—or antidromic—opposite to

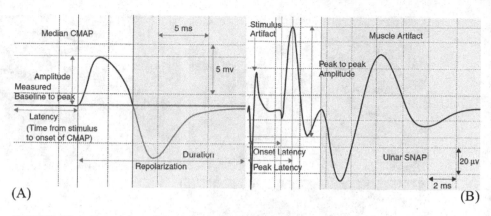

**FIGURE 58.1** Examples of Median Nerve CMAP (A) and SNAP (B).

physiologic conduction. The most common motor NCS are orthodromic, and stimulation is proximal and recorded over the most distal muscle innervated by the muscle of interest. Sensory NCS are typically antidromic, and stimulation is placed proximally over the sensory nerve and recorded distally (in contrast with physiologic transmission toward the spinal cord). Normal values are available based on a standard placement of the stimulation and recording sites.

Different CMAP waves can be obtained based on the type of stimulation (e.g., supramaximal, submaximal), the direction of the stimulation (orthodromic or antidromic), and the location being studied. The M wave or motor response is obtained by supramaximal orthodromic stimulation of a peripheral nerve recorded distally at the muscle endpoint. An F wave is a late response obtained by using supramaximal antidromic stimulation of motor neurons. The H wave, thought to be due to a spinal reflex, is commonly obtained from the calf muscles using submaximal stimulation to evaluate S1 radiculopathy. The blink reflex (Rl and R2 waves) is a brain stem reflex typically obtained by stimulating the supraorbital branch of the trigeminal nerve to the orbicularis oculi. Examples of a CMAP (m wave) and SNAP are shown in Figure 58.1.

## Basic Nerve Conduction Studies Standard Placements
### Median Motor Nerve to Abductor Pollicis Brevis (Figure 58.2)

Active electrode: Abductor pollicis brevis
Reference electrode: First metacarpophalangeal joint.
Ground electrode: Dorsum of the hand
Temperature probe: Dorsum of the hand
Stimulation points: 1—8 cm from recording site; 2—above elbow by the medial border of the biceps

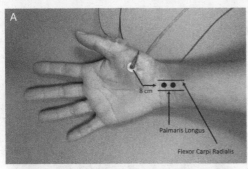
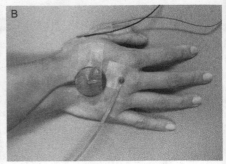
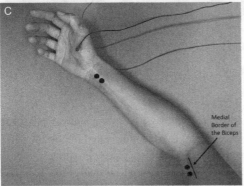

**FIGURE 58.2** Median motor nerve to abductor pollicis brevis.

## Median Sensory Nerve to Index Finger (Figure 58.3)

Active electrode: ring electrode placed distal to the base of second digit and proximal to the PIP joint

Reference electrode: Ring electrode placed 4 cm distal to the active electrode

Ground electrode: Dorsum of the hand

Temperature probe: Dorsum of the hand

Stimulation point: 14 cm proximal to active electrode over the median nerve

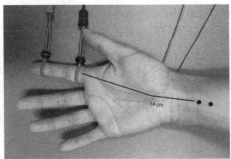

**FIGURE 58.3** Median sensory nerve to index finger.

### Ulnar Motor Nerve to Abductor Digiti Minimi (Figure 58.4)

Active electrode: Abductor digiti minimi (ADM)
Reference electrode: Fifth metacarpophalangeal joint
Ground electrode: Dorsum of the hand
Temperature probe: Dorsum of the hand
Stimulation points: 1—8 cm from recording site; 2—below ulnar groove; 3—above ulnar groove

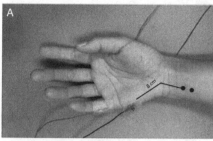
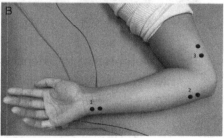

**FIGURE 58.4** Ulnar motor nerve to abductor digiti minimi.

### Ulnar Motor Nerve 2-Channel to Abductor Digiti Minimi and First Dorsal Interosseus (Figure 58.5)

Active electrode 1: ADM reference electrode: fifth metacarpophalangeal joint
Active electrode 2: First dorsal interosseus (FDI) reference electrode: thumb IP joint
Ground electrode: Dorsum of the hand
Temperature probe: Dorsum of the hand
Stimulation points: 1—8 cm from recording site; 2—below ulnar groove; 3—above ulnar groove

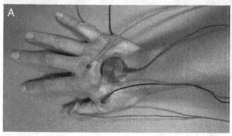
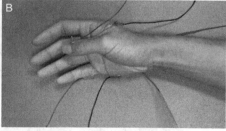

**FIGURE 58.5** Ulnar motor nerve 2-channel to abductor digiti minimi and first dorsal interosseous.

### Ulnar Sensory Nerve to Fifth Digit (Figure 58.6)

Active electrode: Ring electrode slightly distal to the base of the fifth digit
Reference electrode: Ring electrode placed 4 cm distal to the active electrode
Ground electrode: Dorsum of the hand
Temperature probe: Dorsum of the hand
Stimulation point: 14 cm proximal to active electrode over the ulnar nerve

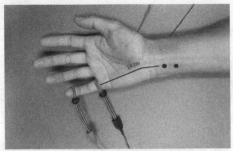

**FIGURE 58.6** Ulnar sensory nerve to fifth digit.

## Fibular Motor Nerve to Extensor Digitorum Brevis (Figure 58.7)

Active electrode: Extensor digitorum brevis (EDB)
Reference electrode: Fifth metatarsophalangeal joint
Stimulation sites: 1—8 cm from recording site; 2—posterior and inferior to the fibular head; 3—popliteal fossa
Ground electrode: Dorsum of the foot
Temperature probe: Dorsum of the foot

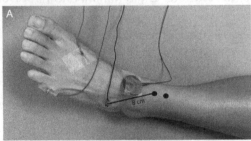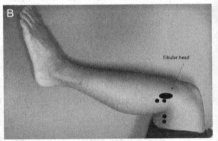

**FIGURE 58.7** Fibular motor nerve to extensor digitorum brevis.

## Tibial Motor Nerve to Abductor Hallucis (Figure 58.8)

Active electrode: Abductor hallucis (medial foot)
Reference electrode: First metatarsophalangeal joint

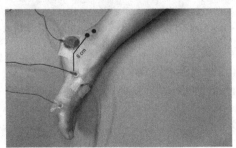

**FIGURE 58.8** Tibial motor nerve to abductor hallucis.

Ground electrode: Dorsum of the foot or between stimulation and recording sites
Temperature probe: Dorsum of the foot
Stimulation points: 1—8 cm from the active electrode; 2—popliteal fossa (not shown)

## Sural Sensory Nerve (Figure 58.9)

A 3-cm bar electrode placed posterior to the lateral malleolus with the reference electrode distally. Stimulation point: 14 cm from recording site midline or slightly lateral to the midline of the posterior lower leg.
Ground electrode: Between stimulation point and bar electrode
Temperature probe: Dorsum of the foot

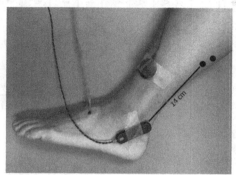

**FIGURE 58.9** Sural sensory nerve.

## H-Reflex (S1 Radiculopathy) (Figure 58.10)

Active electrode: Midpoint between the posterior calcaneus and the popliteal crease
Reference electrode: Over posterior calcaneous
Ground: Between stimulation site and recording electrode
Temperature probe: Dorsum of the foot
Submaximal stimulation, cathode proximal at the popliteal crease

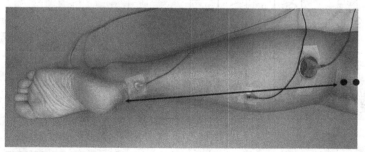

**FIGURE 58.10** H-reflex.

## Nerve Conduction Studies Reference Values (Tables 58.1–58.4)

## TABLE 58.1 MOTOR NERVE REFERENCE VALUES

| NERVE (MUSCLE STUDIED) | AGE | DISTAL LATENCY (MS)*/ GENDER | AGE | AMPLITUDE (MV)** | SITE | AGE/HEIGHT | CONDUCTION VELOCITY (M/S)** |
|---|---|---|---|---|---|---|---|
| Median (APB) 8 cm | All | 4.5 | All | 4.1 | | All | 49 |
| | 19–49 | 4.6 M | 19–39 | 5.9 | | 19–39 | 49 M |
| | | 4.4 F | 40–59 | 4.2 | | | 53 F |
| | 50–79 | 4.7 M | | | | 40–79 | 47 M |
| | | 4.4 F | 60–79 | 3.8 | | | 51 F |
| Ulnar (ADM) 8 cm | All | 3.7 | All | 7.9 | Below elbow | All | 52 |
| | | | | | Across elbow | All | 43 |
| | | | | | Above elbow | All | 50 |
| Fibular/ Peroneal (EDB) 8 cm | All | 6.5 | All | 1.3 | | All | 38 |
| | | | 19–39 | 2.6 | Ankle to the fibular head | 19–39, <5'7" | 43 |
| | | | | | | 19–39, >5'7" | 37 |
| | | | 40–79 | 1.1 | | 40–79, <5'7" | 39 |
| | | | | | | 40–79, >5'7" | 36 |
| | | | | | Across fibular head | -- | 42 |

**TABLE 58.1 MOTOR NERVE REFERENCE VALUES** (continued)

| NERVE (MUSCLE STUDIED) | AGE | DISTAL LATENCY (MS)*/ GENDER) | AGE | AMPLITUDE (MV)** | SITE | AGE/HEIGHT | CONDUCTION VELOCITY (M/S)** |
|---|---|---|---|---|---|---|---|
| Tibial (AH) 8 cm | All | 6.1 | All | 4.4 | | All | 39 |
| | | | 19–29 | 5.8 | | 19–49, <5'3" | 44 |
| | | | | | | 19–49, 5'3"–5'7" | 42 |
| | | | 30–59 | 5.3 | | 19–49, ≥5'7" | 37 |
| | | | | | | 50–79, <5'3" | 40 |
| | | | 60–79 | 1.1 | | 50–79, 5'3"–5'7" | 37 |
| | | | | | | 50–79, ≥5'7" | 34 |

*Upper limits: 97th percentile of the observed differences distribution. **Low limits: 3rd percentile of the observed differences distribution.

ADM, abductor digiti minimi; AH, abductor hallucis; APB, abductor pollicis brevis; EDB, extensor digitorum brevis.

*Source:* Shan Chen, et al. AANEM Practice Topic:: Electrodiagnostic reference values for upper and lower limb nerve conduction studies in adult populations. *Muscle Nerve.* 2016;54: 371–377.

### TABLE 58.2 ACCEPTABLE AMPLITUDE/CONDUCTION VELOCITY DROP

| NERVE | SITE | AMP DROP | CV DROP |
|---|---|---|---|
| Ulnar motor | Across elbow | | 15 m/s or 23% |
| Fibular motor | Ankle to the below fibular head | 32% | -- |
| | Across fibular head | 25% | 6 m/s or 12% |
| Tibial motor | Ankle to knee | 10.3 mV or 71% | -- |

AMP, amplitude; CV, conduction velocity.

### TABLE 58.3 SENSORY NERVE REFERENCE VALUES

| NERVE | AGE | ONSET LATENCY (MS) | PEAK LATENCY (MS) | BMI | AMPLITUDE (μV)* | |
|---|---|---|---|---|---|---|
| | | | | | ONSET TO PEAK | PEAK TO PEAK |
| Superficial Radial (10 cm) | All | 2.2 | 2.8 | All | 7 | 11 |
| Median (second digit, wrist 14 cm, palm 7 cm) | All | 3.3 (wrist) | 4.0 (wrist) | All | 11 (wrist) | 13 (wrist) |
| | | 1.6 (palm) | 2.3 (palm) | | 6 (palm) | 8 (palm) 19 |
| | 19–49 | | | <24 | 17 | |
| | | -- | -- | ≥24 | 11 | 13 |
| | 50–79 | -- | -- | <24 | 9 | 15 |
| | | -- | -- | ≥24 | 7 | 8 |
| Ulnar (fifth digit, 14 cm) | All | 3.1 | 4.0 | All | 10 | 9 |
| | 19–49 | -- | -- | <24 | 14 | 13 |
| | | | | ≥24 | 11 | 8 |
| | 50–79 | -- | -- | <24 | 10 | 13 |
| | | | | ≥24 | 5 | 4 |
| MABC (10 cm) | -- | -- | 2.6 | -- | 4 | 3 |
| LABC (10 cm) | -- | -- | 2.5 | -- | 5 | 6 |
| Sural (14 cm) | -- | 3.6 | 4.5 | -- | 4 | 4 |

*The lower limits of onset-to-peak and peak-to-peak amplitudes are shown as mean – 2 SD, showing the statistically significant effects of age and BMI on the amplitudes of the median and ulnar sensory nerves at the wrist ($p < .01$).

BMI, body mass index.

## TABLE 58.4 MEDIAN AND ULNAR LATENCY DIFFERENCES

| MEDIAN–ULNAR (WRIST) | SENSORY (14 CM) | | MOTOR (8 CM)* | |
| | ONSET | PEAK | AGE | |
| --- | --- | --- | --- | --- |
| Changes in latencies (ms)* | 0.5 | 0.4 | All | 1.5 |
| | | | 19–49 | 1.4 |
| | | | 50–79 | 1.7 |

*Upper limits of normal is the 97th percentile of the observed differences distribution. These values only apply if the median is greater than the ulnar value, look up the normals if ulnar sensory is greater than the median. The ulnar motor latency should not be longer than the median. If it is, then ulnar pathology at the wrist may be present.

Electrode placement: Ground electrode always placed between the stimulating and recording electrodes. Temperature above 32 °C for the upper extremities and above 31 °C for the lower extremities, measured at the dorsum of the hands and feet.

Acknowledgments: This document represents the collaborative efforts of the AANEM Normative Data Task Force led by Dr. Timothy Dillingham based on data provided by Dr. Ralph Buschbacher and other's publications. Thanks also to Drs. Ileana Howard and Gautam Malhotra and the AANEM staff Shirlyn A. Adkins, JD and Whitney Lutteke for their help in creating the charts.

## NEEDLE EMG

Needle electromyography is a critical diagnostic technique to assess physiological changes in muscle fibers as a result of either a primarily peripheral nervous system or muscle disease. The needle serves as an electrode to record electrical activity occurring in the muscle at rest (spontaneous activity) and to also record MUAPs during muscle contraction. The electromyographer is able to analyze and interpret those potentials and learn significant information about the function of both nerves and muscles.

Both muscle and nerve have resting transmembrane potentials that are stable due to positively charged ions on the outside of the membranes and negatively charged ions on the inside. When a muscle fiber is depolarized, ions redistribute along the inside and outside of the membranes resulting in a muscle fiber action potential that can be recorded extracellularly. During electromyography, the needle electrode is placed as close as possible to a contracting motor unit; the resulting potential that is seen is called a MUAP. The MUAP is a summation and average of the individual muscle fiber action potentials in the vicinity of the needle electrode recording surface. In general, in the absence of a pathologic process, when the muscle is at rest and the needle electrode is not being moved, no electrical activity should be recorded by the needle electrode.

Two electrodes (active and reference) must be present in the field of the depolarizing muscle fiber, the potential is measured as the difference between the two sites. The ground electrode serves as a common point of reference for both active and reference electrodes. In clinical practice, two major types of needles are available (monopolar and concentric) and based on the recording characteristic of each produce slightly different appearances of

MUAPs. When a monopolar needle is used, it serves as the active recording electrode and a reference electrode is placed on the skin near the needle insertion site. The concentric needle is designed with both the recording electrode and the reference electrode built into the needle. Due to the design, concentric needle recorded MUAPs will have smaller amplitudes, slightly shorter durations, and increased phases compared to those recorded by monopolar needles.[4]

During a study, the electromyographer must be able to recognize and analyze various EMG waveform parameters in order to accurately diagnose diseases. Being able to differentiate normal from abnormal spontaneous activity, accurately analyze MUAPs, and recognize that different muscle recruitment patterns are all critical parts of the needle examination.

Fibrillations and positive sharp waves are examples of abnormal spontaneous activity that are important to recognize when diagnosing either muscle or nerve diseases. Additional types of spontaneous activity include complex repetitive discharges, myotonia, and myokymia. During MUAP analysis, there are generally five components of the MUAP that should be evaluated: rise time, phases/turns, duration, amplitude, and stability. Based on those MUAP parameters, a muscle can generally be classified as normal, neuropathic, or myopathic. Generally, MUAPs with large amplitude, long duration, and polyphasicity are associated with neuropathic processes while small amplitude, short duration, and polyphasic MUAPs are associated with myopathic processes. Lastly, recruitment of muscle fibers must be addressed and is classified into four general categories: normal, early (increased), reduced, or central.[5]

### Indications and Application Guidelines

Electromyography is a diagnostic tool that serves as an extension of the physical examination and provides supporting data to confirm or exclude a clinical diagnosis. Results of an electrodiagnostic study should not be seen as a binary result (normal or abnormal), but rather it should be seen as providing additional layers of information regarding the health of the peripheral nervous and muscular systems (see Box 58.1)

### Absolute and Relative Contraindications

There are few absolute contraindications to electromyography in a consenting patient; however, consideration of patient characteristics influencing the risk of examination versus potential

## BOX 58.1

### SUMMARY: UTILITY OF ELECTRODIAGNOSTIC TESTING

- Confirm suspected clinical diagnosis
- Exclude competing diagnoses
- Interrogate the integrity of the peripheral nervous system
- "Localize the lesion" or clarify the site of pathology
- Characterize the pathologic disease process (e.g., demyelinating, axonal)
- Determine the extent of the disease process
- Identify healthy or unaffected nerves and/or muscles
- Assist in predicting prognosis for recovery
- Assist in predicting results of epidural steroid injection or surgery

benefit should be performed to minimize harm. Serious complications from electrodiagnostic studies are extremely rare and include hematoma, pneumothorax, and cellulitis.[2]

Patients presenting for EMG should be queried about use of anticoagulants, and a recent international normalized ratio (INR) may help stratify risk for patients on warfarin. While no clear guidelines exist for safe levels of anticoagulation to minimize the risk of bleeding and hematoma, reasonable caution must be taken in these individuals when performing studies in deep, non-compressible muscles or body regions prone to compartment syndrome (for example, in the posterior compartment of the calf). Further risk/benefit analysis may be indicated for a patient found to have supratherapeutic anticoagulation prior to proceeding with electrodiagnostic studies.

Pneumothorax is a reported complication associated with the needle examination of muscles around the thorax—such as the rhomboids, serratus anterior, diaphragm, thoracic paraspinals, and trapezius. The use of ultrasound may confer increased safety during electrodiagnosis in this body region.

The risk of skin infection following EMG may be lower following the advent of single-use needle electrodes; however, care should be taken in patients with significant medical comorbidities that may predispose to poor healing, such as diabetes and peripheral vascular disease. In addition, needle examination should not be performed directly in an area with a suspected or actual skin infection.

Needlestick injury is common and likely underreported. Universal precautions must be taken to avoid the transmission of bloodborne pathogens, and clinicians who sustain needlestick injury should be encouraged to seek medical attention in a timely manner for risk stratification to determine the need for postexposure prophylaxis.

## EMG STUDY DESIGN

Most electrodiagnostic studies require a combination of both NCS and needle electromyography in order to fully evaluate for both peripheral nervous system and muscle diseases. All electrodiagnostic evaluations should start with a thorough history and physical examination. Based on the history and physical, imaging, further information from the referring provider, and previous electrodiagnostic studies, the clinician can then develop an appropriate differential diagnosis. The electrodiagnostic study is then designed to help narrow the differential as much as possible. Needle electromyography is particularly helpful in localizing a process in the peripheral nervous system, detecting axon loss in peripheral nervous system conditions, and identifying muscle disease processes. It is also critical to remember that the electrodiagnostic study is very dynamic, and the study that is designed at the onset is often modified as information is obtained during the electrodiagnostic testing.

### Example Presentations: Suspected Radiculopathy

Patients with suspected radiculopathy are often referred to electrodiagnostic laboratories. Patients generally present with low back pain as well as radiating pain, sensory complaints, and weakness. While NCS is helpful in these presentations to potentially rule or generalized peripheral neuropathies or focal nerve entrapments, the needle EMG remains the most useful part of the electrodiagnostic examination to confirm the presence of a motor radiculopathy.

The general approach to evaluate for radiculopathy is to sample multiple muscles from various myotomes and peripheral nerves. Weak muscles should be included in the evaluation as well as the paraspinal muscles in most cases. In general, a thorough evaluation of a limb for radiculopathy should include at least five muscles and the corresponding paraspinal muscles. The strongest evidence of radiculopathy occurs when needle electromyography reveals abnormalities in multiple muscles from the same myotome but different peripheral nerves. For example, if abnormalities are noted in the tibialis anterior, tensor fascia lata, and mid or lower lumbar paraspinals, this would provide strong evidence of an L5 motor radiculopathy. It is important to note that needle electromyography is not able to detect sensory-predominant radiculopathies.[3]

### Example Presentation: Painless Weakness

When patients present with muscle weakness without significant pain or sensory complaints, anterior horn cell disease, pure motor neuropathies, neuromuscular junction disorders, or myopathic processes must be considered. Again, history and physical examination with additional focus on family history and bulbar or respiratory symptoms is critical. For all of these disease processes, sensory NCS would be expected to be normal. Careful motor NCS, including proximal studies or repetitive stimulation as appropriate based on history and physical examination, should identify motor neuropathy or neuromuscular junction disorders. A properly designed needle electromyography study is critical to the appropriate diagnosis. In designing the needle electromyography portion of the study to detect a myopathic process, one must ensure sufficient sampling of upper and lower limbs that include both proximal and distal muscles. The thoracic paraspinal should be done in the evaluation of myopathies due to their proximal location. An additional consideration in the detection of myopathies is to use quantitative needle analysis. The subtle finding of myopathy may be missed using semiquantitative methods. Needle electromyography study design for evaluation of motor neuron diseases requires evaluation of muscles in four regions of the body (bulbar, cervical, thoracic, and lumbar). There are various criteria for the electrodiagnostic classification of motor neuron disease that all involve some combination of abnormal spontaneous activity, acute and chronic neuropathic MUAPS changes, and abnormal recruitment in the various body regions described earlier.

### Muscles to Consider in the EMG Evaluation: Innervation and Roots (Table 58.5)

Table 58.5 is available online only in the digital product, see access information via the following url located under the References heading.

## ACKNOWLEDGMENTS

The authors would like to acknowledge Amanda Wise, DO, and Xiaomeng Li, MD, PharmD for their assistance with the chapter.

## REFERENCES

The full list of references and Table 58.5 appear in the digital product found on http://connect
.springerpub.com/content/book/978-0-8261-6226-7/part/part04/chapter/ch58

# ERGONOMICS

DEBRA CHERRY AND DUANE ROBINSON

## CORE DEFINITIONS

Ergonomics is the study of physical and cognitive demands of work to ensure a safe and productive workplace.[1] UpToDate defines ergonomics as follows[2]:

"Ergonomics is defined as the science related to humans and their work, embodying anatomic, physiologic, and mechanical principles affecting the efficient use of human energy. Safe lifting techniques, proper posture, appropriate seating position, and adaptive equipment are only a few of the many examples of ergonomics in the workplace."

## SCIENTIFIC BACKGROUND

Physical stressors associated with musculoskeletal disorders include awkward postures, repetitive motions, application of sustained or high force, and vibration (Table 59.1).

**TABLE 59.1 ERGONOMIC RISK FACTORS FOR MUSCULOSKELETAL DISORDERS**

| MUSCULOSKELETAL DISORDERS | Risk Factors |
|---|---|
| NECK | Posture, repetition of forceful movements, forceful movements[3]; keyboard position close to the body, low work task variation, self-perceived medium/high muscular tension[4] |
| SHOULDER | Posture, repetition, and force[3,5] |
| ELBOW | Strong forces, posture, force with repetition[3,6] |
| HAND AND WRIST TENDONITIS | Repetition, force, and posture, and these in combination[3,7] |
| CTS | Repetition, force, vibration, and these factors in combination[3,8] |
| HAVS | Vibration[3] |
| LOW BACK MSDS | Heavy physical work, lifting, forceful movement, awkward postures, whole-body vibration[3,9] |

CTS, carpal tunnel syndrome; HAVS, hand-arm vibration syndrome; MSDs, musculoskeletal disorders.

---

The full list of resources and references appears in the digital product found on http://connect .springerpub.com/content/book/978-0-8261-6226-7/part/part04/chapter/ch59

## INDICATIONS

Computer workstations, use of hand tools, lifting/pushing/pulling such as warehouse work, and manual handling of patients are especially suitable for an ergonomic evaluation. Many employers and insurance companies will provide an ergonomist evaluation to suggest environmental modifications for individuals to minimize physical stressors while performing their job.

## PREVENTION OF MUSCULOSKELETAL DISORDERS

### Neck

Workers should maintain their neck in a neutral position and avoid prolonged positioning of the neck in extension or flexion. When possible, position workpieces at a level where the neck does not need to be flexed, extended, or rotated. For office workers, this may simply involve positioning a computer monitor at a height conducive to a neutral neck position. For tradesmen, such as welders, workpieces should be positioned in a similar manner to promote good neck posture. Work involving raising the hands above the shoulders can cause neck pain and should be limited or avoided through the use of engineering controls or administrative, exposure duration limiting, controls.

*Example:* A 53-year-old woman, 5'3" in height, presents with unbearable neck pain while using her home computer to complete vocational retraining, which is provided under her worker's compensation claim. Her physician writes a prescription for an ergonomic evaluation of the home workstation, a benefit that is provided by the worker's compensation insurance carrier, and faxes the prescription to the vocational rehabilitation counselor assigned to this case. The ergonomist finds that the standard desk height of 29 inches is too high for this woman to achieve a neutral posture, and her chair is not adjustable, forcing her to hold her neck in extension and shrug her shoulders while typing. With an adjustable chair and a keyboard tray, she is able to place her workstation components in the optimal position (Figure 59.1) and her neck strain is alleviated.

### Shoulder

A shoulder injury is reduced by designing work to prevent sustained shoulder elevation, abduction, flexion, or external rotation. Work above shoulders should be eliminated by engineering controls or minimized. Small loads carried with the arm at extremes of abduction or flexion place increased stress on the shoulder due to the long lever arm involved and so can cause injury when these postures are sustained.

*Example:* A 55-year-old female sonographer, 5'6" in height, presents with chronic shoulder pain from performing portable, bedside abdominal sonograms, particularly on obese patients. She is holding the arm in abduction while applying pressure with the transducer. The employer provides an ergonomic evaluation, which recommends adjusting the bed height to position the patient below the sonographer's arm and turning the monitor rather than rotating the sonographer's arm. These adjustments reduce but do not eliminate shoulder symptoms. Other adjustments include reducing the total number of sonograms per shift and distributing the more difficult sonograms to other technicians.

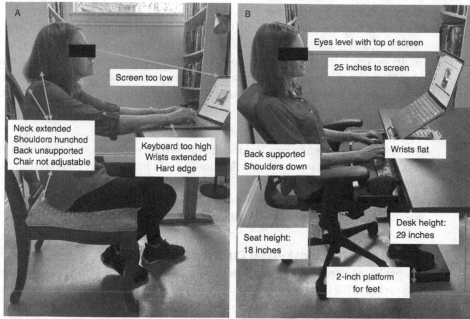

**FIGURE 59.1** Suboptimal positioning of workstation components for a woman who is 5'3" in height sitting at a standard height desk (A) and optimal positioning of workstation components (B).

## Elbow

Reducing elbow injury requires limiting high-force gripping, pinching, and repeated forceful wrist or finger flexion. Exercises that strengthen forearm musculature can aid prevention. Hand tools and processes can be designed to avoid the need for high force exertion of the muscles of the forearm, particularly where impact or throwing is involved. Prolonged elbow flexion should be avoided to prevent cubital tunnel syndrome. Pressure on the ulnar groove should be avoided as well.[10]

*Example:* A 40-year-old trucker presents with elbow pain consistent with lateral epicondylitis. He is responsible for loading and strapping down the loads on his truck about five to six times per day with 10+ straps, using ratcheting with a lever arm to tighten the straps. His employer declines the recommended ergonomic evaluation. While an onsite evaluation is not possible, the patient is directed to the "Keep Trucking Safe" website (www.keeptrucking-safeblog.org/keep-trucking-safe-website-2) for ergonomic tips, the "Be a Pro" strapping tips at www.cdc.gov/niosh/nioshtic-2/20044716.html, and occupational therapy.

## Hand and Wrist Tendonitis

Prolonged forceful gripping and repeated wrist motion should be reduced. Ergonomic modifications that promote a neutral position of the wrist are recommended. Dental hygienists are particularly at risk for wrist pain from chronic repetitive movements, awkward and static positions, sustained grasp on instrument handles, and extended use of vibratory instruments.[11]

## Carpal Tunnel Syndrome

To prevent carpal tunnel syndrome (CTS), the worker should avoid repeated, repeated and sustained, and forceful gripping. Repeated wrist and finger motions, positioning of the wrist in flexion or extension for long periods, or direct pressure on the area of the carpal tunnel should also be avoided. Tools that augment grip or pinch force should be used. Leaning rests or tool holders/positioners that support the weight of tools in the hands should be used.[12]

## Hand-Arm Vibration Syndrome

Prevention recommendations include the following: Avoidance of power tools with high levels of handle displacement or acceleration, use of administrative controls to limit the total time spent using hand tools per day (American College of Government Industrial Hygienists thresholds), and use of vibration-reducing tool holders, antivibration gloves, or tape on the handles. Use of power tools during cold weather should also be avoided.[1]

## Low Back Musculoskeletal Disorders

Proper lifting posture is key to prevention and generally allows the load to be kept as close as possible to the back, provides a broad base of support for good balance, permits the lifter to see ahead and avoid obstacles, employs neutral spine posture, and avoids trunk rotation, flexion, and extension. The National Institute for Occupational safety and Health (NIOSH) lifting equation can be used to calculate parameters for a safe lift. This equation takes into account the need for significant load control, hand position, how far the object to be lifted is away from the worker's body, load weight, and frequency of lifting. An application for smartphones to perform this calculation is available for download from the NIOSH website; the app returns a lifting index that is ideally lower than 1.0 for a safe lift.[13] The maximum weight to lift under ideal conditions is approximately 25 kg or 55 lbs. Oregon Occupational Safety and Health Administration (OSHA) has a lift calculator that returns the weight in pounds that is safe to lift under variable conditions.[14]

NIOSH also publishes advice on pushing and pulling. When pushing or pulling is required, the area ahead should be level, offers traction, and clear. Braking should be available if the surface to be traversed is not level. It is recommended that loads are pushed, rather than pulled. The coefficient of friction between the floor and the sole of the shoes should be at least 0.8 wherever heavy loads are moved. If the load does not start to move when a reasonable amount of force is applied, additional manpower or mechanical help is recommended. Cart handles should be positioned at about hip height. Two vertical handles, or two sets of handles at different heights, allow workers of different stature to grasp the load at optimal points.[1]

## BASIC ORDER SETS

A physician may recommend an ergonomic evaluation by writing a prescription. These can be a provider to worker's compensation claim manager or vocational rehabilitation counselors. It is important to include the worker's compensation claim number on the prescription and notify the employer as authorization may be required. Some large companies perform ergonomic assessments internally by request regardless of worker's compensation status.

With the patient's permission, a prescription or request for ergonomic evaluation may be sent to a risk manager, environmental services, or human resources department. In some instances, workers prefer that the physician NOT contact their employer, and the worker's wishes must be respected.

If an onsite ergonomic evaluation is not available, physical therapy may be prescribed to include simulation of job tasks with ergonomics training. Work conditioning typically includes 2 hours per day for 4 weeks of exercise with job simulation tasks. Work hardening programs rely on interdisciplinary services provided 8 hours per day for 4 weeks including exercise, job simulation tasks, goal setting, and other services such as vocational counseling.

## RESOURCES AND REFERENCES

The full list of resources and references appears in the digital product found on http://connect .springerpub.com/content/book/978-0-8261-6226-7/part/part04/chapter/ch59

# EXERCISE PRESCRIPTION

MARK E. SEDERBERG AND CINDY LIN

## CORE DEFINITIONS

**Physical activity (PA):** Any bodily movement produced by skeletal muscles that require energy expenditure.

**Exercise:** Structured and planned PA with the purpose of increasing an individual's health, physical performance or fitness, or for enjoyment.

**Aerobic exercise:** Exercise providing cardiovascular conditioning that predominantly utilizes aerobic energy production. Typically, this consists of sustained repetitive movements such as running, walking, hand cycling, biking, swimming, or rowing.

**High-intensity interval training (HIIT):** A type of exercise that involves repeated bouts of high-intensity effort at >80% max heart rate (HR), followed by a lower-intensity recovery period at 40% to 50% max HR. This is often done in the "sprint interval training method" with 30 to 60 seconds of near-full effort, followed by 4 to 5 minutes of recovery, repeated three to –five times. Another common method is the 1:1 method, which involves equal time high intensity and low intensity (i.e., 2 min high-intensity cycling followed by 2 min low-intensity cycling). HIIT generally should not be prescribed to a patient that is sedentary at baseline without medical clearance. Studies indicate that HIIT provides similar or superior health benefits compared to classic aerobic exercise and can be accomplished in a shorter workout duration.[1]

**Balance (neuromotor) training:** Static or dynamic exercises designed to improve an individual's stability and body control while standing or sitting. These types of exercises can be helpful to prevent falls in older adults or those with mobility impairments.[2] Examples include Tai Chi, yoga, Pilates, or sustained single-leg standing balance. Higher-level dynamic multiplanar or sports-specific balance exercises can also be useful as part of sports performance training or rehabilitation for injury prevention.[2]

**Muscle strengthening exercises:** Exercises designed to increase the power, endurance, and strength of targeted muscles or muscle groups by contraction against an external force. This force can be from free weights, gravity, or water resistance among others. Strengthening exercises typically involve an isotonic contraction, wherein muscle tone or tension remains constant as the muscle length changes. Types of isotonic contraction include concentric, shortening of the agonistic muscle, and eccentric, lengthening of the agonistic muscle. Additionally, strengthening can occur with an isometric contraction where there is no change in

The full list of resources and references appears in the digital product found on http://connect .springerpub.com/content/book/978-0-8261-6226-7/part/part04/chapter/ch60

the length of the muscle, or with isokinetic contraction, where the rate of muscle shortening is constant regardless of the force exerted by the muscle.

## CLINICALLY RELEVANT SCIENTIFIC BACKGROUND

Exercise is effective for both the prevention and treatment of numerous acute and chronic medical conditions, with selected chronic conditions highlighted in Table 60.1. However, only half of the general American adult population meets the recommended weekly aerobic exercise and only 20% meet both the aerobic and muscle-strengthening guidelines.[9] The effects of inadequate PA are estimated to be responsible for 10% of premature deaths in the United States.[10] The 2018 PA guideline released by the United States Department of Health and Human Services, along with the American College of Sports Medicine (ACSM), notes that while different age groups and health conditions have distinct abilities and specialized exercise needs, essentially everyone benefits from exercise.[11] See Table 60.2 for exercise guidelines for specific populations.

**TABLE 60.1 BENEFITS OF EXERCISE IN THE PREVENTION AND TREATMENT OF SELECTED CHRONIC HEALTH CONDITIONS[3]**

| MEDICAL CONDITION | BENEFIT OF EXERCISE |
|---|---|
| Dementia | Reduced risk of the onset of vascular dementia, Alzheimer's disease (28% reduced risk)[4] |
| Parkinson's disease | Improved walking speed and economy, gait function, balance, ease of ADLs[3] |
| Multiple sclerosis | Improve mobility, fatigue, quality of life, muscle strength, ability to carry our ADLs[3] |
| Obesity | Exercise role in weight loss is controversial. Exercise associated with the reduction of fat mass and abdominal obesity. Counteracts muscle mass loss during dieting. May help prevent weight gain[3] |
| Type 2 diabetes mellitus | Reduces risk of onset by 46%.[5] Significant improvement in glucose control, decreased risk of diabetes-related complications[3] |
| Hypertension | Prevents hypertension. In hypertensive individuals, reduction of both systolic and diastolic blood pressure of 7.4 and 5.8 mmHg, respectively[3] |
| Coronary artery disease | Reduced mortality, hospital admissions. Reduce cholesterol and triglyceride levels[3] |
| Heart failure | Increased quality of life, beneficial effect on New York Heart Association class, decreased heart-related hospitalizations[3] |
| Chronic obstructive pulmonary disease | Increased quality of life, decreased dyspnea, increased exercise capacity, decreased hospitalizations[3] |

*(continued)*

**TABLE 60.1 BENEFITS OF EXERCISE IN THE PREVENTION AND TREATMENT OF SELECTED CHRONIC HEALTH CONDITIONS[3] (continued)**

| MEDICAL CONDITION | BENEFIT OF EXERCISE |
| --- | --- |
| OA | Decrease pain (short and long term), increased level of function with knee and hip OA. Increased balance and gait speed[3] |
| Osteoporosis | Decreases risk of acquiring.[6] Increases bone marrow density if already osteoporotic. Increases balance and strength, decreases the risk of fall/fracture.[3] |
| Chronic low back pain | Decreases pain. Increases working capacity[3] |
| Cancer | Protective incidence of breast, colon, prostate, endometrial cancers. Decreased recurrence or death from breast and colon cancer. Improved quality of life in those with cancer[3] |
| Asthma | Decrease frequency and severity of asthma attacks[3] |
| Depression | Decreases incidence.[7] Reduces in the severity of depressive symptoms. Prevents relapse[8] |
| Anxiety | Reduction of symptoms of anxiety[3] |

ADL, activities of daily living; OA, osteoarthritis.

**TABLE 60.2 SUMMARY OF THE 2018 UNITED STATES DEPARTMENT OF HEALTH AND HUMAN SERVICES AND AMERICAN COLLEGE OF SPORTS MEDICINE PHYSICAL ACTIVITY GUIDELINES[11]**

| GROUP | SPECIAL NOTES | AEROBIC EXERCISE | MUSCLE STRENGTHENING EXERCISE |
| --- | --- | --- | --- |
| Ages 3–5 | Should be physically active throughout the day and avoid inactivity | | |
| Ages 6–17 | 60 minutes or more of moderate-to-vigorous physical activity daily, with bone-strengthening activity at least 3 days a week | Most of the 60 minutes or more per day should be aerobic physical activity and should include a vigorous-intensity physical activity at least 3 days a week | As part of their 60 minutes or more of daily physical activity, children and adolescents should include muscle-strengthening physical activity at least 3 days a week |
| Adults | Move more and sit less throughout the day. Additional health benefits are gained by engaging in physical activity beyond the equivalent of 300 minutes of moderate-intensity physical activity a week | At least 150–300 minutes/week of moderate-intensity, or 75–150 minutes/week of vigorous-intensity aerobic physical activity, or an equivalent combination of the two | Moderate or greater intensity muscle strengthening that involves all major muscle groups on 2 or more days a week |

(continued)

**TABLE 60.2 SUMMARY OF THE 2018 UNITED STATES DEPARTMENT OF HEALTH AND HUMAN SERVICES AND AMERICAN COLLEGE OF SPORTS MEDICINE PHYSICAL ACTIVITY GUIDELINES**[11] (*continued*)

| GROUP | SPECIAL NOTES | AEROBIC EXERCISE | MUSCLE STRENGTHENING EXERCISE |
|---|---|---|---|
| Older adults | Include multicomponent physical activity that includes balance training as well as aerobic and muscle-strengthening activities | Same as adults. However, if they cannot do 150 minutes of moderate-intensity aerobic activity a week because of chronic conditions, they should be as physically active as their abilities and conditions allow | Same as adults |
| Adults with chronic illness or disability | Adults with chronic conditions or symptoms should be under the care of a health care provider for monitoring | Same as adults. If unable, they should engage in regular PA according to their abilities and should avoid inactivity | Same as adults |
| Pregnancy and postpartum | Women who habitually engaged in a vigorous-intensity aerobic activity or who were physically active before pregnancy can continue these activities during pregnancy and the postpartum period. Avoid contact or collision sports, or activities with a high risk of falling | Women should do at least 150 minutes (2 hrs and 30 min) of moderate-intensity aerobic activity a week during pregnancy and the postpartum period | Avoid doing exercises that involve lying on their back after the first trimester of pregnancy because this position can restrict blood flow to the uterus and fetus |

Of equal importance to exercise is how individuals spend their nonexercise waking hours, which vastly outweigh their time exercising. When this predominantly consists of sedentary behaviors such as prolonged sitting at a desk or vehicle, energy expenditure is low. There is an almost dose-dependent association between daily sitting time and mortality from cerebrovascular disease and all-cause mortality, with the strongest association among those sitting greater than 6 hours per day, and those that do not achieve ACSM exercise guidelines.[12] Interventions such as using a sit-to-stand desk or moving around at least 5 minutes each hour to interrupt prolonged sedentary time is advisable.[13]

## INDICATIONS AND APPLICATION GUIDELINES

### Exercise Prescription Components

The acronym FITT (frequency, intensity, time, type) is used to describe the four components of an exercise prescription, similar to the detail provided for a medication prescription. Refer to the ACSM guidelines to aid in prescription writing.[13] Another component to an exercise prescription may include a daily step count goal. Studies currently recommend a goal for adults of 7,000 to 10,000 steps per day.[14] For those that are more sedentary, increasing the number of daily steps the patient is previously taking by just 2,000 to 2,400 seems to decrease cardiovascular risk.[15,16]

## Frequency

For aerobic exercise, the prescription should specify the number of sessions per week. For those with time constraints, there is also evidence that short bouts of PA, that is, 10 minutes at a time throughout the day give many of the same benefits as a single equivalent session of sustained exercise.[17] All healthy adults aged 18 to 65 years should participate in moderate-intensity aerobic PA for a minimum of 30 minutes on 5 days per week, or vigorous-intensity aerobic activity for a minimum of 20 minutes on 3 days per week.

With muscle strengthening exercises, major muscle groups should be exercised two to three times per week. 48 hours of rest are advised between sessions for each muscle group to allow for adequate recovery.

## Intensity

There are numerous ways to describe aerobic exercise intensity. Two that are easy for patients to utilize are HR and rating of perceived exertion (RPE).

*HR:* HR is an objective measure of exercise intensity. This can be measured manually or with activity trackers. Intensity is typically measured as a percentage of the maximum HR, estimated as 220 beats per minute minus the age. Low-intensity exercise is 40% to 50% max HR, moderate-intensity exercise 50% to 75% max HR, and vigorous exercise 70% to 85% max HR. Note that HR may not be an accurate measure in individuals taking a beta-blocker.

*RPE:* This uses a subjective measure of how hard a person feels they are exerting themselves. The ACSM guidelines use a conversational RPE scale to define their aerobic exercise as "moderate intensity" or "vigorous intensity." This is a useful measure, as it requires no equipment, minimal training, and gives the patient a sense of control on their exercise intensity. The prescriber should ensure that the patient understands what the prescribed intensity means. "Moderate intensity" describes an exercise in which you are breathing harder than normal and could talk but not sing. "Vigorous intensity" means it would be difficult to carry on a conversation.[13]

Muscle-strengthening intensity is measured in pounds or kilograms, or with a more individualized measure, percent one-repetition maximum (1-RM). The 1-RM is defined as the greatest amount of weight that can be moved through a full range of motion with correct posture in a controlled manner. The %1-RM should be inversely related to the number of repetitions performed.

## Time

The length of time an activity or exercise is performed. This is typically expressed in minutes for aerobic exercise. Especially for the exercise-naïve, adding in a rate of progression in time may help improve motivation and avoid injury. A common recommendation is increasing the duration by 5 to 10 minutes every 1 to 2 weeks until reaching the targeted exercise time goal.[13]

For muscle strengthening exercises, this is expressed in repetitions (reps) and sets. A rep is performing a single exercise once (such as one bicep curl). A set is a group of reps performed without stopping. The optimal number of reps, sets, and time of rest between sets depends on the muscle strengthening goals. A common starting routine would include two to four sets of 8 to 12 reps with a rest period of 2 to 3 minutes between sets. However, in the untrained, there are benefits with even one set.[13] This would likely be performed with weights about 60% to 80% 1-RM. Increasing reps to 15 to 30, with no more than two sets or 50% 1-RM targets muscle endurance rather than strength.[13]

## Type

The type of exercise prescribed should be one that the individual has the ability, access, and motivation to perform. The type could include walking, hand cycling, biking, rowing, water aerobics, hiking, a home exercise video, tennis, or yoga. Take into consideration any medical conditions the patient has along with the ACSM exercise guidelines in selecting an activity.

For muscle strengthening, there are many types of resistance such as body weight, elastic bands, weight machines, or free weights.

## SAMPLE ORDER SET

### For a 65-Year-Old Sedentary Male With Diabetes Type II and Right Knee Osteoarthritis

Frequency: Aerobic—5 days per week; muscle training 2 days per week.

Intensity: Aerobic—moderate intensity; muscle training 60% 1-RM, RPE moderate intensity—"talk but not sing" during exercise.

Type: Aerobic: cycling and/or water aerobics in a heated pool; muscle training: free weights targeting major muscle groups including the gluteal, quads, hamstrings.

Time: Aerobic—30 minutes per session, ok to start in 10-minute bouts if not exercising regularly at baseline. Muscle training: two to four sets of 8 to 12 reps for each muscle group.

## ADDITIONAL RESOURCES

For those that are new to exercise, education and supervision by a qualified exercise health professional can increase compliance and may increase safety and confidence.[13] This could include physical and occupational therapists, certified personal trainers, or athletic trainers. Seek out community resources in your area such as the YMCA, community centers, and other group exercise locations that may have helpful and appropriate classes and equipment.

## RESOURCES AND REFERENCES

The full list of resources and references appears in the digital product found on http://connect.springerpub.com/content/book/978-0-8261-6226-7/part/part04/chapter/ch60

# NEUROPSYCHOLOGICAL EVALUATION

NICKOLAS A. DASHER AND KRISTINA E. PATRICK

## CORE DEFINITIONS

Neuropsychological evaluation is a method for objective investigation of brain-related effects on cognitive, motor, behavior, and emotional functioning. It employs multiple lines of inquiry (e.g., interview, record review, testing) but is predicated primarily on use of validated tests that measure a person's cognitive functioning in comparison to expectation based on normative standards corrected for age and, when appropriate, education, gender, and other demographic factors. The resulting pattern of a patient's neuropsychological profile is interpreted in the context of their broader medical and psychosocial history to assist with diagnosis, intervention plans, and community integration (e.g., return to work or school).

## NEUROCOGNITIVE SCREENING

The use of brief, cognitive screening tests has become increasingly common in clinical practice, both in outpatient and inpatient settings. Some commonly utilized measures are described as follows.

**Mini-mental status examination (MMSE):** The MMSE includes items to address orientation, memory, attention, naming, verbal comprehension, and visuospatial ability in individuals 18 to 85 years of age. It is scored on a range of 0 to 30, with a score >23 considered within normal limits.[1] Significant limitations of the MMSE are its poor sensitivity for detecting mild cognitive impairment (MCI) and lack of items to assess executive function.

**Montreal cognitive assessment (MoCA):** The MoCA was developed to address limitations of the MMSE and includes similar domains as well as items to assess for higher-level executive and language abilities.[2] It is also scored on a range of 0 to 30, with a score >25 considered within normal limits. Compared to the MMSE, the MoCA has demonstrated greater sensitivity to detect MCI and executive weaknesses across a broader range of patient populations.[3-5]

**Cognitive and linguistic scale (CALS):** The CALS[6] is a 20-item quantitative scale with scores ranging from 20 to 100 that was developed to quantify cognitive and linguistic changes

---

The full list of resources and references appears in the digital product found on http://connect .springerpub.com/content/book/978-0-8261-6226-7/part/part04/chapter/ch61

following pediatric, traumatic, or acquired brain injury during inpatient rehabilitation. It is administered serially and can be used with patients acutely following injury to document recovery.

**National Institutes of Health (NIH) toolbox:** The NIH Toolbox is a multidimensional set of brief royalty-free computerized measures assessing cognitive, emotional, motor, and sensory functions that have been normed and validated in a broad sample of the U.S. population.[7] Though primarily used in research thus far, the NIH Toolbox is becoming increasingly utilized in clinical care.

While cognitive screening measures can provide useful information about a patient's abilities, they are not a substitute for comprehensive neuropsychological evaluation in making neurocognitive diagnoses and recommendations. Performance can vary considerably based on demographic factors. For minority or lower educated patients, screening measures are likely to result in a higher rate of false-positive errors.[8] In contrast, limited score variance can increase risk of ceiling effects, which are especially inflated for highly educated individuals with strong verbal abilities.[8] Therefore, it should not be assumed that a person scoring within normal limits on a screening measure is cognitively intact. In addition to reporting the scores, it is recommended that providers also describe the areas of observed difficulties and place greater emphasis on the patient's subjective report in documentation.

## NEUROPSYCHOLOGICAL EVALUATION INDICATIONS

While cognitive screening measures have utility in identifying patients with potential cognitive impairment, they should not be used for diagnostic and treatment planning purposes given their poor sensitivity and specificity compared to that of a comprehensive neuropsychological examination.[9] A comprehensive neuropsychological evaluation can be several hours long and includes a clinical interview, testing of several domains of function including intellectual ability, verbal skills, visual-spatial skills, memory, attention, executive functions, motor skills, academic skills, emotional–behavioral functioning, and adaptive skills; review of medical and educational records; and interactive feedback with the patient, family, and/or referring provider. A comprehensive evaluation is appropriate when there is a question regarding the etiology of cognitive decline or concern about a patient's functional abilities or capacity. Specifically, a neuropsychological evaluation is especially helpful for the following.

### Differential Diagnosis

There is significant overlap between presenting cognitive difficulties and underlying neurological or psychological etiologies. A neuropsychological evaluation is effective for differentiating between neurodegenerative diseases[10] as well as mood versus organic factors.[11]

### Understanding the Impact of Medical Condition and Treatment on Functioning

Neuropsychological evaluation can provide information regarding functional impairments stemming from a patient's medical condition(s) as well as iatrogenic effects of treatment. Neuropsychologists can interpret a patient's deficits in the context of expected profiles consistent with specific disorders or side effects of treatments. This information is valuable for guiding clinical care.

### Establish and Track Cognition Preintervention and Postintervention and Treatment

Neuropsychological evaluation is frequently utilized to document baseline neurocognitive functioning prior to surgery or treatment changes including those for epilepsy,[12] brain cancer,[13] organ transplant,[14] and deep brain stimulation.[15] This evaluation can serve to help localize areas of neurological abnormalities associated with functional deficits; provide information about lateralization of language; identify cognitive, emotional, and behavioral barriers likely to impact treatment adherence; and provide information regarding prognosis for neurocognitive outcome following treatment. Repeat neuropsychological evaluation is also typically conducted following surgery to assess for neurocognitive changes and provide recommendations for clinical and educational intervention.

### Provide Recommendations Regarding Functional Abilities and Participation in Work and School

In cases where there is concern that a patient's cognitive status may adversely impact their ability to comprehend and adhere to provider instruction, adequately manage their activities of daily living (e.g., finances, medications, operate a motor vehicle), appropriately participate in learning and educational experiences, and make safe decisions, a neuropsychological evaluation can offer greater insight into these abilities.[16] Testing can also be instrumental in developing a graduated return-to-work plan, particularly in accordance with a vocational counselor and, for students, provide appropriate recommendations for academic interventions and accommodations.

### Assess for Premorbid Factors Contributing to Current Presentation

While it may be apparent what the primary cause of a patient's cognitive impairment is (e.g., traumatic brain injury [TBI]), a neuropsychological evaluation can elucidate other factors contributing to the patient's presentation including learning disability or developmental delays.[16] Understanding the role of premorbid factors can help to guide appropriate expectations in regard to level of recovery after injury or illness.

## TIMING FOR A NEUROPSYCHOLOGICAL EVALUATION

Determining the ideal time to refer for comprehensive testing varies based on several factors including age of the patient, type of brain injury or illness, severity, course of treatment, and the urgency of needing to understand functional abilities (e.g., return to work or school). Brief neurocognitive testing or screening can be beneficial to document the pattern of cognitive impairment and guide early intervention during the acute phase of recovery. More comprehensive neuropsychological evaluation is often valuable following stabilization of recovery when questions remain regarding a patient's cognitive and functional status. Pediatric patients may require earlier and more frequent evaluations due to developmental factors. Younger children may demonstrate greater recovery, particularly of language skills, than adults following brain injury due to greater potential for reorganization of functions while the brain has high plasticity. On the other hand, an early insult can sometimes cause greater damage because the injury interferes with typical brain development. Children with neurological conditions often fall further behind their peers over time because their skills develop at a slower rate than peers. In addition, deficits in higher-level skills (e.g., executive functions) may become more apparent as children get older and demands for these skills increase. Frequent neuropsychological follow-up may be beneficial for documenting changes in neurocognitive status that correspond with development, consideration of expected age-related gains, and updating developmentally appropriate recommendations for clinical and educational intervention. The type of injury or illness and severity also affect consideration for neuropsychological evaluation referral.

## Mild Traumatic Brain Injury and Concussion

Neurocognitive deficits following concussion typically abate after 1 to 3 weeks. In most cases, full cognitive recovery is expected. For the small percentage of patients whose symptoms persist, a biopsychosocial model has been proposed to explain etiology of symptoms.[17] The concussion starts as a biological event, and persistent symptoms are explained by psychological factors (e.g., adjustment to restrictions, misattribution of symptoms, expectations regarding recovery, secondary gain), social factors (e.g., decreased involvement in social and recreational activities, missed schoolwork), and physical changes (e.g., deconditioning from reduced exercise, sleep disruption, or hypersomnolence). Targeted neuropsychological evaluation can be beneficial for identifying factors contributing to persistent post-concussive symptoms, determining symptom validity, identifying factors that may contribute to secondary gain, providing psychoeducation to patients and caregivers, and generating recommendations for treatment.[18] If further treatment is necessary, brief cognitive behavioral therapy with a focus on altering negative belief patterns, building coping skills, and gradually increasing activity has been shown to reduce post-concussive symptoms.[19,20]

## Moderate-to-Severe Traumatic Brain Injury

Sequelae and degree of cognitive recovery remain highly individualized after moderate-to-severe TBI, but in general, the majority of recovery occurs within the first year after injury, with variable degrees of continued recovery in the second year.[21] Further cognitive recovery 3+ years after injury is rare, but functional improvements via developing accommodation and compensation strategies are common. The utility of a neuropsychological evaluation will depend on functional state and goals of the patient, but it is generally recommended that comprehensive testing be conducted at 4 to 6 months post-injury to address degree of recovery and/or after 1 year to predict the level of likely recovery, identify areas in need of further rehabilitation, and develop accommodations for functional difficulties at work, school, and home. Motor and basic cognitive difficulties tend to improve in the early stages of recovery, but higher-order cognitive difficulties and emotional/behavioral symptoms are more likely to persist long term and often become more apparent when the patient transitions from a highly structured environment (e.g., inpatient rehabilitation unit) to a less structured and more demanding environment (e.g., home, work, school).

## Stroke

The sequelae of cognitive recovery following stroke depend on size and location of lesion, but in general, it is most rapid in the first 3 to 6 months, less pronounced in 6 to 12 months, and often plateaus after a year.[22] Bedside or brief assessment is recommended during the acute and subacute stages to identify deficits for rehabilitation. Once recovery has plateaued, degrees of persistent cognitive impairment are not uncommon, so more comprehensive testing can be helpful at this stage, particularly if deficits are more subtle in order to develop accommodations and therapies to mitigate functional difficulties.

## Brain Tumor and Cancer

Cognitive impairment can result from brain tumor and treatments, including surgery, chemotherapy, and radiotherapy. If possible, neurocognitive testing is recommended prior to treatment in order to establish comparative baseline to track changes after intervention.[13,23] Baseline cognitive functioning can also assist with predicting mortality risk for patients with recurrent tumor.[24] For patients currently undergoing chemotherapy and radiation, unless there is a great deal of urgency (e.g., need for immediate return to work or school), it is advised that testing wait until treatment has been completed in order to minimize the impact of fatigue and other treatment effects on performance. Ideal timing for post-treatment neuropsychological evaluation largely depends on the patient's cognitive state and functional concerns. It is recommended that providers be as specific as possible in the referral regarding the questions to address with testing, including, (a) Has there been cognitive decline as a result of tumor, treatment, or both? (b) Are cognitive deficits related to tumor/treatment or emotional distress? and (c) Would the patient benefit from cognitive rehabilitation or need accommodations with return to school or work. Pediatric patients require more frequent neuropsychological follow-up because they are more likely to experience neurocognitive late effects from treatment.[25] In particular, intrathecal methotrexate and cranial radiation have been shown to slow the rate of development of white matter, which impacts processing speed and acquisition of new skills. Children treated at younger age and with higher doses of radiation are at higher risk for experiencing neurocognitive difficulties.

## FACTORS TO ADDRESS PRIOR TO A NEUROPSYCHOLOGICAL EVALUATION

While the presence of transient psychosomatic factors does not affirmatively contraindicate a neuropsychological evaluation, reasonable efforts should be made to stabilize acute emotional distress and pain prior to comprehensive testing. Their presence increases the likelihood of patients performing poorer or more inconsistent than would be typically expected, leading to unreliable or even invalid findings, which could limit formulation of firm impressions in their cases. Another important consideration is whether the patient has a sleep disorder. Obstructive sleep apnea (OSA) and sleep fragmentation are associated with a range of cognitive impairments in attention, processing speed, and memory, particularly in older populations, and to a degree can remain persistent as a result of chronic hypoxemia and neurovascular damage.[26] A dose–response relationship between continuous positive airway pressure (CPAP) adherence and levels of cognitive improvements has been well documented in approximately two-thirds of treated patients, so it is advised that patients with untreated OSA be adherent to their CPAP for at least 1 month prior to a neuropsychological evaluation.[27] It is also helpful to rule out situational or transient factors that may be explaining cognitive complaints. For instance, if a child is experiencing difficulty in school following frequent absences, academic accommodations and interventions should be provided before referring for a neuropsychological evaluation. Finally, it is important to assess the patient's history of previous testing. Practice effects have the potential to obscure true deficits or declines that would otherwise be detected. It is advised that for patients who have not otherwise experienced a major illness or event since testing that could result in deterioration of function, and that they not be referred for repeat testing until 9 to 12 months of previous assessment.[28]

## RESOURCES AND REFERENCES

The full list of resources and references appears in the digital product found on http://connect.springerpub.com/content/book/978-0-8261-6226-7/part/part04/chapter/ch61

# ORTHOSES

MARK S. HOPKINS AND MARLÍS GONZÁLEZ-FERNÁNDEZ

## CORE DEFINITIONS

An orthosis is a device, applied to the exterior of the body, for the purpose of supporting, correcting, aligning, or improving the function of moveable parts of the body or reducing pain of the head, spine, or extremities.[1,2]

Generally, orthoses are organized into lower limb, upper limb, and spinal categories. Further subcategories are based on the joints affected.

Orthosis users are a heterogeneous group and not easily categorized by diagnosis alone. Therefore, in many cases, the focus of orthotic prescription is on orthosis design and function and less on the underlying etiology and diagnosis. Evaluation for orthoses involves a functional assessment and the establishment of reasonable functional goals, anticipated outcomes, and duration of use.

## INDICATIONS AND USE GUIDELINES

### Lower Limb Orthoses

The prescription and design of a lower limb orthosis begins with a clear diagnosis and physical examination including functional assessment and gait analysis. The orthotist will determine the joint to control (ankle/foot, knee, and/or hip), construction and materials (custom fabricated vs. prefabricated; metal, plastic, and hybrid), straps and fitting modifications, and recommendations for appropriate footwear.

### Foot Orthoses

Foot orthoses (FOs) are employed to directly support and align the foot to prevent or correct foot deformities and, thereby, improve the function of the foot and lower limb. FOs can reduce stress on the foot, ankle, knee, hip, pelvis, and spine by correcting faulty alignments and properly controlling the motion within the foot; support the longitudinal and transverse arches of the foot; provide relief for painful areas; provide an even distribution of the weight-bearing stresses over the entire plantar surface of the foot; and equalize leg length discrepancy.

FOs can be either prefabricated or customized and are made with a wide range of materials. FOs can be generally described as either accommodative or corrective/functional with further classification into soft, semirigid, or rigid subcategories. The detailed design of

---

The full list of references appears in the digital product found on http://connect.springerpub.com/content/book/978-0-8261-6226-7/part/part04/chapter/ch62

the foot orthosis includes (a) posting or wedging under the rearfoot, forefoot, or both, (b) metatarsal arch support, (c) reliefs or cutouts for painful areas, and (d) forefoot extension modifications.

## Ankle Foot Orthoses

The general indications for an ankle foot orthoses (AFOs) are (a) motor control deficits of the lower limb and resultant functional deficits (safety, mobility limitations, and gait inefficiency); (b) foot, ankle, or knee instability causing pain, deformity, or limited function; (c) immobilization required for pain control, fracture stabilization, burns, trauma, or wound management; and (d) foot/ankle joint contracture management. The orthosis includes the foot and ankle and therefore has lever arms extending proximal and distal to the ankle joint. The length of the lever arm, the ankle joint control, and the materials used to fabricate the AFO determine the control.

Traditional AFOs (Figure 62.1A) are made of two metal sidebars and joints connected proximally by a leather-covered calf band and attached distally to the shoe. Molded plastic AFOs (Figure 62.1B) are intended to be in contact with the limb for more control, are lighter weight, and allow for easier use with more than one shoe. The ankle joint control provided by an AFO can be considered to either limit or assist motion and can be constructed either with or without an ankle joint.

Common nonarticulated AFOs include solid ankle and posterior leaf spring (PLS). PLS AFOs assist dorsi-flexion (DF) during swing phase with limited restriction of stance phase motion. Common articulated designs include free motion in the sagittal plane for frontal plane control only, DF assist, and limited motion. The addition of straps and padding to the orthosis allows for more aggressive control of instability either due to weakness or due to ROM limitations from spasticity or contracture.

The supramalleolar AFO with a short proximal lever arm is used for frontal and transverse plane control of the subtalar, midtarsal, and forefoot. The floor reaction AFO (Figure 62.1C) uses a DF stop and a molded pretibial shell to create a knee extension stabilizing force for patients with knee buckling from quadriceps weakness or other pathology. Myoelectric

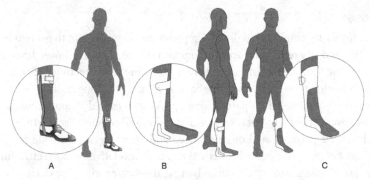

**FIGURE 62.1** (A) Metal, (B) plastic, (C) floor reaction ankle foot orthoses.

*Source*: Reprinted from González-Fernández M, Friedman J. *Physical Medicine and Rehabilitation Pocket Companion*. Demos Medical Publishing; 2011.

orthoses (e.g., Walk-aid or Bioness L300) provide functional electrical stimulation (FES) foot drop correction and may be used as an AFO replacement for some cases of upper motor neuron-related DF paralysis or weakness resulting in foot drop.

Many AFO designs are now fabricated with composite materials that allow for a broader range of material characteristics over traditional metal or thermoplastics. Ultralightweight; increased stiffness, strength, and durability; and the possibility of dynamic response from material deflection are possible with composite materials such as carbon fibers and epoxy resins. Many of these AFOs are available in prefabricated modules that allow for custom fitting to the individual for fit and function optimization. Custom-fabricated AFOs using composite materials are also an option particularly when a prefabricated orthosis cannot be custom fitted for proper fit and function.

## Knee Orthoses

Knee orthoses (KOs) are prescribed for support of the tibiofemoral and/or patellofemoral joints. Common designs include neoprene sleeves with buttress pads to control for patellar tracking dysfunction and rigid frame style orthoses with medial and lateral joints for triplanar control. A commonly prescribed KO is the compartment unloader style. This KO creates a varus or valgus thrust to open either the lateral or medial compartment of the arthritic knee for pain relief. This type of KO is fabricated as a rigid frame with one or two knee joints and an adjustable alignment feature for frontal plane thrust control.

## Knee Ankle Foot Orthoses

Knee ankle foot orthoses (KAFOs) provide support for the lower limb with indications which mirror not only that of the AFO but also with direct knee control (Figure 62.2A). Mechanical knee joints can either be built as double upright systems (medial and lateral) or as a single upright system with a single knee joint, most commonly on the lateral side of the knee. The long mechanical lever arms of the KAFO allow for direct control of the knee joint for frontal plane (varus/valgus), sagittal plane (flexion/hyperextension), or transverse plane (rotation) limits. Foot and ankle control options remain the same as for the AFO (articulated or nonarticulated; free motion, DF assist, or limited motion). Knee joints can be organized as either single axis or polycentric and knee-buckling prevention. The majority of knee joints have a 0° stop built into the design to prevent hyperextension. Joints most commonly provide a static lock mechanism, floor reaction effect often with posterior offset axes of rotation, or stance control which allow selective lock and unlock during the stance and swing phases, respectively. New stance control orthotic knee joints with electronic and microprocessor control are now available which allow for more customization of walking control for individual users. This includes the options to allow for controlled knee flexion under a load and various modes which the user can select. Construction techniques include traditional all metal and leather systems with shoe attachment, molded plastic, and hybrid combinations of metal and plastic construction including the aforementioned composite materials. KAFOs are typically custom due to the complexity of crossing multiple joints and maintaining accurate orthosis and anatomic joint alignment.

As the KAFO is concerned with direct control of the knee, the first decision is the knee joint control mechanism. The ankle joint and knee joint controls should be considered as a system balancing stability and mobility with the goal of providing the least restrictive device

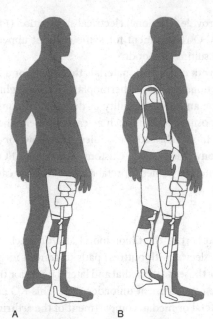

A       B

**FIGURE 62.2** (A) Knee ankle foot orthosis, (B) RGO.

*Source*: Reprinted from González-Fernández M, Friedman J. *Physical Medicine and Rehabilitation Pocket Companion*. Demos Medical Publishing; 2011.

possible. Knee joint control, ankle joint control, construction, additional straps, and the appropriate footwear make the basic prescription.

## Hip Knee Ankle Foot Orthoses and Hip Orthoses

Orthoses that cross the hip joint fall into one of two categories those that extend to the foot and ankle (HKAFOs) and those that do not (hip orthoses [HOs]). The general design of the HKAFO mirrors that of the KAFO but with the addition of a hip joint, pelvic band, and pelvic belt. This addition allows for direct control of hip instability either in the frontal plane to reduce lateral trunk lean (Trendelenburg's gait or gluteus medius lurch compensation) or in the sagittal plane to limit posterior lean of the trunk. Transverse plane or rotational control is inherent in the design of the HKAFO with pelvic connection proximally and foot/ankle leverage distally. Unilateral HKAFOs are prescribed for significant paralysis and instability of the entire lower limb and require a high level of custom fitting and user training.

Unilateral abduction HOs may be prescribed to limit hip flexion, adduction, and internal rotation following total hip arthroplasty. The RGO (Figure 62.2B) is a bilateral HKAFO with a molded spinal extension and mechanical reciprocating leg assist system mounted posterior and proximal to the hip joints. The user creates the reciprocal pattern by unloading one limb and extending the trunk with the assist of the arms pushing on an assistive device (walker or bilateral crutches). This pattern is an alternative to a swing to or swing through pattern for clients with paraplegia. Full ROM, intact skin, spasticity, orthostatic hypotension, osteoporosis, and upright posture need to be assessed in advance.

## Upper Limb Orthoses

Upper limb orthoses are provided based on the duration of anticipated use, materials and fabrication techniques, integration of the orthosis into a therapeutic care plan, referral patterns, preferences, and professional availability. In general, orthotists provide devices that are intended for long-term use and those that require more complex construction (e.g., high-temperature plastics and metals). Orthoses fabricated from low-temperature thermoplastics, directly molded to the client's limb, and fully integrated into a specific therapy treatment program are primarily the responsibility of physical or occupational therapists.

## Hand Orthosis

Hand orthoses are designed to maintain the palmar arch, keep the thumb in opposition, maintain the web space, or act as a vehicle for the attachment of other orthotic systems and assistive devices. Features of the HO may include an opponens bar, thumb adduction stop, metacarpophalangeal extension stops, interphalangeal joint extension assists, and molded palmar arch support. HOs are often designed to immobilize a specific joint to assist with healing after trauma or overuse injury. The orthosis may be prefabricated or custom fabricated and composed of a wide array of materials.

## Wrist Hand Orthosis

Wrist hand orthoses (WHOs) have many of the features of the HO but extend across the wrist for more control of the hand and direct control of the wrist. WHOs may be categorized as static or dynamic. Prefabricated gauntlet-style WHOs are commonly prescribed for overuse injuries and soft tissue trauma. Static, palmar wrist cock-up WHOs (Figure 62.3A) are a very common orthosis and are provided for the passive positioning of the hand and wrist following trauma or neurological insult. Support of the hand and wrist

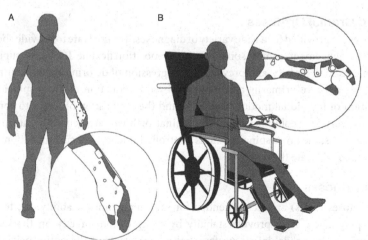

**FIGURE 62.3** (A) Wrist hand orthosis cock-up. (B) Wrist hand orthosis tenodesis.

*Source:* Reprinted from González-Fernández M, Friedman J. *Physical Medicine and Rehabilitation Pocket Companion.* Demos Medical Publishing; 2011.

with a WHO following peripheral nerve injury is common with the design and trim lines specific to the injury and paralysis pattern.

An example of a dynamic orthosis is the tenodesis-style WHO (Figure 62.3B) which assists prehension through a wrist-driven flexor hinge linkage system. Wrist extension provides a metacarpophalangeal flexion force. The tenodesis WHO is indicated in cases of C6 or C7 quadriplegia primarily but could be used for C5-level cases with either a shoulder-operated cable system or other external power sources (e.g., FES, compressed air) to create wrist extension. Myo-orthoses can be used to provide FES-facilitated tenodesis.

## Elbow Wrist Hand Orthoses and Elbow Orthoses

Elbow wrist hand orthoses (EWHOs) are designed to fulfill several functions including positioning the hand in space, providing elbow flexion, contracture management, and postoperative stabilization or immobilization. The orthosis can be prefabricated or custom fabricated; static with a set position for all segments or dynamic with static progressive or dynamic joints or a hybrid construction type; and fabricated from many types of materials. Elbow orthoses (EOs) are commonly prescribed for protection of unstable elbow joints without forearm or wrist deficits.

## Shoulder Elbow Wrist Hand Orthoses

Shoulder elbow wrist hand orthoses (SEWHOs) are often designed for the short-term static immobilization of the shoulder following postoperative reconstruction. One common static and prefabricated SEWHO, often referred to as an "airplane splint," immobilizes the shoulder in abduction and neutral rotation with the elbow at 90° so that the hand is placed out to the side and in front of the body. A dynamic type of SEWHO may be prescribed following brachial plexus injury and is designed to support the flaccid arm and may provide cable-operated elbow flexion through a harness and powered by scapular abduction of the contralateral limb.

## Spinal and Cranial Orthoses

Spinal orthoses are provided for a wide variety of diagnoses. The goals are to provide abdominal support, pain management, control spine position (reposition flexible deformity, support and accommodate fixed deformity, and prevent the progression of deformity), and control spine motion. These goals are primarily accomplished by the reduction of gross spinal motion, the stabilization of individual motion segments, and the application of forces to control the progression of vertebral column deformities. Spinal orthoses are generally categorized by the spinal segments, the gross spinal motions controlled, the level of customization, and the materials used to fabricate the orthosis.

## Sacroiliac Orthoses

Sacroiliac orthoses (SIOs) are recommended for sacroiliac joint instability due to trauma, overuse, or pregnancy. They provide stability by compression directly on the sacrum as the "keystone" of the pelvis, by circumferential compression of the entire pelvis, and by compression and support of lower abdominal muscles. Canvas or other flexible materials are commonly used, and the orthoses are often prefabricated.

## Lumbar Sacral Orthoses

Lumbar sacral orthoses (LSOs) are recommended to manage pathologies in the L2–S1 region. The anterior trim lines extend from the xiphoid process to the symphysis pubis and posteriorly from the inferior angle of the scapula to the sacrococcygeal junction. LSOs can be categorized as either semirigid or rigid. A corset-style LSO is a commonly prescribed semirigid spinal orthosis for the relief of low back pain. The corset may be made of fabric or other flexible materials with adjustable closures to ensure a snug fit and rigid horizontal stays or molded plastic inserts for additional stiffness. The corset increases abdominal compression to provide relief of stress on the posterior spinal musculature and thereby provide pain relief. Rigid spinal orthoses are defined by the plane of motion that is most restricted by the orthosis. For example, the Knight LSO controls motion in the sagittal plane and is composed of a rigid posterior frame with a pelvic band, a thoracic band, and a pair of paraspinal uprights. Custom-molded thermoplastic body jacket-style LSOs are available and provide rigid triplanar motion limitation due to the rigid materials and the intimacy of fit over the pelvis.

## Thoracic Lumbar Sacral Orthoses

Thoracic lumbar sacral orthoses (TLSOs) are recommended to manage pathologies in the T3–S1 region. They have anterior trim lines that extend from the sternal notch to the symphysis pubis and posteriorly from the spine of the scapula to the sacrococcygeal junction. TLSOs can be categorized as either semirigid or rigid. A corset-style TLSO is a commonly prescribed semirigid spinal orthosis for the relief of lumbar and/or thoracic spine pain. Similar to the LSO corset, the TLSO corset relies on abdominal compression to provide relief of stress on the posterior spinal musculature and thereby provide pain relief. They differ in that the TLSO includes a posterior extension to the spine of scapula with shoulder straps used to create an extension force on the thoracic spine and limit flexion. Rigid TLSOs are composed of a rigid posterior frame with a pelvic band, a thoracic band, a pair of paraspinal uprights, an interscapular band, and axillary straps for flexion and extension control. As in the LSO versions, leather-covered metal bands are the traditional materials; however, foam-covered thermoplastic versions are now common. A corset front is also used to create abdominal compression to further support the spine.

Custom-molded thermoplastic body jacket-style TLSOs are available and provide the most effective rigid triplanar motion limitation due to their rigidity and the intimacy of fit over the pelvis and trunk. Hyperextension style TLSOs (e.g., Jewett style) are rigid frame (usually prefabricated) and specifically designed for T10–L2 anterior compression fractures to prevent flexion and allow extension of the thoracolumbar spine using a classic three-point pressure system with contact at the sternum, pubic, and thoracolumbar areas. The goal of scoliosis TLSOs is to prevent the progression of spinal deformity. They achieve this goal through end point control, transverse loading, and curve correction. There are several versions of low-profile TLSOs designed for scoliosis management including Boston, Rosenberger, Miami, Lyonnaise, and Wilmington. Compliance with wearing times and routine follow-ups for adjustments are critical for curve stabilization.

## Cervical Thoracic Lumbar Sacral Orthoses

Cervicothoracic lumbosacral orthoses (CTLSOs) provide control of the entire spine for stabilization following multilevel trauma or post-surgical reconstruction. The Minerva-style orthosis can be entirely custom fabricated or can be the combination of a custom-fabricated TLSO with a prefabricated cervical extension. The Milwaukee CTLSO consists of a custom-molded pelvic section, metal frame superstructure, and neck ring, with lateral straps and pads used for the treatment of idiopathic scoliotic curves with an apex at T7 or superior or for cases of Scheuermann's kyphosis.

## REFERENCES

The full list of references appears in the digital product found on http://connect.springerpub.com/content/book/978-0-8261-6226-7/part/part04/chapter/ch62

# SPECIALTY BEDS

HOLLY VANCE

## CORE DEFINITIONS

Support surfaces are an essential part of pressure injury prevention and also wound healing.[1] The National Pressure Injury Advisory Panel (NPIAP) Support Surface Standards Initiative has defined the terms relevant to support surfaces (Table 63.1)[2]

## CLINICALLY RELEVANT SCIENTIFIC BACKGROUND

Until recently, not much research has been done to help clinicians specify a particular brand or type of support surface. In 2001, a support standards initiative was begun in partnership with the NPIAP intended to develop consistent terminology, test methods, and reporting standards for surfaces.[3,4] It has evolved into the Support Surface Standards Initiative (S3I) affiliated with ANSI/RESNA to become the official standards body for the United States.[4] Additionally, in 2015, multiple expert clinicians from the Wound Ostomy Continence Nurses Society (WOCN) developed and published a support surface algorithm intended to guide clinicians in selecting support surfaces based on the needs of individual patients.[5] It was validated by consensus and is the first evidence- and consensus-based algorithm geared to selection of support surfaces.[5] Found online and in print, the algorithm provides a step-by-step guide to choosing the most appropriate support surface for patients.[5]

## INDICATIONS

Specialized support surfaces are intended for those with pressure injuries or other wounds, at risk for pressure injuries, incontinence, or mobility issues.[6] Please note that specific support surfaces have absolute contraindications and should be considered carefully when assessing the patient's needs (Table 63.2).[6] Special consideration should be given to the location and condition of wounds, a patient's activity, ability to turn and reposition, risk for falls and entrapment, size and weight, weight capacity of the bed frame and mattress, and the patient's response to the support surface.[6] Additional considerations include the ability of facilities to access specialized support surfaces and also the patient's ability and resources to obtain a particular support surface in the outpatient setting.[6]

---

The full list of resources and references appears in the digital product found on http://connect.springerpub.com/content/book/978-0-8261-6226-7/part/part04/chapter/ch63

**TABLE 63.1 TERMS AND DEFINITIONS AS DESCRIBED BY THE NATIONAL PRESSURE INJURY ADVISORY PANEL SUPPORT SURFACE STANDARDS INITIATIVE[2]**

| TERM | DEFINITION |
|---|---|
| Active support surface | Type of support surface that is powered and capable of changing its load distribution (or weight dispersal) properties, with or without applied load. |
| Air fluidized | Support surface feature that produces a fluid state, providing pressure redistribution, by forcing air through a granular medium (e.g., silicone beads). |
| Alternating pressure | Support surface feature that produces cyclic changes in loading and unloading to provide pressure redistribution. These cyclic changes are characterized by amplitude, duration, frequency, and rate of change parameters. |
| Basic/Standard hospital mattress | Term used to describe a facility's mattress; varies between hospitals. It is generally assumed that this is a nonpowered foam or spring mattress. |
| Bottoming out | Occurs when the support surface becomes deformed beyond critical immersion and there is loss of effective pressure redistribution. |
| Critical immersion | Point at which deformation of the support surface has gone beyond threshold and results in increased concentration and localized pressure. |
| Elastic foam | Polymer with a broad range of weight capacity and resiliency for comfort and cushioning; typically includes interconnected and open cell structures. Elasticity allows the foam to resist deformation and return to its original shape after the force causing deformation has been removed. |
| Envelopment | Ability of a support surface to conform or mold around irregularities of the body without a major increase in pressure. |
| Fatigue | Reduced ability of the surface or its components to function as specified. |
| Friction | Parallel resistance to motion relative to the common boundary between two surfaces (e.g., skin sliding against a sheet when moving a patient up in bed). |
| Gel | Ranging from hard to soft, gel is a network of solid aggregates, colloidal dispersions, or polymers which may display elastic properties. |
| Immersion | Depth of penetration (sinking) into the surface, allowing for pressure redistribution over the surrounding area rather than directly over a bony prominence. |
| Integrated bed system | Combination of bed frame and support surface as a single unit that is unable to function separately. |
| Life expectancy | Time period over which a product is effectively able to fulfill its designated purpose. |

(continued)

**TABLE 63.1 TERMS AND DEFINITIONS AS DESCRIBED BY THE NATIONAL PRESSURE INJURY ADVISORY PANEL SUPPORT SURFACE STANDARDS INITIATIVE[2] (*continued*)**

| TERM | DEFINITION |
|---|---|
| Low air loss | Support surface that uses air flow to assist in microclimate management of the skin. |
| Mattress | Support surface designed for the full body, intended to be positioned directly on an existing bed frame. |
| Mechanical load | Distribution of force across a surface. |
| Microclimate | Regarding support surfaces, this refers to temperature and humidity at the interface of the skin/body and support surface. |
| Multi-zoned surface | Support surface wherein different segments of the surface can have differing pressure redistribution abilities. |
| Nonpowered | Support surface that does not use or require an external source of energy to operate. |
| Overlay | Support surface designated for placement directly over an existing support surface. |
| Powered | Support surface that requires or uses external energy sources for operation. |
| Pressure | Force per unit area applied perpendicular to the area of interest. |
| Pressure redistribution | Support surface ability to distribute load over the body's contact areas. |
| Pulsation | Support surface feature providing repeating higher and lower pressures leading to cyclic changes in surface stiffness. These typically have shorter inflation and deflation durations and have higher frequency and lower amplitude compared to alternating pressure. |
| Reactive support surface | Support surface, powered or nonpowered, that changes load distribution properties only in response to an applied weight or load. |
| Shear stress | Force per unit area applied parallel to the perpendicular area of interest. |
| Support surface | Pressure redistribution specialty device designed for management of tissue loads, microclimate, and/or other therapeutic functions. Includes but is not limited to mattresses, integrated bed systems, mattress replacements or overlays, seat cushions, and seat cushion overlays. |
| Therapeutic working load (Weight range) | Rated weight range intended for the features of a support surface to function at. |
| Viscoelastic foam (Memory foam) | Porous polymer which conforms in proportion to the applied load (weight). Dampened elastic properties are exhibited when load is applied. |
| Zone | Segment with one pressure redistribution ability. |

*Source*: Adapted from the National Pressure Injury Advisory Panel Support Surface Initiatives Standard (S3I). For more in-depth list of terms refer to: https://cdn.ymaws.com/npiap.com/resource/resmgr/s3i_terms-and-defs-feb-5-201.pdf

TABLE 63.2 SUPPORT SURFACES, INDICATIONS, AND CONTRAINDICATIONS[5-7]

| TYPE OF SUPPORT SURFACE | INDICATIONS | ABSOLUTE CONTRAINDICATIONS |
|---|---|---|
| *Reactive (e.g., foam)* Changes load distribution properties only in response to an applied weight or load Can be powered or nonpowered | Patients without wounds or moisture issues Used with caution in patients with minor moisture issues, such as with Braden subscale score of 2 or less Okay for use in patients with unstable spines | Weight limitations— ensure they are on a surface appropriate to their weight and girth |
| *Alternating pressure* Produces cyclic changes in loading and unloading to provide pressure redistribution Changes load distribution properties with or without an applied load | For use in patients at risk for pressure injury but without moisture issues | Unstable spine Cervical or skeletal traction Weight limitations— ensure they are on a surface appropriate to their weight and girth |
| *Low air loss* Provides air flow that assists with microclimate management Slow continuous air flow is provided through a pump, and as the patient lies on the mattress, their weight is evenly distributed, providing pressure redistribution | For use in patients with moisture and incontinence issues Used with caution in patients who are combative/ restless/agitated | Unstable spine Cervical or skeletal traction Weight limitations— ensure they are on a surface appropriate to their weight and girth |
| *Air fluidized* Contains silicon beads that behave like fluid once air is pumped through the beds and allows the patient to "float" with one-third of their body above the surface and the remaining two-thirds immersed in the surface | For use in patients with complicated wounds or wounds on multiple turning surfaces. Used with caution in patients who are combative/ restless/agitated Used with caution in patients requiring frequent head of bead elevation or have a need for aggressive pulmonary toilet Used with caution in patients with claustrophobia or at risk for delirium | Unstable spine Cervical or skeletal traction Weight limitations— ensure they are on a surface appropriate to their weight and girth Trendelenburg positioning is not possible in this type of surface |

A skin and pressure injury risk assessment should be performed on every patient when considering a support surface.[5] Commonly used assessments include the Braden scale and the Norton scale, pressure injury risk assessment scales that can aid clinicians in choosing the appropriate support surface.[5,8] The WOCN algorithm is based on the Braden scale.[5]

Minimizing the number and type of layers between the patient and support surface is important.[1,5,7] The maximum number of recommended layers by the NPIAP and WOCN is three, including sheets and body-worn absorptive products.[7] It is also important to ensure that the type of layer is compatible with the mattress, for instance, a diaper with a plastic backing is not recommended for use with a patient on a low air loss or air-fluidized bed, as the plastic backing blocks the air flow of the surface and negates the therapeutic effect.[7]

The specific support surface chosen for a patient should be based on a direct clinical assessment. For more in-depth information and assistance in choosing the best surface for a specific patient consider referring to the WOCN support surface algorithm.[5]

## SPECIALTY BED SAMPLE ORDER SET

ADULT Pressure and Moisture Management

Pressure Redistribution Bed

Indications: Risk of pressure injury or treatment of existing pressure injuries. Provides specialized pressure redistribution mattress. Mattress is spine safe. If patient has a moisture or incontinence problem, order a low air loss mattress replacement. For tall patients (over 7") order extender. Contraindications: Weight limit of 550 lbs/ 249 kg.

Bariatric Pressure Redistribution Bed

Indications: Weight >500 lbs ~227 kg or patients who would benefit from a wider turning surface. If patient has a moisture or incontinence problem, order a low air loss mattress replacement (bariatric).

Low Air Loss Mattress Replacement—Normal Weight

Indications: Risk of pressure injury or treatment of existing pressure injuries and has a moisture or incontinence problem. Contraindications: Unstable spine, cervical or skeletal traction. Weight Limit: 300 lbs ~135 kg.

Low Air Loss Mattress Replacement—Bariatric

Indications: Patients who are >300 lbs ~135 kg on acute care bed and are at risk of pressure injury or treatment of existing pressure injuries and have a moisture or incontinence problem. Contraindications: Unstable spine, cervical or skeletal traction. Weight limit: 1,000 lbs ~454 kg. Requires a bariatric bed frame.

Air-Fluidized Bed

Indications: Flap protocol with attending approval. Patients with complex wounds or wounds on multiple turning surfaces. Contraindications: Unstable spine, cervical or skeletal traction. Weight limit: 350 lbs ~158 kg.

## RESOURCES AND REFERENCES

The full list of resources and references appears in the digital product found on http://connect .springerpub.com/content/book/978-0-8261-6226-7/part/part04/chapter/ch63

# TRACHEOSTOMY

ALBA AZOLA AND DOMINIQUE VINH

## CORE DEFINITIONS

A tracheostomy is an opening in the trachea that allows ventilation. This opening is created surgically (tracheotomy), usually by a horizontal incision between the second and third tracheal ring. Tracheotomies may also be performed percutaneously with bronchoscopic or ultrasound guidance. When compared to surgical tracheostomies, percutaneous tracheostomies have been associated with improved outcomes including reduced wound infection and scarring.[1]

When caring for a patient with a tracheostomy, it is vital to understand the reason for the tracheostomy, this will guide decision-making and management in the rehabilitation setting. Having a tracheostomy may impair the patient's ability to communicate, swallow, and their sense of smell; basic and safe modifications can be implemented to support rehabilitation efforts.[2]

The basic indications for performing a tracheotomy include the following:

1. Acute respiratory failure and need for prolonged mechanical ventilation: Most common indication, two-thirds of all cases.[3] Assist with the weaning from ventilator support by reducing dead space during ventilation.
2. Upper airway obstruction: In the presence of stridor, air hunger, retractions, and severe sleep apnea that have failed medical management and are not surgical candidates or refuse other surgical modalities.[4]
3. Assist with clearance of secretions: Particularly in setting of increased aspiration of upper airway secretions or deficient clearance of lower respiratory tract secretions.

## PHYSIOLOGIC CHANGES ASSOCIATED WITH TRACHEOSTOMY

### Increased Secretions

When a tracheostomy is placed, the flow of air through the entire upper airway is bypassed. One of the main functions of the upper airway (i.e., nasal cavity and pharynx) is to humidify and heat the air before entering the trachea and lungs. When dry air enters directly into the

---

The full list of references appears in the digital product found on http://connect.springerpub.com/content/book/978-0-8261-6226-7/part/part04/chapter/ch64

trachea, it results in irritation of the respiratory mucosa and increased mucus production of the respiratory epithelium. Mucus plugs are the most common culprit of obstruction of the tracheostomy tube. Humidified air via tracheostomy collar should be provided for patients who have tracheostomies and who are not being capped or have a humidifying valve in place.

### Impaired Speech and Swallowing

Voice sounds in speech are produced by the vibration of the vocal folds generated by the airflow during expiration. When a tracheostomy tube is large or has an inflated cuff, such that it occupies the entire diameter of the trachea, it prevents airflow to generate vibrations of the vocal folds. Deflating the tracheostomy cuff or downsizing the tracheostomy will allow air to reach the glottis and allow or improve voice sound production. A speaking valve (e.g., Passy-Muir valve) is a one-way valve that allows air in through the tracheostomy and seals the tracheostomy during expiration so that the air travels out through the upper airway (Figure 64.1). In patients where a speaking valve does not allow for sound production, airway evaluation by an otolaryngologist is warranted to rule out a subglottic obstruction.

### Decreased Perception of Smell

Another effect of bypassing the upper airway is decreased perceived sense of smell; this is a bothersome symptom to patients and can result in decreased appetite.[5]

## ASSESSMENT AND MANAGEMENT

### Tracheostomy Tube Types

Clear documentation of the patient's tracheostomy type, whether cuffed or uncuffed, and size is important. Adult sizes typically used are four (small female) through eight (large male). Some brands do come on half sizes (Figure 64.2).

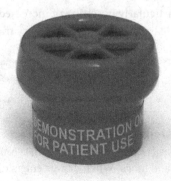

**FIGURE 64.1**  Speaking valve.

*Source*: Courtesy of Terbergen.

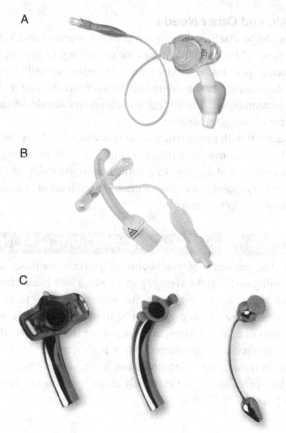

**FIGURE 64.2** Common tracheostomy type. (A) Shiley; (B) Portex; (C) Jackson.

*Sources*: (A) ©2021 Medtronic. All rights reserved. Used with the permission of Medtronic. (B) Courtesy of Smiths Medical. (C) Provided courtesy of Premier.

The most common types of tracheostomy devices include:

**Shiley®**: Most common, made of polyvinyl chloride (PVC), has inner cannula that can be removed and cleaned, single patient use (Figure 64.2). May be cuffed (air filled) or uncuffed. Extended length (XLT) at proximal or distal flange is available.

**Portex™ Bivona®**: Made out of silicone with an internal coil, for softness and flexibility, thus, the shape adapts to the airway. The balloon is tight to shaft and should be filled with water not saline as this may damage the cuff. Also available with air or foam cuff.

**Jackson**: Least commonly used. Made out of metal, extremely durable, cuffless can be sterilized and used on different patients. Requires special adaptor for connecting to the ventilator. May be preferred for some patients who require chronic ventilation or who have difficulty managing secretions.

## Suctioning, Humidified Air, and Other Needs

Patients with tracheostomy should be discharged with a suctioning machine and kits. The patient and caregivers should be taught proper techniques for suctioning. Other important equipment includes a humidifier, a spare tracheostomy tube in same size, as well as one size down as in case of accidental decannulation, the stoma may become smaller and a smaller tracheostomy tube will allow recannulation. The patient and caregivers should be familiar with daily care and tracheostomy exchange procedure.

The patient should also be familiar with the instructions of how and when to use one-way speaking valves and caps and how to remove them if there is difficulty with breathing while they are on. Again, decreased tolerance of capping in a patient previously able to tolerate warrants airway evaluation by otolaryngology to assess for granulation tissue obstructing the airway or the presence tracheal or subglottic stenosis.

## DECANNULATION—IMPLICATIONS AND PROCEDURES

Accidental decannulation in the majority of tracheostomy patients (without airway obstruction) is not a life-threatening event. In the average patient with a well-healed tract, the tracheostomy tube can be easily replaced. If resistance is met while attempting to place the tracheostomy tube, a one size smaller tracheostomy should be used to establish the airway. If there is a concern for formation of a false passage, and the patient is in acute respiratory distress, endotracheal intubation should be performed. In a patient with upper airway obstruction requiring tracheostomy accidental decannulation is an airway emergency as airway obstruction makes endotracheal intubation extremely difficult or in some cases (i.e., severe subglottic stenosis) not possible.

## Decannulation Protocols

Specific details of decannulation protocols vary, but the general principles are similar. The first step is confirmation of airway and lack of obstruction. A consultation with otolaryngology for airway evaluation, flexible endoscopic nasopharyngoscopy, and retrograde view through the tracheostomy stoma to ensure that there is no airway obstruction prior to closing the stoma may be necessary. Once cleared, daytime capping trials may be initiated. If daytime capping trial is tolerated, overnight capping trial with continuous pulse oximetry should be performed. If no desaturations are recorded, the tracheostomy may be removed and the stoma allowed to close. Typically, stoma closure will take 1 to 2 weeks. An occlusive dressing and applying pressure over the stoma while speaking to prevent air leak will aid closure. Compromised nutritional status may also delay the healing and closure of the stoma. If the stoma fails to close in 12 weeks referral to otolaryngology for airway evaluation is needed as persistent stoma may be related to existing airway obstruction.

## REFERENCES

The full list of references appears in the digital product found on http://connect.springerpub.com/content/book/978-0-8261-6226-7/part/part04/chapter/ch64

# URODYNAMICS

CRISTINA L. SADOWSKY, ALBERT C. RECIO, AND PHILIPPINES G. CABAHUG

## CORE DEFINITIONS

Urodynamic studies (UDS) are functional tests utilized to describe the function of the lower urinary tract.

UDS assess the two primary bladder functions: storage and elimination.[1] A comprehensive UDS tests several parameters to include:

1. Uroflowmetry: Measures the flow rate and volume at which the bladder empties.
2. Cystometric study: Measurement of the urine volume and pressures inside the bladder during filling.
3. Electromyography: Records the electrical activity of the pelvic floor muscle.
4. Leak point pressure: Measurement taken of the bladder pressure at the point where leakage occurs; it tests the amount of abdominal pressure required to drive fluid across the urethral sphincter.
5. Urethral pressure profile: The fluid pressure needed to open a closed urethra; it is employed to assess sphincter closure pressure and urethral competence during filling, voiding, and abdominal pressure.
6. Pressure flow studies: Begins when the "permission to void" is given and ends when the individual considers voiding has finished; includes uroflowmetry measures.
7. Video urodynamic tests using ultrasound or x-rays (optional): If available, UDS done under fluoroscopy allows for evaluation of vesicoureteral reflux, location of bladder outlet obstruction, and assessment of other bladder anomalies such as bladder diverticulum and stones.

### Important Measurements During Urodynamic Studies

*Filling rate of the bladder during cystometry:* (a) Physiological filling rate (less than the predicted maximum calculated as body weight (kilogram) divided by 4 (milliliter/minute); (b) nonphysiological filling rate (greater than the predicted maximum).[2]

*Bladder sensation (mL):* (a) The first sensation of bladder filling, which is felt when the patient first becomes aware of bladder filling (it is vague sensation, felt in the lower

---

The full list of resources and references appears in the digital product found on http://connect.springerpub.com/content/book/978-0-8261-6226-7/part/part04/chapter/ch65

pelvis, which waxes and wanes, and could be easily ignored for few minutes; 150–175 mL); (b) first desire to void, a familial constant sensation that would lead the patient to void in the next convenient moment, but still voiding can be delayed (it is felt in the lower abdomen and gradually increases with bladder filling; 250–275 mL); and (c) strong desire to void, a persistent desire to void without fear of leakage and felt in the perineum or urethra (400–430 mL).

*Bladder compliance:* Defined as the relationship between the change in bladder volume and change in detrusor pressure as a measure for the distensibility of the bladder. Compliance = change vol/change Pdet. Compliance reflects the amount of fluid in the bladder to increase the bladder pressure by 1 cm $H_2O$ (mL per cm $H_2O$). Normal bladder compliance values vary between 30 and 100 mL/cm $H_2O$; in patients with neurogenic bladder, values of 13 to 40 mL/cm $H_2O$ have been associated with a high risk of upper urinary tract complications.

*Cystometric capacity:* The bladder volume at the end of filling cystometry, when "permission to void" is given; normal cystometric capacity varies widely but is normally between 300 and 500 mL, with higher values in men than in women.

*Abdominal pressure ($P_{abd}$):* Tthe steady-state pressure within the abdominal cavity; recorded with rectal catheter. Initial resting abdominal and bladder pressures are 5 to 20 cm $H_2O$ in the supine position, 15 to 40 cm $H_2O$ in the sitting position, and 30 to 50 cm $H_2O$ in the standing position.

*Vesical pressure ($P_{ves}$):* The pressure exerted on the contents of the bladder. Vesical pressure is the sum of the intra-abdominal pressure from outside the bladder and the detrusor pressure exerted by the bladder wall musculature; recorded with urethral catheter.

*Detrusor pressure ($P_{det}$):* The component of vesical pressure created by the tension (active and passive) exerted by the bladder wall; calculated (not measured) by subtracting abdominal pressure ($P_{abd}$) from vesical pressure ($P_{ves}$). $P_{det}$ in an empty bladder that varies between 0 and 10 cm $H_2O$ in 90% of cases. Normal $P_{det}$ during bladder filling at a rate of 50 to 60 mL/s should be <20 cm $H_2O$.

*Maximum urethral pressure (MUP):* Maximum pressure of the urethral pressure profile (10–25 cm $H_2O$) Maximum urethral closure pressure (MUCP): maximum difference between urethral pressure and intravesical pressure (20–90 cm $H_2O$ in men, 20–75 cm $H_2O$ in women).

*Urine flow rate (mL/s) and volume:* Voided volume is normally >150 mL (commensurate with the amount of volume instilled into the bladder during the cystometric/filling phase); maximum flow rate (Qmax) should be >15 mL/s in men (assigning normal values in females is more difficult), and the curve of the flow should be bell shaped.

*Post-void residual measurement:* Amount of urine left in the bladder after voiding (normal <50 mL).

*Detrusor leak point:* Measurement of the detrusor pressure when leakage starts in the absence of detrusor contractions or increased abdominal pressure (normal <40 cm $H_2O$).

*Abdominal/Valsalva leak point:* Intravesical pressure at which urine leakage occurs because of increased abdominal pressure in the absence of detrusor contraction; it measures the ability of the urethra to resist an increase in abdominal pressure. It should be tested during cystometry after the bladder has been filled to at least 150 to 200 mL.

## INDICATIONS

UDSs are indicated in the evaluation of neurogenic bladder and bladder incontinence.

## COMPLICATIONS

The most common complications of UDS include urinary tract infections, pain, increased spasticity, and trauma-related to catheterization.

### Possible Urodynamic Studies Outcomes in Neurogenic Bladder Related to Spinal Cord Injury

Detrusor overactivity: Is a urodynamic observation characterized by involuntary detrusor contractions during the filling phase which may be spontaneous or provoked.[3]

Detrusor hyper-reflexia: Involuntary, uninhibited detrusor contractions

Detrusor areflexia: Acontractility due to an abnormality of nervous control.

Detrusor–sphincter dyssynergia: Failure of the external urethral sphincter to relax during micturition; also, intermittent or continuous involuntary contraction of the urethral sphincter during detrusor contractions; it is typical in patients with suprasacral spinal cord injury. The term detrusor–sphincter dyssynergia cannot be used in the absence of neurologic disease.

## BASIC ORDER SET

The European Association of Urology (EAU) Guidelines on Urological Infections suggests considering antibiotic prophylaxis prior to UDS in high-risk patients, including those with a history of prior urogenital infection. So, consider:

1. Urine analysis and culture 14 days prior to the procedure
2. Start antibiotics if:
   - Bacteriuria and pyuria identified: 5 to 7 days prior to UDS
   - Bacteriuria only: 3 days prior to UDS
   - Clean urine specimen: 1 day prior to UDS
3. Last antibiotic dose should be day of procedure

## RESOURCES AND REFERENCES

The full list of resources and references appears in the digital product found on http://connect .springerpub.com/content/book/978-0-8261-6226-7/part/part04/chapter/ch65

# WHEELCHAIRS

ERIN MICHAEL, ELIZABETH FARRELL, MEREDITH LINDEN, PHILIPPINES G. CABAHUG,
CRISTINA L. SADOWSKY, AND ALBERT C. RECIO

## CORE DEFINITIONS

Individuals living with significant lower limb dysfunction, most prominently those with spinal cord injury (SCI), often rely on wheelchairs both for independence with mobility and for health optimization. These wheelchairs are considered complex rehab technology (CRT) different from off-the-shelf durable medical equipment (DME), as CRT is "(1) designed, manufactured, individually configured, adjusted or modified for a specific individual to meet the individual's unique medical, physical or functional needs and capacities; (2) serves a medical, physical or functional purpose that is not useful to a person in the absence of disability, illness, injury or other medical condition; and (3) requires certain services to ensure appropriate design, configuration, and use."[1] Specialized CRT ensures that users achieve maximal functional independence with mobility while minimizing the secondary complications.

Physical medicine and rehabilitation physicians have a pivotal role in helping individuals with SCI-related paralysis, and other disabling conditions receive the most appropriate wheelchair and seating system. This chapter describes different types of wheelchairs and seating systems, reviews indications for a seating clinic referral, and outlines the process for prescribing CRT.

### Wheelchairs and Seating Systems

A prescription for CRT includes a power or manual wheelchair (MWC) base and additional critical components, including the seating system or accessories. These items are highly customized and should be prescribed for individual users. The prescribing physician should strive to attain the most appropriate justifiable wheelchair and components for each individual, in collaboration with a seating specialist and a supplier. Power wheelchairs (PWCs) are differentiated into different "Groups" based on performance requirements and MWCs are differentiated into "K-Codes" by weight and axle adjustability.[2,3]

### Power Wheelchair Groups

A higher PWC group indicates higher performance. Group 2 PWCs offer limited power seat functions and do not offer drive wheel suspension. This category of PWC is not considered

---

The full list of resources and references appears in the digital product found on http://connect
.springerpub.com/content/book/978-0-8261-6226-7/part/part04/chapter/ch66

CRT and does not require evaluation by a specialized seating therapist. They are the least costly category of PWC; however, they do not adequately meet the medical and functional needs of special populations.

Groups 3 and 4 PWCs offer multiple power seat functions required for pressure relief, position changes, and improved self-care. They also possess improved drive wheel suspension with vibration dampening which is critical for patients experiencing pain and spasticity. Groups 3 and 4 PWCs best meet the needs for most individuals with SCI or others with similar disability. A specialized evaluation from a seating therapist is required to procure Groups 3 and 4 PWCs.

Research supports the necessity of using multiple power seat functions—tilt, recline, and power elevating leg rests—in combination—for optimal pressure relief, edema management,[4,5] and pain management.[5] This combination also improves the user's ability to perform self-care tasks, including dressing and bladder management from the wheelchair. Fewer transfers throughout the day may result in decreased pain, decreased risk of pressure injuries from sheering during transfers, and reduced caregiver burden.

Clinical research also shows that chronic, daily exposure to whole-body vibration from wheelchair use is linked to detrimental health outcomes, including low back pain, neck pain, shoulder pain, muscle fatigue, and nerve damage.[6,7] Vibration may also be linked to increased risk of peripheral or cardiovascular disease and multiple cancers.[7] The addition of drive wheel suspension in the Group 3 and 4 PWC results in vibration dampening and decreases the users' overall exposure.

## Manual Wheelchair Classes

MWCs are classified by frame weight and designated by K-Codes, ranging from K0001 to K0009.[3] The two codes most commonly prescribed for the full-time wheelchair user with SCI are K0004 (high-strength lightweight, less than 34 lbs) and K0005 (ultralightweight, less than 30 lbs). Many ultralightweight frames now weigh less than 20 lbs, due to innovation of materials including aluminum, titanium, and carbon fiber.

The most impactful difference between these codes is freedom of rear axle adjustability. The K0004 axle is only adjustable in one plane. Due to limited adjustability, this makes the K0004 the least costly alternative. The K0005 axle is fully adjustable in both the horizontal and vertical planes. Additionally, camber can be added through the K0005 axle. Camber brings the top of the wheel closer to the user for improved efficiency of propulsion.

The MWC user is at high risk for upper extremity pain and pathology. To reduce risk, SCI clinical practice guidelines[8] recommend that the full-time user be provided with "a high-strength, fully customizable MWC made of the lightest possible material." These guidelines also indicate that the rear axle should be "as far forward as possible without compromising stability of the user" and the rear wheel positioned so that when the user's hand is at the top dead center of the hand rim their elbow is in 100° to 120° of flexion.[8] Poor axle position can adversely impact energy expenditure, rolling resistance, push frequency, and chair footprint.[9] Proper wheel position can only be achieved with a fully adjustable axle, as attaining this position is based on the individual, making the K0005 the appropriate equipment to meet the user's medical and functional needs.

## Manual Wheelchair Configuration

The way in which an MWC is configured has significant impact on the user's independence with functional mobility. Specifically, wheel size and position play an important role in maneuverability and stability of the chair.

Rear wheel position impacts upper limb health, as noted previously. It also impacts overall chair stability and user functionality. A more forward wheel results in improved ease of performing wheelies and takes weight off the smaller front caster wheel. This allows the user to navigate variable terrain more effectively. A more rearward wheel position creates more chair stability and may be beneficial for the newer user.

Front wheel or caster size also impacts functionality of the chair. A smaller wheel turns easier but has higher rolling resistance and can easily get stuck in crevasses. A larger wheel turns more slowly but negotiates terrain better. A good compromise is a 4- to 5-inch wheel with wider tire.

Camber brings the top of the wheel closer to improve efficiency and reduce shoulder abduction during propulsion. This is particularly important in the pediatric population. It also improves overall lateral stability of the chair by creating a wider base of support. Camber does add width—1 inch for each degree—to the chair, which could create access issues.

This further emphasizes the importance of selecting an MWC with greater adjustability and promotes justification of a K0005 over a K0004 wheelchair in special populations.

## Power Assist and Power Add-on

Power assist or power add-on systems can be added to an MWC to supplement the push or turn the MWC into a PWC. Motors may be in the wheel hubs or added to the rear axle of the chair. With power assist, ability to propel is still generally necessary, while with power add-on, a joystick becomes the drive control. Such systems may be appropriate for the person who cannot functionally propel, due to upper extremity strength limitations, poor endurance, or upper extremity pain but requires the transportability and reduced weight of an MWC. Such systems should be ruled out if the user cannot perform effective pressure relief.

## Seating Systems

The "Seating System" refers to the cushion and backrest. It can comprise many additional components, including headrests, chest straps, pelvic belts, and lower extremity positioners. Seating systems provide skin protection, postural support, pain reduction, stability enhancement, and functional reach improvement. An improper seating system can cause skin breakdown, postural deformity, pain or even loss of independence, or poor participation.[9] Appropriate seating system selection requires a thorough, collaborative evaluation and product trials.

## INDICATIONS FOR SEATING CLINIC REFERRAL

The process of obtaining a new wheelchair and seating system begins with a physician referral to a specialized seating clinic. Indications that a seating clinic evaluation is warranted include the following:

- Poor posture when seated in the wheelchair
- Poor fit due to growth or weight gain/loss
- Pain
- Skin breakdown
- Inadequate function in the wheelchair
- Poor condition of the user's wheelchair and seating system
- Decline in the individual's function, including frequent falls in the ambulatory individual or declining gait speed
- Increased time or inability to participate in activities of daily living (ADLs) within the home

The wheelchair itself should provide the user with the highest possible level of independence with mobility. An effective seating system provides neutral spinal and pelvic alignment, effective support of upper and lower extremities, and adequate pressure relief. A wheelchair should fit as an extension of the person's body. Poor posture in the wheelchair can result in pain, loss of function, pressure injury, skin breakdown, organ dysfunction, and fixed postural abnormalities. A wheelchair user should be referred to a specialized seating clinic if their current wheelchair is no longer meeting their mobility needs.

## Documentation

Proper medical documentation is critical in order to obtain a wheelchair and seating system. Inaccurate or incomplete documentation in the medical record could cause significant delays in ordering much-needed equipment. Medicare as well as some additional third-party payers have specific documentation requirements which must be met before CRT can be ordered.

Medicare requires that a face-to-face (FTF) mobility evaluation with the prescribing physician take place prior to ordering a power mobility device. A power mobility device includes PWCs or power assist/add-on to a MWC. Functional assessment of the individual's mobility needs must be well documented in the medical record. The documentation must also reflect that the mobility evaluation was the primary reason for the visit, although the physician is able to provide other medical advice and interventions during the visit.

The FTF appointment must include the following components: height and weight, upper extremity and lower extremity strength and range of motion, cardiopulmonary examination, and neurological examination. During the FTF visit, the physician must explain why a less costly alternative, such as a MWC or an assistive device, is insufficient to meet the individual's in-home mobility needs and how a power mobility device will allow them to achieve at least one of the necessary ADLs within the home.

This FTF appointment must have occurred within a specific time frame prior to ordering the power mobility device. It can occur either before or after the therapist's evaluation. The timeline of the FTF visit is subject to change. It is advised that the physician communicate with the equipment supplier regarding specific timeline requirements.

While an FTF appointment is not required for MWC prescription at this time, medical documentation must support the need for this device. The most recent physician's visit note should document impairments and mobility limitations that necessitate the full-time use of an MWC. This note should also document and rule out less costly alternatives, such as bracing and/or an assistive device. Once the clinical documentation is received by the CRT supplier, they will send the physician a corresponding detailed order to finalize the process, as required by the payer. This must be reviewed and signed by the physician and returned to the supplier in a timely manner. Inadequate or delayed documentation may prevent insurance approval.

## RESOURCES AND REFERENCES

The full list of resources and references appears in the digital product found on http://connect .springerpub.com/content/book/978-0-8261-6226-7/part/part04/chapter/ch66

# INDEX